Mosby's Guide to
PHYSICAL
EXAMINATION

Mosby's Guide to
PHYSICAL EXAMINATION

HENRY M. SEIDEL, M.D.

Associate Dean for Student Affairs, Associate Professor of Pediatrics,
The Johns Hopkins University School of Medicine, Baltimore, Maryland

JANE W. BALL, R.N., C.P.N.P., Dr. P.H.

Project Coordinator, Pediatric Emergency Medical Services Training Program,
Children's Hospital, National Medical Center, Washington, D.C.

JOYCE E. DAINS, R.N., Dr. P.H.

Assistant Professor, School of Nursing,
University of Texas Health Science Center at Houston, Houston, Texas

G. WILLIAM BENEDICT, M.D., Ph.D.

Assistant Professor,
The Johns Hopkins University School of Medicine, Baltimore, Maryland

Original illustrations by
George J. Wassilchenko

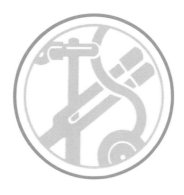

The C. V. Mosby Company

ST. LOUIS   WASHINGTON, D.C.   TORONTO   1987

MOSBY

A TRADITION OF PUBLISHING EXCELLENCE

Senior Editor: Barbara Ellen Norwitz
Developmental Editor: Sally Adkisson
Project and Developmental Editor: Lin A. Dempsey
Manuscript Editor: Daphna Gregg
Production: Jeanne A. Gulledge, Susan Trail, Celeste Clingan, Mary G. Stueck
Art Director: Kay Michael Kramer
Design: Diane M. Beasley

Printed in the United States of America

The C.V. Mosby Company
11830 Westline Industrial Drive, St. Louis, Missouri 63146

Library of Congress Cataloging in Publication Data
Mosby's guide to physical examination.

 Bibliography: p.
 Includes index.
 1. Physical diagnosis. I. Seidel, Henry M. II. Title:
Guide to physical examination. [DNLM: 1. Physical
Examination—methods. WB 205 M894]
RC76.M63 1987   616.07′54   86-28456
ISBN 0-8016-0440-0

TS/VH/VH 9 8 7 6 5 4 3 2   03/C/363

Preface

This text has been designed and written for students who are learning to perform physical examinations. We believe this book will be a valuable resource as you learn to perform this integral aspect of your future practice, that of interviewing the patient, collecting the history, performing the physical examination, and making a clinical judgment about your patient's health care needs.

We have made an attempt to focus your attention on the patient as an individual, rather than a collection of body parts and systems. This effort begins with the interview, in which you are guided to consider the patient's motives in seeking health care at a particular time and the manner in which the problem is interfering with daily life. Although subsequent chapters are organized by body parts or systems, we have tried to sensitize you to the concerns of the patient during each portion of the examination. In each chapter our intent is to guide you in your approach to the patient, suggesting adaptations for different ages and conditions.

A special feature of this book is the inclusion within each chapter of appropriate modifications in approach, techniques, and findings for the examination of newborns and infants, children and adolescents, and older adults. In many chapters, examination findings for the pregnant woman have also been included.

The basis of all good physical examination is complete and accurate historical (subjective) information obtained from the patient or family member. Chapter 1 offers guidelines for the development of a rapport with the patient, consideration of verbal and nonverbal cues to health problems, and the outline of a comprehensive health history for various age groups.

Chapter 2 offers an overview of examination techniques and equipment used during the physical examination. Beginning with Chapter 3, each chapter has been divided into four major units: Anatomy and Physiology, Review of Related History, Examination and Findings, and Common Abnormalities. Each unit begins with information about the adult patient and is followed by adaptations or special considerations when the patient is an infant, child, adolescent, pregnant woman, or older adult.

Anatomy and Physiology of each system or body part provides important landmarks for the physical examination and an understanding of the physiologic basis of findings. The Review of Related History provides a more intensive focus of inquiry when a system-specific problem is identified during the interview or examination. The Examination and Findings section is organized by equipment needed, the approach to the patient, procedures for the examination, and expected findings. In many cases, unexpected findings and their possible associated disorders are included. You will note that, throughout this text, we have avoided the terms "normal" and "abnormal" in the description of physical findings. It is our belief that these terms connote a value judgment that the new learner has not yet had an opportunity to appreciate. It is our hope that use of other terminology will enable the student to better understand the range of findings considered normal and abnormal. Common Abnormalities, disease states associated with the system or body part, appear at the end of each chapter. The cluster of symptoms and related data for each abnormality will be useful to you as you begin clinical decision making. The information provided about each of these disorders should be supplemented by other textbooks.

The book concludes with chapters designed to help you put the information into practice. Suggestions for the sequence of the physical examination, integrating all systems, are provided for each age group. This is followed by guidelines for recording the collected subjective and objective patient data in an organized way and for beginning the process of clinical decision making.

The book is richly illustrated, enhancing the text. Throughout are photographs and drawings that demonstrate underlying anatomic structures, proper techniques of examination, and expected and unexpected findings. In addition, there are numerous tables that summarize information provided and assessment tools that are frequently used in practice.

We have made every attempt to provide you with a comprehensive guide to the physical examination for patients of all ages. It is our hope that you will find this a useful text as you learn the physical examination procedures and that it will serve as a resource reference in your practice.

Henry M. Seidel
Jane W. Ball
Joyce E. Dains
G. William Benedict

Acknowledgments

The development of a new textbook requires the creativity, expertise, and dedication of many persons. Special thanks go to Barbara Norwitz, our Editor, who offered us the opportunity to write the book, and for her inspiration, guidance and support; to Sally Adkisson, our Developmental Editor, for her direction, editorial sense, and commitment to details; to Lin Dempsey, for her forbearance in editing and reediting the manuscript; and to George Wassilchenko, who brought the book to life and inspired us with his illustrations. And finally, the love and support of each of our families created the climate for the production of this book.

In addition, we wish to offer many thanks to . . .
Jeffrey Marc Miller
William A.H. Sammons, M.D.
Evangeline Soulikas
Zuhair A. Kareem
Homer Pilgrim
Augusta Tucker Townsend
Mary Ann Knott
Nancy Hutton Wissow, M.D.
Stephen Josef Wissow
Mary Joyner
Alice Lee
Virginia Winstead
Roberta Preston
Patricia Heid
Jean Wheeler

And a special "thank you" to the staff of The Johns Hopkins University and Hospital for their patience and support.

Contents

Mosby's Guide to
PHYSICAL EXAMINATION

The History and Interviewing Process

The purpose of this book is to offer instruction in acquiring information about the well and the sick as they seek health and medical care. It is not easy to get the sense of another person or fully appreciate someone else's orientation in the world. The images we each receive from the external world are probably much the same. However, the way in which we make those images a part of our experience and our base of information varies enormously. If we are to keep our interpretations from being misinterpretations and our perceptions from being misperceptions, we must make every effort to sense the world of the individual patient as that patient senses it.

The primary objective of interacting with a patient is to find out what is at the root of that person's concern and to do something about it. The search is for matters of concern at all times, whether there is a chief complaint or a simply stated request for a check-up. If you do not keep constant the need to identify the patient's underlying worries, believe them, and try to deal with them, you will probably not be of much help. And you need to understand what the patient expects of you.

The diagnostic process involves identifying and evaluating the common and the rare, understanding as much as possible the threats to the smooth flow of the patient's life, and recognizing and localizing findings that may be aberrations. The history and physical examination not only begin the diagnostic process, they are the hub around which diagnosis and treatment revolve. Your approach must be orderly; random approaches often result in random solutions, seriously limiting the likelihood of successful outcomes. Order, however, does not imply rigidity.

You have to be compulsive as you compile information, giving careful attention to the obvious so that you understand it and record it precisely, while maintaining your sensitivity to the less obvious, "soft" clues that are almost always to be found in the history or physical examination. The ability to do this well distinguishes the good clinician.

Communicating with the Patient

Factors that Enhance Communication

From the start, there are several points to keep in mind. A clinician's stiffly formal demeanor inhibits the patient's ability to communicate, whereas a too casual, laid back attitude fails to instill confidence. Because the patient may search for meaning in everything you say, avoid being careless with words. What may seem innocuous to you may not be to the patient. You should begin to understand the intellectual and emotional constraints on the way you ask questions and convey information. Similarly, your face need not be a mask, but avoid the extremes of reaction—startle, surprise, laughter, grimacing—as the patient provides information.

Sometimes you will be concerned about the patient's ability to understand what you try to convey and what you are seeking to discover, but do not ever allow yourself to discount the patient's experience and the information he or she provides.

The patient's associations may be important, and you must allow freedom for the patient to pursue them. Be flexible! Ask open-ended questions in the beginning. Later, as information accumulates, it will be necessary to know precise, measurable details, and you must become more specific. But early in the interview it is entirely appropriate to let the patient tell you what the experience was like. The patient's or observer's description of the experience should be heard and recorded. This will be helpful in the future for others who are involved with the patient to have a sense of how the patient and the family responded to the experience.

Open-endedness cannot be allowed to go on forever, of course. Gentle guidance is helpful ("But now we must look further at another part of the story"). You cannot assume that a verbose tale is the complete story. You must be certain that you have asked all the questions you need.

Your questions must be clearly understood. Define any words the patient cannot understand, but do not use so many technical terms that the definitions become confusing. Be clear and explicit; use the patient's terms if possible, but you must not be patronizing. Meet the level of your patient's ability to understand. (There can be traps in this, however. A professional colleague who is a patient may not be familiar with the jargon of your particular discipline.)

Resist the tendency to be manipulative. Avoid leading questions. For example, ask how often something happened, allowing the patient to define *often,* rather than, "It didn't happen too often, did it?" Pursue the information with short, uncomplicated questions using understandable language. Ask one question at a time, avoiding a barrage of questions that prohibit the patient from being expansive or that limit the patient to simple yes or no answers. It is often better to say, "Tell me about . . . ," rather than, "Is it . . . ?" Always be adaptable to the patient's language. If a patient uses a term to describe an event, adopt that term as you attempt to explore further.

Sometimes you will be confused by what the patient tells you. Recognize the confusion as a piece of information and begin to clarify if you can. The confusion may be a clue to a patient's underlying emotional or organic difficulty.

If the patient makes a reference that is not immediately relevant to your purposes, be flexible enough to clarify at least the nature of the irrelevancy. This allows you to make a decision on the need for further exploration. Although too many digressions can lead to an infinity of misspent time, paying attention to a digression of the moment may save a lot of time later on.

Some apparent irrelevancies may provide important background information. A parent, for example, may have died of cancer. The fact itself may not be important at that moment, but the patient's response to the fact and the intensity of feeling associated with it can give important shape to your approaches. Such an understanding is vital to your pursuit of diagnosis and management. Thus no history is complete without information about the patient's past and present life situation, reaction to earlier events, and coping methods.

Never assume a patient's every question requires an encyclopedic answer. Be sensitive to the extent of an answer that is being sought.

Learn to be sensitive to the subtle as well as the obvious in the question; learn to

Fig. 1-1
The interviewing process.

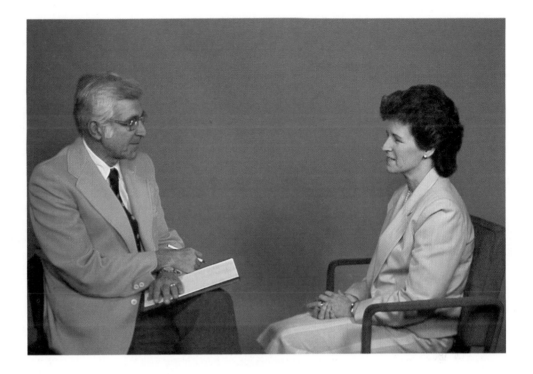

go far enough but not too far. Your sensitivity must include choosing your words carefully. Most lay people think *tumor* is synonymous with *cancer* and will often interpret your use of the word *nervous* to mean that they have emotional problems. Obviously you can paralyze your spontaneity in too precise choice of words, but you do need to exercise care. If the patient seems to ask a leading question, one you do not feel prepared to answer at the moment, it is possible to say, "Why do you ask?" to seek better understanding of the direction of the patient's thinking. Children need age-appropriate responses to their questions.

It is easy to be too directive about certain issues. Avoid that trap! When the patient asks for advice, be sure you understand the patient's experience and attitudes. Try for an interchange that allows the patient to come to a decision as free as possible of the imposition of your value judgment. To the extent that you can avoid this, you remain a health professional and avoid becoming preacher. The competent health professional understands that value judgments are not necessarily imbued with wisdom.

The American Board of Internal Medicine has suggested the following questions that might be asked by an interviewer who gives full concern to the patient's feelings and needs. Rarely, if ever, would one patient be asked all of these questions; exactly which ones are appropriate must be determined by each patient's particular situation. For example, questions about a living will would alarm a patient seeking a routine checkup but may relieve a patient hospitalized with a life-threatening disease.

1. What do you think is causing your symptoms?
2. What is your understanding of your diagnosis?
   Its importance? Its need for management?

3. How do you feel about your illness? Frightened? Threatened? As a wage earner? As a family member? Angry that you are afflicted?
4. Do you believe treatment will help?
5. How are you coping with your illness?
   Crying? Drinking more? Tranquilizers? Talking more? Less? Changing lifestyles?
6. Do you want to know all details about your diagnosis and its effect on your future?
7. How important is "doing everything possible"?
   How important is "quality of life"?
   Have you prepared a living will?
8. Do you have people you can talk with about your illness?
9. Is there anyone else we should contact about your illness or hospitalization? Family members? Friends? Employer? Hospital chaplain, minister, priest, rabbi? Attorney?
10. Do you want or expect emotional support from the health care team?
11. Are there financial questions about your medical care that trouble you? Insurance coverage? Tests or treatment you may not be able to afford? Timing of payments required from you?
12. How would you like to be addressed?
13. If you have had previous hospitalizations, does it bother you to be seen by teams of doctors, nurses, and medical students on rounds?
14. How private a person are you?
    Are you concerned about the confidentiality of your medical records?
    Would you prefer to talk to an older/younger, male/female physician?
    Are there medical matters you do not wish disclosed to others?
    Would you prefer to give your history so no one else can hear?*

Moments of Tension

Curiosity about You

Patients are aware that you are a person with a life of your own. All of them will at one time or another have some curiosity about aspects of your experience.

Sometimes you will be asked about yourself. You need not violate your personal life. Often a direct answer, unvarnished by detail, will suffice to satisfy the patient's curiosity, prevent great invasion into your personal life, but communicate nevertheless that you are not completely isolated. You may find it comfortable to chat about certain, sometimes relevant aspects of your own experience. You may, for example, respond to an inquiry that you are married, but you need not give extended detail about your spouse.

Silence

We are always confounded by silence, and most of us feel the need to fill it with some kind of chatter. Be gentle and do not force. You may have to edge the patient along with an open-ended question ("What seems to worry you?") or a mild nudge ("And after that?").

*From A guide to awareness and evaluation of humanistic qualities in the internist, June 1985, American Board of Internal Medicine.

Crying

People will cry. Let them. Let the moment pass at the patient's pace. Wait to resume your question until the patient is ready. If you become aware that the patient needs to cry but is suppressing it, give permission. Offer a tissue or simply say, "I know you're feeling badly. It's all right to cry." Such a moment often generates greater warmth between you and the patient. You have shared something; and you have respected the patient's need. The patient has sensed your feelings of caring, and the relationship has grown.

Compassionate Moments

Do not hesitate to say that you feel for the patient, that you are sorry for something that happened and that you know it may have been painful. Be open and direct about a tender circumstance. It is alright to bring things out in the open as long as your guiding hand is gentle and you are not too aggressive or insistent. Sometimes you state the obvious and you confront it. Sometimes you make an inference and hope that you guessed right in bringing the patient's feelings to the surface. When you are uncertain, ask ("How are you feeling? Are you as bothered by all this as I think you are?").

Seduction

There are limits to your expressions of warmth and cordiality. You are a professional and you must behave professionally. The insecure, dependent patient is sometimes seductive and often too readily susceptible to manipulation. You must not, either intentionally or unintentionally, fall into the seductive trap of playing to feelings of insecurity and dependence. The behavior of such patients can be a most serious problem. Such a situation can be averted by being courteously calm and firm from the start delivering the clear—and immediate—message that the relationship is and must remain professional.

Anger

Sometimes those patients who are angriest and most hostile are the ones who need you the most. Nevertheless, it is difficult to understand anger and hostility. We are all to some extent intimidated by it. You can deal with it by confronting it. It is alright to say, "I know you're angry. Won't you tell me why? I want to hear." You may sometimes be aware that you have made the patient angry by being late for the interview, by taking too long, by in some way getting in the way of the patient's life or concerns. You will only add to the anger by pretending that it does not exist. Face it head on. Acknowledge it and, if it is appropriate, apologize. Happily, the anger generally will not last long. As with crying, the patient should be given the opportunity to express the feeling and to find that you will not shrink away from it. Generally, you can continue on a better footing after anger is vented than before.

Dissemblance

Patients may not always tell the whole story. They may be hiding something, either purposely or unconsciously. Neither push too hard when you think this is happening nor neglect it. Allow the interview to go on and then come back to it with gentle questioning. Ultimately you can say, "I think that you may be more concerned than you are saying;" or, "I think that you're worried about what we might find out." You should be satisfied that you have learned all that is necessary. But satisfaction may not come in one sitting. You may have to pursue it later that day or the next or, perhaps, with other members of the family.

Knowing Yourself

Knowing and understanding yourself is important. If you are to be successful you must understand what bias you bring to each interaction with the patient. You will respond differently to children and the aged, to men and women, to blacks and whites, to rich and poor. You must know why and how. For example, if a patient makes you angry, why should that be? Your own disenchantment of the moment? Some underlying frustration in your life? Does your hostile response to someone in need evolve from a conflict of values or an absence of trust? Whatever the reason, you must understand it before you displace anger to the patient and harm the relationship, perhaps making it difficult to continue. This unhappy circumstance may evolve because the patient may suggest, either obviously or subtly, an absence of trust. Or you might be rushed, frustrated, or already angry for reasons extraneous to the moment. All of us want to be liked by our patients, and if we sense that this is not forthcoming, we are apt to react with some degree of hostility. This dangerous moment can be avoided if you understand yourself and if you have the maturity and personal security to respond to that understanding.

Always keep in mind the role of your own feelings and behavior. In all this, an appreciation of reality and the wish to be caring are much supported by a leavening of gentle humor.

CHILDREN

Children are like other people. They want to have attention paid to them. They do not want to be patronized, and they love it when you get down on the floor and play with them. They have anxieties and fears that must be anticipated and eased. Talk with them, hold them, reassure them, include them! And when they are old enough, allow them to be heard fully. The older the child, the more productive it becomes to include him or her in the interview, asking questions directly of the child.

The older child and the adolescent require a particular alertness on your part. Their hesitancies or passive, sometimes vaguely hostile, silences may suggest that they would prefer to be alone with you, free of a parent. Be sensitive to these clues and respect the need for separation. This is perhaps easier with adolescents, but the need for privacy also exists among older, preadolescent children. In general, be aware that it often helps to separate the child from the parent in order to get a more complete history.

In the best of circumstances, adolescents are sometimes reluctant to talk. Give clear evidence of your respect for their need for confidence and for their burgeoning adulthood. It is helpful in the beginning to talk about their lives and about what is going on around them. It rarely pays to force conversation, because they will not readily respond to confrontation. On the other hand, you will often sense a palpable need to talk and an inability to get the words out. Silences can be long, sometimes sheepish, occasionally angry, most often unproductive of an eventual forcing of talk. Many of us have found it helpful to have a few cards with subjects common to teenagers noted on them. Simply ask the patient to look at the cards and to indicate silently the ones that note the subjects of present concern. Then you can say the necessary words, phrase the appropriate questions, and make the transition to a verbal discussion reasonably comfortable.

Fig. 1-2
Interviewing a child with his parent.

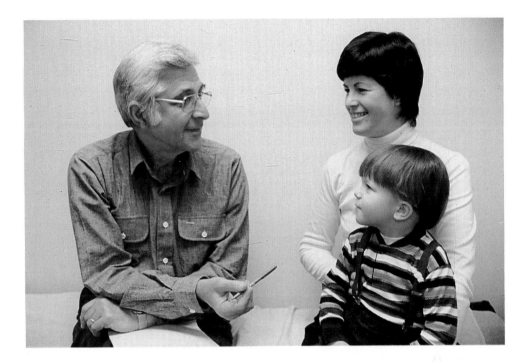

OLDER ADULTS

Individual variations in knowledge, experience, cognitive abilities, and personality all affect the interview process with older adults, just as with younger adults. Age-related physiologic changes that could be impediments to the interview process may be present in some older adults. Remember, however, that people age at different rates and that chronologic age alone is a poor benchmark for determining the presence of those changes. Avoid falling into the stereotyping trap of assuming that all older adults, by virtue of their age, experience all of the so called normal changes associated with aging.

Some older adults may have sensory losses, in both perception and reception, that make communication more difficult. Some degree of hearing loss is not uncommon, thus necessitating some special considerations. Position yourself so that the patient can see your face. Speak clearly and slowly, taking care not to avert your head while you are talking. (Shouting only magnifies the problem by distorting consonants and vowels.) In some instances, a written interview may ultimately be less frustrating to both you and the patient. If this becomes necessary, tailor the process to include only the most pertinent questions, because this method can be tedious and exhausting for patients.

Conversely, impaired visual perception and light-dark adaptation can adversely affect the interview if written interview forms are used. Provide the patient with a well illuminated environment and a light source that does not glare or reflect in the eyes.

Some older adults may be confused or experience memory loss, particularly for recent events. Take the extra time that you need with these patients. Ask short (but not leading) questions, and keep your language simple. Consult other family members to clarify discrepant information or to fill in the gaps.

Approach each patient as an individual. It is certainly important to be knowledgeable about physiologic and psychologic changes associated with aging, and it is

Fig. 1-3
Interviewing an older adult.

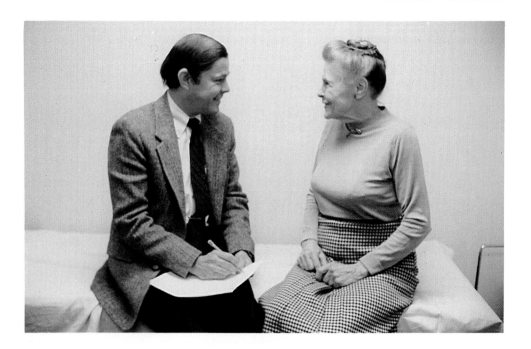

appropriate to anticipate what effect these changes may have on the interview. It is equally important, however, to appreciate that not all adults experience the same changes, or at the same rate, and that some areas do not decline with age. The older patient brings to the interview a lifetime of experience that may be a source of richness, wisdom, meaning, and perspective. Do not discount it.

PATIENTS WITH HANDICAPS

Patients with serious and handicapping physical or emotional disorders—the deaf, the blind, the depressed, the psychotic, the mentally retarded, the brain-injured—must all be respected and your approach adapted to their needs. Patients who are emotionally restricted may not be able to give an effective history, but they must be respected and the history should be obtained from them to the extent possible. Their points of view and their attitudes matter. Still, when necessary, the family, other health professionals involved in care, and the patient's record must be queried in order to get the complete story. Nevertheless, every patient must be fully respected and fully involved to the limit of emotion, mental capacity, or physical handicap.

Some of the most common communication barriers can be overcome if you keep the following in mind:
- Families are, happily, often available.
- Translators may be found for language barriers most of the time.
- The deaf often read, write, and read lips, but you must speak slowly and enunciate each word clearly and in full view; a translator who signs may be available.
- The blind usually can hear; talking louder to make a point does not help. Remember, however, that you must always make vocal what you are trying to communicate; gestures will not help.

The History

Taking the history usually begins your relationship with the patient. A prime objective is to identify those matters the patient defines as problems. You must be aware of the hidden as well as the obvious concerns, and you need to assure, to the extent possible, accuracy. You have to develop a sense of the patient's reliability as an interpreter and reporter of events. Sometimes you will realize that the patient is suppressing some information either purposely or without realizing it, underreporting other experiences, or giving them a context that is less intense than you might feel appropriate. You will find yourself in a constant state of subjective evaluation as the history goes along. Indeed, some circumstances that worry you might not be seen by the patient as unusual, which is all the more reason to seek understanding of the patient's perspective. Your attitude of friendliness and obvious respect will go a long way in the pursuit of information and in assuring your patient's help in obtaining it.

Setting for the Interview

The large university teaching hospital, the setting in which most health professionals are educated, is in some ways a disadvantageous setting to begin your accomodation to patient care. You must not allow the profusion of technical competence and the variety of skills to obscure the essential interactions that must take place between you and the patient. There are really few extra aids you need to extend your senses. Even in an empty space, the interview can be a rich and positive interchange, an experience that is rewarding to the patient and to you.

Obviously, the setting in which you take the history must be as comfortable as possible. Often the space provided is small and rather barren. The colors are frequently not warm and the chairs straightbacked and uncomfortable. No matter; you are the focal point of warmth and attention. You can assure that there are no bulky desks or tables between you and the patient. Have a clock placed (preferably behind the patient's chair) where you can see it without obviously looking at your watch. Sit comfortably and at ease, maintaining eye contact and a conversational tone of voice. Your manner can manifest interest that assures the patient that you care and that relieving the patient's worry or pain is your prime—in fact, your only—concern at the moment.

You can accomplish this only with a discipline that allows you to concentrate on the matter at hand, giving it for that moment primacy in your life, and dispelling both personal and professional distractions.

Structure of the History

Your purpose in taking the history is to establish a relationship with the patient and to learn about the patient. The process by which you do this has an organization that has been widely accepted for decades. The structure includes:

Chief complaint
Present problem
Past medical history
Family history
Social and experiential history
Systems review

The chief complaint is a brief statement of the reason the patient offers for the visit. It is always important, however, to go beyond the obvious reason and to probe for underlying concerns. If the patient has a sore throat, why is he or she worried about it? Is it the pain and fever, or is it the concern caused by past experience with a friend or relative who developed rheumatic heart disease?

Understanding the present problem requires a step by step revelation of the circumstances that surround the primary reason for the patient's visit. The medical history goes beyond this to an exploration of the patient's overall health before the present problem, including all of the patient's past medical and surgical experiences. Then the patient's family requires attention: its health, past medical experience, illnesses, social experiences, deaths, and genetic and environmental circumstances that have influenced the patient's life. A careful inquiry about the personal and social experience of the patient should include work habits and the multiplicity of relationships in the family, school, and workplace. Finally, the systems review takes a different tack in that it requires a detailed review of possible complaints in each of the body's systems, looking for complementary or seemingly unrelated symptoms that may not have surfaced during the rest of the history.

Although there must be a structure to the history taking, rigidity is not necessary. You should be flexible, but you must be compulsive about achieving as many of your goals as possible and sensitive to nuance in pursuing each suggestion, however subtle, that there may yet be a nugget of information to be found.

Leave opportunity for give and take, for the patient to ask questions and to explore feelings. You need not allow the patient to ramble; gentle constraint is most often recognized and successful.

Taking the History

Introduce yourself to the patient, clearly stating your name and your role in the process. If you are still a student, do not mask the fact. You must then be certain that you understand the patient's full name and that you pronounce it correctly.

Address the patient properly (Mr., Miss, Mrs., Ms.) and repeat the name at appropriate times. Avoid the familiarity of using a first name when you do not expect familiarity in return. Never use a surrogate term for the patient's name; for example, when the patient is a child, do not address the parent as "mother" or "father."

By this time you should be seated at any easy distance from the patient, comfortably and without any furniture barriers between you. Unless you have known the patient in the past and know that there is no matter of great urgency, proceed with reasonable dispatch, asking the patient to state the reason for the visit. Listen; do not be too directive at this point. Let the patient spill it all out and, after the first flow of words, begin to shape the direction of the interview. Begin to probe for what Feinstein calls the "iatrotropic stimulus," the stimulus to seek health care. If, indeed, 100 people wake up with a sore throat and 97 go to work and 3 seek care, what underlying dimension prompted those decisions?

This is the point at which you begin to give structure to the present problem, giving it a chronologic and sequential framework, fleshing out the bare bones of the chief complaint, probing for the underlying concerns. Unless there is some obvious urgency, go slowly, hear the full story, and refrain from striking out too quickly on what seems the obvious course of questioning. The patient will take clues from you on the amount of leisure you will allow; you must walk a fine line between permitting this leisure and meeting the obvious time constraints of your profession.

You do not need a lot of time to let the patient know that you have *enough* time. Lean back, fix your attention on the patient and *listen;* avoid interrupting unless you really have to, and do not anticipate the next question before you have heard the complete answer.

Once you have understood the patient's chief complaint and present problem and have obtained a sense of possible underlying concerns, it is time to go on to other segments of the history—the family and medical histories, emotional concerns, and social accompaniments to the present. Remember that nothing in the patient's experience is isolated. There are aspects of the present illness that require careful integration with the medical and family history. Keep in mind that the life of the patient is not constructed according to your outline, that many factors give shape to the present illness, and that any one chief complaint may involve more than one illness.

As the interview proceeds, thoroughly explore each positive response with these relevant questions:

Where: Where are symptoms located, as precisely as possible? If they seem to move, what is the range of their movement? Where is the patient when the complaint occurs—at work or play, active or resting, in the city or country?

When: Everything happens in a chronologic sequence. When did it begin, does it come and go? If so, how often and for how long? What time of day? What day of the week?

What: What does it mean to the patient? What is its impact? What does it feel like? What is its quality and intensity? Has it been bad enough to interrupt the flow of the patient's life, or has it been dealt with rather casually? What happened contemporaneously that might be related?

How: The background of the symptom becomes important in answering the "how" question. How did it come about? What is the ambiance of the complaint? Are other things going on at the same time, such as work, play, mealtime, or sleep? Is there illness in the family? Have there been similar episodes in the past? Is there concern about similar symptoms in friends or relatives? Are there companion complaints? How is the patient coping? Are there social supports? Remember that nothing ever happens in isolation.

Why: Of course, the answer to "why" is the solution to the problem. All other questions lead to this one.

When these questions are kept in mind, you will be able to define what you have heard as clearly as possible. You can place it in a context appropriate to the patient's age and sex. You will also be able to determine the size of a complaint—that is, how intense it is, how frequently it occurs, and how much it affects the patient's life.

As the interview approaches its end, it is possible to return to the more free-flowing, less structured style that might have dominated as the patient first described the present problem. It is a time to review the discussion and ask the patient to supply any missing details; to express concern; and to summarize your understanding in a way that communicates your need for thoroughness and your wish to devote whatever time is necessary.

Try to verify that the patient understands the circumstance and treatment and that the patient and family seem to be coping. Repeat instructions, if there are any, and ask to hear them back. Always discuss and explain the next step, whether it is the appointment time, methods of keeping in touch, exchange of telephone numbers, or planning for the physical examination that will follow the interview.

GENERAL GUIDELINES FOR HISTORY TAKING

- Ensure the patient's physical comfort—and yours.
- Provide good lighting.
- Maintain privacy, using available curtains and shades.
- Provide relative quiet. If the setting is a hospital room, turn off the television set (it is distracting to speak with a patient whose eyes are constantly darting up to the television).
- Do not overtire the patient by trying to do it all at one time. Come back later if possible. If it is during an office or clinic visit, let the circumstance guide the length of the initial interview; it may be appropriate to schedule completing the history at a later date.
- Always give the patient a chance to state what is primary in his or her mind.
- Do not pursue the specific, and do not attempt precise descriptions until all of the patient's general concerns have been fully stated.
- Arrive at a judgment of the patient's ability to be perceptive and articulate.
- Particularly in the early stages of an interview, the clinician should offer thoughtful, respectful silence with gentle encouragement to talk and should listen with obvious intent.
- Save directive approaches for later in the interview. (Ultimately it is essential to be precise about each finding and to establish the sequence of events.)
- If the patient is very talkative or too silent, offer some guidance. Sometimes these verbal behaviors offer a clue to a neurologic disturbance or a neurotic need.
- Symptoms can have multiple causes, so do not home in on a possible cause too quickly.
- A chief complaint or a report of a symptom of any kind very often carries with it a hidden concern. Look for underlying and unstated worries. Never trivialize any finding or concern.
- Define any symptom, concern, or finding by as many of the following dimensions as are appropriate: Where is it? What is it like? How bad is it? How long ago was it noted? Does it come and go? In what situation does it happen? Does anything make it better or worse? What else happens along with it?
- In asking direct questions, avoid a manner that suggests you want only a yes or no answer. If you maintain eye contact, occasionally nod your head, and simply say "Indeed" or "Let me hear more," the patient will often continue to talk and give a complete answer.
- Make notes sparingly; jot down enough key words to help you record the history later, but do not be so intent on note taking that it distracts the patient or interferes with listening and observing.
- At the end of your meeting, give the patient an opportunity for review and necessary elaboration. This takes time, but it provides important clues to understanding and management. It may reveal the psychosocial needs of the patient more clearly, may provide insights that will help your decision making, and leaves the patient more satisfied with the interview.

Outline of Clinical History

The following outline is offered as a g
It should not set limits or indicate a
elaborated are indicated in subsequ
tion) offers guidelines for recordi

CHIEF COMPLAINT. In the b
the question, "What problem o
current illness should next b
present?" or "When did thes
status, previous admissions
record.

PRESENT PROBLEM OR ILLNESS. No
applicable to all cases. You will probably find tha
tion the patient on the details of the current problem in.
the chief complaint. Others find it is of more value to obtain u.
and family history before returning to the present. The specific order u.
ing is not critical. What is important is that you obtain the needed informatio.
organize it before finally recording it. At times it is helpful to let the patient sketch
an outline of the present problem and then go back to fill in all the pertinent details.
This has the advantage of allowing the patient to voice the relative importance of
the features surrounding the problem. At other times experience will dictate that
you must obtain the details by specific questions. Nevertheless, leading questions
should be avoided.

The state of health immediately before onset of the present problem should be
determined, and a complete description of the earliest symptoms must be obtained.
"When did you last feel well?" may help define the time of onset. In acute infections
or intoxication, inquiry should be made concerning a possible exposure and incu-
bation period. When the present problem has progressed in attacks separated by
disease-free intervals, it is necessary to obtain the history of a typical attack (onset,
duration, and associated symptoms such as pain, chills, fever, jaundice, and hematuria). You should ask about inciting, exacerbating, or relieving factors, such as
specific activities or positions, diet, and medications. The date at which the patient
had to stop work or school or was restricted to home or bed should be noted. How
the illness affects the patient's usual lifestyle (marriage, leisure activities, ability to
perform tasks or to cope with stress) should be determined. You should try to find
out if the patient feels the problem is becoming better, worse, or remaining stable.
If the problem is long-standing, ask what prompted the patient to seek medical
attention at this particular time. The course of the disease should be developed in
chronologic order up to the present. When there is a conspicuous disturbance of a
particular organ or system, direct questions should be asked regarding all possible
symptoms referrable to this system.

At the end of your questions regarding the present problem, review the chronologic course of events and ask the patient to confirm or correct the information
obtained. If there is more than one important present problem, this process should
be repeated for each problem. In the written history, it is wise to give a specific
number and brief title to each problem. Either here, or in the summary at the end of
the written history, problems can be listed according to order of apparent importance.

PAST MEDICAL HISTORY

A. General health and strength
B. Childhood illnesses: measles, mumps, whooping cough, chickenpox, smallpox, scarlet fever, acute rheumatic fever, diphtheria, poliomyelitis
C. Major adult illnesses: tuberculosis, hepatitis, diabetes, hypertension, myocardial infarction, tropical or parasitic diseases, other infections; any non-surgical hospital admissions
D. Immunizations: smallpox, polio, diphtheria, pertussis and tetanus toxoid, influenza, cholera, typhus, typhoid, last PPD or other skin tests; unusual reactions to immunizations; tetanus or other antitoxin made with horse serum
E. Surgery: dates, hospital, diagnosis, complications
F. Serious injuries: resulting disability; if the present problem has potential medicolegal relation to an injury, give full documentation
G. Medications: current and recent medications, including dosage, both prescription and home remedy
H. Allergies: especially to medications, but also to environmental allergens and foods
I. Transfusions: reactions; date and number of units transfused

FAMILY HISTORY. Ask if there are any members of the patient's family who have illnesses with features similar to the patient's illness. Determine the health or cause of death of parents and siblings, with ages at death. Establish whether there is a history of heart disease, high blood pressure, cancer, tuberculosis, stroke, diabetes, gout, kidney disease, thyroid disease, asthma and other allergic states, blood diseases, sexually transmitted diseases, or any other familial disease. Determine the age and health of spouse and children.

If there is a hereditary disease in the family, such as hemophilia, inquire into the condition of the grandparents, aunts, uncles, and cousins. A pedigree diagram is often helpful in recording this information.

PERSONAL AND SOCIAL HISTORY

A. Personal status: birthplace, where raised, home environment as youth (e.g., parental divorce or separation, socioeconomic class, cultural background), education, position in family, marital status, general life satisfaction, hobbies, interests
B. Habits: diet, regularity of eating and sleeping, exercise (quantity and type), quantity of coffee, tea, tobacco, alcohol; illicit drugs (frequency, type, and amount)
C. Home conditions: housing, economic condition, type of health insurance if any, pets and their health
D. Occupation: description of usual work and present work if different; conditions and hours, physical or mental strain; duration of employment, present and past exposure to heat and cold, industrial toxins (especially lead, arsenic, chromium, asbestos, beryllium, poisonous gases, benzene, and polyvinyl chloride or other carcinogens); any protective devices required
E. Environment: travel and other exposure to contagious diseases, residence in tropics, water and milk supply, other sources of infection if applicable
F. Military record: dates and geographic area of assignments
G. Religious preference: determine any religious proscriptions concerning medical care

REVIEW OF SYSTEMS. It is probable that all of the questions in each system will not be included every time you take a history. Nevertheless, some questions regarding each system should be included in every history. These essential questions are listed in bold type in the outline that follows. More comprehensive and detailed questions relating to each system are listed afterward and should be included whenever the patient gives positive responses to the first group of questions for that system. Keep in mind that these lists do not represent an exhaustive enumeration of questions that might be appropriate within an organ system. Even more detailed questions may be required depending on the patient's problem.

A. **General constitutional symptoms:** fever, chills, malaise, fatigability, night sweats; weight (average, preferred, present, change, appetite)
B. **Skin:** rash or eruption, itching, pigmentation or texture change; excessive sweating, abnormal nail or hair growth
C. **Skeletal:** joint stiffness, pain, restriction of motion, swelling, redness, heat, bony deformity
D. **Head**
   1. General: frequent or unusual headaches, dizziness, syncope, severe head injuries
   2. Eyes: visual acuity, blurring, diplopia, photophobia, pain, recent change in appearance or vision; glaucoma, use of eye drops or other eye medications; history of trauma or familial eye disease
   3. Ears: hearing loss, pain, discharge, tinnitus, vertigo
   4. Nose: sense of smell, frequency of colds, obstruction, epistaxis, postnasal discharge, sinus pain
   5. Throat and mouth: hoarseness or change in voice; frequent sore throats, bleeding or swelling of gums; recent tooth abcesses or extractions; soreness of tongue or buccal mucosa, ulcers; disturbance of taste
E. **Endocrine:** thyroid enlargement or tenderness, heat or cold intolerance, unexplained weight change, diabetes, polydipsia, polyuria, changes in facial or body hair, increased hat and glove size, skin striae
   1. Males: onset of puberty, erections, emissions, testicular pain, libido, infertility
   2. Females:
      a. Menses: onset, regularity, duration of flow, dysmenorrhea, last period, intermenstrual discharge or bleeding, itching, date of last Pap smear, age at menopause, libido, frequency of intercourse, sexual difficulties
      b. Pregnancies: number, miscarriages, abortions, duration of pregnancy in each and any complication during any pregnancy or postpartum period; use of oral or other contraceptives
      c. Breasts: pain, tenderness, discharge, lumps, mammograms
F. **Respiratory:** pain relating to respiration, dyspnea, cyanosis, wheezing, cough, sputum (character and quantity), hemoptysis, night sweats, exposure to TB; date and result of last chest x-ray
G. **Cardiac:** chest pain or distress, precipitating causes, timing and duration, relieving factors, palpitations, dyspnea, orthopnea (number of pillows needed), edema, claudication, hypertension, previous myocardial infarction, estimate of exercise tolerance, past ECG or other cardiac tests
H. **Hematologic:** anemia, tendency to bruise or bleed easily, thromboses, thrombophlebitis, any known abnormality of blood cells, transfusions
I. **Lymph nodes:** enlargement, tenderness, suppuration

  J. **Gastrointestinal:** appetite, digestion, intolerance for any class of foods, dysphagia, heartburn, nausea, vomiting, hematemesis, regularity of bowels, constipation, diarrhea, change in stool color or contents (clay-colored, tarry, fresh blood, mucus, undigested food), flatulence, hemorrhoids, hepatitis, jaundice, dark urine; history of ulcer, gallstones, polyps, tumor; previous x-rays (where, when, findings)

  K. **Genitourinary:** dysuria, flank or suprapubic pain, urgency, frequency, nocturia, hematuria, polyuria, hesitancy, dribbling, loss in force of stream, passage of stone; edema of face, stress incontinence, hernias, sexually transmitted disease (inquire what kind and symptoms, and list results of STS, if known)

  L. **Neurologic:** syncope, seizures, weakness or paralysis, abnormalities of sensation or coordination, tremors, loss of memory; unusual frequency, distribution, or severity of headaches, serious head injury in past

  M. **Psychiatric:** depression, mood changes, difficulty concentrating, nervousness, tension, suicidal thoughts, irritability, sleep disturbances

CONCLUDING QUESTIONS. At the conclusion of obtaining the history, ask the patient, "Is there anything else that you think would be important for me to know?" If several complaints are mentioned and discussed in the history, it is often useful to ask, "What problem concerns you most?" In certain situations, such as vague, complicated, or contradictory histories, it may be helpful to ask, "What do you think is the matter with you?"

CHILDREN

The history for an infant or child will be modified according to age. It is a good idea to remember that the following is just an outline.

CHIEF COMPLAINT. The history may be taken from a parent or other responsible adult. However, the child should be included as much as possible as appropriate for his or her age. The latent fears underlying any chief complaint of both parents and children should also be explored. Note the relationship of the person providing the history for the child.

PRESENT PROBLEM OR ILLNESS. The degree and character of the reaction to the problem on the part of parent and child should be noted.

PAST MEDICAL HISTORY
A. General health and strength: depending on the age of the patient or the nature of the problem, different aspects of the history assume or lose importance; reserve detailed questioning for those aspects most pertinent to the age of the child
B. Mother's health during pregnancy
 1. General health as related by the mother
 2. Specific diseases or conditions; infectious disease (approximate gestational month), weight gain, edema, hypertension, proteinuria, bleeding (approximate time), eclampsia
 3. Medications, hormones, vitamins, special or unusual diet, general nutritional status
 4. Quality of fetal movements and time of onset
 5. Emotional and behavior status (attitudes toward pregnancy and children)
 6. Radiation exposure

C. Birth
1. Duration of pregnancy
2. Place of delivery
3. Labor (spontaneous or induced); duration, analgesia or anesthesia, complications
4. Delivery: presentation, forceps or spontaneous, complications
5. Condition of infant, time of onset of cry, Apgar scores if available
6. Birth weight
D. Neonatal period
1. Congenital anomalies: baby's condition in hospital, oxygen requirements, color, feeding characteristics, vigor, cry; duration of baby's stay in hospital and whether infant was discharged with mother; prescriptions such as bilirubin lights or antibiotics
2. First month of life: jaundice, color, vigor of crying, bleeding, convulsions, or other evidence of illness
E. Feeding
1. Bottle or breast: reason for changes, if any; type of formula used, amounts offered and consumed, frequency of feeding and weight gain
2. Present diet and appetite, age of introduction of solids, age when child achieved three feedings per day; present feeding patterns, elaborate on any feeding problems; age weaned from bottle or breast; daily intake of milk; food preference; ability to feed self
F. Development: these are commonly used developmental milestones. The list should be enlarged when indicated. Parents may have baby books, which can stimulate recall; photographs may be helpful
1. Age when able to:
   a. hold head erect while in sitting position
   b. roll over from front to back and back to front
   c. sit alone and unsupported
   d. stand with support and alone
   e. walk with support and alone
   f. use words
   g. talk in sentences
   h. dress self
2. Age when toilet trained; approaches to and attitudes about toilet training
3. School: grade, performance, problems
4. Dentition: age of first teeth, loss of deciduous teeth, and eruption of first permanent teeth
5. Growth: height and weight in a sequence of ages; changes in rates of growth or weight gain
6. Sexual: present status; in female, time of development of breasts, nipples, sexual hair, menstruation (description of menses); in male, development of pubic hair, voice changes, acne, emissions
G. Illnesses: immunizations, communicable diseases, accidents, hospitalizations

FAMILY HISTORY. Obtain a maternal gestational history, listing all pregnancies together with the health status of living children. For deceased children include date, age, cause of death, and dates and duration of pregnancies in the case of miscarriages. Inquire about the mother's health during pregnancies and age of parents at the birth of this child. Are the parents cousins or otherwise related?

PERSONAL AND SOCIAL HISTORY

A. Personal status: school adjustment, masturbation, nail biting, thumb sucking, breath holding, temper tantrums, pica, tics, rituals; reactions to prior illnesses, injuries, or hospitalization

B. Home conditions: father's occupation, mother's occupation, the principal care-taker(s) of child, parents divorced or separated; educational attainment of parents; cultural heritage; food prepared by whom; adequacy of clothing; dependence on relief or social agency; number of rooms in house and number of persons in household; sleep habits, sleeping arrangements available for the child

REVIEW OF SYSTEMS. In addition to the usual concerns, inquire about any past testing of the child. Ask about the following:

Skin—eczema, seborrhea, "cradle cap"

Ears—otitis media (frequency, laterality)

Nose—snoring, mouth breathing, allergic reaction

Teeth—dental care

OLDER ADULTS

Older adults can present a special challenge in organizing the information obtained from the history. They may have multiple health problems that are often chronic, progressive, debilitating, and overlapping with the process of aging. Disease symptoms may be less dramatic in older patients, producing vague or nonspecific signs and symptoms. Confusion, for example, may be the only symptom of an infection or a cerebrovascular accident. Pain is often an unreliable symptom, because some older patients seem to lose pain perception and experience pain in a different manner from the classic expectations. The excruciating pain usually associated with pancreatitis, for example, may be perceived by the older patient as a dull ache, and myocardial infarction can occur without the cardinal symptom of pain. Conversely, older patients have a higher risk of developing painful conditions or injuries. Since many conditions may be present simultaneously, the cause of pain may be difficult to isolate.

Some patients fail to report symptoms, because they are afraid that the complaint will be attributed to old age or feel that nothing can be done. They may have lived with a chronic condition for so long that they have incorporated the symptoms as part of their expectation of daily living.

The tendency for multiple problems to be treated with multiple drugs places the older patient at risk for iatrogenic disorders. A complete medication history is essential, with special attention to interactions of drugs, diseases, and the aging process.

Functional assessment should be included as part of the older patient's history. In the review of systems, include questions that address functional capacity in the following areas:

Self-care activities	Instrumental activities
Walking	Driving a car
Getting out of bed	Using public transportation
Bathing	Dialing a telephone
Combing hair	Hanging up clothes
Shaving	Obtaining groceries
Dressing	Preparing meals
Eating (chewing)	Taking medications as prescribed
Getting to bathroom by self	

Other dimensions of functional capacity that should also be explored include social resources, economic resources, recreational activity, sleep patterns, environmental control, and use of the health care system. The interrelationship of physical health, mental health, social situation, and the environment is particularly evident in the older population.

· · ·

Once the history has been taken, it is necessary to move on to the physical examination—the laying on of hands. The bulk of the remaining chapters in this book discuss the many parts of the physical examination. The chapters are necessarily segmented and do not reflect the natural flow that you will develop with experience. No matter; by the last chapter we will bring it all together and, by then, you should be ready to move on to the next step of responsibility in your clinical experience.

Examination Techniques and Equipment

This chapter provides an overview of the techniques of inspection, palpation, percussion, and auscultation that are used throughout the physical examination. In addition, general use of the equipment for performing these techniques is discussed. Specific details regarding utilization of each of the techniques and the equipment as they relate to specific parts of the examination can be found in appropriate chapters.

Examination Techniques

Inspection

Inspection is the process of observation. Your eyes and nose are sensitive tools for gathering data throughout the examination. Take time to practice and develop this skill. Challenge yourself to see how much information can be collected through inspection alone. As the patient enters the room, for example, observe the gait and stance, and the ease or difficulty with which undressing and getting onto the examining table is accomplished. These observations alone will reveal a great deal about the patient's neurologic and musculoskeletal integrity. Is eye contact made? Is the demeanor appropriate for the situation? Is the clothing appropriate for the weather? The answers to these questions provide clues to the patient's emotional and mental status. Color and moisture of the skin or unusual odor can alert you to the possibility of underlying disease. These preliminary observations require only a few seconds, yet they provide basic information that can influence the rest of the examination.

Unlike palpation, percussion, and auscultation, inspection can continue throughout taking the history and during the physical examination. With this kind of continuity, what you see about the patient and the patient's demeanor is constantly subject to confirmation or dispute. Be aware of both the patient's verbal statements and body language right up to the end of the appointment. At that point, the stance, stride, strength of a handshake, and eye contact can tell you a great deal about the patient's perception of the consultation.

Some general guidelines will be helpful as you proceed through the examination and inspect each area of the body. Adequate lighting is essential. The primary lighting can be either daylight or artificial light, as long as the light is direct enough to reveal color, texture, and mobility without distortion from shadowing. Secondary, tangential lighting from a lamp that casts shadows is also important for observing contour and variations in the body surface. Inspection should be unhurried. Give yourself time to tune into what you are inspecting. Pay attention to detail and note your findings. An important rule to remember is that you have to expose what you want to inspect. All too often exposure is compromised for modesty, at the cost of important information. Part of your job is to look and observe critically.

Knowing what to look for is, of course, essential to the process of focused attention. The ability to narrow or widen your perceptual field selectively will come with time and experience, but it begins right now and develops only through practice.

Palpation

Palpation involves the use of your hands and fingers to gather information through the sense of touch. Certain parts of your hands and fingers are better than others for specific types of palpation. The palmar surface of the fingers and finger pads is more sensitive than the finger tips and is used whenever discriminatory touch is needed for determining position, texture, size, consistency, masses, fluid, and crepitus. The ulnar surface of the hand and fingers is the most sensitive area for distinguishing vibration. The dorsal surface of the hands is best for estimating temperature. Of course, this estimate provides only a crude measure and is best used to detect temperature differences in comparing parts of the body.

Specific techniques of palpation are discussed in more detail as they occur in each part of the examination. Palpation may be either light or deep and is controlled by the amount of pressure applied with the fingers or hand. For light palpation press in to a depth up to 1 centimeter and for deep palpation press in about 4 centimeters. Light palpation should always precede deep palpation, since the latter may elicit tenderness or disrupt tissue or fluid, thus obviating your ability to gather information through light palpation. Short fingernails are essential to avoid discomfort or injury to the patient.

Touch is in many ways therapeutic, and palpation is the actuality of the "laying on of hands." It is the moment at which we begin our physical invasion of the patient's body. Our much repeated advice that your approach be gentle and your hands be warm is not only practical but symbolic of your respect for the patient and for the privilege the patient gives you.

Percussion

Percussion involves striking one object against another, thus producing vibration and subsequent sound waves. In the physical examination your finger functions as a hammer, and the vibration is produced by the impact of the finger against underlying tissue. Sound waves are heard as percussion tones (called resonance) that arise from vibrations 4 to 6 centimeters deep in the body tissue. The degree of percussion tone is determined by the density of the medium through which the sound waves travel. The more dense the medium, the quieter the percussion tone. The percussion tone over air is loud, over fluid less loud, and over solid areas soft. The degree of percussion tone is classified and ordered as follows:

Tympany
Hyperresonance
Resonance
Dullness
Flatness

Tympany is the loudest, flat the quietest. Quantification of the percussion tone is difficult, especially at first. As points of reference, the gastric bubble is considered to be tympanic, air-filled lungs (as in emphysema) to be hyperresonant, healthy lungs to be resonant, the liver to be dull, and muscle to be flat. Degree of percussion is more easily distinguished by listening to the sound change as you move from one area to another. Since it is easier to hear the change from resonance to dullness

Fig. 2-1
Percussion technique: tapping interphalangeal joint. Only the middle finger of the nondominant hand should be in contact with the skin surface.

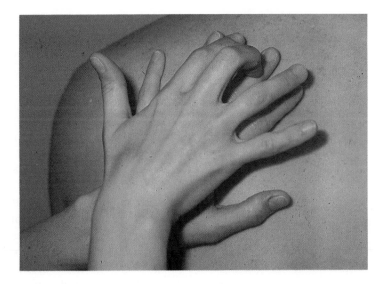

rather than from dullness to resonance, proceed with percussion from areas of resonance to areas of dullness. A partially full milk carton is a good tool for practicing percussion skills. Begin with percussion over the air-filled space of the carton, appreciating its resonant quality. Work your way downward and listen for the change in sound as you encounter the milk. This principle applies in percussion of body tissues and cavities.

The techniques of percussion are the same, regardless of the structure you are percussing. Immediate (direct) percussion involves striking the finger or hand directly against the body. A more refined variant of the technique, called mediate or indirect percussion, is used by most clinicians. In this technique the finger of one hand acts as the hammer and a finger of the other hand acts as the striking surface. To perform indirect percussion place your nondominant hand on the surface of the body with the fingers slightly spread. The distal phalanx of the middle finger should be placed firmly on the body surface with the other fingers resting gently. Snap the wrist of your other hand downward, and with the tip of the middle finger sharply tap the interphalangeal joint of the finger that is on the body surface (Fig. 2-1). You may tap just distal to the interphalangeal joint if you choose, but decide on one and be consistent because the sound varies from one to the other.

Several points are essential to note in developing the technique of percussion. The downward snap of the striking finger originates from the wrist and not the forearm or shoulder. The tap should be sharp and rapid; once the finger has struck, the wrist snaps back, quickly lifting the finger to prevent dampening the sound. The tip and not the pad of the plexor finger is used (hence short fingernails are again a necessity). Percuss one location several times to facilitate interpretation of the tone. Like other techniques, percussion must be practiced to obtain the skill needed to produce the desired result. In learning to distinguish between the tones, it may be helpful to close your eyes to block out other sensory stimuli, concentrating exclusively on the tone you are hearing.

The fist may also be used in percussion. Fist percussion is most commonly used to elicit tenderness arising from the liver, gallbladder, or kidneys. In this technique, use the ulnar aspect of the fist to deliver a firm blow to the area. Too gentle a blow will not produce enough force to stimulate the tenderness, but too hearty a blow can create unnecessary discomfort even in a well patient. Practice on yourself or a colleague until you achieve that desired middle ground.

Auscultation

Auscultation involves listening for sounds produced by the body. Some sounds, such as speech, are audible to the unassisted ear. Most other sounds require a stethoscope to augment the sound. Specific types of stethoscopes, their use, and desired characteristics are discussed in the section on stethoscopes in this chapter.

Although what you are listening for will depend on the specific part of the examination, there are some general principles that apply to all auscultory procedures. Auscultation should be carried out in a quiet environment. Listen not only for the presence of sound but also its characteristics: intensity, pitch, duration, and quality. The sounds are often subtle or transitory, and you must listen intently in order to hear the nuances. Closing your eyes may help you focus on the sound and narrow your perceptual field to prevent distraction by visual stimuli. Try to target and isolate each sound, concentrating on one sound at a time. Take enough time to identify all the characteristics of each sound. Auscultation should be carried out last, after other techniques have provided information that will assist in interpreting what you hear. Too often the temptation is to rush right in with the stethoscope, thus missing the opportunity to gather data that would be useful.

One of the most difficult achievements in auscultation is learning to isolate sounds. You cannot hear everything all at once. Whether it is a breath sound or a heartbeat or the sequence of respirations and heartbeats, each segment of the cycle must be isolated and listened to specifically. After the individual sounds are identified, they are put together. Do not anticipate the next sound; concentrate on the one at hand.

Measurement of Pulse, Respiration Rate, and Blood Pressure

The triad of pulse, respiration, and blood pressure is often considered to be the baseline indicator of a patient's health status. They may be measured early in the physical examination or integrated into separate aspects of the examination.

The pulse may be palpated in several different areas. However, the radial pulse is most often used as the screening measure for heart rate, which is the number of cardiac cycles per minute. With the pads of your second and third fingers, palpate the radial pulse on the flexor surface of the wrist laterally. Count the pulsations, also noting the rhythm, amplitude, and contour. A detailed discussion of evaluation of arterial pulses is found in Chapter 9, Heart and Blood Vessels, in the section on the peripheral vascular system.

Respirations are measured by inspection. Observe the rise and fall of the patient's chest and the ease with which breathing is accomplished. Count the number of respiratory cycles (inspiration and expiration) that occur in 1 minute to determine the respiratory rate. Also observe the regularity and rhythm of the breathing pattern. Note the depth of respirations and whether the patient uses accessory muscles. A more thorough evaluation of respiration is detailed in Chapter 8, Chest and Lungs.

Fig. 2-2
Select the appropriate size
blood pressure cuff.

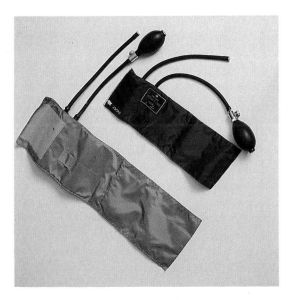

Table 2-1
Guidelines for Blood Pressure
Cuff Widths in Children*

Age	Cuff Width in Centimeters
Newborn	2.5-3
Infants (less than 1 year)	4-5
Children 1 to 4 years	6-7
Children 5 to 10 years	8-10
Children over 10 years	10-12

*Adapted from Whaley, L., and Wong, D.: Nursing care of infants and children, ed. 2, St. Louis, 1983, The C.V. Mosby Co.

Blood pressure is a peripheral measurement of cardiovascular function. Indirect measures of blood pressure are made with a stethoscope and an aneroid or mercury sphygmomanometer. Electronic sphygmomanometers, which do not require the use of a stethoscope, are also available. Each sphygmomanometer is composed of a cuff with an inflatable bladder, a pressure manometer, and a rubber hand bulb with a pressure control valve to inflate and deflate the bladder. The electronic sphygmomanometer senses vibrations and converts them into electrical impulses. The impulses are transmitted to a device that translates them into a digital readout. The instrument is relatively sensitive and is also capable of simultaneously measuring the pulse rate.

Cuffs are available in a number of sizes; the appropriate size is determined by the size of the patient's limb (Fig. 2-2). For adults choose a width that is one third to one half the circumference of the limb. The length of the bladder should be twice the width (about 80% of the limb circumference), not quite enough to completely encircle the limb. For children the cuff width should cover approximately two thirds of the upper arm or thigh (Table 2-1). For both adults and children cuffs that are too wide will underestimate blood pressure, and those that are too narrow will give an artificially high measurement.

Other pointers for using blood pressure equipment are:
- If you are using a mercury sphygmomanometer, keep the manometer vertical and make all readings at eye level.
- If you are using an aneroid instrument, position the dial so that it faces you directly. An aneroid manometer becomes inaccurate with repeated use and needs calibrating periodically.
- If the patient has an obese arm, substitute a larger cuff, using the cuff size principles to choose the appropriate size. If a sufficiently large cuff is unavailable, a standard cuff can be wrapped around the forearm and a stethoscope placed over the radial artery.
- Avoid slow or repeated inflation of the cuff, which can cause venous congestion and result in inaccurate readings. If repeated measurements are needed, wait at least 15 seconds between readings, with the cuff fully deflated. You can also remove the cuff and elevate the arm for 1 or 2 minutes.

The specific technique for measuring blood pressure is described in Chapter 9, Heart and Blood Vessels.

Some particularly sensitive examiners with a gentle touch can judge blood pressure by feeling the pulse. We all can do this when there is an obvious "bound" or "leap." You can use your finger to compress the pulse and make a judgment about the blood pressure from the amount of exertion required to shut off the beat.

Measurement of Height and Weight

Height and weight of adults are measured with a standing platform scale with a height attachment. The scale uses a system of adding and subtracting weight in increments as small as 0.25 pounds or 0.1 kilograms to counterbalance the weight placed on the scale platform. The scale is calibrated each time it is used.

Calibrate the scale to zero before the patient mounts the platform by moving both the large and small weights to zero. The balance beam should be made level and steady by adjusting the calibrating knob. The height attachment is pulled up, and the head piece is positioned at the patient's crown (Fig. 2-3).

Electronic scales are becoming more common. The weight is electronically calculated and provided as a digital read-out. These scales are automatically calibrated each time they are used.

The infant platform scale is used for measuring weights of infants and small children (Fig. 2-4). It works the same as the adult scale but can measure in ounces and grams. The scale has a platform with curved sides in which the child may sit or lie.

Infant heights can be measured by using an infant measuring board that comes with a rigid headboard and movable footboard (Fig. 2-5). The measuring board is placed on the table so that the head- and footboards are perpendicular to the table. The infant lies supine on the measuring board with the head against the headboard. The footboard is moved until it touches the bottom of the infant's feet.

An infant can also be measured by placing the baby on a pad, putting one pin into the pad at the top of the head and another at the heel of the extended leg. The length is then measured from pin to pin.

Once a child is able to stand erect without support, a stature measuring device is used to measure height. The device consists of a movable headpiece attached to a rigid measurement bar and platform. A tape measure attached to the wall and a movable headpiece can also be used (Fig. 2-6).

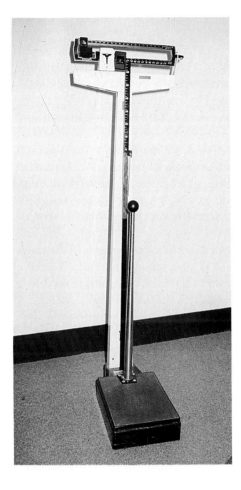

Fig. 2-3
Platform scale with height
attachment.

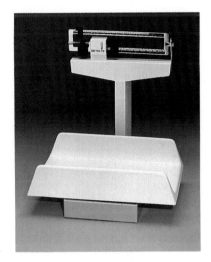

Fig. 2-4
Infant platform scale.

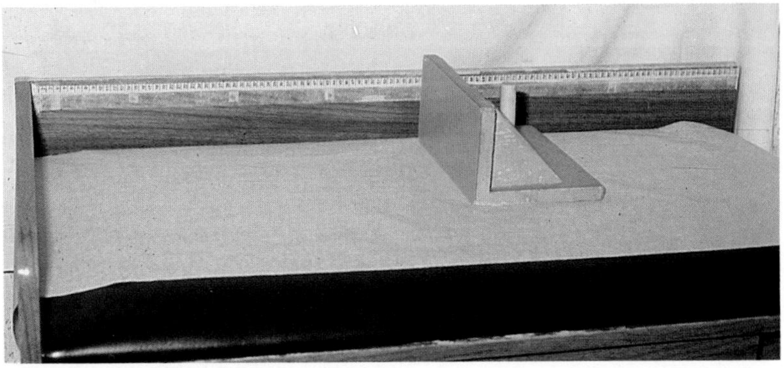

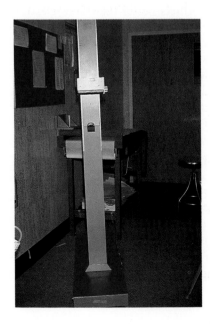

Fig. 2-6
Device to measure height
of children.

Fig. 2-5
Device to measure length of infant.

Instrumentation

Stethoscope

Auscultation of most sounds requires a stethoscope. Three basic types are available: acoustic, magnetic, and electronic. The acoustic stethoscope is a closed cylinder that transmits sound waves from the source along its column to the ear (Fig. 2-7). The rigid diaphragm has a natural frequency of around 300 Hz. It screens out low pitched sounds, and best transmits high pitched sounds such as the second heart sound. The bell endpiece, with which the skin acts as the diaphragm, has a natural frequency varying with the amount of pressure exerted. It transmits low-pitched sounds when very light pressure is used. With firm pressure, it converts to a diaphragm endpiece. The chestpiece contains a closure valve so that only one endpiece, either the diaphragm or bell, is operational at any one time (thus preventing inadvertent dissipation of sound waves).

The magnetic stethoscope has a single endpiece that is a diaphragm. It contains an iron disk on the interior surface behind which is a permanent magnet. A strong spring keeps the diaphragm bowed outward when it is not compressed against a body surface. Compression of the diaphragm activates the air column as magnetic attraction is established between the iron disk and the magnet. Rotation of a frequency dial adjusts for high, low, and full frequency sounds.

The electronic stethoscope picks up sound vibrations transmitted to the surface of the body and converts them into electrical impulses. The impulses are amplified and transmitted to a speaker where they are reconverted to sound.

The most commonly used of the three types is the acoustic stethoscope, which comes in several models. The ability to auscultate accurately depends in part on the quality of the instrument, so it is important that the stethoscope have the following characteristics:

- The diaphragm and bell are heavy enough to lie firmly on the body surface.
- The diaphragm cover is rigid.
- The bell is large enough in diameter to span an intercostal space in an adult and deep enough so that it will not fill with tissue.
- A rubber or plastic ring is around the bell edges to ensure secure contact with the body surface.
- The tubing is thick, stiff, and heavy, which conducts better than thin, elastic, or very flexible tubing.
- The length of the tubing is between 30.5 and 40 cm (12 to 18 inches) in order to minimize distortion.
- The earpieces fit snugly and comfortably. Some instruments have several sizes of earpieces and some have hard and soft earpieces. The determining factors are how they fit and feel. The earpieces should be large enough to occlude the meatus, thus blocking outside sound; if they are too small they will slip into the ear canal and be painful.
- Angled binaurals point the earpieces toward the nose so that sound is projected toward the tympanic membrane.

To stabilize the stethoscope when it is in place, hold the endpiece between the second and third fingers, pressing the diaphragm firmly against the skin (Fig. 2-8). Since the bell functions by picking up vibrations, it must be positioned so that the vibrations are not dampened. Place the bell evenly and lightly on the skin, making sure there is skin contact around the entire edge. To prevent extraneous noise, avoid touching the tubing with your hands or allowing the tubing to rub against any surfaces.

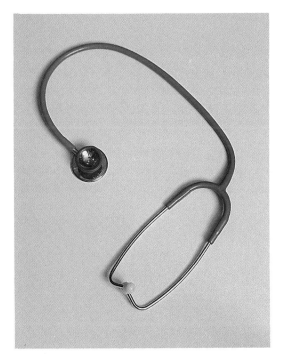

Fig. 2-7
Acoustic stethoscope.

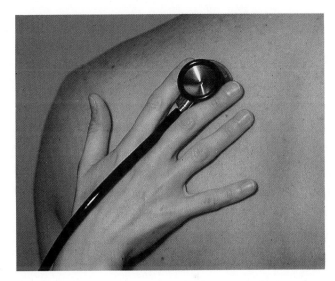

Fig. 2-8
Proper technique for holding the stethoscope.

Many pediatric specialists have found that a tiny, virtually weightless doll clinging to the structure of a stethoscope provides a diversion for the young child without interfering with the examination. Decoration and color will not interfere with what you hear.

Ophthalmoscope

The ophthalmoscope has a system of lenses and mirrors that enables visualization of the interior structures of the eye (Fig. 2-9). A light source in the instrument provides illumination through various apertures while you focus on the inner eye. The large aperture, which is used most often, produces a large round beam. The various apertures, described in Table 2-2, are selected by rotating the aperture selection dial.

The lenses in varying powers of magnification are used to bring the structure under examination into focus by converging or diverging light. On the front of the ophthalmoscope is an illuminating lens indicator that displays the number of the lens positioned in the viewing aperture. The number, ranging from about −20 to +40, corresponds to the magnification power of the lens (diopters). The positive numbers (plus lenses) are shown in black, the negative numbers (minus lenses) in red (Fig. 2-10). Clockwise rotation of the lens selector brings the minus sphere

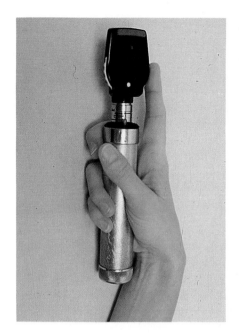

Fig. 2-9
Ophthalmoscope. Index finger is
placed on lens selection disk.

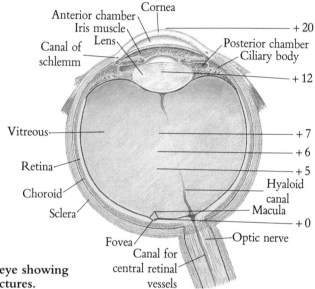

Fig. 2-10
Longitudinal cross-section of eye showing
lens diopters to focus eye structures.

Table 2-2
Apertures of the
Ophthalmoscope

Aperture	Examination Use
Small aperture	Small pupils
Red-free filter	Produces a green beam for examination of the optic disc for pallor and minute vessel changes
Slit	Examination of the anterior eye and determination of the elevation of lesions
Grid	Estimation of the size of fundal lesions

lenses into place. Counterclockwise rotation brings the plus sphere lenses into place. The system of plus and minus lenses can compensate for myopia or hyperopia in both the examiner and the patient. There is no compensation for astigmatism.

The ophthalmoscope head is seated in the handle by fitting the adapter of the handle into the head receptacle and pushing downward while turning the head in a clockwise direction. The two pieces will lock into place.

Turn on the ophthalmoscope by depressing the on/off switch and turning the rheostat control clockwise to the desired intensity of light. Turn the instrument off when you have finished using it to preserve the life of the bulb.

A more detailed discussion of the actual ophthalmoscopic examination is provided in Chapter 6, Eyes.

Snellen Visual Acuity Chart

The Snellen alphabet chart is used for a screening examination of far vision (Fig. 2-11, *A*) The chart contains letters of graduated sizes with standardized numbers at the end of each line of letters. These numbers indicate the degree of visual acuity when read from a distance of 20 feet. The "E" chart can be used in the same way for illiterate or non-English-speaking patients and for children (Fig. 2-11, *B*) Variations of the chart with geometric patterns rather than letters are also available.

Test visual acuity for each eye, using the standardized numbers on the chart. Visual acuity is recorded as a fraction, with the numerator of 20 (the distance

A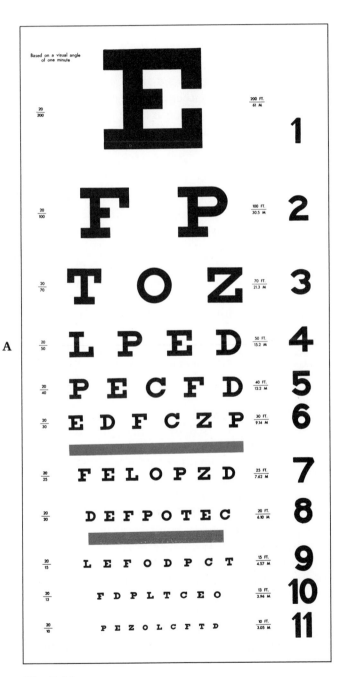

B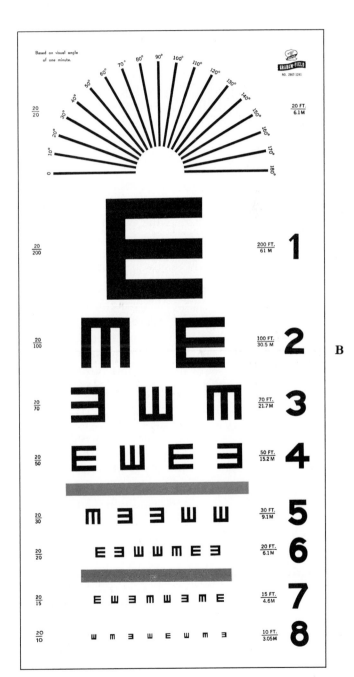

Fig. 2-11
A, Snellen and, **B,** "E" charts for testing distant vision.

between the patient and the chart) and the denominator as the distance from which the person with normal vision could read the lettering. The larger the denominator, the poorer the vision. The standard used for normal vision is 20/20. Measurement of less than 20/20 indicates either a refractive error or an optic disorder. Record the smallest complete line that the patient can read accurately without missing any letters. If the patient is able to read some but not all letters of the next smaller line, indicate this by adding the number of letters read correctly on that next line, for example 20/25 +2. This would indicate that the patient read all of the letters in the 20/25 line correctly and also two of the letters of the 20/20 line correctly.

Near Vision Charts

To assess near vision a specially designed chart such as the Rosenbaum or Jaeger charts can be used, or simply use newsprint. The Rosenbaum chart (Fig. 2-12) contains a series of numbers, Es, Xs, and Os in graduated sizes. Test and record vision for each eye separately. Acuity is recorded as either distance equivalents such as 20/20 or Jaeger equivalents such as J-2. Both these measures are indicated on the chart. If newsprint is used, the patient should be able to read it without difficulty.

Otoscope

The otoscope provides illumination for examining the external auditory canal and the tympanic membrane (Fig. 2-13). The otoscope head is seated in the handle in the same manner as the ophthalmoscope and is turned on the same way. An attached speculum narrows and directs the beam of light. Select the largest size speculum that will fit comfortably into the patient's ear canal. A glass plate magnifies and acts as a viewing window. In many models the glass plate slides aside, allowing insertion of a cerumen spoon or forceps while the otoscope remains in place. Chapter 7 (Ears, Nose, and Throat) discusses the specific techniques of examination.

The otoscope can also be used for the nasal examination if a nasal speculum is not available. Use the shortest, widest speculum and insert it gently into the patient's naris.

Pneumatic Attachment

The pneumatic attachment for the otoscope is used to evaluate the fluctuating capacity of the tympanic membrane. A short piece of rubber tubing is attached to the head of the otoscope. A handbulb attached to the other end of the tubing, when squeezed, produces puffs of air that causes the tympanic membrane to move. If no handbulb is attached, place the open end of the tubing in your mouth and puff and suck into the tubing to produce the same effect.

Nasal Speculum

The nasal speculum is used with a penlight to visualize the lower and middle turbinates of the nose (Fig. 2-14). Be sure that the patient is in a comfortable position. The head may need to be supported, or you can have the patient lie down. You will need to tilt the patient's head at various angles for a complete nasal examination. Stabilize the speculum with your index finger to avoid contact of the blades with the nasal septum, which can cause discomfort. The blades are opened by squeezing the handles of the instrument.

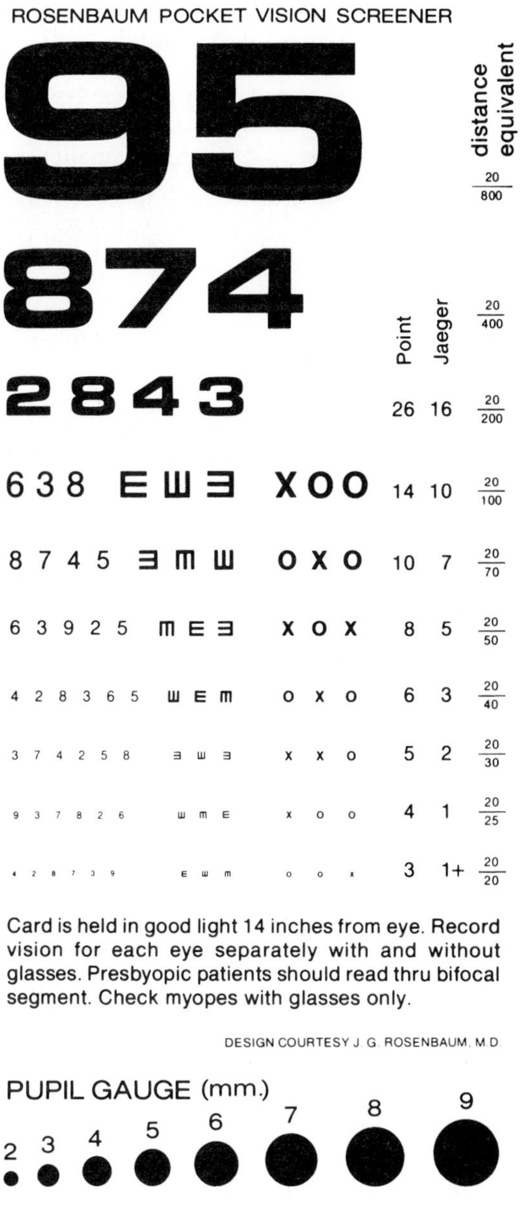

ROSENBAUM POCKET VISION SCREENER

							Point	Jaeger	distance equivalent
95									$\frac{20}{800}$
874									$\frac{20}{400}$
2 8 4 3							26	16	$\frac{20}{200}$
6 3 8	E Ш Ǝ	X O O					14	10	$\frac{20}{100}$
8 7 4 5	Ǝ Ш Ш	O X O					10	7	$\frac{20}{70}$
6 3 9 2 5	Ш Ǝ Ǝ	X O X					8	5	$\frac{20}{50}$
4 2 8 3 6 5	Ш Ш Ш	O X O					6	3	$\frac{20}{40}$
3 7 4 2 5 8	Ǝ Ш Ǝ	X X O					5	2	$\frac{20}{30}$
9 3 7 8 2 6	Ш Ш Ш	X O O					4	1	$\frac{20}{25}$
4 2 8 7 3 9	Ш Ш Ш	O O X					3	1+	$\frac{20}{20}$

Card is held in good light 14 inches from eye. Record vision for each eye separately with and without glasses. Presbyopic patients should read thru bifocal segment. Check myopes with glasses only.

DESIGN COURTESY J. G. ROSENBAUM, M.D.

PUPIL GAUGE (mm.)

2 3 4 5 6 7 8 9

Fig. 2-12
Rosenbaum chart for testing near vision.

Fig. 2-13
Otoscope with various size specula and pneumatic attachment.

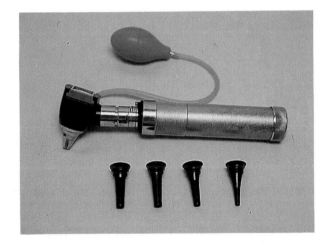

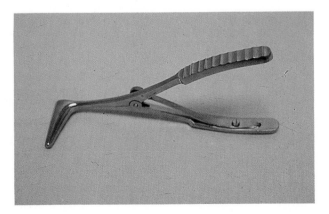

Fig. 2-14
Nasal speculum.

Tuning Fork

Tuning forks are used in screening tests for auditory function and for vibratory sensation as part of the neurologic examination (Fig. 2-15) As tuning forks are activated, vibrations are created that produce a particular frequency of sound wave, expressed as cycles per second (cps) or Hertz. Thus a fork of 512 Hz vibrates 512 cycles per second.

For auditory evaluation use a fork with a frequency of 500 to 1000 Hz, because it can estimate hearing loss in the range of normal speech, approximately 300 to 3000 Hz. Forks of lower frequency can cause you to overestimate bone conduction and can be felt as vibration as well as heard. Activate the fork by gently stroking the prongs or tapping them against the knuckles of your hand, so that they ring softly (Fig. 2-16). Because touching the tines will dampen the sound, the fork must be held at the base. Hearing is tested at near threshold level, which is the lowest intensity of sound at which an auditory stimulus can be heard. Striking the prongs too vigorously results in a loud tone that is above the threshold level and will require time to quiet to a tone appropriate for auditory testing. The specific tuning fork tests for hearing are described in Chapter 7, Ears, Nose, and Throat.

For vibratory sensation, use a fork of lower frequency. The greatest sensitivity to vibration occurs when the fork is vibrating between 100 and 400 Hz. Activate the tuning fork by tapping it against the heel of your hand and apply the base of the fork to a bony prominence. The patient feels the vibration as a buzzing or tingling sensation. The specific areas of testing are described in Chapter 17, Neurologic System and Mental Status.

Percussion (Reflex) Hammer

The percussion hammer is used to test deep tendon reflexes. Hold the hammer loosely between thumb and index finger, so that as you tap the tendon, the hammer moves in a swift arc and in a controlled direction. Use a rapid downward snap of the wrist, tap quickly and firmly, and then snap your wrist back so that the hammer does not linger on the tendon (Fig. 2-17). The tap should be brisk and direct. Practice this action to achieve smooth, rapid, and controlled motion. You can use either the pointed or flat end of the hammer. The flat end is more comfortable when striking the patient directly; the pointed end is useful in small areas, such as your finger placed over the patient's biceps tendon. Chapter 17 (Neurologic System and Mental Status) contains a detailed discussion of evaluation of deep tendon reflexes.

Your finger can also act as a reflex hammer, which can be particularly useful when you are examining the very young. Certainly it is less threatening to a child than a hammer. There are many pediatric specialists who let the child hold the hammer while they use their fingers.

Neurologic Hammer

A variant of the percussion hammer, the neurologic hammer is also used for testing deep tendon reflexes (Fig. 2-18). In addition, the hammer has two features that make it a multipurpose neurologic instrument. The base of the handle unscrews, revealing a soft brush. A tiny knob on the head also unscrews, to which is attached a sharp needle. These additional implements can be used to determine sensory perception as part of the neurologic examination. To avoid the possibility of infection, be sure that you clean the needle with a bacteriostatic solution before each use, although many practitioners advise against using this needle at all. The procedure for testing sensory perception is described in detail in Chapter 17, Neurologic System and Mental Status.

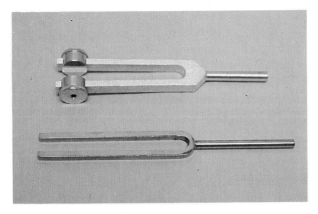

Fig. 2-15
Tuning forks for auditory
screening and testing
vibratory sensation.

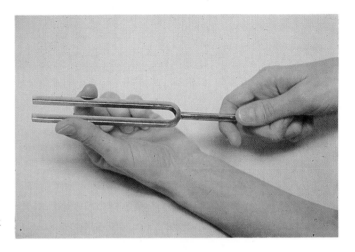

Fig. 2-16
Stroking the tuning fork
to activate it.

Fig. 2-17
A, Reflex hammer. **B,** Use
a rapid downward snap
of the wrist.

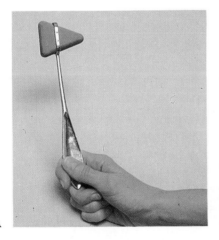

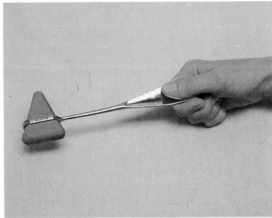

A

B

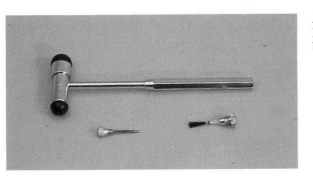

Fig. 2-18
Neurologic hammer. Note the
brush and needle.

Tape Measure

A tape measure 7 to 12 mm wide is used for determining circumference, length, and diameter. It may be helpful to have one that measures in both inches and millimeters. Tape measures are available in a variety of materials. It should be nonstretchable for accuracy and pliable for circumference measurement. Since it is placed against the skin, beware of edges that are sharp and can cut.

When measuring make sure that the tape is not caught or wrinkled beneath the patient. Pull the tape closely but not tightly enough to cause depression of the skin when measuring circumference.

When monitoring serial measures, such as head circumferences or abdominal girth, it is important to place the tape measure in the same position each time. If serial measures are made over a period of days, an easy way to assure accurate placement is to mark with pen the borders of the tape at several intervals on the skin. Subsequently, the tape can be placed within the markings. Accurate placement of the tape for specific measurements is described in Chapter 3 and related chapters.

Transilluminator

Transilluminators consist of a strong light source with a narrow beam. The beam is directed to a particular body cavity and is used to differentiate between various media present in that cavity. Light is differentially transmitted by air, fluid, and tissue, which allows you to detect the presence of fluid in sinuses, the presence of blood or masses in the scrotum, and abnormalities in the cranium of infants.

Specific transilluminating instruments are available, or a flashlight with a rubber adapter can be used (Fig. 2-19). In either case, transillumination should be performed in a darkened room. Place the beam of light directly against the area to be observed, shielding the beam with your hand if necessary. Watch for the red glow of light through the body cavity. Note the presence or absence of illumination and any irregularities.

Fig. 2-19
Transilluminators. Watch for the red glow. *Left,* Chun gun. *Right,* Flashlight with transilluminator attachment.

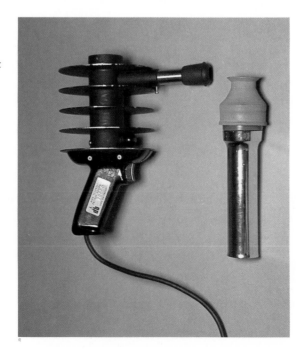

Fig. 2-20
Vaginal specula. From left to right: **A,** Short-billed pediatric, pediatric, small Pederson, Pederson, small Graves, large Graves, plastic Graves. **B,** Short-billed pediatric, pediatric, small Pederson, Pederson, small Graves, large Graves.

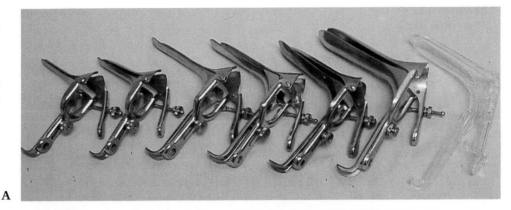

A

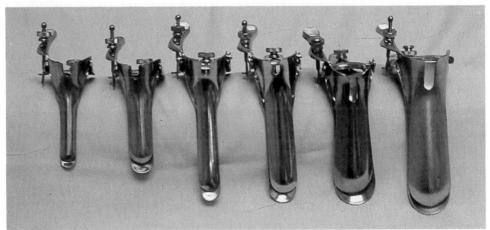

B

Vaginal Speculum

Vaginal specula are composed of two blades and a handle. There are three basic types of vaginal specula, which are used to view the vaginal canal and cervix. The Graves speculum is available in a variety of sizes with blades ranging from 3.5 to 5 inches in length and 0.75 to 1.25 inches in width. The blades are curved with a space between the closed blades. The bottom blade is about 0.25 inch longer than the top blade to conform with the longer posterior vaginal wall and to aid in visualization. The Pederson speculum has blades that are as long as those of the Graves speculum but are both narrower and flatter. It is used for women with small vaginal openings. Pediatric or virginal specula are smaller in all dimensions, with short, narrow, flat blades (Fig. 2-20).

Specula are available in either disposable plastic or reusable metal. The metal speculum has two positioning devices. The top blade is hinged and has a positioning thumbpiece lever attached. When you press down on the thumbpiece, the distal end of the blade rises, thus opening the speculum. The blade can be locked in an open position by tightening the thumbscrew on the thumbpiece. The degree of opening of the proximal end of the blades is controlled by moving the top blade up or down; it is locked in place by another thumbscrew, which is on the handle.

The plastic speculum operates differently from the metal one. The bottom blade is fixed to a posterior handle, and the top blade is controlled by an anterior lever handle. As you press on the lever, the distal end of the top blade elevates. At the same time the base of the speculum also widens. The speculum is locked into position with a catch on the lever handle that snaps into place in a positioning groove.

You will need to become familiar with and practice with both types of specula in order to feel comfortable with them. Do not wait until you are in the process of doing your first examination or you are likely to be embarrassed and cause discomfort to the woman by your initial clumsiness in handling (or mishandling) the instrument.

The procedure for performing the speculum examination is described in detail in Chapter 12, Female Genitalia and Pregnancy.

Goniometer

The goniometer is used to determine the degree of joint flexion and extension. The instrument consists of two straight arms that intersect and can be angled and rotated around a protractor, which is marked with degrees (Fig. 2-21). Place the center of the protractor over the joint and align the straight arms with the long axis of the extremity. The degree of angle flexion or extension is indicated on the protractor. The specific joint examinations are discussed in Chapter 16, Musculoskeletal System.

Wood's Lamp

The Wood's lamp contains a light source with a wavelength of 360 nm (Fig. 2-22). This is the black light that causes certain substances to fluoresce when exposed to the light. It is used primarily to determine the presence of fungi on skin lesions. Darken the room, turn on the Wood's lamp, and shine it on the area or lesion you are evaluating. Yellow-green fluorescence indicates the presence of fungi.

WHAT EQUIPMENT DO YOU NEED TO PURCHASE?

Students are confronted by a large number and variety of pieces of equipment that are necessary to perform physical examination. A frequently asked question is, "What do I *really* need to buy?" The answer to that depends somewhat on where you will be practicing. If you are in a clinic setting, for example, wall mounted ophthalmoscopes and otoscopes are provided. This is not necessarily true in a hospital setting.

The following list is intended only as a guideline to the equipment that you will use most often and should personally own.

Stethoscope
Ophthalmoscope
Otoscope
Ruler
Tape measure
Reflex hammer
Tuning forks: 500–1000 Hz for auditory screening, 100–400 Hz for vibratory sensation
Penlight
Near vision screening chart

Calipers for Skinfold Thickness

Skinfold thickness calipers are designed to measure the thickness of subcutaneous tissue at certain points of the body (Fig. 2-23). Specifically calibrated and tested calipers are used, such as the Lange and Herpenden models. The skinfold is pinched up, so that the sides of the skin are parallel. Place the caliper edges at the base of the fold, being careful not to capture bone or muscle. Tighten the calipers so that they are grasping the skinfold but not compressing it. The specific technique for triceps skinfold thickness measurement is described in Chapter 3, Growth and Measurement.

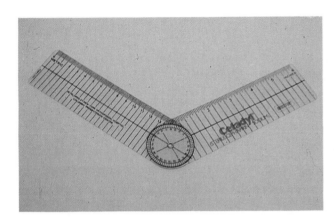

Fig. 2-21
Goniometer.

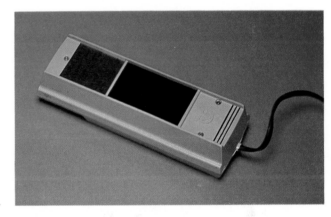

Fig. 2-22
Wood's lamp.

Fig. 2-23
Triceps skinfold caliper.
Grasp the handle and
depress lever with thumb.

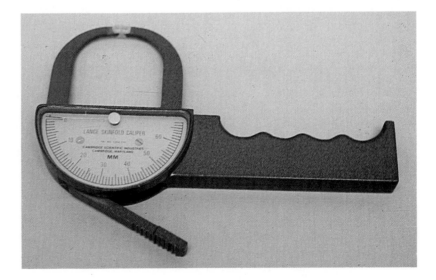

Growth and Measurement

Weight and body composition offer much information about an individual's health status, often providing a clue to the presence of disease when out of balance. The care of children is exciting because of the constancy of change that is explicit in growth and development. Children just do not stay the same. Measuring their weights and heights, giving careful attention to the sequence of their achievements, is gratifying as you get to know a child over time. When all goes well and the child grows and develops as you would wish, there is great pleasure. But, when all is not well, your careful attention and early detection can often correct or at least ameliorate a problem.

The focus of this chapter is evaluation of an individual's anthropometric parameters and the examination for growth, gestational age, and pubertal development. Neurologic and motor development of children are discussed in Chapters 16 (Musculoskeletal System) and 17 (Neurologic System and Mental Status).

Anatomy and Physiology

Growth, the increase in size of an individual or single organ, is dependent on a sequence of endocrine, genetic, constitutional, environmental, and nutritional influences. Through the biologic process of development and maturation, individual organ systems acquire function.

Endocrine Influences

The growth process requires the interaction and balance of many hormones for normal growth and development to proceed (Fig. 3-1).

Growth hormone, secreted by the pituitary gland, acts primarily during late infancy and adulthood to stimulate DNA synthesis and increase cell numbers. Insulin, in concert with growth hormone, assists growth by promoting protein (cytoplasm) accumulation in the cell and cell proliferation. Thyroxin, secreted by the thyroid gland, greatly influences fetal and neonatal growth. Thyroxin enhances skeletal growth and development, promotes sexual maturation, and influences mental development.

The gonads begin to secrete testosterone and estrogen during puberty. Testosterone enhances muscular development and sexual maturation and promotes bone maturation and epiphyseal closure. Estrogen stimulates the development of female secondary sexual characteristics and linear growth by the acceleration of skeletal maturation and epiphyseal fusion. It also stimulates the growth and differentiation of the genitalia during the fetal period. Androgens, secreted by the adrenal glands, promote masculinization of the secondary sex characteristics and skeletal maturation.

Fig. 3-1
Hormones affecting growth during childhood and the age at which they are most influential.
Redrawn from Hughes, 1984.

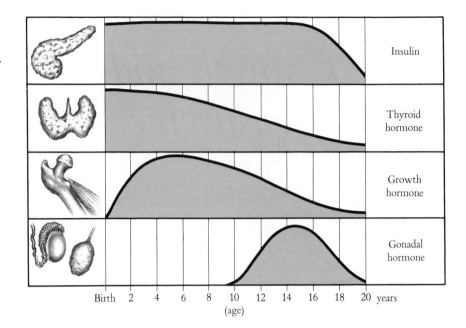

The developmental changes of puberty are caused by the interaction of the hypothalamus, pituitary gland, and gonads. Gonadotropin-releasing hormone, secreted by the hypothalamus, stimulates the pituitary to secrete follicle-stimulating hormone (FSH) and luteinizing hormone (LH). These hormones, in turn, act on the gonads to stimulate germ cell maturation and the synthesis of sex steroid hormones. The adolescent growth spurt results from the synergistic action of the sex steroids and growth hormone when other endocrine functions are normal.

Differences in Growth by Organ System

Each organ and organ system has its particular period of rapid growth, marked by rapid cell differentiation and changes in form, that is influenced by the physical and environmental factors to which it is exposed. As individuals, each of us has a unique growth timetable and final growth outcome. However, the sequential patterns are consistent for all of us, unless some external environmental or inherent pathophysiologic process intervenes (Figs. 3-2 and 3-3).

General growth encompasses most body measurements and organ growth, specifically the musculoskeletal system, liver, and kidneys. Their growth approximates the growth curves described for stature.

Skeletal growth is considered complete when the epiphyses of long bones have completely fused. The mean age for this event (± 2 years) in males is 17.5 years and in females is 15.5 years, 2 years after menarche. However, skeletal growth continues until 30 years of age with the apposition of bone to the upper and lower surfaces of the vertebral bodies. The increase in stature is only 3 to 5 mm during this time. Stature is stationary between the ages of 30 to 45 years and then begins to decline (Tanner, 1978).

Weight is closely related to growth in stature and organ development. Growth and development are influenced by nutritional adequacy, which contributes to the number and size of adipose cells. The number of adipose cells increases throughout childhood. Sex-related differences in fat deposition appear in infancy and continue through adolescence.

Lymphatic tissues (lymph nodes, spleen, tonsils, adenoids, and blood lympho-cytes) are small in relation to total body size but are well developed at birth. These tissues grow rapidly to reach adult dimensions by 6 years of age. By age 10 to 12 the lymphatic tissues are at their peak, about double adult size. During adolescence, they decrease in size until stable adult dimensions are reached.

Fig. 3-2
Rates of growth in various tissues between fetal development and adolescence.
Redrawn from Smith, 1977.

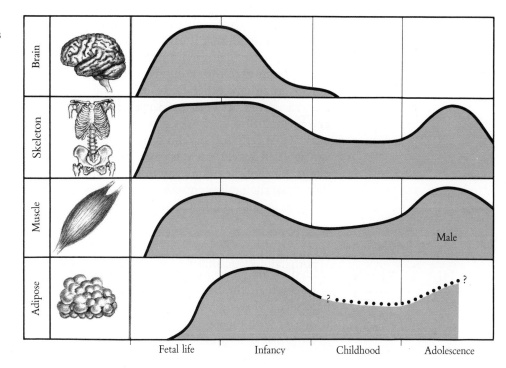

Fetal life   Infancy   Childhood   Adolescence

Fig. 3-3
Growth rates for the body as a whole and three specialized tissues between birth and adulthood. *General* is the body as a whole, including external dimensions, and the respiratory, digestive, renal, circulatory, and musculoskeletal systems. *Lymphatic* includes the thymus, lymph nodes, and intestinal lymph masses. *Neural* includes the brain, dura, spinal cord, optic apparatus, and head dimensions. *Genital* includes the reproductive organ systems.
From Whaley and Wong, 1983.

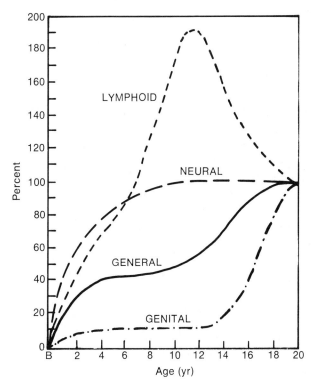

The reproductive organs, both internal and external, have a slow prepubertal growth. With the interaction of the hypothalamus, pituitary, and gonadal hormones, the reproductive organs double in size during adolescence, achieving maturation and function.

The brain is a marvelous organ, so fully developed at an early age that it provides infants and young children opportunities to sense and appreciate the world and to learn an enormous amount. We often fail to appreciate the sophistication of that brain in the body of a baby or a toddler. At some subconscious level we do not expect it to do all that it can, and we tend to underestimate the ability of the very young to sense their environment.

The brain with the skull, eyes, and ears, completes physical development more quickly than any other body part. The most rapid and critical period of brain growth occurs between conception and 2 years of age. Most of the neurons are present by 18 to 20 weeks gestation, and two thirds of brain cells are present at birth. Glial cells and myelin continue to develop after birth, and by 10 months of age new cell development is complete. Cell size continues to increase, and at 2 years of age, 80% of the brain growth is completed (Trauner, 1979). During adolescence the size of the head increases because of development of air sinuses and thickening of the scalp and skull, not because of brain growth.

INFANTS AND CHILDREN

As the child grows from infancy to adulthood, the change in body proportions is related to the pattern of skeletal growth (Fig. 3-4).

Growth of the head predominates during the fetal period. Fetal weight gain naturally follows growth in length, but weight reaches its peak during the third trimester with the increase in organ size (Fig. 3-5). The birth weight of the infant is in large part determined by the mother's prepregnancy weight, weight gained during pregnancy, placental function, and gestational age (Fig. 3-6).

During infancy the growth of the trunk predominates, and weight gain velocity proceeds at a rapid but decelerating rate. The fat content of the body increases slowly during early fetal development, and then rapidly accelerates during infancy until approximately 9 months of age.

Fig. 3-4
Changes in body proportions from 8 weeks of gestation through adulthood.

Redrawn from Crouch and McClintic, 1976.

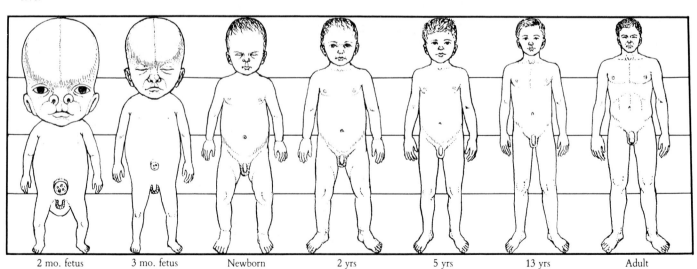

| 2 mo. fetus | 3 mo. fetus | Newborn | 2 yrs | 5 yrs | 13 yrs | Adult |

TIMETABLE OF HUMAN PRENATAL DEVELOPMENT
1 to 6 weeks

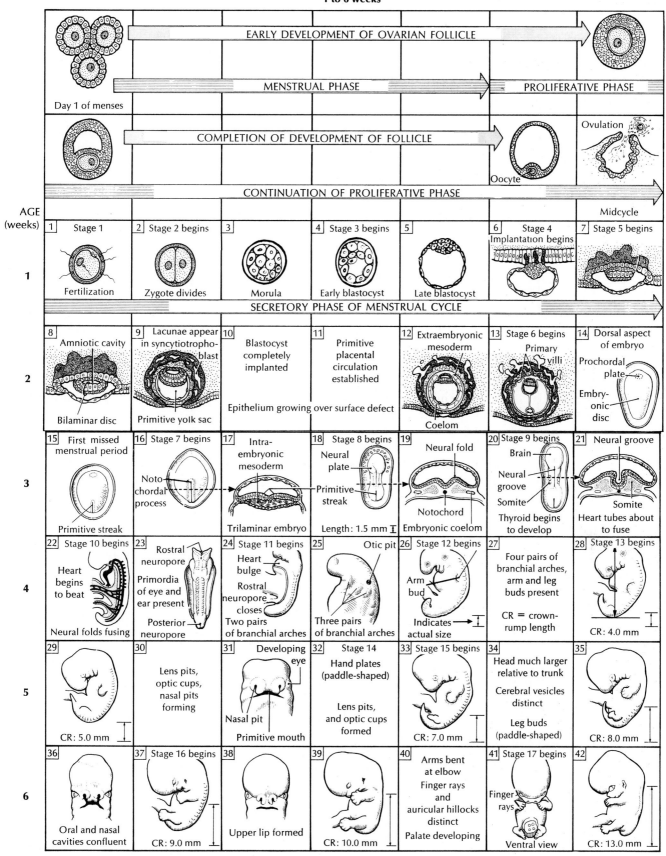

Fig. 3-5

Timetable of human prenatal development.

From Moore, K.L.: "The Developing Human. Clinically Oriented Embryology," 3rd ed., 1982. Courtesy W.B. Saunders Company, Philadelphia, Pennsylvania.

Continued.

TIMETABLE OF HUMAN PRENATAL DEVELOPMENT
7 to 38 weeks

Fig. 3-5, cont'd
Timetable of human prenatal development.

From Moore, K.L.: "The Developing Human. Clinically Oriented Embryology," 3rd ed., 1982. Courtesy W.B. Saunders Company, Philadelphia, Pennsylvania.

The legs are the fastest growing body part during childhood, and weight is gained at a steady rate. Fat tissue increases slowly until 7 years of age, at which time a prepubertal fat spurt occurs prior to the true growth spurt.

The trunk and the legs elongate during adolescence. During this period about 50% of the individual's ideal weight is gained, as the skeletal mass and organ systems double in size. It is during adolescence that males develop broader shoulders and greater musculature than females, while females develop a wider pelvic outlet. Males have a slight increase in body fat during early adolescence, and then have a proportionate gain in lean body tissue. Females have a persistent increase in fat tissue throughout adolescence occurring after the peak growth spurt (Peck and Ullrich, 1985).

PREGNANT WOMEN

Progressive weight gain is expected during pregnancy, but the amount will vary among women. The growing fetus accounts for only 5 to 10 lb of the total weight gained. The remainder results from an increase in maternal tissues (placenta, amniotic fluid, uterus, blood and fluid volume, breasts, and fat reserves) (Fig. 3-7).

Desirable weight gain follows a curve through the trimesters of pregnancy. The rate of weight gain is slow during the first trimester, rapid during the second trimester, and less rapid during the third trimester. Maternal tissue growth accounts for most of the weight gained in the first and second trimesters, while fetal growth accounts for weight gained during the third trimester.

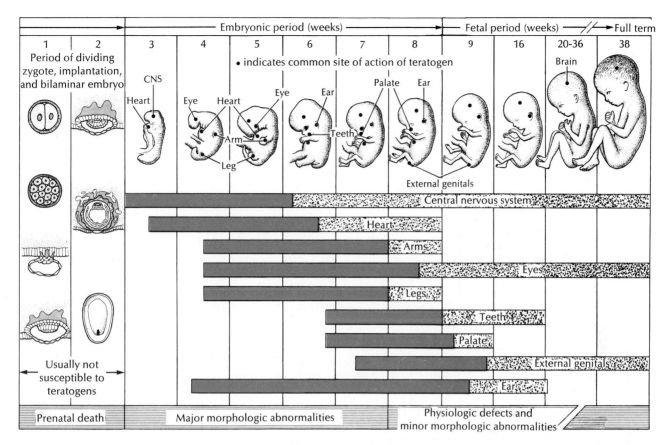

Fig. 3-6
**Sensitive, or critical, periods in human development. Solid red denotes highly sensitive periods;
stippled red indicates stages that are less sensitive to teratogens.**
From Moore, K.L.: "The Developing Human. Clinically Oriented Embryology," 3rd ed., 1982. Courtesy W.B. Saunders Company.

Fig. 3-7
**Weight gain during
pregnancy and tissue
growth contributing to the
total weight gained.**
From Schneider, 1983.

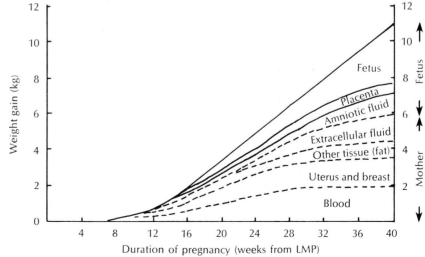

OLDER ADULTS   Stature declines in the older adult, beginning at approximately 50 years of age. Women lose an average of 4.9 cm whereas men lose an average of 2.9 cm (Malasanos, et al., 1986). This is caused by a thinning of the intervertebral disks and by the development of kyphosis.

Muscle mass decreases by 30% to 40% between 30 and 80 years of age; however, exercise contributes to a slower reduction of muscle mass. This decline in lean body mass is accompanied by an increase in body fat, so that the total body weight tends to remain constant with aging. There is a reduction in size and weight of various organs associated with aging, especially the liver, lungs, and kidneys. The bones decrease in density and weight by 12% in men and 25% in women (Malasanos, et al., 1986).

Review of Related History

General Considerations

1. Nutrition: usual caloric intake, calories adequate or excessive for maintenance of weight; proportion fat, protein, carbohydrate in diet
2. Usual weight and height
3. Chronic illness: gastrointestinal, renal, pulmonary, cardiac, cancer, infections, or allergies
4. Medications: steroids, diet pills, laxatives

Present Problem

1. Weight gain or loss: time period; sudden or gradual; related to dieting; change in life-style, eating pattern, appetite, activity, or stress
2. Vomiting or diarrhea: frequency, consistency, time period, able to keep food down, self-induced, signs of dehydration, association with chronic illness
3. Noticeable change in body proportions or fat distribution: coarsening facial features, enlarging hands and feet, moon facies, or trunk-girdle fat distribution rather than a generalized fat distribution (may indicate endocrine pathology)
4. Excessive concern with losing weight: never thin enough, weight goal, fasting, bulimia, body image, clothing size, amenorrhea
5. Pregnancy: date of last menstrual period, prepregnancy weight, weight gain pattern, following established weight gain curve for gestational course, dietary intake

Past Medical History

1. Chronic illness
2. Previous weight loss or gain efforts

Family History

1. Obesity
2. Constitutionally short or tall stature, precocious or delayed puberty
3. Genetic or metabolic disorder: cystic fibrosis, mucopolysaccaridosis, dwarfism

INFANTS

1. Estimated gestational age, birth weight
2. Following an established percentile growth curve
   a. Unexplained changes in length, weight, or head circumference
   b. Poor growth: falling 1 or more standard deviations off growth curve pattern, below 5th percentile for weight and height, infant small for gestational age, quality of mother–infant interaction
3. Development: achieving milestones at appropriate ages
4. Nutrition: dietary intake and calories adequate for growth
5. Congenital anomaly or chronic illness: heart defect, hydrocephalus, microcephalus, malabsorption syndrome, urinary tract infection

CHILDREN AND ADOLESCENTS

1. Sexual maturation of girls: early (before 8 years) or delayed (beyond 13 years) signs of breast development and pubic hair, age at menarche
2. Sexual maturation of boys: early (before 9 years) or delayed (beyond 14 years) signs of genital development and pubic hair
3. Short stature: not growing as fast as peers, change in shoe and clothing size in past year, extremities short or long for size of trunk, size of head disproportionate to body, height of parents
4. Tall stature: growing faster than peers, height of parents, signs of sexual maturation

OLDER ADULTS

1. Nutrition: weight gain or loss, income adequate for nutritional purchases, "meals on wheels" participant, social interaction with meals, number of meals a day
2. Chronic debilitating illness: problems with meal preparation, problems eating

Examination and Findings

EQUIPMENT

- Standing platform scale with height attachment
- Skinfold thickness calipers
- Measuring tape
- Infant scale
- Recumbent measuring board (for infants)
- Stature measuring device (for children)

Weight and Standing Height

To measure weight, have the patient stand in the middle of the scale platform while you balance the scale. Move the largest weight to the 50-lb or 10-kg increment under the patient's weight. Adjust the smaller weight to balance the scale. Read the weight to the nearest 0.1 kg or ¼ lb. Weight variations occur during the day and from day-to-day with changes in fluid and intestinal contents of the body. When monitoring a patient's weight daily or weekly, weigh the patient at a consistent time of day.

To measure height, have the patient stand erect with back to scale. Pull up the height attachment and position the headpiece at the patient's crown. Make the reading at the nearest centimeter or ½ in.

Table 3-1

*Elbow Breadth Measurements Associated with Medium Size Frames for Men and Women at Various Ages. Measurements Lower Than Ranges Given Indicate a Small Frame, While Higher Measurements Indicate a Large Frame**

	Men		Women	
Age (yrs)	Elbow Breadth (cm)		Age (yrs)	Elbow Breadth (cm)
18–24	>6.6–<7.7		18–24	>5.6–<6.5
25–34	>6.7–<7.9		25–34	>5.7–<6.8
35–44	>6.7–<8.0		35–44	>5.7–<7.1
45–54	>6.7–<8.1		45–54	>5.7–<7.2
55–74	>6.7–<8.1		55–74	>5.8–<7.2

Adapted from Frisancho, 1984.
*Data from the National Health and Nutrition Examination Survey (NHANES) I (1971 to 1974) AND NHANES II (1976 to 1980) conducted by the National Center for Health Statistics (NCHS).

Table 3-2

*Selected Percentiles of Weight and Triceps Skinfold Thickness by Height in U.S. Men, Age 25 to 54 Years, With Small, Medium, and Large Frames**

Height		Weight (kg)					Triceps (mm)						
In	Cm	5	15	50	85	95	5	10	15	50	85	90	95
Small Frames, Men													
62	157	46	52	64	71	77				11			
63	160	48	53	61	70	79			6	10	17		
64	163	49	55	66	76	80		5	5	10	16	18	
65	165	52	58	66	77	84	4	5	6	11	17	19	21
66	168	56	59	67	78	84	5	6	6	11	18	18	20
67	170	56	62	71	82	88	5	6	6	11	18	20	22
68	173	56	62	71	79	85	5	6	6	10	15	16	20
69	175	57	65	74	84	88		6	6	11	17	20	
70	178	59	67	75	87	90			7	10	17		
71	180	60	70	76	79	91			7	10	16		
72	183	62	67	74	87	93				10			
73	185	63	69	79	89	94							
74	188	65	71	80	90	96							
Medium Frames, Men													
62	157	51	58	68	81	87				15			
63	160	52	59	71	82	89				11			
64	163	54	61	71	83	90		6	6	12	18	20	
65	165	59	65	74	87	94	5	7	8	12	20	22	25
66	168	58	65	75	85	93	5	6	7	11	16	18	22
67	170	62	68	77	89	100	5	7	7	13	21	23	28
68	173	60	66	78	89	97	4	5	7	11	18	20	24
69	175	63	68	78	90	97	5	6	7	12	18	20	24
70	178	64	70	81	90	97	5	6	7	12	18	20	23
71	180	62	70	81	92	100	4	5	7	12	19	21	25
72	183	68	74	84	97	104	5	7	7	12	20	22	26
73	185	70	75	85	100	104	6	7	8	12	20	24	27
74	188	68	77	88	100	104		6	9	13	21	23	
Large Frames, Men													
62	157	57	66	82	99	108							
63	160	58	67	83	100	109							
64	163	59	68	84	101	110							
65	165	60	69	79	102	111				14			
66	168	60	75	84	103	112		9		14	30		
67	170	62	71	84	102	113		7	7	11	23	27	
68	173	63	76	86	101	114		9	10	14	22	23	
69	175	68	74	89	103	114	6	7	8	15	25	29	31
70	178	68	74	87	106	114	7	7	7	14	23	25	30
71	180	73	82	91	113	123	6	8	10	15	25	27	31
72	183	73	78	91	109	121	5	6	7	12	20	22	25
73	185	72	79	93	106	116	5	6	7	13	19	22	31
74	188	69	82	92	105	120			8	12	19		

Adapted from Frisancho, 1984.
*Data from the NHANES I (1971 to 1974) and NHANES II (1976 to 1980), conducted by the NCHS.

Measurement of the elbow breadth provides an estimate of frame size. Have the patient extend the right arm and flex the elbow to 90 degrees. The patient's fingers should be pointing up with the palm turned laterally. Facing the patient, place skinfold calipers, held on the same plane as the upper arm, on the two most prominent bones of the elbow to measure the elbow breadth. (Sliding calipers may be needed if the skinfold calipers do not extend to the breadth of the elbow.) Read the patient's measurement in centimeters and compare it with the table of elbow breadth measurements for age and sex (Table 3-1).

Table 3-3
Selected Percentiles of Weight and Triceps Skinfold Thickness by Height for U.S. Women, Age 25 to 54 Years, With Small, Medium, and Large Frames*

Height		Weight (kg)					Triceps (mm)						
In	Cm	5	15	50	85	95	5	10	15	50	85	90	95
Small Frames, Women													
58	147	37	43	52	58	66		12	13	24	30	33	
59	150	42	44	53	63	72	8	11	14	21	29	36	37
60	152	42	45	53	63	70	8	11	12	21	28	29	33
61	155	44	47	54	64	72	11	12	14	21	28	31	34
62	157	44	48	55	63	70	10	12	14	20	28	31	34
63	160	46	49	55	65	79	10	11	13	20	27	30	36
64	163	49	51	57	67	74	10	13	13	20	28	30	34
65	165	50	53	60	70	80	12	13	14	22	29	31	34
66	168	46	54	58	65	74			12	19	30		
67	170	47	52	59	70	76				18			
68	173	48	53	62	71	77				20			
69	175	49	54	63	72	78							
70	178	50	55	64	73	79							
Medium Frames, Women													
58	147	41	50	63	77	79			20	25	40		
59	150	47	52	66	76	85	15	19	21	30	37	40	40
60	152	47	52	60	77	85	14	15	17	26	35	37	41
61	155	47	51	61	73	86	11	14	15	25	34	36	42
62	157	49	52	61	73	83	12	14	16	24	34	36	40
63	160	49	53	62	77	88	12	13	15	24	33	35	38
64	163	50	54	62	76	87	11	14	15	23	33	36	40
65	165	52	55	63	75	89	12	14	15	22	31	34	38
66	168	52	55	63	75	83	11	13	14	22	31	33	37
67	170	54	57	65	79	88	12	13	15	21	29	30	35
68	173	58	60	67	77	87	10	14	15	22	31	32	36
69	175	49	60	68	79	87		11	12	19	29	31	
70	178	50	57	70	80	87				19			
Large Frames, Women													
58	147	56	67	86	105	117							
59	150	56	67	78	105	116				36			
60	152	55	66	87	104	116				38			
61	155	54	66	81	105	115		25	26	36	48	50	
62	157	59	65	81	103	113	16	19	22	34	48	48	50
63	160	58	67	83	105	119	18	20	22	34	46	48	51
64	163	59	63	79	102	112	16	20	21	32	43	45	49
65	165	59	63	81	103	114	17	20	21	31	43	46	48
66	168	55	62	75	95	107	13	17	18	27	40	43	45
67	170	58	65	80	100	114	13	16	17	30	41	43	49
68	173	51	66	76	104	111		16	20	29	37	40	
69	175	50	68	79	105	111			21	30	42		
70	178	50	61	76	99	110				20			

Adapted from Frisancho, 1984.
*Data from the NHANES I (1971 to 1974) and NHANES II (1976 to 1980), conducted by the NCHS.

Once the frame size has been determined, the appropriateness of the patient's weight for height and frame can be evaluated (Tables 3-2 and 3-3). It will be necessary to convert the patient's weight to kilograms to utilize the tables.

Triceps Skinfold Thickness

The measurement of skinfold or fatfold thickness provides another parameter to evaluate the nutritional status of the patient. The jaws of skinfold thickness calipers must be correctly placed to get an accurate reading.

To determine the site of the triceps skinfold thickness measurement, have the patient flex the left arm at a right angle. Position yourself behind the patient and make a horizontal mark halfway between the tips of the olecranon and acromial processes on the posterior aspect of the arm. Then draw a line along the vertical plane of the arm to cross the midpoint. Allowing the patient's arm to hang relaxed, use your thumb and forefinger to grasp and lift the triceps skinfold about ½ in proximal to the marked cross. Make sure you feel the main bulk of the triceps muscle, identifying the muscle's subcutaneous interface between your fingers deep to the skinfold. (If you do not feel the muscle bulk, you may be too medial or lateral to the muscle mass and need to reposition your fingers.) Place the caliper jaws at the marked cross on each side of the raised skinfold, but not so tight as to cause an indentation (Fig. 3-8). Make two readings, with the gauge at eye level, to the nearest millimeter at the same site and derive an average.

Fig. 3-8
Placement of calipers for triceps skinfold thickness measurement.

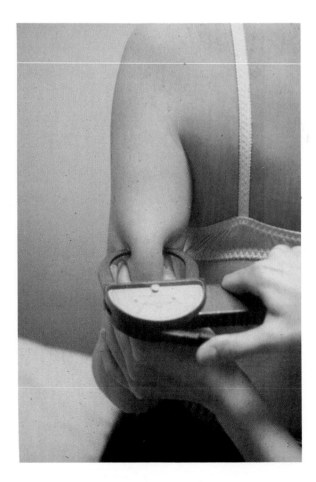

Since approximately 50% of the body fat is present in the subcutaneous tissue layers, a correlation exists between the triceps skinfold thickness and the body's fat content. Therefore the triceps skinfold measurement may be used in the diagnosis of obesity. Compare the patient's measurement with the percentiles of triceps skinfold thickness by age and sex (Tables 3-2 and 3-3).

INFANTS

A baby born at term who is as big as you expect—and as proportioned as you expect—not too big and not too small, and is free of a history of pre- or perinatal difficulty obviously has the best chance for an undisturbed neonatal and infancy period. Distortions of the expected during the first few days of life must always be given serious attention and must always be considered clues to potential problems. This is true whether it is a distortion of a measurement or a subjective impression on physical examination of the baby's vibrancy and interest in life, particularly in feeding.

Recumbent Length

Recumbent length is the measurement of choice for infants between birth and 24 to 36 months of age (Fig. 3-9). Place the infant supine on the measuring board, having the parent hold the infant's head against the headboard. Hold the infant's legs straight at the knees, and place the footboard against the bottom of the infant's feet. Read the length measurement to the nearest ½ cm or ¼ in. Compare the infant's length to the population standard, using the appropriate growth curve for sex and age, and identify the infant's percentile placement (Fig. 3-10).

At birth, healthy term newborns have length variations between 45 to 55 cm (18 to 22 in). *Text continued on p. 58.*

Fig. 3-9
Measurement of infant length.

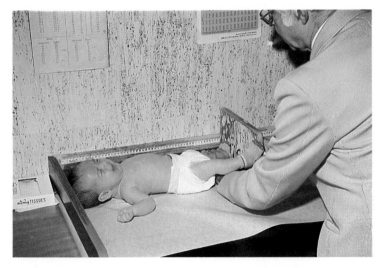

Fig. 3-10
Physical growth curves for children: birth to 36 months. A, Boys.

Courtesy Ross Laboratories, Columbus, Ohio.

A

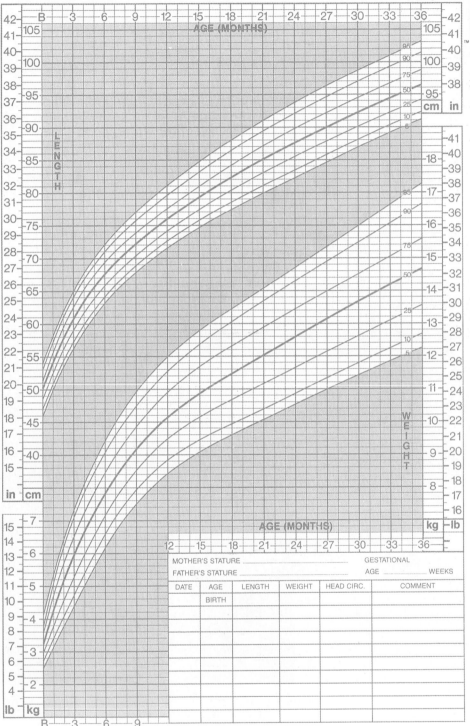

Fig. 3-10, cont'd
For legend see opposite page.

BOYS: BIRTH TO 36 MONTHS
PHYSICAL GROWTH
NCHS PERCENTILES*

NAME_____ RECORD #_____

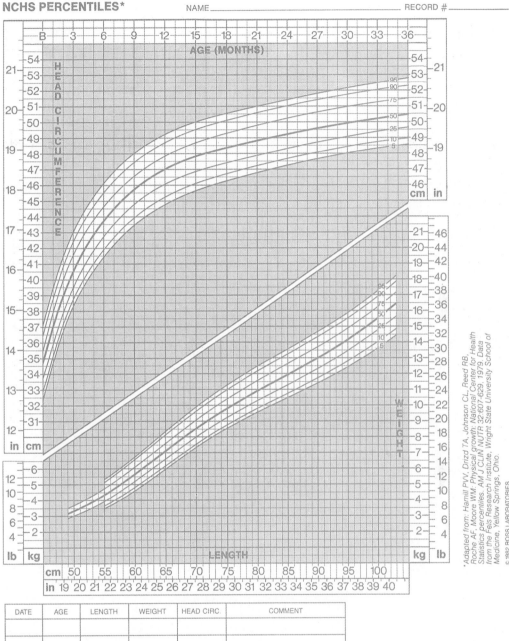

DATE	AGE	LENGTH	WEIGHT	HEAD CIRC.	COMMENT

*Adapted from: Hamill PVV, Drizd TA, Johnson CL, Reed RB, Roche AF, Moore WM: Physical growth: National Center for Health Statistics percentiles. AM J CLIN NUTR 32-607-629, 1979. Data from the Fels Research Institute, Wright State University School of Medicine, Yellow Springs, Ohio.

© 1982 ROSS LABORATORIES

Fig. 3-10, cont'd
Physical growth curves for children: birth to 36 months. B, Girls.

Courtesy Ross Laboratories, Columbus, Ohio.

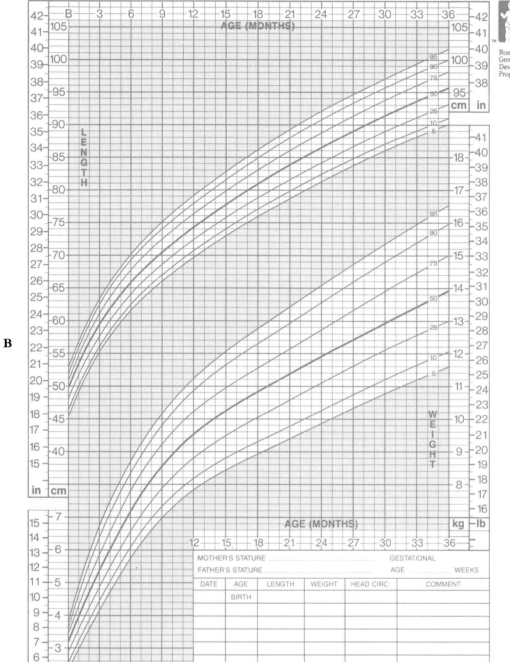

GIRLS: BIRTH TO 36 MONTHS
PHYSICAL GROWTH
NCHS PERCENTILES*

*Adapted from: Hamill PVV, Drizd TA, Johnson CL, Reed RB, Roche AF, Moore WM: Physical growth: National Center for Health Statistics percentiles. AM J CLIN NUTR 32:607-629, 1979. Data from the Fels Research Institute, Wright State University School of Medicine, Yellow Springs, Ohio.

Fig. 3-10, cont'd
For legend see opposite
page.

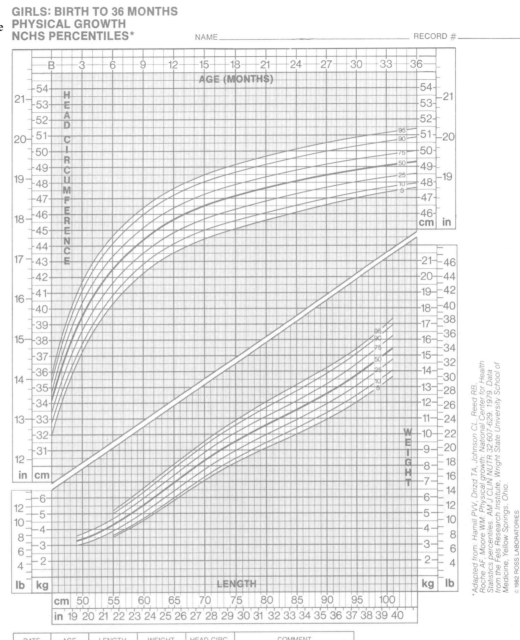

GIRLS: BIRTH TO 36 MONTHS
PHYSICAL GROWTH
NCHS PERCENTILES*

NAME _____ RECORD # _____

DATE	AGE	LENGTH	WEIGHT	HEAD CIRC.	COMMENT

*Adapted from: Hamill PVV, Drizd TA, Johnson CL, Reed RB,
Roche AF, Moore WM. Physical growth: National Center for Health
Statistics percentiles. AM J CLIN NUTR 32.607-629, 1979. Data
from the Fels Research Institute, Wright State University School of
Medicine, Yellow Springs, Ohio.

© 1982 ROSS LABORATORIES

ROSS LABORATORIES
COLUMBUS, OHIO 43216
Division of Abbott Laboratories, USA   ROSS

G106/JUNE 1983   LITHO IN USA

Weight

Use an infant scale, measuring weight in ounces or grams for infants and small children (Fig. 3-11). Distract the infant and balance the scale as you would for a standing scale. Read the weight to the nearest 10 gm or ½ oz when the infant is most still. Plot the infant's weight on the appropriate growth curve for age and sex, comparing the infant's weight to the population standard. Identify the infant's percentile placement.

Healthy term newborns vary in weight between 2500 and 4000 gm (5 lb 8 oz to 8 lb 13 oz).

Head Circumference

You should measure the head circumference at every health visit for infants until 2 years of age, and then measure the young child's head circumference yearly until 6 years of age. Wrap the measuring tape snugly around the child's head at the occipital protuberance and the supraorbital prominence, to find the point of largest circumference, taking care not to cut the skin (Fig. 3-12). Make the reading to the nearest 0.5 cm or ⅛ in. (Remember to remeasure the head circumference at least one time to check the accuracy of your measurement.)

Plot the infant's head circumference on the appropriate growth curve, comparing the infant's measurement with expected measurements for the population (Fig. 3-10).

Expected head circumferences for term newborns range between 32.5 and 37.5 cm (12½ to 14½ in) with a mean of 33 to 35 cm (13 to 14 in). At 2 years of age the infant's head circumference is two thirds its adult size. A head circumference increasing rapidly and rising above percentile curves suggests increased intracranial pressure. A head circumference growing slowly enough to fall off percentile curves suggests microcephaly.

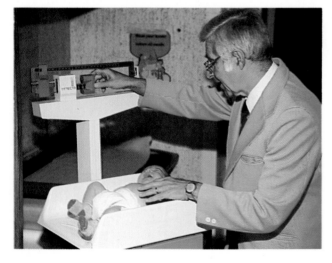

Fig. 3-11
Measurement of infant weight.

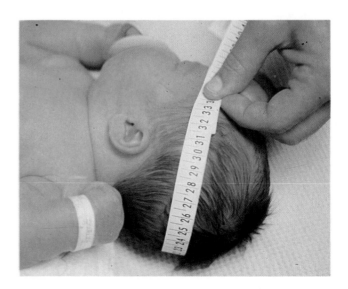

Fig. 3-12
Appropriate placement of the measuring tape to obtain the head circumference.

Fig. 3-13
Measurement of infant chest circumference.

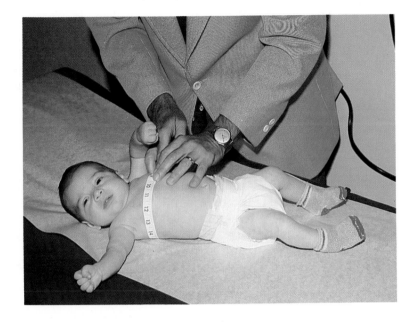

Chest Circumference

While the chest circumference is not used universally, it is a useful measurement for comparison with the head circumference when you suspect a problem in either head size or chest size. Wrap the measuring tape around the infant's chest at the nipple line, firmly but not tight enough to cause an indentation of the skin (Fig. 3-13). The chest circumference measurement is ideally taken midway between inspiration and expiration and read to the nearest 0.5 cm or ⅛ in.

The newborn's head circumference may equal or exceed its chest circumference by 2 cm (¾ in) for the first 5 months of age. Between the ages of 5 months and 2 years, the infant's chest circumference should closely approximate the head circumference. After 2 years of age the chest circumference should exceed the head circumference, because the chest grows faster than the head (Table 3-4).

Table 3-4
Average Chest and Head Circumference for U.S. Children at Specific Ages

Age	Chest Circumference (cm)	Head Circumference (cm)	
		Males	Females
Birth	35	35.3	34.7
3 months	40	40.9	40.0
6 months	44	43.9	42.8
12 months	47	47.3	45.8
18 months	48	48.7	47.1
2 years	50	49.7	48.1
3 years	52	50.4	49.3

Data from Lowrey, 1986, and Waring and Jeansonne, 1982.

Gestational Age

Gestational age is an indicator of a newborn's maturity. It is determined by calculating the number of completed weeks since the first day of the mother's last menstrual period to the date of birth. An estimate of gestational age is used for evaluating an infant's developmental progress and for differentiating between preterm newborns who are appropriately sized and term newborns who are small for gestational age.

The Dubowitz Clinical Assessment is a standardized tool that uses a newborn's physical and neuromuscular characteristics within 48 hours of birth to establish or confirm the newborn's gestational age. The Dubowitz Scoring Criteria includes 11 physical characteristics and 10 neuromuscular signs. Fig. 3-14 provides directions and criteria for scoring each characteristic. Sum the neonate's score for each criteria and compare the total with the table of scores to determine the gestational age. The assessment is accurate within 2 weeks of the assigned gestational age.

The gestational age of 37 to 41 weeks, which is considered *term,* is associated with the best health outcomes. Infants born before 37 weeks gestation are *preterm,* while infants born after 41 completed weeks of gestation are *postterm.*

External sign	Score*				
	0	1	2	3	4
Edema	Obvious edema of hands and feet; pitting over tibia	No obvious edema of hands and feet; pitting over tibia	No edema		
Skin texture	Very thin, gelatinous	Thin and smooth	Smooth; medium thickness. Rash or superficial peeling	Slight thickening. Superficial cracking and peeling especially of hands and feet	Thick and parchmentlike; superficial or deep cracking
Skin color	Dark red	Uniformly pink	Pale pink; variable over body	Pale; only pink over ears, lips, palms, or soles	
Skin opacity (trunk)	Numerous veins and venules clearly seen, especially over abdomen	Veins and tributaries seen	A few large vessels clearly seen over abdomen	A few large vessels seen indistinctly over abdomen	No blood vessels seen
Lanugo (over back)	No lanugo	Abundant; long and thick over whole back	Hair thinning especially over lower back	Small amount of lanugo and bald areas	At least ½ of back devoid of lanugo
Plantar creases	No skin creases	Faint red marks over anterior half of sole	Definite red marks over > anterior ½; indentations over < anterior ⅓	Indentations over > anterior ⅓	Definite deep indentations over > anterior ⅓
Nipple formation	Nipple barely visible; no areola	Nipple well defined; areola smooth and flat, diameter <0.75 cm	Areola stippled, edge not raised, diameter <0.75 cm	Areola stippled, edge raised, diameter >0.75 cm	
Breast size	No breast tissue palpable	Breast tissue on one or both sides, <0.5 cm diameter	Breast tissue both sides; one or both 0.5-1 cm	Breast tissue both sides; one or both >1 cm	
Ear form	Pinna flat and shapeless, little or no incurving of edge	Incurving of part of edge of pinna	Partial incurving whole of upper pinna	Well-defined incurving whole of upper pinna	
Ear firmness	Pinna soft, easily folded, no recoil	Pinna soft, easily folded, slow recoil	Cartilage to edge of pinna, but soft in places, ready recoil	Pinna firm, cartilage to edge; instant recoil	
Genitals					
Male	Neither testis in scrotum	At least one testis high in scrotum	At least one testis right down		
Female (with hips ½ abducted)	Labia majora widely separated, labia minora protruding	Labia majora almost cover labia minora	Labia majora completely cover labia minora		

Fig. 3-14

Scoring system of physical and neurologic signs for assessment of gestational age.
From Dubowitz, 1970.

Examination and Findings

Posture: Observed with infant quiet and in supine position. Score 0: Arms and legs extended; 1: beginning of flexion of hips and knees, arms extended; 2: stronger flexion of legs, arms extended; 3: arms slightly flexed, legs flexed and abducted; 4: full flexion of arms and legs.

Square window: The hand is flexed on the forearm between the thumb and index finger of the examiner. Enough pressure is applied to get as full a flexion as possible, and the angle between the hypothenar eminence and the ventral aspect of the forearm is measured and graded according to diagram (Fig. 15-3). (Care is taken not to rotate the infant's wrist while doing this maneuver.)

Ankle dorsiflexion: The foot is dorsiflexed onto the anterior aspect of the leg, with the examiner's thumb on the sole of the foot and other fingers behind the leg. Enough pressure is applied to get as full flexion as possible, and the angle between the dorsum of the foot and the anterior aspect of the leg is measured.

Arm recoil: With the infant in the supine position the forearms are first flexed for 5 seconds, then fully extended by pulling on the hands, and then released. The sign is fully positive if the arms return briskly to full flexion (Score 2). If the arms return to incomplete flexion or the response is sluggish it is graded as Score 1. If they remain extended or are only followed by random movements the score is 0.

Leg recoil: With the infant supine, the hips and knees are fully flexed for 5 seconds, then extended by traction on the feet, and released. A maximal response is one of full flexion of the hips and knees (Score 2). A partial flexion scores 1, and minimal or no movement scores 0.

Popliteal angle: With the infant supine and his pelvis flat on the examining couch, the thigh is held in the knee-chest position by the examiner's left index finger and thumb supporting the knee. The leg is then extended by gentle pressure from the examiner's right index finger behind the ankle and the popliteal angle is measured.

Heel to ear maneuver: With the baby supine, draw the baby's foot as near to the head as it will go without forcing it. Observe the distance between the foot and the head as well as the degree of extension at the knee. Grade according to diagram (Fig. 15-3). Note that the knee is left free and may draw down alongside the abdomen.

Scarf sign: With the baby supine, take the infant's hand and try to put it around the neck and as far posteriorly as possible around the opposite shoulder. Assist this maneuver by lifting the elbow across the body. See how far the elbow will go across and grade according to illustrations (Fig. 15-3). Score 0: Elbow reaches opposite axillary line; 1: Elbow between midline and opposite axillary line; 2: Elbow reaches midline; 3: Elbow will not reach midline.

Head lag: With the baby lying supine, grasp the hands (or the arms if a very small infant) and pull him slowly towards the sitting position. Observe the position of the head in relation to the trunk and grade accordingly. In a small infant the head may initially be supported by one hand. Score 0: Complete lag; 1: Partial head control; 2: Able to maintain head in line with body; 3: Brings head anterior to body.

Ventral suspension: The infant is suspended in the prone position, with examiner's hand under the infant's chest (one hand in a small infant, two in a large infant). Observe the degree of extension of the back and the amount of flexion of the arms and legs. Also note the relation of the head to the trunk. Grade according to diagram (Fig. 15-3). If score differs on the two sides, take the mean.

Fig. 3-14, cont'd
Scoring system of physical and neurologic signs for assessment of gestational age.
From Dubowitz, 1970.

Score	Weeks of gestation
0-9	26
10-12	27
13-16	28
17-20	29
21-24	30
25-27	31
28-31	32
32-35	33
36-39	34
40-43	35
44-46	36
47-50	37
51-54	38
55-58	39
59-62	40
63-65	41
66-69	42

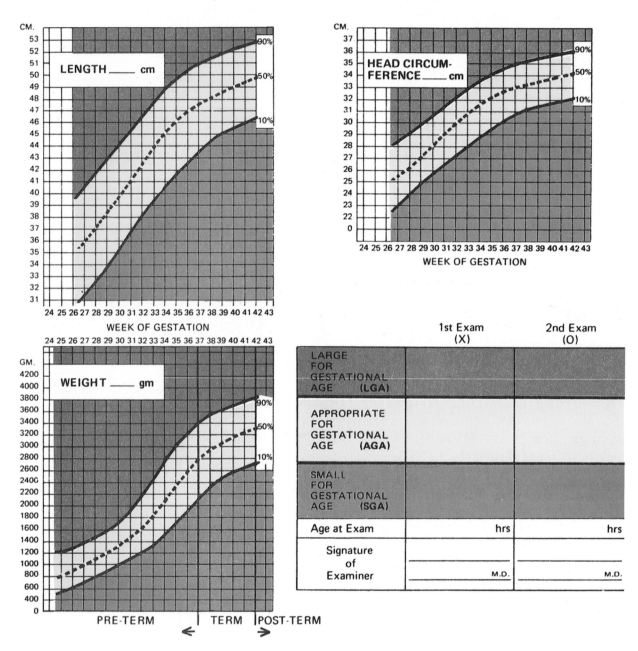

Fig. 3-15
Intrauterine growth curves for length, weight, and head circumference by weeks of gestation.
Modified from Lubchenco, 1966; and Battaglia and Lubchenco, 1967.

Size for Gestational Age

A newborn's fetal growth pattern and size for gestational age can be determined once gestational age is assigned. Standardized intrauterine growth curves are used to plot the newborn's birth weight, length, and head circumference (Fig. 3-15). The infant is then classified as either small, appropriate, or large for gestational age by percentile curve placement for weeks of gestation (Fig. 3-16). The classification system is as follows:

Classification	Weight Percentiles
Appropriate for gestational age (AGA)	10th to 90th
Small for gestational age (SGA)	< 10th
Large for gestational age (LGA)	> 90th

There is an associated risk of morbidity and mortality with small and large for gestational age infants. Risks increase further if the infant is preterm.

Fig. 3-16
Three infants, each 32 weeks gestational age, demonstrating the difference in size between SGA, AGA, and LGA newborns. Birth weights are 600, 1400, and 2750 grams, respectively, from left to right.
From Korones, 1986.

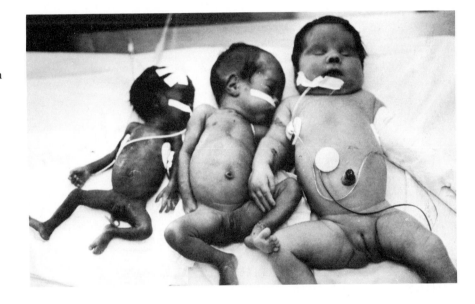

CHILDREN

Stature and Weight

Standing height is obtained beginning at 24 to 36 months when the child is walking well. To get the most accurate measurement, use a freestanding stature measuring device or one that is mounted on the wall. Have the child stand erect with heels, buttocks, and shoulders against the wall, looking straight ahead (Fig. 3-17). The outer canthus of the eye should be on the same horizontal plane as the external auditory canal while you position the headpiece at the crown. The stature reading is made to the nearest 0.5 cm or ¼ in. Table 3-5 lists the expected yearly stature growth, or height velocity, for age and sex.

To calculate height velocity, determine the change in height over a time interval, such as a year. Shorter time intervals may reflect seasonal variations in growth. Make height measurements as close to 12 months apart as possible, no less than 10 months and no more than 14 months. See Fig. 3-18 for the sex-specific height velocity curves.

Fig. 3-17
Measuring the stature of a child.

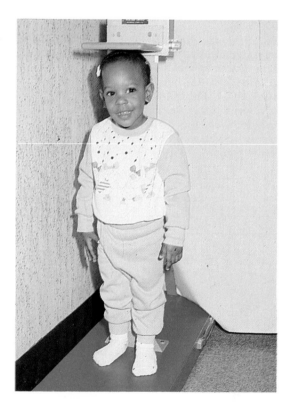

Table 3-5
Expected Height Velocity (Amount of Annual Growth) for Specified Time Intervals During Childhood. Peak Height Velocity During Adolescence is Given for Average Times (13.5 Years in Males and 11.5 Years in Females)

	Height Velocity (cm)	
Age (yrs)	Males	Females
2-3	8.3	8.6
3-4	7.4	7.6
4-5	6.8	6.8
5-6	6.4	6.4
6-7	6.0	6.1
7-8	5.8	5.9
8-9	5.4	5.7
9-10	5.2	5.8
10-11	5.1	6.7
11-12	5.3	8.3
12-13	6.8	5.9
13-14	9.5	3.0
14-15	6.5	0.9
15-16	3.3	0.1
16-17	1.5	
17-18	0.5	

Adapted from Tanner and Davies, 1985.

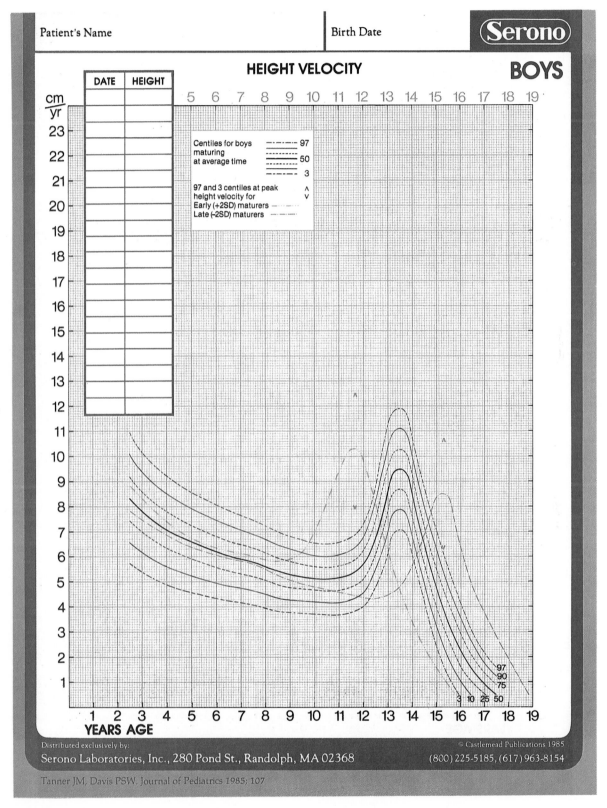

Fig. 3-18
Height velocity growth curves. A, Boys.
From Tanner and Davies, 1985.

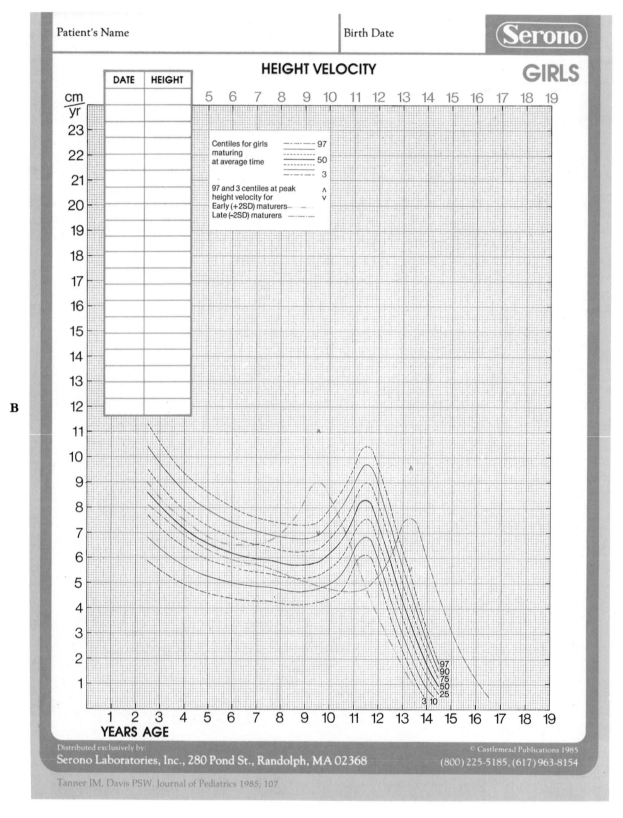

Fig. 3-18, cont'd
High velocity growth curves. B, Girls.
From Tanner and Davies, 1985.

Weigh the young child over 2 years of age on a standing scale, in standard light garments (Fig. 3-19). Read the weight to the nearest 0.1 kg or ¼ lb. Remember to measure the child's head circumference once a year.

Plot the child's height, weight, and head circumference measurements on the appropriate growth curves for sex and age, comparing the child's growth with the population standards (Fig. 3-20). Population standards reflecting various times of the growth spurt for adolescents can be found in Fig. 3-21. The Nellhaus head circumference curve may be used for children older than 3 years (Fig. 3-22).

Over a period of time, interval measurements should demonstrate that the child has established a growth pattern, indicated by consistently following a percentile curve on the growth chart. Children of first generation immigrants may not fit the U.S. population standard, but they should follow a growth pattern consistent with other children, even if it is near or below the 5th percentile. Infants and children who suddenly fall below or rise above their established percentile growth curve should be examined more closely to determine the cause. *Text continued on p. 73.*

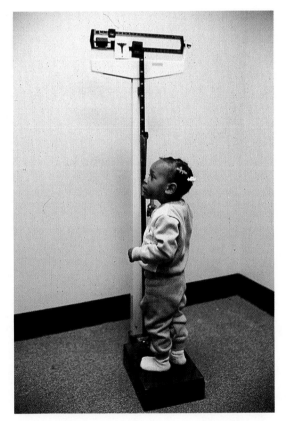

Fig. 3-19
Weighing the child.

Fig. 3-20
Physical growth curves for children, ages 2 through 18 years, for height and weight. A, Boys.

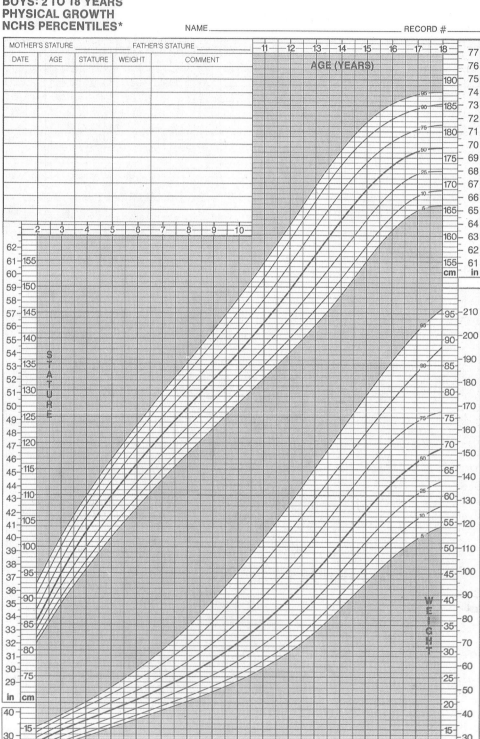

**BOYS: 2 TO 18 YEARS
PHYSICAL GROWTH
NCHS PERCENTILES***

NAME_____ RECORD #_____

Adapted from: Hamill PVV, Drizd TA, Johnson CL, Reed RB, Roche AF, Moore WM: Physical growth: National Center for Health Statistics percentiles. AM J CLIN NUTR 32:607-629, 1979. Data from the National Center for Health Statistics (NCHS) Hyattsville, Maryland.

© 1982 ROSS LABORATORIES

Fig. 3-20, cont'd
Physical growth curves for children, ages 2 through 18 years, for height and weight. **B,** Girls.

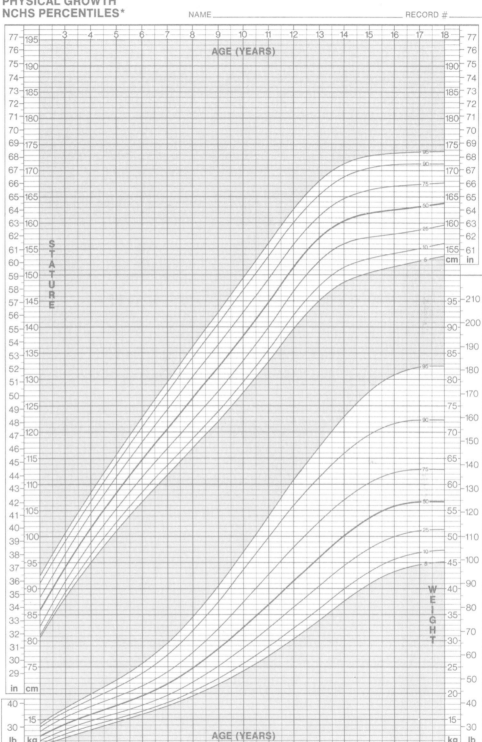

GIRLS: 2 TO 18 YEARS
PHYSICAL GROWTH
NCHS PERCENTILES*

*Adapted from: Hamill PVV, Drizd TA, Johnson CL, Reed RB, Roche AF, Moore WM: Physical growth: National Center for Health Statistics percentiles. AM J CLIN NUTR 32:607-629,1979. Data from the National Center for Health Statistics (NCHS) Hyattsville, Maryland

© 1980 ROSS LABORATORIES

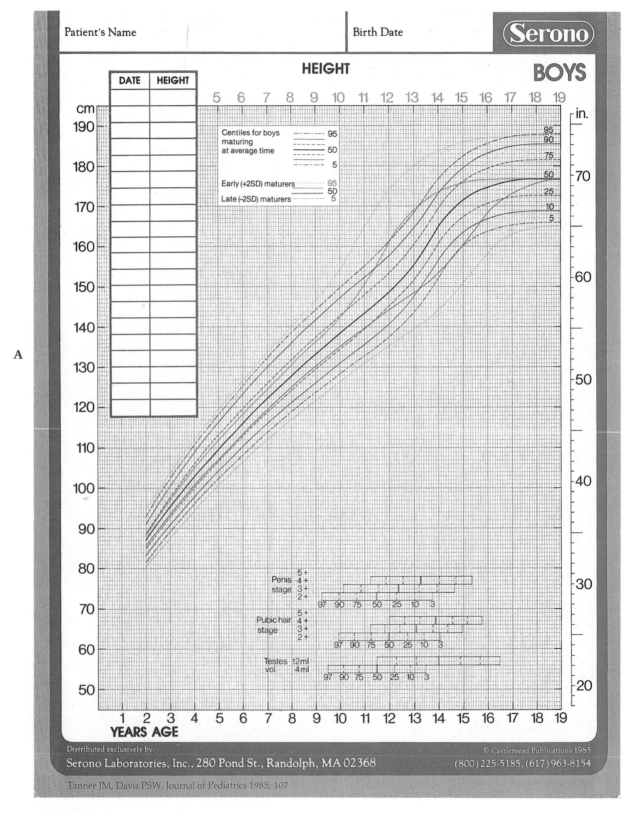

A

Fig. 3-21
Physical growth curves for children and adolescents, 2 through 19 years, for height and sexual development. A, Boys.
From Tanner and Davies, 1985.

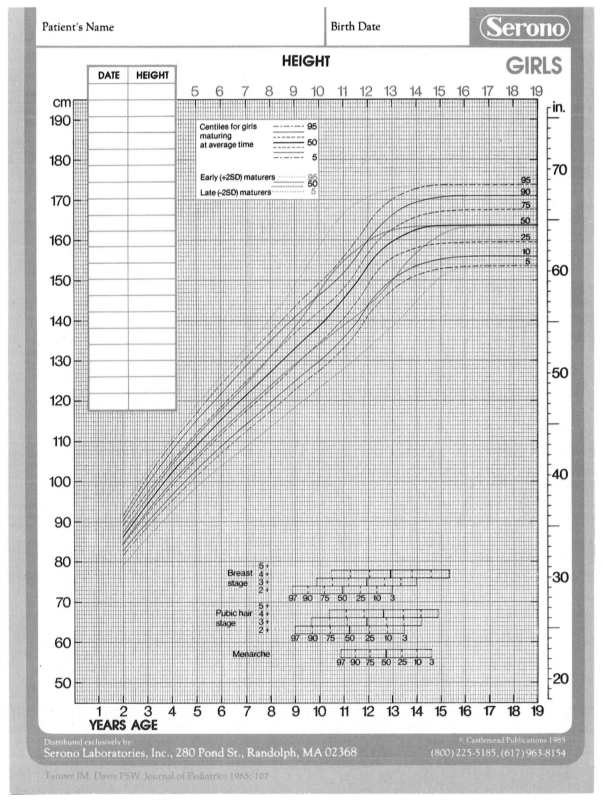

Fig. 3-21, cont'd
Physical growth curves for children and adolescents, 2 through 19 years, for height and sexual development.
B, Girls.
From Tanner and Davies, 1985.

Fig. 3-22
Head circumference growth curves, birth to 18 years. A, Boys. B, Girls.

From Nellhaus, G.: Pediatrics **41**:106, 1968; copyright American Academy of Pediatrics.

A

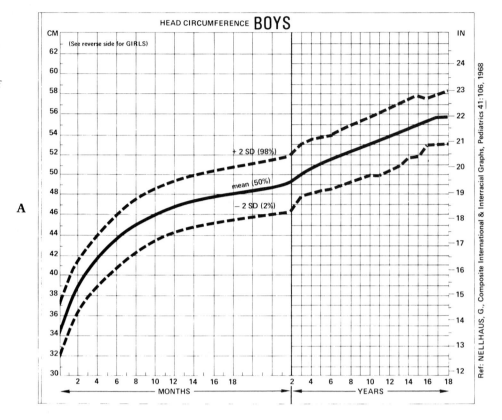

B

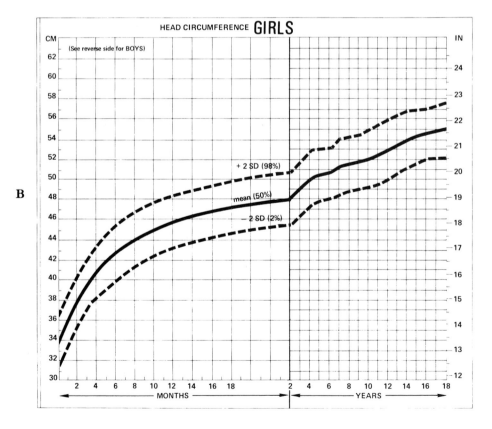

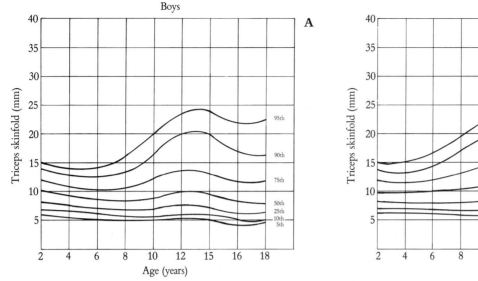

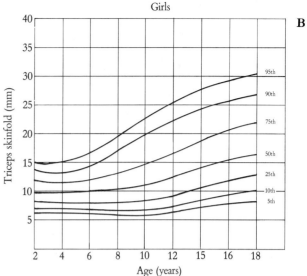

Fig. 3-23
Skinfold thickness curves for children, ages 2 to 18 years.
A, Boys. B, Girls.
Redrawn from Owen, 1982.

Skinfold Thickness

Triceps skinfold thickness measurement is not routinely recommended for children, being reserved for those children who have weight for stature greater than the 90th percentile. It is often difficult to differentiate fatfolds from lean muscle tissue in children. This measurement is more commonly used with adolescents for whom no weight for stature standard currently exists. Using the technique described for adults, take the triceps skinfold measurement. Plot the reading on the sex appropriate standardized curves of triceps skinfold thickness for children and adolescents (Fig. 3-23).

Sitting Height

Take the sitting height measurement and compare it with the total height when a child is suspected of having a growth problem or unusual body proportions. Have the child sit erect at the stature measuring device with buttocks and shoulders against the wall, legs extended and flat against the floor. Position the headpiece at the child's crown while the child looks straight ahead, outer eye canthus and external auditory canal on the same plane. The proportion of sitting height to total body height is then calculated. The expected proportion of sitting height to total height by age (Barness, 1981) is as follows:

Birth	70%
2 years	60%
10 years	52%
Adult	50%

Infantile stature is a sitting height greater than half the standing height, and *adult stature* is a sitting height approximately half that of the standing height. Adult stature in the young child may indicate precocious sexual development or certain types of dwarfism. Infantile stature in the older child may suggest delayed puberty or hypothyroidism.

Arm Span

The arm span measurement, although not routinely obtained, may be useful when evaluating a child with tall stature. Have the child hold his or her arms fully extended from the sides of the body. Measure the distance from the middle fingertip of one hand to that of the other hand. The arm span should equal the child's height or stature. Arm span that exceeds height is associated with Marfan's syndrome.

Mid Upper Arm Circumference

The mid upper arm circumference, not routinely obtained, provides an estimate of muscle mass and available fat and protein stores in the malnourished or chronically ill patient. Place the measuring tape around the patient's upper arm, midway between the tips of the olecranon and acromial processes, the same location where the triceps skinfold thickness measurement is made (Fig. 3-24). Hold the measuring tape snugly, but not tight enough to cause an indentation, and make the reading to the nearest 5 mm (0.5 cm). Compare the measurement with the percentiles of mid upper arm circumference for age and sex to determine the appropriateness of the patient's measurement (Table 3-6).

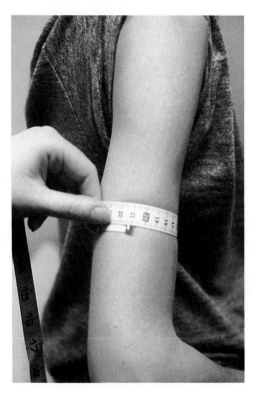

Fig. 3-24
Measurement of mid upper arm circumference.

Table 3-6
Mid Upper Arm
Circumference Percentiles by
Age and Sex

	Mid Upper Arm Circumference Percentiles (mm)				
Age (yrs)	5th	15th	50th	85th	95th
Males					
0.0-0.4	113	120	134	147	153
0.5-1.4	128	137	152	168	175
1.5-2.4	141	147	157	170	180
2.5-3.4	144	150	161	175	182
3.5-4.4	143	150	165	180	190
4.5-5.4	146	155	169	185	199
5.5-6.4	151	159	172	188	198
6.5-7.4	154	162	176	194	212
7.5-8.4	161	168	185	205	233
8.5-9.4	165	174	190	217	262
9.5-10.4	170	180	200	228	255
10.5-11.4	177	186	208	240	276
11.5-12.4	184	194	216	253	291
12.5-13.4	186	198	230	270	297
13.5-14.4	198	211	243	279	321
14.5-15.4	202	220	253	302	320
15.5-16.4	217	232	262	300	335
16.5-17.4	230	238	275	306	326
17.5-24.4	250	264	292	330	354
24.5-34.4	260	280	310	344	366
34.5-44.4	259	280	312	345	371
Females					
0.0-0.4	107	118	127	145	150
0.5-1.4	125	134	146	162	170
1.5-2.4	136	143	155	171	180
2.5-3.4	137	145	157	169	176
3.5-4.4	145	150	162	176	184
4.5-5.4	149	155	169	185	195
5.5-6.4	148	158	170	187	202
6.5-7.4	153	162	178	199	216
7.5-8.4	158	166	183	207	231
8.5-9.4	166	175	192	222	255
9.5-10.4	170	181	203	236	263
10.5-11.4	173	186	210	251	280
11.5-12.4	185	196	220	256	275
12.5-13.4	186	204	230	270	294
13.5-14.4	201	214	240	284	306
14.5-15.4	205	216	245	281	310
15.5-16.4	211	224	249	286	322
16.5-17.4	207	224	250	291	328
17.5-24.4	215	233	260	297	329
24.5-34.4	230	243	275	324	361
34.5-44.4	232	250	286	340	374

Adapted from Frisancho, 1974.

ADOLESCENTS

The changes of puberty do not occur at exactly the same time in each boy and girl, which can cause great concern when they feel they are growing too fast or too slow. This is a good time to share your knowledge about the various rates of speed in human development, reassuring them that almost all of us get there in good time. The Tanner charts are valuable for explaining to older children, particularly adolescents, where they are in reference to others and where they are going. Show them the pictures and talk about it. All adolescents are curious and will gain from your respectful candor.

Assessing growth and development of the older child and adolescent includes evaluating the patient's sexual maturation. In girls breast and pubic hair development are evaluated, and genital and pubic hair development are evaluated in boys. The expected stages of pubertal changes for each secondary sexual characteristic are described in Figs. 3-25 to 3-28.

A sexual maturity rating (SMR) may be assigned, or each secondary sexual characteristic may be rated separately, to determine the child's pubertal development. The SMR is calculated by averaging the girl's stage of pubic hair and breast

Fig. 3-25
Pubic hair development in males.
From Tanner, 1962.

DEVELOPMENT	STAGE	DESCRIPTION
	1	None; preadolescent
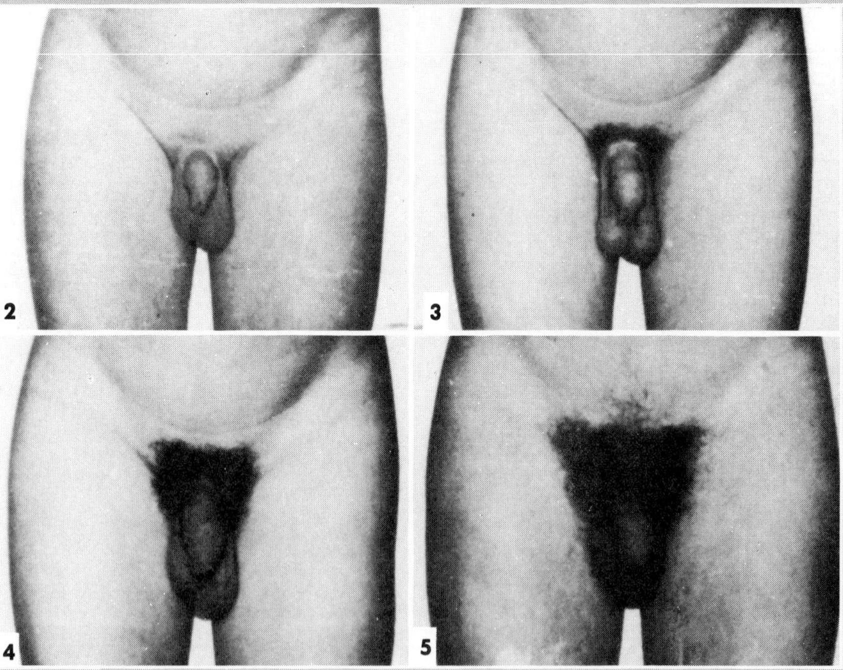	2	Scant, long, slightly pigmented
	3	Darker, starting to curl, small amount
	4	Resembles adult, but less quantity; coarse, curly
	5	Adult distribution, spread to medial surface of thighs

DEVELOPMENT	STAGE	DESCRIPTION

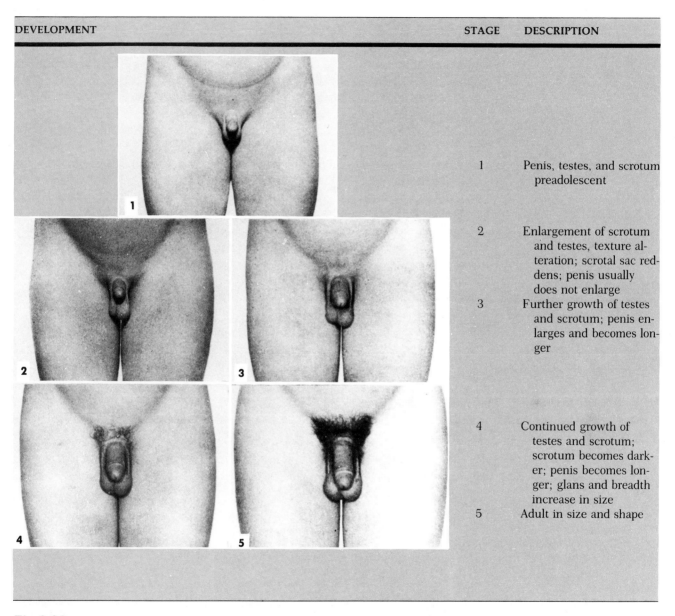

1 — Penis, testes, and scrotum preadolescent

2 — Enlargement of scrotum and testes, texture alteration; scrotal sac reddens; penis usually does not enlarge

3 — Further growth of testes and scrotum; penis enlarges and becomes longer

4 — Continued growth of testes and scrotum; scrotum becomes darker; penis becomes longer; glans and breadth increase in size

5 — Adult in size and shape

Fig. 3-26
Penis and testes/scrotum development in males.
From Tanner, 1962.

development and the boy's stage of pubic hair and genital development. The stage of each secondary sexual characteristic is then related to the timing of other physiologic events occurring during puberty.

The stage of breast and pubic hair development in the female is related to her chronologic age, age at menarche, and evidence of the height spurt. Breasts begin development before pubic hair appears in two thirds of girls. The breasts do not always develop at the same rate, so some asymmetry is common. Menarche generally occurs in SMR 4 or breast stage 3 to 4. The peak height velocity usually occurs before menarche. Development of breast tissue or pubic hair in prepubertal girls younger than 8 years old should be further investigated for cause. These physiologic events may be plotted on a standardized growth curve.

The stage of genital and pubic hair development in the male is related to his age and evidence of the height spurt. External genital changes usually precede pubic hair development. Ejaculation generally occurs at SMR 3, with semen appearing between SMR 3 and 4. The peak height velocity usually occurs later, in SMR 4 or genital development stage 4 to 5. Development of genitals or pubic hair in prepubertal boys younger than 9 years old should be further investigated for cause. These events may be plotted on a standardized growth curve.

Delayed onset of adolescence, in which the secondary sexual characteristics begin development at a later than average age, is often a normal variant in both boys and girls. It is accompanied by a lag in stature growth. Parents often had a similar adolescent pattern. Once pubertal changes begin, the sequence of development is the same as for other adolescents, but it may occur over a shorter time span.

Fig. 3-27
Pubic hair development in females.
From Tanner, 1962.

DEVELOPMENT	STAGE	DESCRIPTION
	1	None; preadolescent
	2	Sparse, lightly pigmented, straight along medial border of labia
	3	Darker, beginning to curl, increased amount
	4	Coarse, curly, abundant amount but less than adult
	5	Adult female triangle, spread to medial surface of thighs

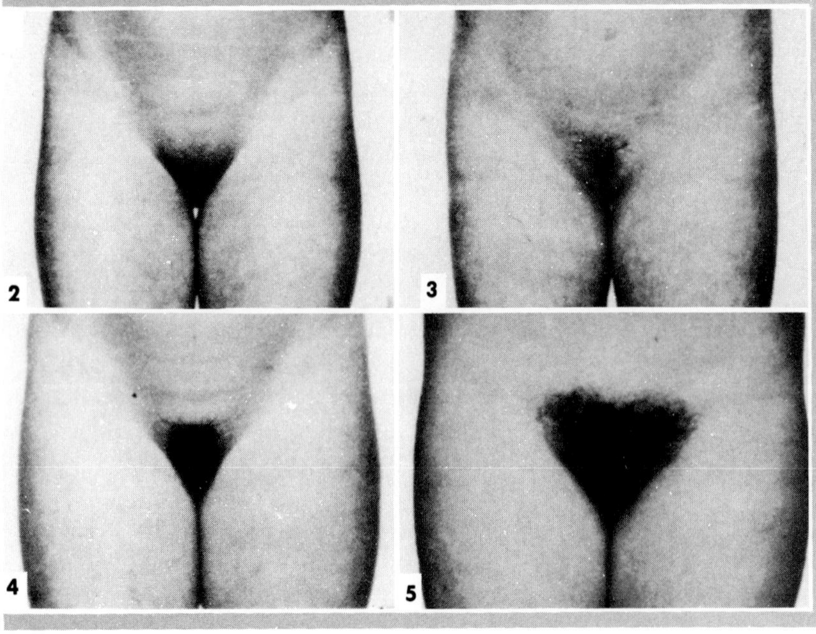

STAGE	BREAST DEVELOPMENT	DEVELOPMENT DESCRIPTION
1		Preadolescent
2		Breast and papilla elevated as small mound; areolar diameter increased
3		Breast and aerola enlarged; no contour separation
4		Areola and papilla form secondary mound
5		Mature; nipple projects areolar part of general breast contour

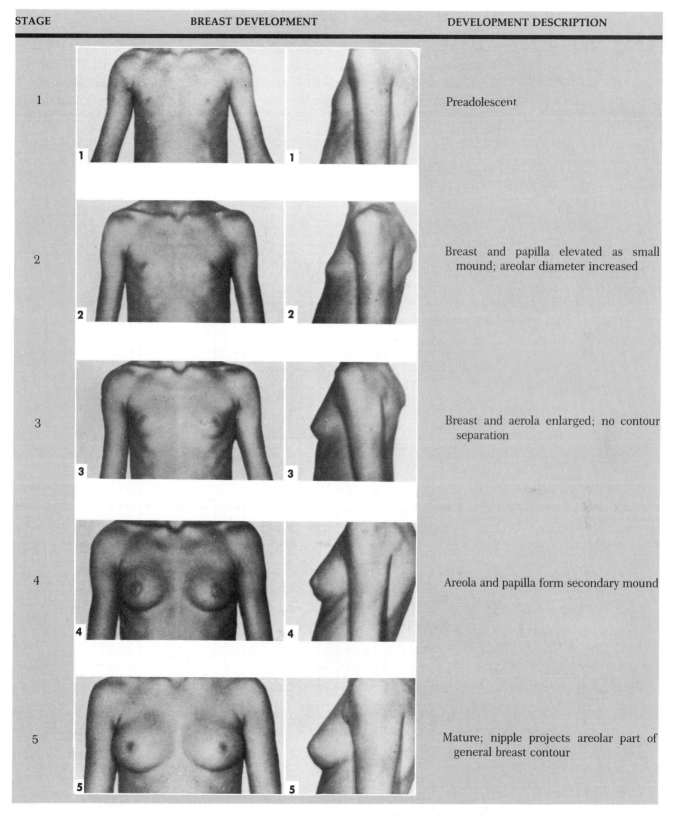

Fig. 3-28
Maturational sequence in girls.
From Tanner, 1962.

PREGNANT WOMEN

Weight gain during pregnancy should be calculated from the woman's prepregnant weight. Plot the weight gain on the prenatal weight gain grid for completed weeks of gestation (Fig. 3-29). Continue monitoring the woman's weight throughout the pregnancy, noting any variation from the expected weight gain by trimester. The woman with appropriate prepregnant weight for height should gain 10 to 14.5 kg (22 to 32 lb) over the entire pregnancy.

Fig. 3-29
Prenatal weight gain curve by weeks of gestation.

From Committee on Maternal Nutrition, Food and Nutrition Board–National Research Council, National Academy of Sciences, 1970.

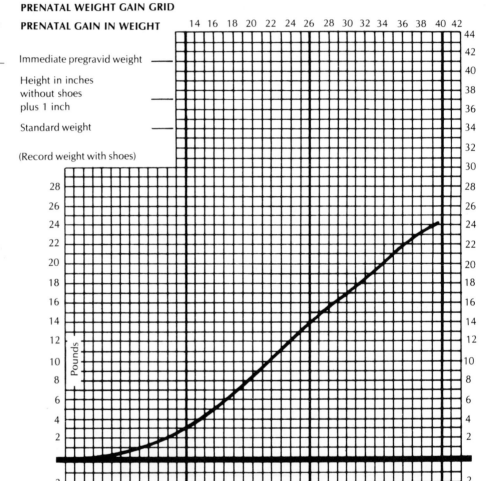

PRENATAL WEIGHT GAIN GRID

PRENATAL GAIN IN WEIGHT

Immediate pregravid weight ____

Height in inches
without shoes
plus 1 inch ____

Standard weight ____

(Record weight with shoes)

OLDER ADULTS Measurement procedures for the older adult are the same used for the general population. Compare the individual's triceps skinfold thickness with his height in the appropriate sex and frame size categories to determine the appropriateness of the patient's weight (Tables 3-7 and 3-8).

Table 3-7
Selected Percentiles of Weight and Triceps Skinfold Thickness for Height in U.S. Men, Age 55 to 74 Years, with Small, Medium, and Large Frames *

Height In	Height Cm	Weight (kg) 5	15	50	85	95	Triceps (mm) 5	10	15	50	85	90	95
Small Frames, Men													
62	157	45	56	61	68	77			6	9	12		
63	160	47	51	62	71	79		5	5	10	16	17	
64	163	47	54	63	72	80	4	4	4	9	20	21	22
65	165	48	59	70	80	90	5	6	7	11	18	19	24
66	168	51	59	68	77	84	5	6	7	11	16	20	20
67	170	55	61	69	79	88	5	6	6	10	15	17	25
68	173	54	58	70	79	86		5	5	10	15	17	
69	175	56	63	75	81	88			8	10	15		
70	178	57	63	76	83	89				11			
71	180	59	65	69	85	91				9			
72	183	60	66	76	86	92							
73	185	62	68	78	88	94							
74	188	63	69	77	89	95							
Medium Frames, Men													
62	157	50	59	68	77	85			5	12	25		
63	160	51	60	70	80	87		7	7	11	20	23	
64	163	55	62	71	82	91	5	6	6	10	17	20	26
65	165	56	64	72	83	89	5	6	7	11	17	19	24
66	168	57	66	74	83	89	6	6	7	12	18	19	22
67	170	59	66	78	87	94	5	6	7	12	18	20	23
68	173	62	68	78	89	101	6	7	8	12	18	21	23
69	175	62	68	77	90	99	5	6	7	12	19	22	25
70	178	62	71	80	90	101	6	7	7	11	18	19	21
71	180	68	72	84	94	101	5	6	6	11	16	17	20
72	183	66	69	81	96	101		6	8	11	19	20	
73	185	68	79	88	93	103			8	13	16		
74	188	69	76	95	98	104				11			
Large Frames, Men													
62	157	54	63	77	91	100							
63	160	55	64	80	92	101				15			
64	163	57	65	77	94	102				21			
65	165	58	73	79	89	103			11	14	22		
66	168	59	73	80	101	105		7	8	13	21	25	
67	170	65	73	85	103	112	6	8	9	16	21	25	27
68	173	67	73	83	95	111	6	7	8	13	20	21	23
69	175	65	74	84	96	105	6	7	8	12	18	20	23
70	178	68	77	87	102	117	5	6	8	14	22	25	31
71	180	65	70	84	102	111		6	6	13	18	22	
72	183	67	81	90	108	112		8	8	13	23	26	
73	185	68	76	88	105	113				11			
74	188	69	78	89	106	114				12			

Adapted from Frisancho, 1984.
*Data from NHANES I (1971 to 1974) and NHANES II (1976 to 1980), conducted by the NCHS.

Table 3-8
Selected Percentiles for Weight and Triceps Skinfold Thickness by Height in U.S. Women, Age 55 to 74 Years, with Small, Medium, and Large Frames*

Height		Weight (kg)					Triceps (mm)						
In	Cm	5	15	50	85	95	5	10	15	50	85	90	95
Small Frames, Women													
58	147	39	48	54	63	71		14	16	21	31	34	
59	150	41	48	55	66	74	11	13	15	21	30	31	33
60	152	43	47	54	67	73	10	11	13	20	29	31	35
61	155	43	45	56	65	71	10	12	14	22	29	29	32
62	157	47	52	58	67	73	11	11	12	21	29	30	32
63	160	42	49	58	67	74		12	13	20	29	30	
64	163	43	49	60	68	75		12	13	21	27	29	
65	165	43	49	60	69	75				18			
66	168	44	50	68	70	76				23			
67	170	45	51	61	71	77							
68	173	45	51	61	71	77							
69	175	46	52	62	72	78							
70	178	47	52	63	73	79							
Medium Frames, Women													
58	147	40	49	57	72	85	5	13	17	28	40	40	41
59	150	47	52	62	74	86	12	15	18	26	34	38	41
60	152	47	52	65	76	86	13	17	18	25	33	34	38
61	155	49	54	64	78	86	13	16	18	25	35	37	42
62	157	49	54	64	78	88	13	15	17	24	33	36	39
63	160	52	55	65	79	89	12	14	16	24	32	35	38
64	163	51	57	66	78	87	12	14	16	25	33	34	37
65	165	54	59	67	78	88	14	16	17	24	33	35	39
66	168	54	57	66	79	88	12	13	16	24	33	33	36
67	170	51	61	72	82	89		17	17	27	35	35	
68	173	52	59	70	83	90				25			
69	175	53	60	72	84	91							
70	178	54	61	73	85	92							
Large Frames, Women													
58	147	53	63	92	95	104				45			
59	150	54	63	78	95	105				36			
60	152	54	69	78	87	105		25	26	35	44	45	
61	155	64	69	79	94	106	18	22	24	33	40	44	46
62	157	59	63	82	93	111	19	24	24	32	40	43	50
63	160	61	67	80	100	118	20	24	25	33	41	43	45
64	163	60	67	77	97	119	18	22	23	29	42	46	50
65	165	60	69	80	98	111	15	17	20	30	43	44	46
66	168	57	63	82	98	109		18	18	27	35	40	
67	170	58	68	80	105	109			22	32	44		
68	173	58	68	79	100	110				26			
69	175	59	69	85	101	110							
70	178	60	69	85	101	111							

Adapted from Frisancho, 1984.
*Data from NHANES I (1971 to 1974) and NHANES II (1976 to 1980), conducted by the NCHS.

Common Abnormalities

Obesity

Exogenous obesity is a generalized, sex-related distribution of excess fat tissue associated with excessive caloric intake. It is characterized by thick skin, pale striae, preservation of muscle strength, and no evidence of osteoporosis (Fig. 3-30, A).

In *endogenous obesity* excess fat tissue is distributed to certain regions of the body, such as the trunk or girdle area, and is associated with a metabolic or endocrine disorder (Fig. 3-30, B).

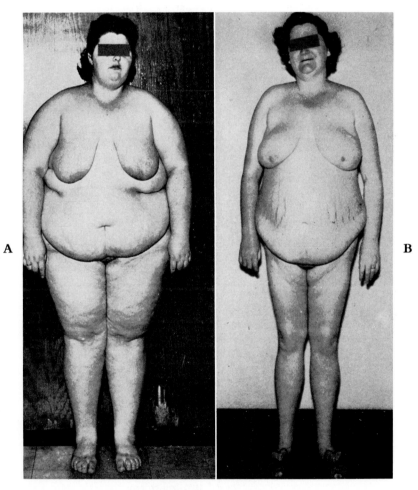

A   B

Fig. 3-30
A, Fat distribution associated with exogenous obesity (female pattern). **B,** Fat distribution associated with endogenous obesity (Cushing's syndrome).
From Prior et al., 1981.

Weight Loss

Cachexia is a severe weight loss and wasting resulting from a debilitating disease process. It is accompanied by sunken eyes, drooping eyelids, weakness, and temporal muscle atrophy (Fig. 3-31).

Anorexia nervosa is a syndrome of severe weight loss and wasting resulting from self-starvation that primarily occurs in adolescent and young adult women. It is characterized by a weight loss of 25% or more, amenorrhea, constipation, preoccupation with food, abdominal pain, and intolerance to cold.

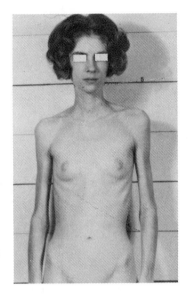

Fig. 3-31
Wasting associated with anorexia nervosa.
From Ezrin et al., 1979.

Metabolic Disorders

Acromegaly

Gradual marked enlargement and elongation of the bones of the face, jaw, and extremities are indicative of acromegaly. This disorder is associated with a pituitary tumor causing excessive production of growth hormone in middle aged adults. It is characterized by facial feature exaggeration and massive hands and feet, but no change in height (Fig. 3-32).

Fig. 3-32
Acromegaly. Note the coarse facial features, prominent forehead, large nose, and large jaw with prognathism.
Reprinted by permission of Elsevier Science Publishing Co., Inc., from Mazzaferri, E.L.: Endocrinology case studies, ed. 2, Flushing, N.Y., copyright 1975 by Medical Examination Publishing Co., Inc.

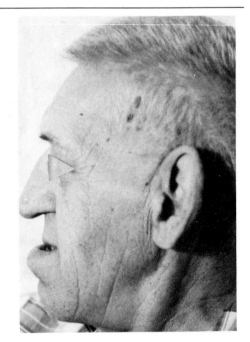

Cushing's Syndrome

This disorder results from a chronic excess cortisol production by the adrenal cortex or from the long term administration of large doses of glucocorticoids. Cushing's syndrome is seen most commonly with steroid therapy. However, on rare occasions it is the result of an adrenal malignancy in the very young. It is characterized by muscle weakness, oligomenorrhea or decreased testosterone levels, and abnormally pigmented, fragile skin. There is a redistribution of fat tissue to include a pendulous pad of fat on the chest and abdomen covered with striae, supraclavicular fat pads, moon facies, and thin extremities (Fig. 3-33).

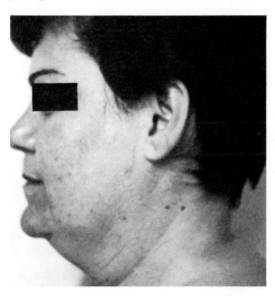

Fig. 3-33
Cushing's syndrome. The characteristic appearance of this syndrome is the round "moon" face with prominent jowls, preauricular fat, and hyperpigmentation and the "buffalo hump" in the low posterior cervical area.
Reprinted by permission of Elsevier Science Publishing Co., Inc., from Mazzaferri, E.L.: Endocrinology case studies, ed. 2, Flushing, N.Y., copyright 1975 by Medical Examination Publishing Co., Inc.

CHILDREN

Congenital Hypothyroidism (Cretinism)

This condition leads to dwarfism and mental retardation, beginning in the fetal period, unless treatment is instituted shortly after birth. The neonate appears normal but develops a stocky build, stubby hands, a broad flat nose, puffy facial features, a large tongue, and poor muscle tone if untreated (Fig. 3-34).

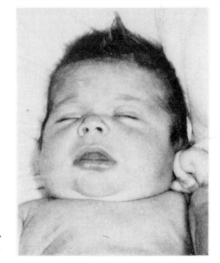

Fig. 3-34
Cretinism (congenital hypothyroidism).
From Jolly, H.: Diseases of children, ed. 4, Oxford, 1981 Blackwell Scientific Publications, Ltd.

Failure to Thrive

The failure of an infant to grow at rates considered appropriate for the population often occurs without organic cause. It may be related to chronic disease, inadequate calories and protein in the diet, improper feeding methods, intrauterine growth retardation, or emotional deprivation. The infant who fails to thrive may be the victim of congenital disorders of the brain, heart, or kidney. These are easy to discover. It is also possible that there are social and emotional causes. An emotionally deprived infant, one who is hungry for affection, will not grow. Growth hormone will be absent in that child. Once the child is given attention, holding, rocking, physical and emotional warmth, the growth hormone will be produced and the child will grow.

Achondroplasia

This genetic disorder causes abnormalities in endochondral ossification. It is characterized by dwarfism with short curved arms and legs, dorsal kyphosis and lumbar lordosis, and a normal sized head and trunk (Fig. 3-35).

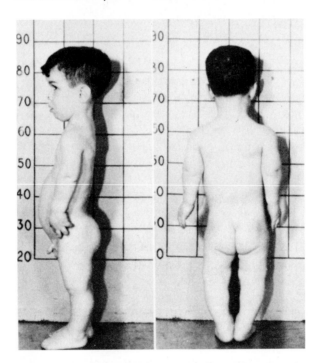

Fig. 3-35
Achondroplasia.
From McKusick, 1972.

Hypopituitary dwarfism

A growth hormone deficiency results in a child with short stature appearing younger than his or her chronologic age. Growth occurs normally for the first 1 or 2 years and then slows markedly, leading to dwarfism unless identified early and treated.

Pituitary Gigantism

Excessive stature growth with normal proportions during early childhood is associated with overproduction of growth hormone caused by a pituitary tumor. Headaches and other symptoms of increased intracranial pressure may be present.

Morquio's Syndrome

This genetic mucopolysaccharidosis disorder causes dwarfism with skeletal abnormalities such as pectus carinatum, crouching posture, and prominent joints. The child appears normal at birth, but the defect becomes apparent by 2 years of age (Fig. 3-36).

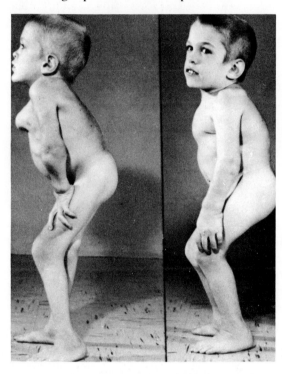

Fig. 3-36
Morquio's syndrome.
From Goodman and Gorlin, 1977.

Premature Pubarche

The early development of sexual hair without signs of sexual maturation is more common in females than males. Pubescence usually occurs at the expected time.

Precocious Puberty

Sexual development with all pubertal changes occurs prior to age 8 in females and age 9 in males. It is usually idiopath-ic, but it may be related to organic brain lesions or McCune-Albright syndrome (Fig. 3-37).

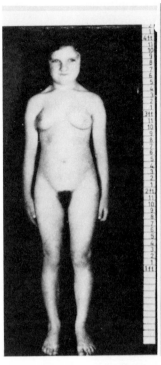
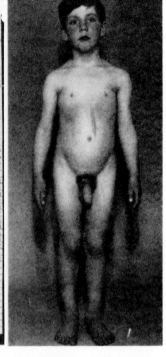

Fig. 3-37
A, Constitutional sexual precocity in a 5-year-old girl. **B,** Constitutional sexual precocity in a 5-year-old boy.

From Jolly, H.: Diseases of children, ed. 4, Oxford, 1981, Blackwell Scientific Publications, Ltd.

Turner's Syndrome

This abnormality of sex chromosomes produces a phenotypic female, usually identified during adolescence because of the absence of sexual development. Some of the following characteristics may be present in any affected child: webbed neck, increased carrying angle of the elbow, shield chest deformity with hypoplastic nipples, short stature, and congenital anomalies of heart or urinary tract (Fig. 3-38).

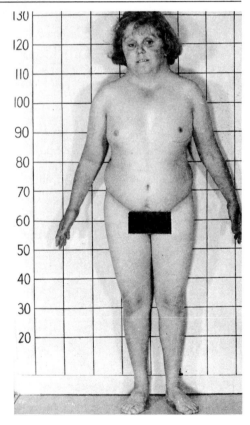

Fig. 3-38
Turner's syndrome.

From Goodman and Gorlin, 1977.

CHAPTER

4

Skin, Hair, and Nails

Anatomy and Physiology

Skin provides an elastic, rugged, self-regenerating, protective covering for the body. But it has another important function: the skin and its appendages are our primary physical presentation to the world.

The skin is a stratified structure composed of several layers that are functionally related. Fig. 4-1 shows the main structural components and their approximate spatial relationships. The anatomy of the skin varies somewhat from one part of the body to another.

Skin structure and physiologic processes allow several integral functions:

- Protects against microbial and foreign substance invasion and minor physical trauma
- Retards body fluid loss by providing a mechanical barrier
- Regulates body temperature through radiation, conduction, convection, and evaporation
- Provides sensory perception via free nerve endings and specialized receptors
- Produces vitamin D from precursors in the skin
- Contributes to blood pressure regulation through constriction of skin blood vessels
- Repairs surface wounds by exaggerating the normal process of cell replacement
- Excretes sweat, urea, and lactic acid
- Expresses emotions

Fig. 4-1
Anatomic structures of skin.

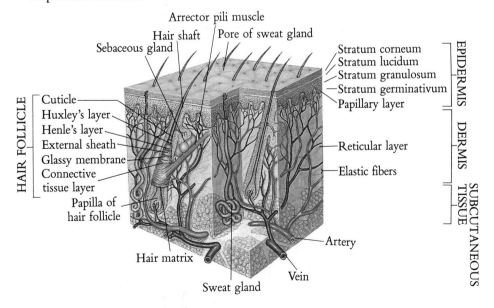

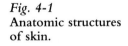

Epidermis

The epidermis, the outermost portion of the skin, consists of two major layers: the stratum corneum, which protects the body against harmful environmental substances and restricts water loss, and the cellular stratum in which the keratin cells are synthesized. The basement membrane lies beneath the cellular stratum and connects the epidermis to the dermis. The epidermis is avascular and depends on the underlying dermis for its nutrition.

The stratum corneum consists of closely packed dead squamous cells that contain the waterproofing protein keratin and form the protective barrier of the skin. These keratin cells are formed in the deepest sublayer of the cellular stratum, the stratum germinativum. The keratinocytes mature as they make their way to the surface through the stratum spinosum and stratum granulosum to replace the cells in the stratum corneum. This basal cell layer also contains melanocytes, the cells that synthesize melanin, which gives the skin its color. An additional sublayer of the cellular stratum, the stratum lucidum, is present only in the thicker skin of the palms and soles and lies just below the stratum corneum.

Dermis

The dermis is the richly vascular connective tissue layer of the skin that supports and separates the epidermis from the cutaneous adipose tissue. Upward projecting papillae penetrate the epidermis and provide nourishment for the living epidermal cells. Elastin, collagen, and reticulin fibers provide resilience, strength, and stability. Sensory nerve fibers located in the dermis form a complex network to provide sensations of pain, touch, and temperature. The dermis also contains autonomic motor nerves that innervate blood vessels, glands, and the arrectores pilorum muscles.

Hypodermis

The dermis is connected to underlying organs by the hypodermis, a subcutaneous layer that consists of loose connective tissue filled with fatty cells. This adipose layer generates heat and provides insulation, shock absorption, and a reserve of calories.

Appendages

The epidermis invaginates into the dermis at myriad points and forms the following appendages: eccrine sweat glands, apocrine sweat glands, sebaceous glands, hair, and nails.

The eccrine sweat glands open directly onto the surface of the skin and regulate body temperature through water secretion. The glands are distributed throughout the body except for the lip margins, eardrums, nail beds, inner surface of the prepuce, and glans penis.

The apocrine glands are specialized structures found only in the axillae, nipples, areolae, anogenital area, eyelids, and external ears. These glands are larger and located more deeply than the eccrine glands. In response to emotional stimuli, the glands secrete a white fluid containing protein, carbohydrate, and other substances. Secretions from these glands are odorless. Bacterial decomposition of apocrine sweat produces the characteristic adult body odor.

The sebaceous glands secrete sebum, a lipid-rich substance that keeps the skin and hair from drying out. Secretory activity, which is stimulated by sex hormones (primarily testosterone), varies according to hormonal levels throughout the life span.

Hair is formed by epidermal cells that invaginate into the dermal layers. Hair consists of a root, a shaft, and a follicle (the root and its covering). The papilla, a

Fig. 4-2
Anatomic structures of nail.
From Thompson et al., 1986.

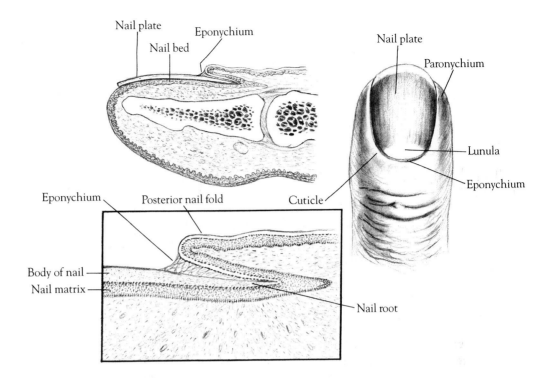

loop of capillaries at the base of the follicle, supplies nourishment for growth. Melanocytes in the shaft provide its color. Adults have two kinds of hair: vellus and terminal. Vellus hair is short, fine, soft, and nonpigmented. Terminal hair is coarser, longer, thicker, and usually pigmented. Each hair goes through cyclic changes: anagen (growth), catagen (atrophy), and telogen (rest), after which the hair is shed. Males and females have about the same number of hair follicles that are stimulated to differential growth by hormones.

The nails are epidermal cells converted to hard plates of keratin. The highly vascular nail bed lies beneath the plate, giving the nail its pink color. The white crescent-shaped area extending beyond the proximal nail fold marks the end of the nail matrix, the site of nail growth. The stratum corneum layer of skin covering the nail root is the cuticle, or eponychium, which pushes up and over the lower part of the nail body. The paronychium is the soft tissue surrounding the nail border. Fig. 4-2 shows the structures of the nail.

INFANTS AND CHILDREN

The skin of infants and children appears smoother than that of an adult, partly because of the relative absence of coarse terminal hair and partly because the skin has not been subjected to years of exposure to the elements. Desquamation of the stratum corneum may be present at birth or very shortly after. The degree of desquamation varies from mild flakiness to shedding of large sheets of cornified epidermis. Vernix caseosa, a mixture of sebum and cornified epidermis, covers the infant's body at birth.

The newborn's body, particularly the shoulders and back, is also covered with fine, silky hair called lanugo. This hair is shed within 10 to 14 days. Some newborns are bald, while others have an inordinate amount of head hair. Either way, most of the hair is shed by about 2 to 3 months of age to be replaced by more permanent hair with a new texture and often a different color.

The eccrine sweat glands begin to function after the first month of life. Apocrine function has not yet begun, giving the skin a less oily texture and resulting in the characteristic inoffensive perspiration.

ADOLESCENTS

During adolescence the apocrine glands enlarge and become active, causing increased axillary sweating and consequently a characteristic adult body odor. Sebaceous glands increase sebum production in response to increased hormone levels, primarily androgen, giving the skin an oily appearance and predisposing the individual to acne.

Coarse terminal hair appears in the axillae and pubic areas of both female and male adolescents and on the face of males. Hair production is one response to changing androgen levels. Refer to Chapter 3 (Growth and Measurement) for a more thorough discussion of maturational changes during adolescence.

PREGNANT WOMEN

Increased blood flow to the skin, especially the hands and feet, results from peripheral vasodilatation and increased numbers of capillaries. Acceleration of sweat and sebaceous gland activity occurs. Both processes assist in dissipating the excess heat caused by the increased metabolism during pregnancy. Vascular spiders and hemangiomas that are present may increase in size.

The skin thickens and fat is deposited in the subdermal layers. Because of increased fragility of connective tissues, separation may occur with stretching. Hormonal changes also cause increased pigmentation of the face, nipples, areolae, axillae, and vulva.

OLDER ADULTS

Sebaceous and sweat gland activity decreases in older adults, and as a result the skin becomes drier and less perspiration is produced. The epidermis begins to thin and flatten, taking on the look of parchment as the vascularity of the dermis decreases. Epidermal permeability is increased, thus reducing the efficiency of the barrier function of the stratum corneum.

The dermis becomes less elastic, loses collagen and elastic fibers, and shrinks, causing the epidermis to fold and assume a wrinkled appearance. Wrinkling is less marked in individuals with black and yellow skins and in those who are obese.

Cutaneous tissue decreases, particularly in the extremities, giving joints and bony prominences a sharp, angular appearance. There is a deepening of the hollows in the thoracic, axillary, and supraclavicular regions.

Gray hair results from a decrease in the number of functioning melanocytes. Axillary and pubic hair production declines because of reduced hormonal functioning. The density and rate of scalp hair growth (anagen phase) declines with age. The size of hair follicles also changes, and there is a progressive transition of terminal hair into vellus hair on the scalp, causing age-associated baldness in both men and women. The opposite transition, from vellus to terminal, occurs in the hair of the nares and on the tragus of men's ears. Women produce increased coarse facial hair because of higher androgen to estrogen ratios. Both genders experience overall loss of hair from the trunk and extremities. The loss of axillary and pubic hair results from diminished androgen production.

Nail growth slows because of decreased peripheral circulation. The nails, particularly the toenails, become thicker, brittle, hard, and yellowish. They develop longitudinal ridges and are prone to splitting into layers.

Review of Related History

General Considerations

1. Skin care habits: cleansing routine, soaps, oils, lotions or local applications used, cosmetics, home remedies or preparations used, sun exposure patterns, use of sun screen agents, recent changes in skin care habits
2. Hair care habits: cleansing routine, shampoos and rinses used, coloring preparations used, permanents, recent changes in hair care habits
3. Nail care habits: any difficulty in clipping or trimming nails, instruments used
4. Medications: topical or systemic (prescribed or over-the-counter)
5. Exposure to environmental or occupational hazards: dyes, chemicals, plants, toxic substances, frequent immersion of hands in water, frequent sun exposure
6. Recent psychologic or physiologic stress

Present Problem

Skin

1. Changes in skin: dryness, pruritus, sores, rashes, lumps, color, texture, odor, amount of perspiration; changes in wart or mole; lesion that does not heal or is chronically irritated
2. Temporal sequence: date of initial onset, time sequence of occurrence and development, sudden or gradual onset, date of recurrence, if any
3. Symptoms: itching, pain, exudate, bleeding, color changes, seasonal or climate variations
4. Location: skinfolds, extensor or flexor surfaces, localized or generalized
5. Associated symptoms: presence of systemic disease or high fever, relationship to stress or leisure activities
6. Recent exposure to drugs, environmental or occupational toxins or chemicals; to persons with similar skin condition
7. Apparent cause: patient perception of cause
8. Travel history: where, when, length of stay, exposure to diseases, contact with travellers
9. What the patient has been doing for the problem: medications or preparations used (prescribed or over-the-counter), response to treatment, what makes the condition worse or better
10. How the patient is adjusting to the problem

Hair

1. Changes in hair: loss or growth, distribution, texture, color
2. Occurrence: sudden or gradual onset, symmetrical or asymmetrical pattern, recurrence
3. Associated symptoms: pain, itching, lesions, presence of systemic disease or high fever, recent psychologic or physical stress
4. Exposure to drugs, environmental or occupational toxins or chemicals, commercial hair care chemicals
5. Nutrition: dietary changes, dieting, malnutrition
6. What the patient has been doing for the problem: medications or preparations used (prescribed or over-the-counter), response to treatment, what makes the problem worse or better
7. How the patient is adjusting to the problem

Nails

1. Changes in nails: splitting, breaking, discoloration, ridging, thickening, markings, separation from nail bed
2. Associated symptoms: pain, swelling, exudate, presence of systemic disease or high fever, recent psychologic or physical stress
3. Temporal sequence: sudden or gradual onset, relationship to injury of nail or finger
4. Recent exposure to drugs, environmental or occupational toxins or chemicals, frequent immersion in water
5. What the patient has been doing for the problem: medications or preparations used (prescribed or over-the-counter), response to treatment, what makes the problem worse or better

Past Medical History

Skin

1. Previous skin problems: sensitivities, allergic skin reactions, allergic skin disorders (such as infantile eczema), lesions, treatment
2. Tolerance to sunlight
3. Diminished or heightened sensitivity to sensory stimuli
4. Cardiac, respiratory, liver, endocrine, or other systemic diseases

Hair

1. Previous hair problems: loss, thinning, unusual growth or distribution, brittle breakage, treatment
2. Systemic problems: thyroid or liver disorder, any severe illness, malnutrition, associated skin disorder

Nails

1. Previous nail problems: injury; bacterial, fungal, or viral infection
2. Systemic problems: associated skin disorder; congenital anomalies; respiratory, cardiac, endocrine, hematologic, or other systemic disease

Family History

1. Current or past dermatologic diseases or disorders in family members: skin cancer, psoriasis, allergic skin disorders, infestations, bacterial, fungal, or viral infections
2. Allergic hereditary diseases such as asthma or hayfever
3. Familial hair loss or coloration patterns

INFANTS

1. Feeding history: breast or formula, type of formula, what foods introduced and when
2. Diaper history: skin cleansing routines, use of rubber pants, method of cleaning washable diapers
3. Types of clothing and washing practices, soaps and detergents used, new blanket or clothing
4. Bath practices, types of soap, oils, or lotions used
5. Dress habits: amount and type of clothing in relation to environmental temperature

6. Temperature and humidity of the home environment: air conditioning, heating system (drying or humidified)
7. Rubbing head against mattress, rug, furniture, wall

CHILDREN

1. Eating habits and types of food, including chocolate, candy, soft drinks, bubble gum
2. Exposure to communicable diseases
3. Allergic disorders: eczema, urticaria, pruritus, hayfever, asthma, other chronic respiratory disorders
4. Skin injury history: frequency of falls, cuts, abrasions; repeated history of unexplained injuries
5. Chronic manipulation of hair
6. Nail biting

OLDER ADULTS

1. Increased or decreased sensation to touch or the environment
2. Generalized chronic itching: exposure to skin irritants, detergents, lotions with high alcohol content, woolen clothing, humidity of environment
3. Susceptibility to skin infections
4. Healing response: delayed or interrupted
5. Frequent falls resulting in multiple cuts or bruises
6. History of diabetes mellitus or peripheral vascular disease
7. Hair loss history: gradual v sudden onset, loss pattern (symmetrical or asymmetrical)

Examination and Findings

EQUIPMENT

- Ruler
- Wood's lamp
- Flashlight with transilluminator
- Magnifying glass (optional)

Skin

Examination of the skin is performed by inspection and palpation. The most important tools are your own eyes and powers of observation. Sometimes when gross inspection leaves you uncertain, a hand-held magnifying glass may help.

Adequate lighting is essential; daylight provides the best illumination for determinating color variations, particularly jaundice. If daylight is unavailable or insufficient, it should be supplemented with overhead fluorescent lighting. Tangential lighting is helpful in assessing contour, but inadequate lighting can result in inadequate assessment.

Although the skin is commonly observed as each part of the body is examined, it is important to make a brief but careful overall visual sweep of the entire body. This "bird's-eye view" gives a good idea of the distribution and extent of any lesions. It also allows you to observe skin symmetry, detect differences between body areas, and compare sun-exposed to non-sun-exposed areas. You can also be alert for special conditions that require attention as the examination progresses.

Adequate exposure of the skin is necessary. It is essential to remove encumbering clothing and to fully remove drapes or coverings as each section of the body is examined. Make sure that the room temperature is comfortable. Look carefully at areas not usually exposed, such as the axillae, buttocks, perineum, backs of thighs, and inner upper thighs. As the examination is completed for each area, the patient should be redraped or covered.

Begin by inspecting the skin and mucous membranes (especially oral) for color and uniform appearance, thickness, symmetry, hygiene, and the presence of any lesions.

Skin thickness varies over the body, with the thinnest skin on the eyelids and the thickest at areas of pressure or rubbing, most notably the soles, palms, and elbows. Note callousing on the hands or feet.

The range of normal skin color varies from deep to light brown, or whitish pink to ruddy with olive or yellow overtones. While color should assume an overall uniformity, there may be sun-darkened areas and darker skin around knees and elbows. Calloused areas may appear yellow. Vascular flush areas (cheeks, neck, upper chest, and genital area) may appear pink or red, especially with anxiety or excitement. Be aware that skin color may be masked by cosmetics and tanning agents. Look for localized areas of discoloration. Several variations in skin color occur in almost all healthy adults and children, including nonpigmented striae (silver or pink "stretch marks" that occur after parturition or weight gain) (Fig. 4-3); freckles in sun-exposed areas; some birth marks; and some flat and raised nevi in various shades of brown, tan, or near skin color (Fig. 4-4). Adult women will frequently have melasma, areas of hyperpigmentation on the face and neck that are associated with pregnancy or the use of hormones (Fig. 4-5). The absence of melanin will produce patches of unpigmented skin or hair (Fig. 4-6).

Fig. 4-3
Striae.
Courtesy Antoinette Hood, M.D., The Johns Hopkins University School of Medicine, Baltimore.

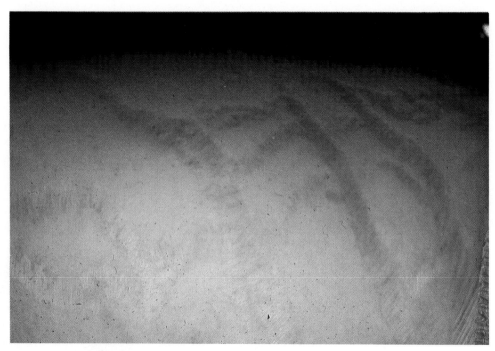

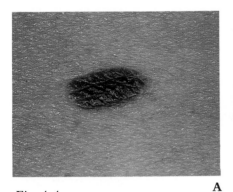 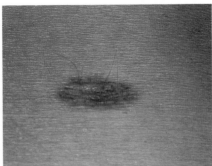 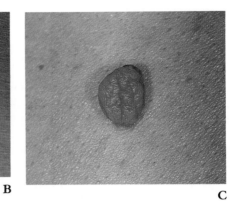

A **B** **C**

Fig. 4-4
Commonly occurring nevi.
A, Junction nevus. Color
and shape of this black
lesion are uniform. **B,**
Compound nevus. Center
is elevated and surrounding
area is flat, retaining
features of a junction
nevus. **C,** Dermal nevus.
Papillomatous with soft,
flabby, wrinkled surface.
From Habif, 1985.

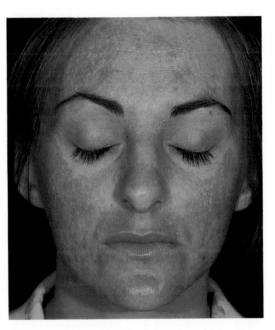

Fig. 4-5
Facial hyperpigmentation:
melasma.
From Habif, 1985.

Fig. 4-6
Vitiligo.
Courtesy Jaime A. Tschen, M.D.
Baylor College of Medicine, Depart-
ment of Dermatology; Houston; from
Thompson et al., 1986.

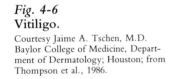

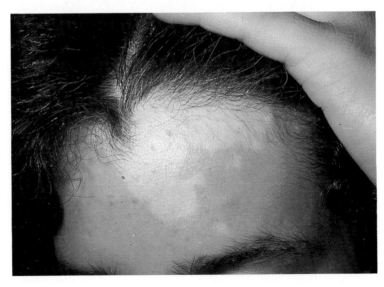

Color hues in dark skinned persons are best seen in the sclera, conjunctiva, buccal mucosa, tongue, lips, nail beds, and palms. Be aware, however, that heavily calloused palms in dark skinned persons will have an opaque yellow cast. Particular variations in skin color may be the result of physiologic pigment distribution. The palms and soles are lighter in color than the rest of the body. Freckling of the buccal cavity, gums, and tongue is common. The sclera may appear yellowish brown (often described as "muddy") or may contain brownish pigment that looks like petechiae. A bluish hue of the lips and gums can be a normal finding in persons with dark skin.

Systemic disorders can produce generalized or localized color changes, which are described in Table 4-1. Localized redness often results from an inflammatory process. Injury, steroids, vasculitis, and several systemic disorders can cause localized hemorrhage into cutaneous tissues, producing red-purple discolorations. The discolorations produced by injury are called ecchymoses; when produced by other causes they are called petechiae if smaller than 0.5 cm in diameter (Fig. 4-7), or purpura if larger than 0.5 cm in diameter (Fig. 4-8). Vascular skin lesions are characterized in Table 4-2.

Table 4-1
Cutaneous Color Changes

Color	Cause	Distribution	Select Conditions
Brown	Darkening of melanin pigment	Generalized	Pituitary, adrenal, liver disease
		Localized	Nevi, neurofibromatosis
White	Absence of melanin	Generalized	Albinism
		Localized	Vitiligo
Red (erythema)	Increased cutaneous blood flow	Localized	Inflammation
		Generalized	Fever, viral exanthems, urticaria
	Increased intravascular red blood cells	Generalized	Polycythemia
Yellow	Increased bile pigmentation (jaundice)	Generalized	Liver disease
	Increased carotene pigmentation	Generalized	Hypothyroidism, increased intake of vegetables containing carotene
	Decreased visibility of oxyhemoglobin	Generalized	Anemia, chronic renal disease
Blue	Increased unsaturated hemoglobin secondary to hypoxia	Lips, mouth, nail beds	Cardiovascular and pulmonary diseases

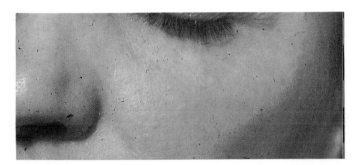

Fig. 4-7
Petechiae.
Courtesy Antoinette Hood, M.D.,
The Johns Hopkins University School
of Medicine, Baltimore.

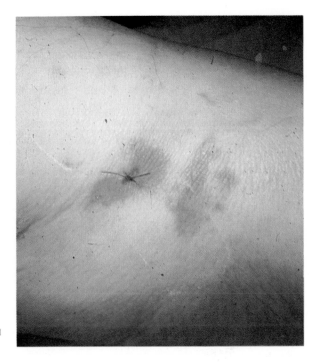

Fig. 4-8
Purpura.
Courtesy Antoinette Hood, M.D.,
The Johns Hopkins University School
of Medicine, Baltimore.

Describe lesions according to characteristics, exudates, pattern of arrangement, location, and distribution:

Characteristics
    Size: measure all dimensions
    Shape or configuration
    Color
    Texture
    Elevation or depression
    Pedunculation
Exudates
    Color
    Amount
    Consistency
Pattern of arrangement
    Annular (rings)
    Grouped
    Linear
    Arciform (bow-shaped)
    Diffuse
Location and distribution
    Generalized or localized
    Region of the body
    Patterns: dermatomal, flexor or extensor, random, relation to clothing lines
        or jewelry
    Discrete or confluent

Tables 4-3 and 4-4 describe the characteristics of primary and secondary lesions. The nomenclature is often used inaccurately; if you are uncertain about a lesion, use the descriptors rather than the name. Be aware that several types of lesions may occur concurrently and that secondary changes may obscure primary characteristics.

Text continued on p. 109.

Table 4-2
Vascular Skin Lesions

Lesion	Characteristics	Cause
Purpura	Red-purple discoloration greater than 0.5 cm diameter	Intravascular defects, infection

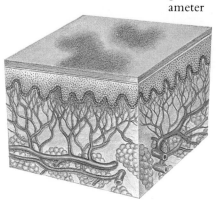

Petechiae	Red-purple discoloration less than 0.5 cm diameter	Intravascular defects, infection

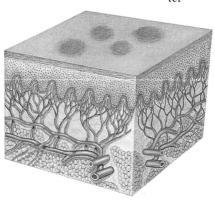

Ecchymoses	Red-purple discoloration of variable size	Vascular wall destruction, trauma, vasculitis

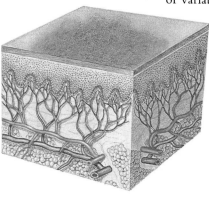

Table 4-2—cont'd
Vascular Skin Lesions

Lesion	Characteristics	Cause
Spider angioma	Red central body with radiating spider-like legs that blanch with pressure to the central body	Liver disease, vitamin B deficiency, idiopathic
Venous star	Bluish spider, linear or irregularly shaped; does not blanch with pressure	Increased pressure in superficial veins
Capillary hemangioma (nevus flammeus)	Red irregular macular patches	Dilation of dermal capillaries

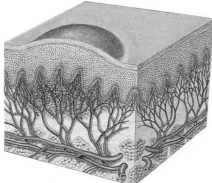

Table 4-3
*Primary Skin Lesions**

Lesion	Description	Examples
Macule	Flat; nonpalpable; circumscribed; less than 1 cm in diameter; brown, red, purple, white, or tan in color	Freckles; flat moles; rubella; rubeola

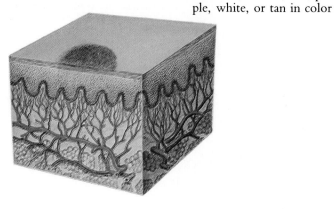

| *Patch* | Flat; nonpalpable; irregular in shape; macule that is greater than 1 cm in diameter | Vitiligo; port-wine marks |

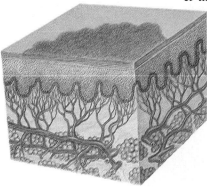

| *Papule* | Elevated; palpable; firm; circumscribed; less than 1 cm in diameter; brown, red, pink, tan, or bluish red in color | Warts; drug-related eruptions; pigmented nevi |

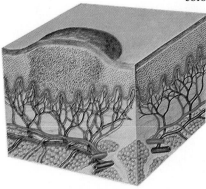

From Thompson et al., 1986.
*Primary skin lesions occur as initial spontaneous manifestations of an underlying pathologic process.

Table 4-3—cont'd
Primary Skin Lesions

Lesion	Description	Examples
Plaque	Elevated; flat topped; firm; rough; superficial papule greater than 1 cm in diameter; may be coalesced papules	Psoriasis; seborrheic and actinic keratoses

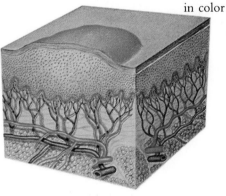

Wheal	Elevated, irregular-shaped area of cutaneous edema; solid, transient, changing; variable diameter; pale pink in color	Urticaria; insect bites

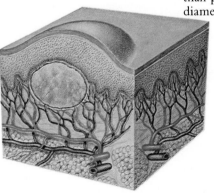

Nodule	Elevated; firm; circumscribed; palpable; deeper in dermis than papule; 1 to 2 cm in diameter	Erythema nodosum; lipomas

Continued.

Table 4-3—cont'd
Primary Skin Lesions

Lesion	Description	Examples
Tumor	Elevated; solid; may or may not be clearly demarcated; greater than 2 cm in diameter; may or may not vary from skin color	Neoplasms

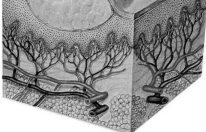

Lesion	Description	Examples
Vesicle	Elevated; circumscribed; superficial; filled with serous fluid; less than 1 cm in diameter	Blister; varicella

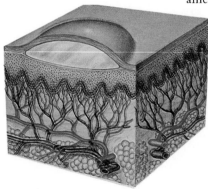

Lesion	Description	Examples
Bulla	Vesicle greater than 1 cm in diameter	Blister; pemphigus vulgaris

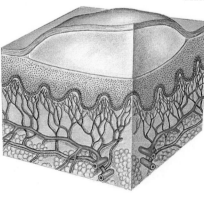

Table 4-3—cont'd
Primary Skin Lesions

Lesion	Description	Examples
Pustule	Elevated; superficial; similar to vesicle but filled with purulent fluid	Impetigo; acne; variola

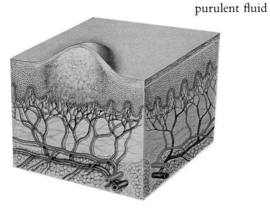

Lesion	Description	Examples
Cyst	Elevated; circumscribed; palpable; encapsulated; filled with liquid or semisolid material	Sebaceous cyst

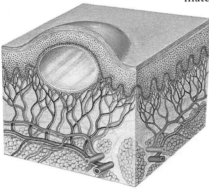

Lesion	Description	Examples
Telangiectasia	Fine, irregular red line produced by dilation of capillary	Telangiectasia in rosacea

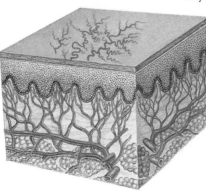

Table 4-4
*Secondary Skin Lesions**

Lesion	Description	Examples
Scale	Heaped-up keratinized cells; flaky exfoliation; irregular; thick or thin; dry or oily; varied size; silver, white, or tan in color	Psoriasis; exfoliative dermatitis

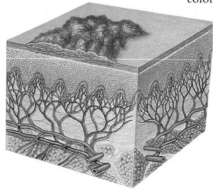

Lesion	Description	Examples
Crust	Dried serum, blood or purulent exudate; slightly elevated; size varies; brown, red, black, tan, or straw in color	Scab on abrasion; eczema

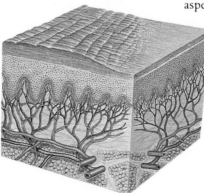

Lesion	Description	Examples
Lichenification	Rough, thickened epidermis; accentuated skin markings caused by rubbing or irritation; often involves flexor aspect of extremity	Chronic dermatitis

From Thompson et al., 1986.
*Secondary lesions are a result of later evolution of a primary lesion or are induced by external trauma to the primary lesion.

Table 4-4—cont'd
Secondary Skin Lesions

Lesion	Description	Examples
Scar	Thin to thick fibrous tissue replacing injured dermis; irregular; pink, red, or white in color; may be atrophic or hypertrophic	Healed wound or surgical incision

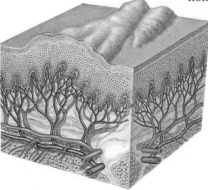

Lesion	Description	Examples
Keloid	Irregularly shaped, elevated, progressively enlarging scar; grows beyond boundaries of wound; caused by excessive collagen formation during healing	Keloid from ear piercing or burn scar

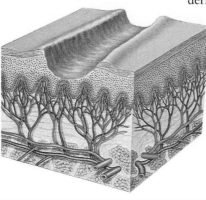

Lesion	Description	Examples
Excoriation	Loss of epidermis; linear or hollowed-out crusted area; dermis exposed	Abrasion; scratch

Continued.

Table 4-4—cont'd
Secondary Skin Lesions

Lesion	Description	Examples
Fissure	Linear crack or break from epidermis to dermis; small; deep; red	Athlete's foot; cheilois

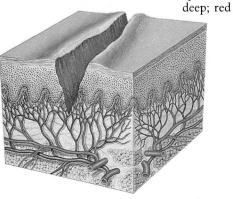

Erosion	Loss of all or part of epidermis; depressed; moist; glistening; follows rupture of vesicle or bulla; larger than fissure	Varicella; variola following rupture

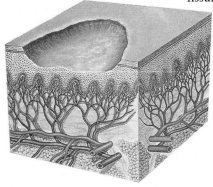

Ulcer	Loss of epidermis and dermis; concave; varies in size; exudative; red or reddish blue	Decubiti; stasis ulcers

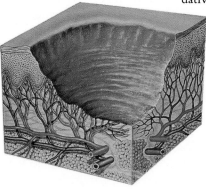

Table 4-4—cont'd
Secondary Skin Lesions

Lesion	Description	Examples
Atrophy	Thinning of skin surface and loss of skin markings; skin translucent and paperlike	Striae; aged skin

A small ruler is necessary for measuring the size of lesions. Examiners frequently rely on household measures such as fruit, vegetables, and coins to estimate the size of lesions, nodules, or eruptions, but the resulting descriptions can be as inaccurate as they are interesting. Subjective estimates should not be used as measures of size; instead, use the ruler and report sizes in centimeters (inches may also be used, but centimeters is the preferred unit of measure). Try to measure size in all dimensions (height, width, depth) when possible.

Use a flashlight for closer inspection of a particular lesion to detect its nuances of color, elevation, and borders. Transillumination may be used to determine the presence of fluid in cysts and masses. Darken the room and place the tip of the transilluminator against the side of the cyst or mass. Fluid-filled lesions will transilluminate with a red glow, whereas solid lesions will not.

The Wood's lamp can be used to distinguish fluorescing lesions. Darken the room and shine the light on the area to be examined. Look for the characteristic blue-green fluorescence that indicates the presence of fungal infection.

As you inspect, palpate the skin for moisture, temperature, texture, turgor, and mobility. Palpation may yield additional data for describing lesions, particularly in relation to elevation or depression.

Minimal perspiration or oiliness should be present. Increased perspiration may be associated with activity, warm environment, obesity, anxiety, or excitement and may be especially noticeable on the palms, scalp, forehead, and in the axillae, usually the dampest area. The intertriginous areas should evidence minimal dampness. Pay particular attention to areas that get little or no exposure to circulating air, such as in the folds of large breasts or obese abdomens or in the inguinal area (Fig. 4-9).

The skin should range from cool to warm to the touch. Use the dorsal surface of your hands or fingers, as these areas are most sensitive to temperature perception. At best, this assessment is a rough estimate of skin temperature; what you are really looking for is bilateral symmetry. Environmental conditions, including the temperature of the examining room, may affect surface temperature.

Fig. 4-9
Examining an intertriginous area. Note fissure and maceration.
From Habif, 1985.

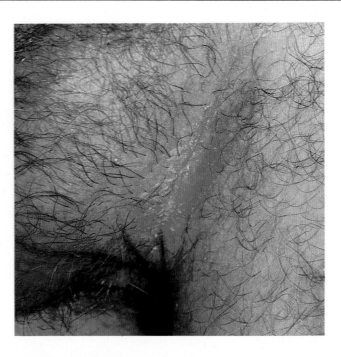

Fig. 4-10
Testing skin turgor.

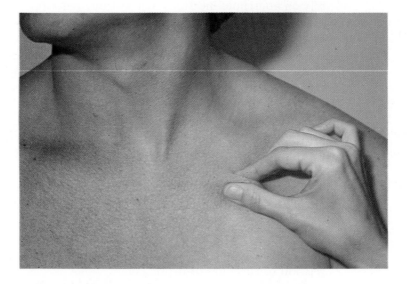

The texture should feel smooth, soft, and even. Roughness on exposed areas or areas of pressure, particularly the elbows, soles, and palms may be caused by heavy or woolen clothing, cold weather, or soap. Extensive or widespread roughness may be the result of a keratinization disorder or healing lesions.

To assess turgor and mobility, gently pinch a small section of skin between the thumb and forefinger and then release the skin (Fig. 4-10). The skin should feel resilient, move easily when pinched, and return to place immediately when released. Turgor will be altered if the patient is substantially dehydrated or if edema is present. Some of the connective tissue diseases, notably the forms of scleroderma, will affect skin mobility.

PATTERNS OF SKIN LESIONS

The patterns of arrangement of skin lesions may be of diagnostic value in many cases. The patterns can sometimes be explained by their pathogenesis. Annular formation indicates a process of extension of the lesion from the initial location to the periphery with clearing in the center. Annular patterns are commonly seen in pityriasis rosea, tinea corporis, tinea cruris, and urticaria. The localization of a number of small primary lesions into groups may be the result of mechanical factors (as in insect bites) or a predisposition of a particular body area to a specific lesion (as in herpes simplex). A linear arrangement may be caused by external factors (as in trauma or contact dermatitis) or determined by developmental origins of the lesions (as in herpes zoster).

Skin lesions may be either generalized or localized, with some disorders producing lesions in characteristic regions of the body. The distribution may provide diagnostic clues. Generalized lesions may be indicative of an underlying systemic disorder, an allergic response, or a genetic disorder. Localized lesions occur frequently as the result of primary irritant or allergic eczematous dermatitis.

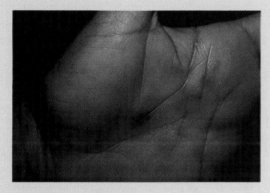

Annular formation of lesions.
Courtesy Stephen B. Tucker, M.D., Department of Dermatology, University of Texas Health Science Center at Houston; from Thompson et al., 1986.

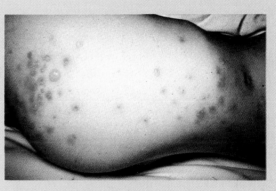

Clustering of lesions.
Reproduced by kind permission of the Wellcome Foundation, Ltd.

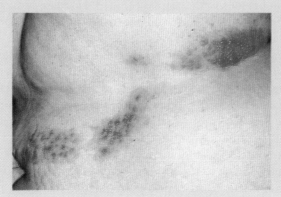

Linear formation of lesions.
From Habif, 1985.

Hair

Palpate the hair for texture, while at the same time inspecting it for color, distribution, and quantity. The scalp hair may be coarse or fine, curly or straight, and should be shiny, smooth, and resilient. Palpate the scalp hair for dryness and brittleness that could indicate a systemic disorder. Color will vary from very light blond to black to gray and may show alterations if rinses or dyes are used.

The quantity and distribution of hair varies according to individual genetic makeup. Hair is commonly present on scalp, lower face, neck, nares, ears, chest, axillae, back and shoulders, arms, legs, pubic area, and around nipples. Note hair loss, which can be either generalized or localized. Look for any inflammation or scarring that accompanies hair loss, particularly when it is localized. Diffuse hair loss usually occurs without inflammation and scarring. The presence of scarring is a helpful symptom in diagnosis. Note whether the hair shafts are broken off or are absent completely.

Genetically predisposed men often display a gradual symmetrical hair loss on the scalp during adulthood as a response to elevated androgen levels. Asymmetrical hair loss may indicate pathology. Women in their 20s and 30s may also develop adrenal androgenic female-pattern alopecia, with a gradual loss of hair from the central scalp.

Fine vellus hair covers the body, while coarse terminal hair occurs on the scalp, pubic, and axillary areas, to some extent on the arms and legs, and in the beard of males. The male pubic hair configuration is an upright triangle with the hair extending midline to the umbilicus. The female pubic configuration is an inverted triangle; the hair may extend midline to the umbilicus. Look for hirsutism in women—growth of terminal hair in a male distribution pattern on the face, body, and pubic area. Hirsutism, by itself or associated with other signs of virilization, may be a sign of an endocrine disorder.

Nails

Inspect the nails for color, length, configuration, symmetry, and cleanliness. The condition of the fingernails can provide important insight to the patient's sense of self. Are they bitten down to the quick? Are they clean? Are they kept smooth and neat, or do they look unkempt? There are, of course, physical clues to pathophysiologic problems in the nails, just as in the hair. The condition of the hair and nails gives a clue about the patient's level of self care and some sense of emotional order and social integration.

The shape and opacity of nails varies considerably among individuals. Nail color should be variations of pink. Pigment deposits or bands may be present in the nail beds of persons with dark skin (Fig. 4-11). The sudden appearance of such a band in whites may indicate melanoma. Yellow discoloration occurs with several nail diseases including psoriasis and fungal infections and may also occur with chronic respiratory disease. Diffuse darkening of the nails may arise from antimalarial drug therapy, candidal infection, hyperbilirubinemia, and chronic trauma, such as occurs from tight-fitting shoes. Green-black discoloration, which is associated with *Pseudomonas* infection, may be confused with similar discoloration caused by injury to the nail bed (subungual hematoma). Pain accompanies a subungual hematoma, whereas pseudomonas infection is painless. Splinter hemorrhages, longitudinal red or brown streaks, may occur with severe psoriasis of the nail matrix or as the result of minor injury to the proximal nail fold. White spots in the nail plate, a common finding, result from cuticle manipulation or other forms of mild trauma. These spots need to be differentiated from longitudinal white streaks or transverse white

Fig. 4-11
Pigmented bands in nails are normal in persons with dark skin.
From Habif, 1985.

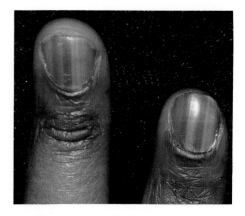

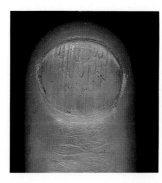

Fig. 4-12
Longitudinal ridging and beading of nail are a common variation of normal.
From Habif, 1985.

bands that are indicative of a systemic disorder. Separation of the nail plate from the bed produces a white, yellow, or green tinge on the nonadherent portion of the nail.

Nail edges should be smooth and rounded. Jagged, broken, or bitten edges or cuticles are indicators of poor care habits and may predispose the patient to localized infection. Peeling nails (from the plate splitting into layers) are usually found in individuals whose hands are subject to repeated water immersion.

The nail plate should appear smooth and flat or slightly curved. Complete absence of the nail (anonychia) may occur as a congenital condition. Look for ridging, grooves, depressions, and pitting. Longitudinal ridging and beading are common normal variants (Fig. 4-12). Longitudinal ridging and grooving may also occur with lichen planus of the nail. Transverse grooves result from repeated injury to the nail, usually the thumb, as with chronic manipulation to the proximal nail fold. The most common cause is picking at the thumb with the index finger. Chronic inflammation, such as occurs with chronic paronychia or chronic eczema, produces transverse rippling of the nail plate. Transverse depressions that appear at the base of the lunula occur following stress that temporarily interrupts nail formation. Involvement of a single nail usually points to injury of the nail matrix. Assure the patient that the nail will grow out and assume normal appearance in about 6 months. Depressions that occur in all the nails are usually in response to systemic disease, including syphilis, disorders producing high fevers, peripheral vascular disease, and uncontrolled diabetes mellitus. Pitting is seen most commonly with psoriasis. Broadening and flattening of the nail plate may be seen in secondary syphilis.

The nail base angle should measure 160 degrees. The best way to observe this is to place a ruler or a sheet of paper across the nail and dorsal surface of the finger and examine the angle formed by the proximal nail fold and nail plate. In clubbing, the angle increases and approaches or exceeds 180 degrees. Clubbing is associated with a variety of respiratory and cardiovascular diseases, cirrhosis, colitis, and thyroid disease (Fig. 4-13).

Examine the proximal and lateral nail folds for redness, swelling, pus, warts, cysts, and tumors. Pain usually accompanies ingrown nails and infections.

The nail plates should feel hard and smooth with a uniform thickness. Thickening of the nail may occur from tight-fitting shoes, chronic trauma, and some fungal infections. Thinning of the nail plate may also accompany some nail diseases.

Gently squeeze the nail between your thumb and the pad of your finger to test for adherence of the nail to the nail bed. Separation of the nail plate from the bed is common with psoriasis, trauma, candidal or pseudomonas infections, and some medications. The nail base should feel firm (Fig. 4-14). A boggy nail base accompanies clubbing.

Fig. 4-13
Finger clubbing. Nail is enlarged and curved.
From Habif, 1985.

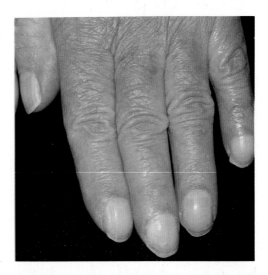

Fig. 4-14
Testing nail bed adherence.

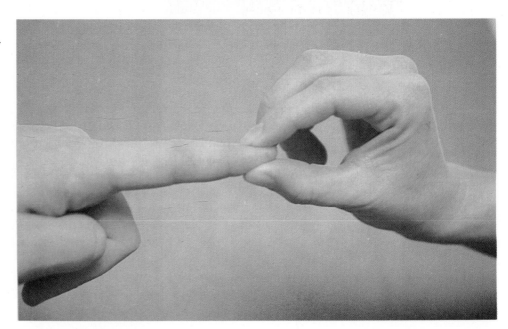

Table 4-5
Nails: Unexpected Findings

Finding and Appearance	Finding and Appearance
Clubbing—early 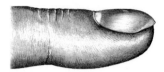	Darkening of nail 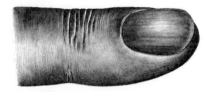
Clubbing—middle 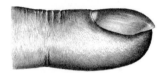	Terry's nails 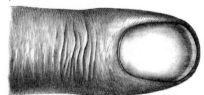
Clubbing—severe 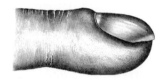	Splinter hemorrhages 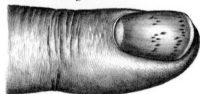
Transverse grooving (Beau's lines) 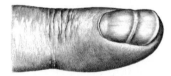	Nail pitting 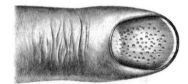
Curvature of nail 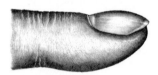	Onycholysis 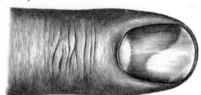
Spoon nail (koilonychia) 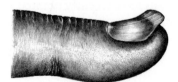	Anonychia (absence of nail) 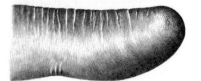
Broadening of nail 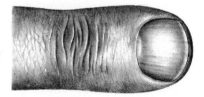	Paronychia 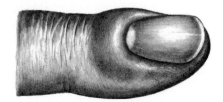

Fig. 4-15
Pink color of newborn.

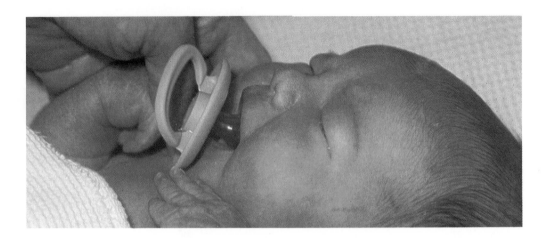

In the first few hours of life the infant's skin may look very red (Fig. 4-15). The more gentle pink coloring that predominates in infancy usually surfaces in the first day after birth. Skin color is partly determined by chubbiness; the less fat, the redder and more transparent the skin. Dark skinned newborns do not always manifest the intensity of melanosis that will be readily evident in 2 to 3 months. The exception in this regard are the nail beds and skin of the scrotum. The normal color changes in newborns are described on p. 117.

Physiologic jaundice may be present to a mild degree in as many as 50% of newborn infants. It usually starts after the first day of life and disappears by the eighth to tenth day but may persist for as long as 3 to 4 weeks. Intense and persistent jaundice should suggest liver disease or severe, overwhelming infection.

The skin of the newborn should be carefully checked for small defects especially over the entire length of the spine, the midline of the head from the nape of the neck to the bridge of the nose, and the neck extending to the ear. This may offer a clue to sinus tracts, brachial clefts, or cysts. The skin should feel soft and smooth.

Inspect the skin for distortions in contour suggestive of hygromas, fluid-containing masses, subcutaneous angiomas, lymphangiomas, nodules, and tumors. Transillumination may help if there is a question regarding the density of the mass or the amount of fluid. The more density and the less fluid, the less the tendency to glow on transillumination.

Turner's syndrome (gonadal dysgenesis caused by absence of an X chromosome, producing an XO karyotype) is frequently associated with congenital lymphedema. Dermatologists have recently pointed out that transient hemangiomas on the feet of infants should make you suspect Turner's syndrome.

All newborn infants are covered to some degree by vernix caseosa, a whitish, moist, cheesy-like substance. Transient puffiness of the hands, feet, eyelids, legs, pubis, or sacrum occurs in some newborns. It has no discernible cause and should not create concern when it disappears within 2 to 3 days.

Cutis marmorata, a mottled appearance of the body and extremities, is part of the newborn's response to changes in ambient temperature, whether cooling or heating. It is more common in premature infants and children with Down's syndrome and hypothyroidism (Fig. 4-16). Cyanosis of the hands and feet (acrocyanosis) may be present at birth in the newborn and may persist for several days or longer if the baby is kept in cool ambient temperatures. It often recurs when the baby is chilled. Generally, when the cyanosis persists, it is more intense in the feet than the hands, and an underlying cardiac defect should be suspected (Fig. 4-17).

NORMAL COLOR CHANGES IN THE NEWBORN

acrocyanosis Cyanosis of hands and feet

cutis marmorata Transient mottling when infant is exposed to decreased temperature

erythema toxicum Pink papular rash with vesicles superimposed on thorax, back, buttocks, and abdomen; may appear in 24 to 48 hours and resolves after several days

harlequin color change Clearly outlined color change as infant lies on side; dependent lower half of body becomes pink and upper half is pale

mongolian spots Irregular areas of deep blue pigmentation, usually in the sacral and gluteal regions; seen predominantly in newborns of African, Asian, or Latin descent

telangiectatic nevi ("stork bites") Flat, deep pink localized areas usually seen in back of neck

From Whaley, L.F., and Wong, D.L.: Nursing care of infants and children, ed. 2, St. Louis, 1983, The C.V. Mosby Co.

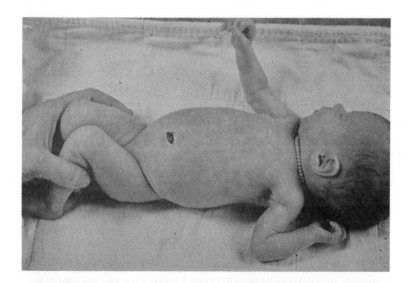

Fig. 4-16
Mottling (cutis marmorata).
Courtesy Mead Johnson & Co., Evansville, IN.

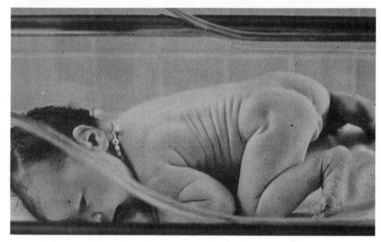

Fig. 4-17
Acrocyanosis of hands and feet in newborn.
Courtesy Mead Johnson & Co., Evansville, IN.

Fig. 4-18
Mongolian spots are
common in babies with
dark skin.

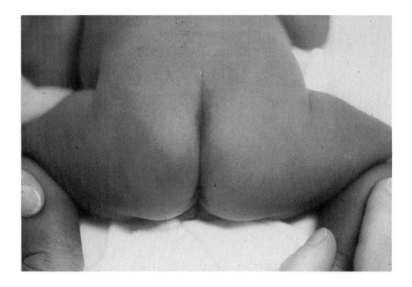

Fig. 4-19
Milia in infant.

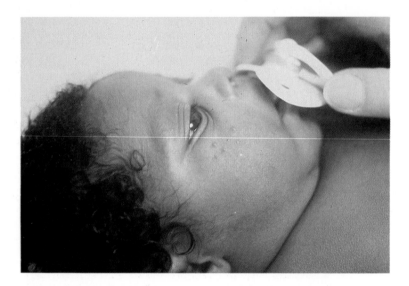

Harlequin dyschronica often occurs in the normal newborn. One half of the body is more red than the other, with a rather sharp demarcation down the midline. The condition is self-resolving and does not last long.

Bluish black to slate gray spots are sometimes seen on the back, buttocks, shoulders, and legs of well babies. These patches, called Mongolian spots, occur most often in babies with dark skin and usually disappear in the preschool years. Mongolian spots are easily mistaken for bruises by the inexperienced examiner (Fig. 4-18).

Milia, small whitish, discrete papules on the face, are commonly found during the first 2 to 3 months of life. The sebaceous glands function in an immature fashion at this age and are easily plugged by sebum (Fig. 4-19).

Sebaceous hyperplasia produces numerous tiny yellow macules and papules in the newborn, probably the result of androgen stimulation from the mother. It frequently occurs on the forehead, cheeks, nose, and chin of the full-term infant. Sebaceous hyperplasia disappears quickly within 1 to 2 months of life.

Fig. 4-20
Testing turgor in infant.

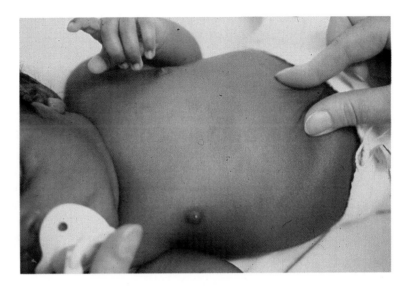

Mothers and fathers sometimes define the excellence of their parenting by the condition of their baby's skin. Diaper rashes are distressing, a false message to the world that parents may not be clean or may not know how to care for the baby. When you notice a skin problem such as diaper rash or impetigo, try to avoid comments or questions that imply that the parent has done something wrong. This, of course, is a guiding principle whenever you are serving children and their parents.

The skin and subcutaneous tissues of an infant and young child, more readily than in the older child and adolescent, can give an important indication of the state of hydration and nutrition. The tissue turgor is best evaluated by gently pinching a fold of the abdominal skin between your index finger and thumb. As with the adult, resiliency will allow it to return to its undisturbed state when released. A child who is seriously dehydrated (more than 3% to 5% of body weight) or very poorly nourished will have skin that retains "tenting" after it is pinched. How quickly the tent disappears provides a clue to the degree of dehydration or malnutrition (Fig. 4-20).

Because the normal range of skin moisture is broad, you need to look at other factors that may suggest a problem. Excessive sweating or dryness alone rarely has pathologic significance in infants or children.

Children with atopic dermatitis or chronic skin changes involving the face will frequently rub their eyes, sufficiently sometimes to cause an extra crease or pleat of skin below the eye. This is known as the Dennie-Morgan fold; it is probably secondary to chronic rubbing and inflammation.

ADOLESCENTS

The examination of the adolescent's skin is the same as that for the adult. The adolescent's skin may have increased oiliness and perspiration, and hair oiliness may also be increased. Increased sebum production predisposes the adolescent to develop acne. Acne is a matter of deep concern to the adolescent. By all means, mention it, and do not hesitate to say quite candidly that you understand how much of a problem it can be. This is a time when you might refer to your own adolescent experience.

As a reflection of maturing apocrine gland function, increased axillary perspiration occurs, and the characteristic adult body odor develops during adolescence.

Hair on the extremities darkens and becomes coarser. Pubic and axillary hair in both males and females develops and assumes adult characteristics. Males develop facial and chest hair that varies in quantity and coarseness. Chapter 3, Growth and Measurement, provides a more thorough discussion of the maturational changes that occur during adolescence.

PREGNANT WOMEN

Striae gravidarum (stretch marks) appear over the abdomen, thighs, and breasts during the second trimester of pregnancy. They fade after delivery but never disappear. Telangiectasias (vascular spiders) may be found on the face, neck, chest, and arms, appearing during the second to fifth month of pregnancy. They usually resolve after delivery. Hemangiomas that were present prior to pregnancy may increase in size, or new ones may develop.

Acne vulgaris may be aggravated during the first trimester of pregnancy but often improves in the third trimester.

OLDER ADULTS

The skin of the older adult may appear more transparent and paler in light skinned individuals. Pigment deposits, increased freckling, and hypopigmented patches may develop, causing the skin to take on a less uniform appearance.

Flaking or scaling, associated with the drier skin that comes with aging, occurs most commonly over the extremities. The skin also becomes thinner—especially over bony prominences, the dorsal surface of hands and feet, forearms, and lower legs—and takes on a parchment-like appearance and texture (Fig. 4-21).

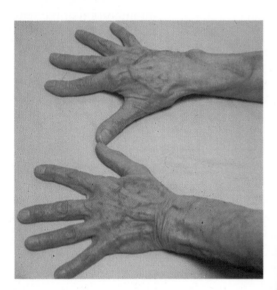

Fig. 4-21
Hands of older adult. Note prominent veins and thin appearance of skin.

Fig. 4-22
Skin hanging loosely, especially around bony prominences.

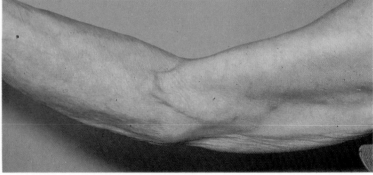

Fig. 4-23
Skin turgor in older adult. Note tenting.

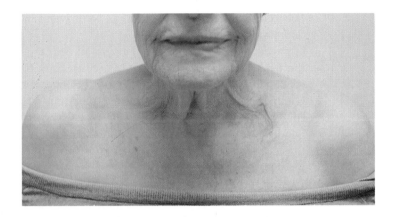

Fig. 4-24
Cherry angioma in older adult.
From Habif, 1985.

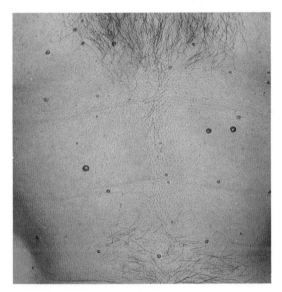

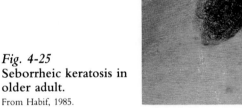

Fig. 4-25
Seborrheic keratosis in older adult.
From Habif, 1985.

The skin often appears to hang loosely on the bony frame as a result of a general loss of elasticity, loss of underlying adipose, and years of gravitational pull (Fig. 4-22). You may observe tenting of the skin when testing for turgor (Fig. 4-23).

Increased wrinkling is evident, especially in areas exposed to sun and in expressive areas of the face. Sagging or drooping is most obvious under the chin, beneath the eyes, in the earlobes, breasts, and scrotum.

Several kinds of lesions may occur on the skin of healthy older adults. The following lesions are considered to be normal findings:

- Cherry angiomas are tiny, bright ruby red, round papules that may become brown with time. They occur in virtually everyone over the age of 30 and increase numerically with age (Fig. 4-24).
- Seborrheic keratoses are pigmented, raised, warty lesions, usually appearing on the face or trunk. These must be distinguished from actinic keratoses, which have malignant potential. Since the lesions may look similar, seek the assistance of an experienced practitioner for differential diagnosis (Fig. 4-25).

- Sebaceous hyperplasia occurs as yellowish flattened papules with central depressions (Fig. 4-26).
- Cutaneous tags (acrochordon) are small, soft tags of skin, usually appearing on the neck and upper chest. They are attached to the body by a narrow stalk (pedunculated) and may or may not be pigmented (Fig. 4-27).
- Cutaneous horns are small, hard projections of the epidermis, usually occurring on the forehead and face (Fig. 4-28).
- Senile lentigines are irregular, round, gray-brown lesions with a rough surface that occur in sun-exposed areas. These are often referred to as "age spots" or incorrectly as "liver spots" (Fig. 4-29).

The hair turns grey or white as melanocytes cease functioning. You will note that the head, body, pubic, and axillary hair thins and becomes sparse and drier. Men may show an increase in coarse aural, nasal, and eyebrow hair; women tend to develop coarse facial hair. Symmetrical balding, usually frontal or occipital, often occurs in men.

The nails thicken, become more brittle, and may be deformed, misshapen, striated, distorted, or peeling. They can take on a yellowish color and may lose their transparency. These changes occur most often in the toenails.

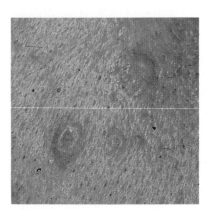

Fig. 4-26
Sebaceous hyperplasia in older adult.
From Habif, 1985.

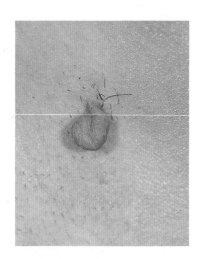

Fig. 4-27
Cutaneous skin tag in older adult.
From Habif, 1985.

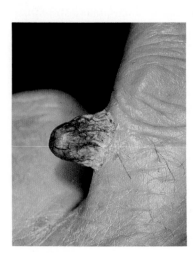

Fig. 4-28
Cutaneous horn.
From Habif, 1985.

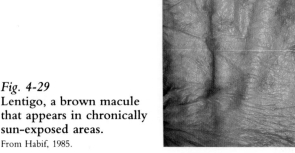

Fig. 4-29
Lentigo, a brown macule that appears in chronically sun-exposed areas.
From Habif, 1985.

Common Abnormalities

Skin

Corn (Clavus)

Corns are flat or slightly elevated, circumscribed, painful lesions with a smooth hard surface. "Soft" corns are caused by the pressure of a bony prominence against softer tissue. They appear as whitish thickenings, commonly between the fourth and fifth toes. "Hard" corns are sharply delineated and have a conical appearance. They occur most often over bony prominences where pressure is exerted, such as from shoes pressing on the interphalangeal joints of the toes (Fig. 4-30).

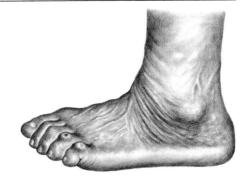

Fig. 4-30
Corn.

Callus

A superficial area of hyperkeratosis is called a callus. Calluses usually occur on the weight-bearing areas of the feet and on the palmar surface of the hands. Calluses are less well demarcated than corns and are usually not tender (Fig. 4-31).

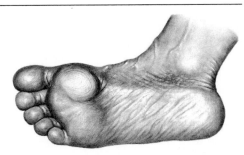

Fig. 4-31
Callus.

Eczematous Dermatitis

The most common inflammatory skin disease is eczematous dermatitis. There are several types, including primary contact dermatitis, allergic contact dermatitis, and atopic dermatitis. The common factor of the various forms is epidermal breakdown, usually as a result of intracellular vesiculation. Eczematous dermatitis has three stages: acute, subacute, and chronic. The acute phase is characterized by erythematous, pruritic, weeping vesicles. Excoriation from scratching predisposes to infection and causes crust formation. Subacute eczema is characterized by erythema and scaling. Itching may or may not be present. In the chronic stage, thick, lichenified, pruritic plaques are present (Fig. 4-32).

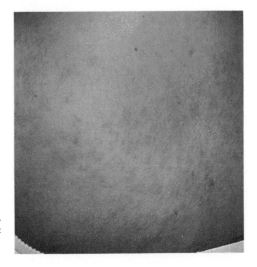

Fig. 4-32
Acute contact dermatitis.

Courtesy Stephen B. Tucker, M.D., Department of Dermatology, University of Texas Health Science Center at Houston; from Thompson et al., 1986.

Furuncle

A furuncle is an acute localized staphylococcal infection. It develops initially as a small perifollicular abscess and spreads to the surrounding dermis and subcutaneous tissue. The initial nodule becomes a pustule surrounded by erythema and edema. The skin is red, hot, and tender. The center of the lesion fills with pus and forms a core that may rupture spontaneously or require surgical incision (Fig. 4-33).

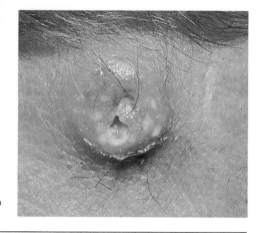

Fig. 4-33
Furuncle.
Courtesy Jaime A. Tschen, M.D., Baylor College of Medicine, Department of Dermatology, Houston; from Thompson et al., 1986.

Folliculitis

Staphylococcal infection of the hair follicle and surrounding dermis produces folliculitis. The primary lesion is a small pustule 1 cm to 2 cm in diameter that is located over a pilosebaceous orifice and may be perforated by a hair. The pustule may be surrounded by inflammation or nodular lesions. After the pustule ruptures, a crust forms (Fig. 4-34).

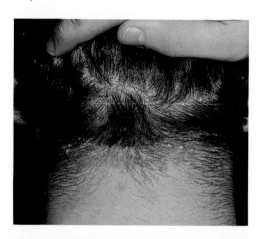

Fig. 4-34
Folliculitis.
From Habif, 1985.

Cellulitis

Diffuse, acute, streptococcal or staphylococcal infection of the skin and subcutaneous tissue is called cellulitis. The skin is red, hot, tender, and indurated. Lymphangitic streaks and regional lymphadenopathy may be present (Fig. 4-35).

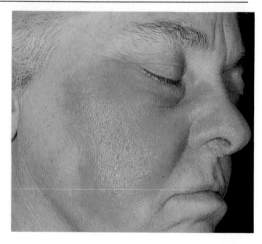

Fig. 4-35
Streptococcal cellulitis—acute phase with intense erythema.
From Habif, 1985.

Tinea (Dermatophytosis)

Tinea is a group of fungal infections that involve the stratum corneum, nails, or hair. The lesions are usually classified according to anatomic location and can occur on nonhairy parts of the body (tinea corporis), on the groin and inner thigh (tinea cruris), scalp (tinea capitis), feet (tinea pedis), and nails (tinea unguium). The lesions vary in appearance and may be papular, pustular, vesicular, erythematous, or scaling. Secondary bacterial infection may be present (Fig. 4-36).

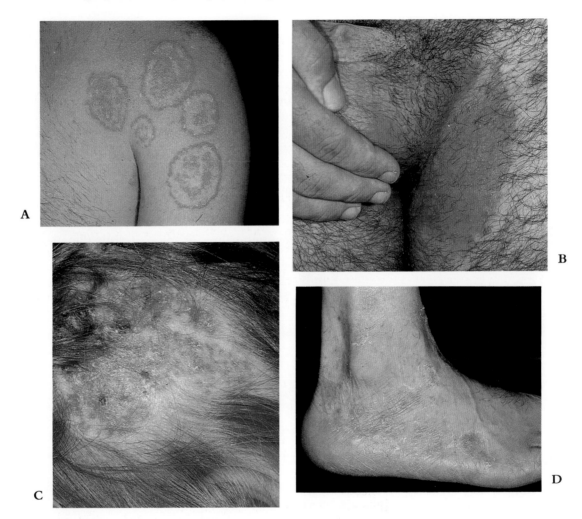

Fig. 4-36
A, Tinea corporis. **B,** Tinea cruris. **C,** Tinea capitis. **D,** Tinea pedis.
From Habif, 1985.

Psoriasis

Psoriasis is a chronic and recurrent disease of keratin synthesis that is characterized by well circumscribed, dry, silvery, scaling papules and plaques. Lesions commonly occur on the back, buttocks, extensor surfaces of the extremities, and the scalp (Fig. 4-37).

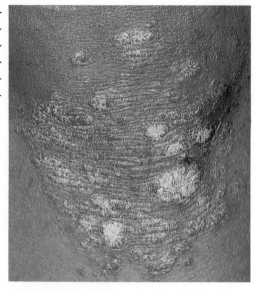

Fig. 4-37
Psoriasis. Note characteristic silvery scaling.
From Habif, 1985.

Drug Eruptions

The most common skin reaction to a drug consists of discrete or confluent erythematous maculopapules on the trunk, face, extremities, palms, or soles of the feet. The rash appears from 1 to several days after starting the drug and fades in 1 to 3 weeks. Pruritus is characteristic (Fig. 4-38).

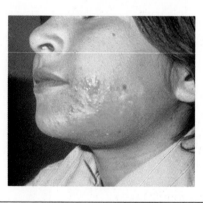

Fig. 4-38
Drug eruption.
From Thompson et al., 1986.

Herpes Zoster (Shingles)

A viral infection, usually of a single dermatome, that consists of red, swollen plaques or vesicles that become filled with purulent fluid. Pain, itching, or burning of the dermatome area usually precedes eruption by 4 to 5 days (Fig. 4-39).

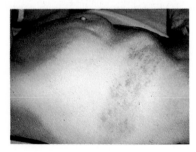

Fig. 4-39
Herpes zoster lesions confined to one dermatome.
Reproduced by kind permission of the Wellcome Foundation, Ltd.

Herpes Simplex

Viral infection by herpes simplex produces tenderness, pain, paresthesia, or mild burning at the infected site prior to onset of the lesions. Grouped vesicles appear on an erythematous base and then erode, forming a crust. Lesions last 2 to 6 weeks. Two different virus types cause the infection. Type 1 is usually associated with oral infection and type 2 with genital infection; however, crossover infections are becoming increasingly common (Fig. 4-40).

A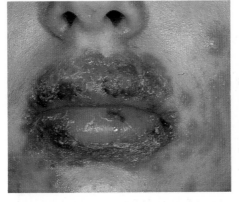

B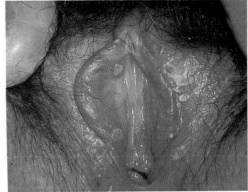

Fig. 4-40
Herpes simplex. A, Oral; **B,** Genital.
From Habif, 1985.

Basal Cell Carcinoma

This most common malignant cutaneous neoplasm is commonly found on the face. Fair skin and solar exposure are risk factors. It occurs in various clinical forms including nodular, pigmented cystic, sclerosing, and superficial (Fig. 4-41).

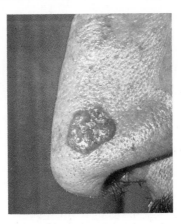

Fig. 4-41
Basal cell carcinoma, the most commonly occurring skin cancer.
Courtesy Gary Monheit, M.D., University of Alabama at Birmingham School of Medicine; from Thompson et al., 1986.

Squamous Cell Carcinoma

This malignant tumor arises in the epithelium. It occurs most commonly in sun-exposed areas, particularly the scalp, back of hands, lower lip, and ear. The lesions are soft, mobile, elevated masses with a surface scale. The base of the lesion may be inflamed (Fig. 4-42).

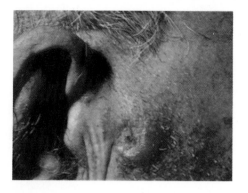

Fig. 4-42
Squamous cell carcinoma.
Courtesy Gary Monheit, M.D., University of Alabama at Birmingham School of Medicine; from Thompson et al., 1986.

Hair

Alopecia Areata

The sudden, rapid, patchy loss of hair, usually from the scalp or face, is called alopecia areata. The hair shaft is poorly formed and breaks off at the skin surface. Regrowth begins in 1 to 3 months. The prognosis for total regrowth is excellent in cases with limited involvement (Fig. 4-43).

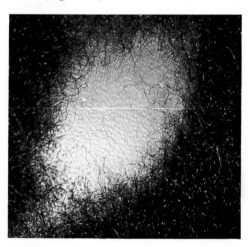

Fig. 4-43
Alopecia areata.
Courtesy Stephen B. Tucker, M.D., Department of Dermatology, University of Texas Health Science Center at Houston; from Thompson et al., 1986.

Scarring Alopecia

This type of alopecia results from skin diseases of the scalp that cause scarring and destruction of hair follicles.

Traction Alopecia

Alopecia can result from prolonged tension of the hair. It can occur from wearing certain hair styles such as braids or using hair rollers and hot combs. The area of loss corresponds directly to the area of stress. The scalp may or may not be inflamed.

Hirsutism

Hirsutism is the growth of terminal hair in women in the male distribution pattern on the face, body, and pubic areas. Hirsutism may or may not be accompanied by other signs of virilization (Fig. 4-44).

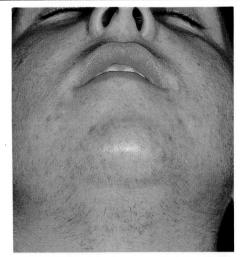

Fig. 4-44
Hirsutism. Coarse facial hair development in adult female.
From Habif, 1985.

Nails: Infections

Paronychia

Inflammation of the paronychium produces redness, swelling, and tenderness at the lateral and proximal nail folds. Purulent drainage often accumulates under the cuticle. It can occur as an acute or chronic process. Chronic paronychia can produce rippling of the nails (Fig. 4-45).

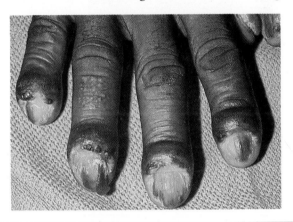

Fig. 4-45
Chronic paronychia with nail dystrophy.
Courtesy Jaime A. Tschen, M.D., Baylor College of Medicine, Department of Dermatology, Houston; from Thompson et al., 1986.

Tinea Unguium

Fungal infection of the nail occurs in four distinct patterns. In the most common form the distal nail plate turns yellow or white as hyperkeratotic debris accumulates, causing the nail to separate from the nail bed (onycholysis). The fungus grows in the nail plate causing it to crumble (Fig. 4-46).

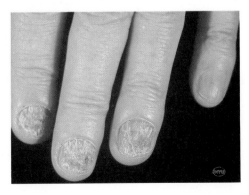

Fig. 4-46
Tinea unguium.
Courtesy American Academy of Dermatology and Institute for Dermatologic Communication and Education, Evanston, IL.

Nails: Injury

Ingrown Nails

Ingrown nails most commonly involve the large toe. The nail pierces the lateral nail fold and grows into the dermis, causing pain and swelling (Fig. 4-47).

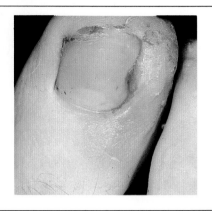

Fig. 4-47
Ingrown toenail. Swelling and inflammation occur at lateral nail fold.
From Habif, 1985.

Subungual Hematoma

Trauma to the nail plate severe enough to cause immediate bleeding and pain produces a subungual hematoma. The amount of bleeding may be sufficient to cause separation and loss of the nail plate. Trauma to the proximal nail fold may also cause bleeding that is not apparent for several days. In either case, the hematoma remains until the nail grows out (Fig. 4-48).

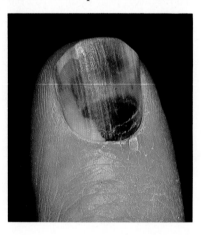

Fig. 4-48
Subungual hematoma.
From Habif, 1985.

Leukonychia Punctata

These white spots appear in the nail plate as a result of minor injury or manipulation of the cuticle. They either spontaneously resolve or grow out (Fig. 4-49).

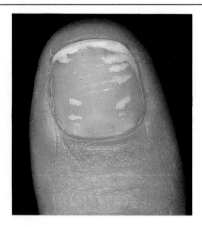

Fig. 4-49
White spots on nail from injury (leukonychia punctata).
From Habif, 1985.

Habit-Tic-Deformity

This abnormality is caused by biting or picking the proximal nail fold of the thumb with the index fingernail. This results in horizontal sharp grooving in a band that extends to the tip of the nail (Fig. 4-50).

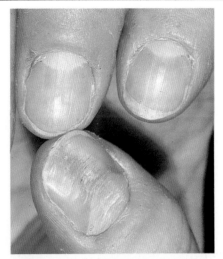

Fig. 4-50
Habit-tic deformity.
From Habif, 1985.

Onycholysis

Onycholysis is loosening of the nail plate with separation from the nail bed that begins at the distal groove (Fig. 4-51).

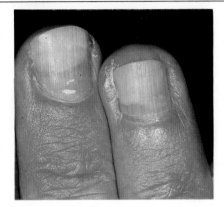

Fig. 4-51
Onycholysis. Separation of nail plate starts at distal groove.
From Habif, 1985.

Curvature

Inward folding of the lateral edges of the nail causes the nail bed to draw up and often become painful. Curvature is most common in the toenails and is thought to be caused by shoe compression (see p. 115).

Nails: Changes Associated with Systemic Disease

Koilonychia
(Spoon Nails)

Central depression of the nail with lateral elevation of the nail plate produces a concave curvature and spoon appearance. This is associated with iron deficiency anemia, syphilis, fungal dermatoses, and hypothyroidism (see p. 115).

Beau's Lines

Transverse depressions in all of the nails appear at the base of the lunula weeks after a stress that temporarily interrupts nail formation. Beau's lines are associated with coronary occlusion, hypercalcemia, and skin disease. The grooves disappear when the nails grow out (Fig. 4-52).

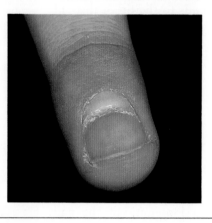

Fig. 4-52
Beau's lines following systemic disease.
From Habif, 1985.

White Banding (Terry's Nails)

Transverse white bands cover the nail except for a narrow zone at the distal tip. The changes are associated with cirrhosis and hypoalbuminemia (Fig. 4-53).

Fig. 4-53
Terry's nails: transverse white bands.
From Habif, 1985.

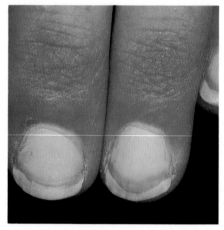

Psoriasis

Psoriasis can produce pitting, onycholysis, discoloration, and subungual thickening. Yellow scaly debris often accumulates, elevating the nail plate. Severe psoriasis of the matrix and nail bed results in grossly malformed nails and splinter hemorrhages (Fig. 4-54).

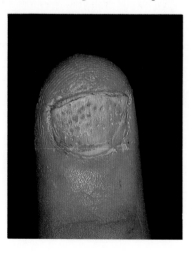

Fig. 4-54
Nail pitting from psoriasis.
From Habif, 1985.

Nails: Periungual Growths

Warts

Warts are epidermal neoplasms caused by viral infection. They can occur at the nail folds and extend under the nail. A longitudinal nail groove may occur from warts located over the nail matrix.

Digital Mucous Cysts

These cysts contain a clear jelly-like substance and occur on the dorsal surface of the distal phalanx. A longitudinal nail groove may occur from cysts located at the proximal nail fold.

CHILDREN

Cafe au Lait Patches

These coffee-colored patches may be either harmless or indicative of underlying disease. The presence of more than five patches with diameters of more than 1 cm in children under age 5 suggests neurofibromatosis (von Recklinghausen's disease). Any cafe au lait patches should be considered suspicious by a beginning practitioner. (Fig. 4-55).

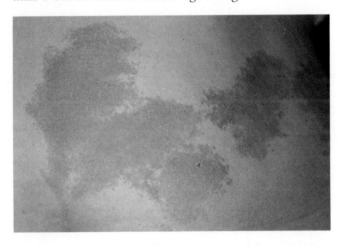

Fig. 4-55
Cafe au lait patches.

Seborrheic Dermatitis

This chronic, recurrent, erythematous scaling eruption is localized in areas where sebaceous glands are concentrated, such as scalp, back, intertriginous, and diaper areas. The scalp lesions are scaling, adherent, thick, yellow, and crusted ("cradle cap") and can spread over the ear and down the nape of the neck. Lesions elsewhere are erythematous, scaling, and fissured (Fig. 4-56).

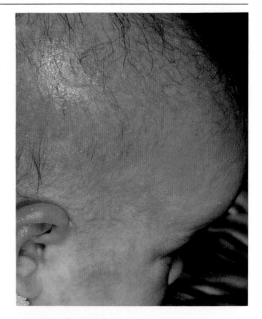

Fig. 4-56
Seborrheic dermatitis.
From Habif, 1985.

Miliaria
("Prickly Heat")

Miliaria is an irregular, red, macular rash caused by occlusion of sweat ducts during periods of heat and high humidity. Overdressed babies are prone to this in the summertime (Fig. 4-57).

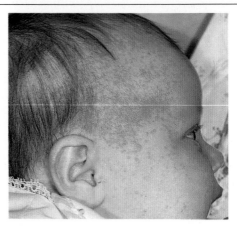

Fig. 4-57
Miliaria in infant.
From Habif, 1985.

Impetigo

This highly contagious staphylococcal and streptococcal infection of the epidermis commonly causes pruritus, burning, and regional lymphadenopathy. The initial lesion is a small erythematous macule that changes into a vesicle or bulla with a thin roof. Crusts with a characteristic honey color form from the exudate as the vesicles or bullae rupture (Fig. 4-58).

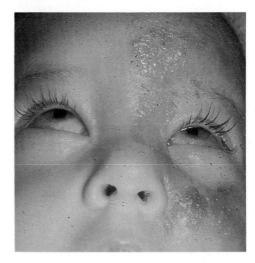

Fig. 4-58
Impetigo. Note characteristic crusting.
Courtesy Antoinette Hood, M.D., Department of Dermatology, School of Medicine, The Johns Hopkins University, Baltimore, MD.

Acne Vulgaris

The inflamed lesions of acne involve stagnation of sebum, and comedon formation in the pilosebaceous follicle, with bacterial invasion. Acne is seen most commonly in adolescents, though it may occur initially or continue into the adult years (Fig. 4-59).

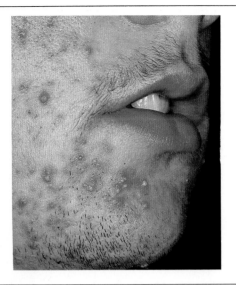

Fig. 4-59
Acne in adolescent.
From Habif, 1985.

Reddened Patchiness

Irregular reddened areas can occur on the nape of the neck, upper eyelids, forehead, and upper lip that suggest a richer capillary bed. These lesions include capillary hemangioma, nevus flammeus, nevus vasculosus, and telangiectatic nevus. They invariably disappear by about 1 year of age, although they may occasionally recur, even in adults (Fig. 4-60).

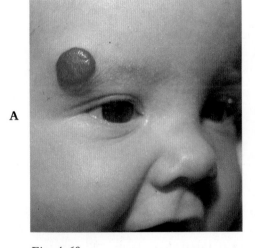

A

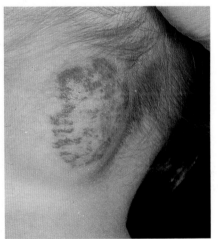

B

Fig. 4-60
A, Strawberry hemangioma in infant. **B,** Cavernous hemangioma in infant.
From Habif, 1985.

Exanthems

Viral or bacterial infections with cutaneous manifestations are common in children. These include "childhood diseases" such as rubella, rubeola, varicella, roseola, scarlet fever, and erythema infectiosum. These exanthems are usually preceded by a prodromal period of systemic symptoms (Fig. 4-61).

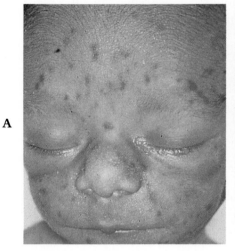
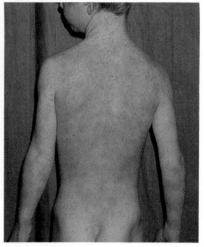

Fig. 4-61
A, Congenital rubella. B, Rubeola.
Courtesy Donald C. Anderson, M.D., Baylor College of Medicine, Houston; from Thompson et al., 1986.

Trichotillomania

Loss of scalp hair can be caused by physical manipulation. Hair is twisted around the finger and pulled or rubbed until it breaks off. The act of manipulation is usually an unconscious habit. The affected area has an irregular border, and hair density is greatly reduced, but the site is not bald (Fig. 4-62).

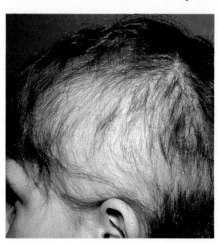

Fig. 4-62
Trichotillomania in young child.
From Habif, 1985.

OLDER ADULTS

Stasis Dermatitis

The lower legs and ankles are affected with erythematous, scaling, weeping patches. Stasis dermatitis is secondary to edema of chronic peripheral vascular disease (Fig. 4-63).

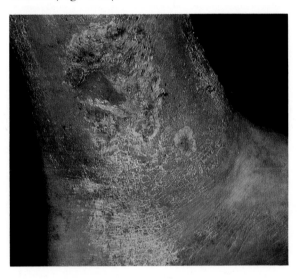

Fig. 4-63
Stasis dermatitis in older adult with impaired peripheral circulation.
From Habif, 1985.

Solar Keratosis (Senile Actinic Keratosis)

This disorder produces a slightly raised erythematous lesion that is usually less than 1 cm in diameter with an irregular, rough surface. The lesion is most common on the dorsal surface of the hands, arms, neck, and face. Solar keratosis occurs secondary to chronic sun damage and has malignant potential (Fig. 4-64).

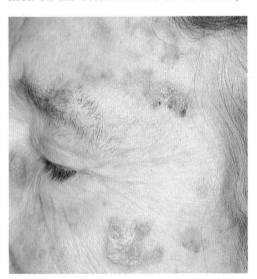

Fig. 4-64
Actinic keratosis in older adult in area of sun exposure.
From Habif, 1985.

Head and Neck

Together the head and neck provide the bony housing and protective cover for the brain, including the special senses of vision, hearing, smell, and taste. Before examining the special senses and the neurologic system, it is important to carefully evaluate the overlying structures.

Anatomy and Physiology

The skull is composed of 7 bones (2 frontal, 2 parietal, 2 temporal, and 1 occipital) that are fused together and covered by the scalp. Bones of the skull are used to identify the location of findings referable to the head (Fig. 5-1). The facial skull has several cavities for the eyes, nose, and mouth. The bony structure of the face is formed from the fused frontal, nasal, zygomatic, ethmoid, lacrimal, sphenoid, and maxillary bones and the movable mandible.

Major landmarks of the face are the palpebral fissures and the nasolabial folds (Fig. 5-2). Facial muscles are innervated by cranial nerves V and VII. The temporal artery is the major accessible artery of the face, passing just anterior to the ear, over the temporal muscle, and onto the forehead.

The structure of the neck is formed by the cervical vertebrae, ligaments, and the sternocleidomastoid and trapezius muscles, which give it support and movement (Fig. 5-3). Mobility is greatest at the level of C4-5 or C5-6. The sternocleidomastoid muscle extends from the upper sternum and anterior third of the clavicle to the mastoid process. The trapezius muscle extends from the scapula and vertebrae to the occipital prominence.

The relationship of these muscles to each other and to adjacent bones creates triangles used as anatomic landmarks. The posterior triangle is formed by the trapezius and sternocleidomastoid muscles and the clavicle (Fig. 5-4). The posterior cervical lymph nodes lie in this triangle.

The anterior triangle is formed by the medial borders of the sternocleidomastoid muscles and the mandible. The hyoid bone, cricoid cartilage, trachea, thyroid, and anterior cervical lymph nodes lie inside this triangle. The carotid artery and internal jugular vein lie deep and run parallel to the sternocleidomastoid muscle along its anterior aspect. The external jugular vein crosses the surface of the sternocleidomastoid diagonally. The hyoid bone lies just below the mandible. The thyroid cartilage is shaped like a shield, its notch on the upper edge marking the level of bifurcation of the common carotid artery. The cricoid cartilage is the uppermost ring of the tracheal cartilages.

Fig. 5-1
Bones of the skull.

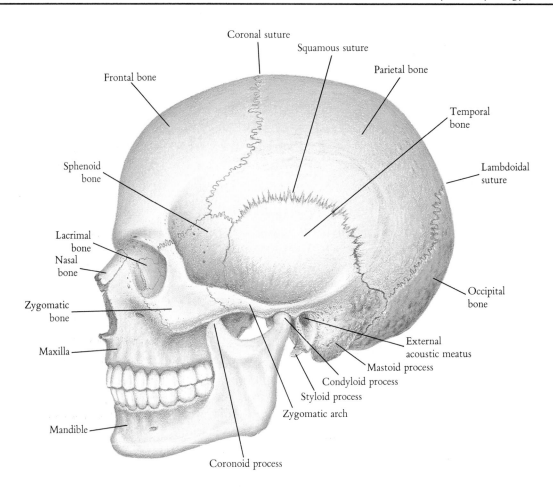

Fig. 5-2
Landmarks of the face.

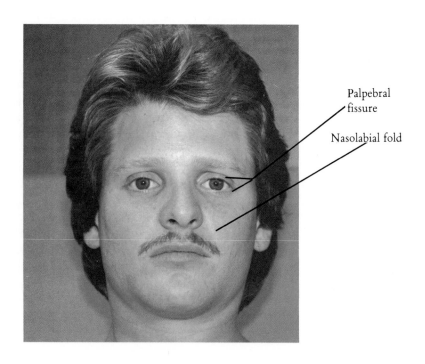

Fig. 5-3
**Underlying structures of
the neck. A, Anterior view.
B, Lateral view.**

A

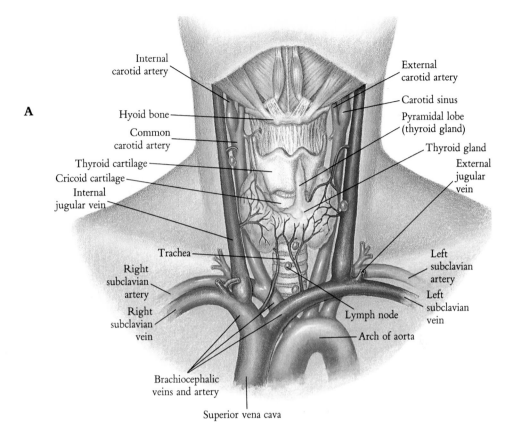

Internal
carotid artery

External
carotid artery

Carotid sinus

Hyoid bone

Common
carotid artery

Pyramidal lobe
(thyroid gland)

Thyroid gland

Thyroid cartilage

External
jugular
vein

Cricoid cartilage

Internal
jugular vein

Trachea

Right
subclavian
artery

Left
subclavian
artery

Left
subclavian
vein

Right
subclavian
vein

Lymph node

Brachiocephalic
veins and artery

Arch of aorta

Superior vena cava

B

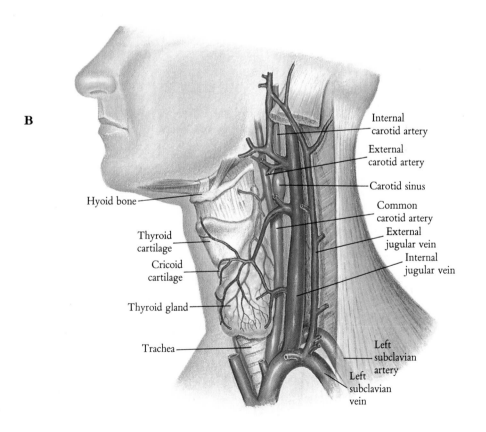

Internal
carotid artery

External
carotid artery

Carotid sinus

Hyoid bone

Common
carotid artery

Thyroid
cartilage

External
jugular vein

Internal
jugular vein

Cricoid
cartilage

Thyroid gland

Trachea

Left
subclavian
artery

Left
subclavian
vein

Fig. 5-4
Anterior and posterior triangles of the neck.

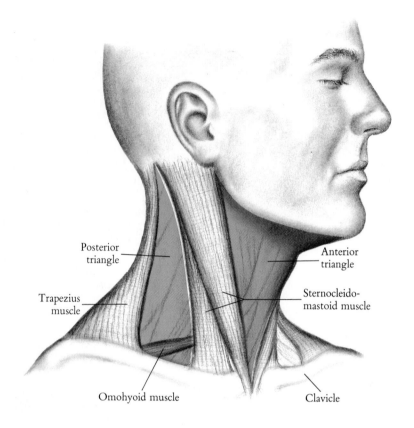

Posterior triangle

Anterior triangle

Trapezius muscle

Sternocleido-mastoid muscle

Omohyoid muscle

Clavicle

The thyroid is the largest endocrine gland in the body, producing two hormones, thyroxine (T_4) and triiodothyronine (T_3). Its two lateral lobes are butterfly shaped and joined by an isthmus at their lower aspect. This isthmus lies across the trachea below the cricoid cartilage. A pyramidal lobe, extending upward from the isthmus slightly to the left of midline, is present in about one third of the population. The lobes curve posteriorly around the cartilages and are in large part covered by the sternocleidomastoid muscles.

INFANTS

The seven cranial bones are soft and separated by the sagittal, coronal, and lambdoidal sutures (Fig. 5-5). The anterior and posterior fontanels are the membranous spaces formed where four cranial bones meet and intersect. Spaces between the cranial bones permit the expansion of the skull to accommodate brain growth. Ossification of the sutures begins after completion of brain growth, at about 6 years of age, and is finished by adulthood. The fontanels ossify earlier, with the posterior fontanel closing by 2 months of age and the anterior fontanel closing by 24 months of age.

The process of birth through the vaginal canal often causes molding of the newborn skull, during which the cranial bones overlap or move to new positions. Within days the newborn skull resumes its appropriate shape and size.

Fig. 5-5
**Fontanels and sutures on
the infant's skull.**

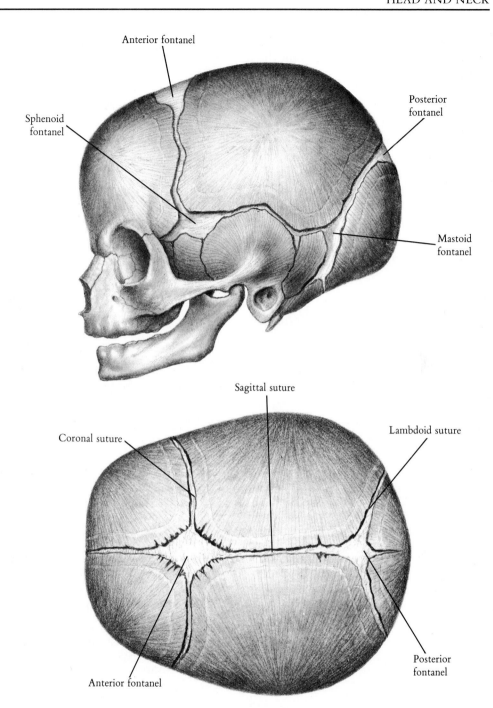

Anterior fontanel

Sphenoid
fontanel

Posterior
fontanel

Mastoid
fontanel

Sagittal suture

Coronal suture

Lambdoid suture

Posterior
fontanel

Anterior fontanel

ADOLESCENTS Subtle changes in facial appearance occur throughout childhood. In the male adolescent the nose and thyroid cartilage enlarge, and facial hair develops, emerging first on the upper lip, then the cheeks, lower lip, and chin.

OLDER ADULTS With aging the rate of T_4 production and degradation gradually decreases, and the thyroid gland becomes more fibrotic.

Review of Related History

General Considerations

1. Employment: risk of head injury, use of helmet, exposure to toxins or chemicals
2. Stress, tension, demands at home, work, or school
3. Potential risk of injury: participation in sports, handrails available, use of seat belts, unsafe environment
4. Nutrition: recent weight gain or loss, food intolerances, eating habits (skip meals)
5. Use of alcohol
6. Medications: anticonvulsants, antiarrhythmics, thyroid, oral contraceptives, cafergot, propranolol, aspirin, or other pain preparations

Present Problem

1. Head injury
   a. Independent observer's description of event
   b. State of consciousness after injury: immediately and 5 minutes later; duration of unconsciousness; combative, confused, alert, or dazed
   c. Predisposing factors: seizure disorder, poor vision, light-headedness, blackouts
   d. Associated symptoms: head or neck pain, laceration, hematoma, local tenderness, change in breathing pattern, blurred or double vision, discharge from nose or ears, nausea or vomiting, urinary or fecal incontinence
2. Headache
   a. Onset: early morning, during night, during day; gradual versus abrupt
   b. Duration: minutes, hours, days, weeks; relieved by medication, sleep, resolves spontaneously; occurs in clusters, headache-free periods
   c. Location: entire head, unilateral, specific site (neck, sinus region, behind eyes, hatband distribution)
   d. Character: throbbing, pounding, boring, shock-like, dull, nagging, constant pressure
      1. Severity: same or different with each event
      2. Visual prodromal event: scotoma, hemianopia, distortion of size, shape, or location
      3. Pain aggravated with movement
   e. Pattern: worse in AM or PM, worse or better as day progresses, occurs only during sleep
      1. Episodes closer together or worsening, lasting longer
      2. Change in level of consciousness as pain increases

   f. Associated symptoms: nausea, vomiting, diarrhea, photophobia, visual disturbance, difficulty falling asleep, increased lacrimation, nasal discharge, tinnitus, paresthesias, mobility impairment

   g. Precipitating factors: fever, fatigue, stress, food additives, prolonged fasting, alcohol, seasonal allergies, menstrual cycle, intercourse, oral contraceptives

   h. Efforts to treat: sleep, pain medication

  3. Stiff neck

   a. Neck injury or strain, head injury, swelling of neck

   b. Fever, bacterial or viral illness

   c. Character: limitation of movement; pain with movement, pain relieved by movement; continuous or cramping pain; radiation patterns to arms, shoulders, hands, or down the back

   d. Predisposing factors: unilateral vision or hearing loss

   e. Efforts to treat: heat, pain medication

  4. Thyroid problem

   a. Change in temperature preference: more or less clothing, different from patient's family

   b. Swelling in the neck; interference with swallowing; redness; pain with touch, swallowing, or hyperextension of the neck

   c. Change in texture of hair, skin, or nails; increased pigmentation of skin at pressure points

   d. Change in emotional stability: increased energy, irritability, nervousness, lethargy, complaisance, disinterest

   e. Increased prominence of eyes, puffiness in periorbital area, blurred or double vision

   f. Change in menstrual flow, bowel habits

Past Medical History

1. Head trauma, subdural hematoma, recent lumbar puncture
2. Radon or radium treatment around head and neck
3. Headaches: migraine, vascular
4. Surgery for tumor
5. Seizure disorder
6. Thyroid dysfunction, surgery

Family History

1. Headaches: type, character, similarity to patient's
2. Thyroid dysfunction

INFANTS

1. Prenatal history: mother's use of drugs or alcohol, treated for hyperthyroidism
2. Birth history: vaginal or cesarean section delivery; presentation, difficulty of delivery, use of forceps (associated with caput succedaneum, cephalhematoma, Bell's palsy, molding)
3. Unusual head shape: bulging or flattening (congenital anomaly or positioning in utero), preterm infant, head held at angle, preferred position at rest
4. Quality of head control

5. Acute illness: diarrhea, vomiting, fever, stiff neck, irritability (associated with meningitis)
6. Congenital anomalies: meningomyelocele, encephalocele, microcephaly, or hydrocephaly
7. Neonatal screening for congenital hypothyroidism

OLDER ADULTS

1. Dizziness with head or neck movement
2. Weakness or impaired balance increasing risk of falling and head injury

Examination and Findings

EQUIPMENT

- **Tape measure**
- **Stethoscope**
- **Cup of water**
- **Transilluminator (electronic or flashlight attachment, for infants)**

Head and Face

Begin examining the head and neck with inspection of head position and facial features, making observations throughout the history and physical examination. The patient's head should be held upright and still. A horizontal jerking or bobbing motion is associated with a tremor, while a nodding movement is associated with aortic insufficiency, especially if nodding is synchronized with the pulse. Holding the head tilted to one side to favor a good eye or ear occurs with unilateral hearing or vision loss, but it is also associated with shortening of the sternocleidomastoid muscle.

Facial features (eyelids, eyebrows, palpebral fissures, nasolabial folds, and mouth) should be inspected for shape and symmetry with rest, movement, and expression. The integrity of cranial nerves V and VII has been partially tested, as detailed in Chapter 17 (Neurologic System and Mental Status). Facial characteristics will vary according to race, sex, and body build. Some slight asymmetry is common.

When facial asymmetry is present, note whether all features on one side of the face are affected or only a portion of the face, such as the forehead, lower face, or mouth. Suspect facial nerve paralysis when the entire side of the face is affected and facial nerve weakness when the lower face is affected. If only the mouth is involved, suspect a problem with the peripheral trigeminal nerve.

Tics, spasmodic muscular contractions of the face, head, or neck, should be noted. They may be associated with pressure on or degenerative changes of the facial nerves, or they may be psychogenic.

Note any change in the shape of the face or unusual features, such as edema, puffiness, coarsened features, prominent eyes, hirsutism, lack of expression, excessive perspiration, pallor, or pigmentation variations. Certain disorders will cause characteristic changes in facial appearance (Table 5-1).

Text continued on p. 153.

Table 5-1
Descriptions of Facies and
Their Associated Disorders

Facies	Associated Disorders
A rounded or "moon" shaped face with thin erythematous skin, hirsutism	Cushing's syndrome, hypercortisolism

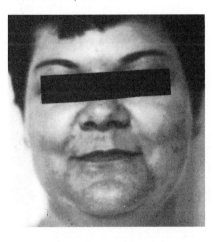

Cushing's syndrome.
Reprinted by permission of Elsevier Science Publishing Co., Inc., from Mazzaferri, E.L.: Endocrinology case studies, ed. 2, Flushing, N.Y., 1975, Medical Examination Publishing Co., Inc.

Sunken appearance of the eyes, cheeks, and temporal areas; sharp nose; dry rough skin	Cachectic facies, wasting diseases

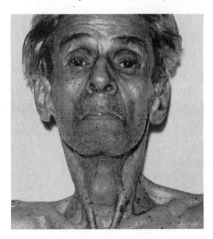

Cachexia.
From Prior et al., 1981.

Dull, puffy, yellowed skin; coarse, sparse hair; temporal loss of eyebrows; periorbital edema	Myxedema, hypothyroidism

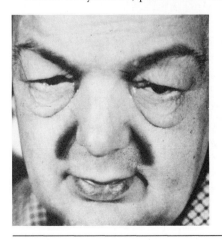

Myxedema.
From Prior et al., 1981.

Continued.

Table 5-1—cont'd
Descriptions of Facies and
Their Associated Disorders

Facies	Associated Disorders
Fine moist skin with fine hair; prominent eyes and lid retraction, staring or startled expression	Hyperthyroidism, Graves disease

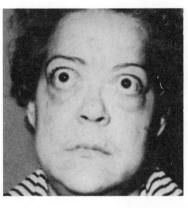

Graves' disease.
From Prior et al., 1981.

Butterfly-shaped rash over malar surfaces and bridge of nose, either a blush with swelling or scaly, red, maculopapular lesions	Systemic lupus erythematosus

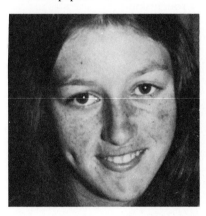

Typical "butterfly" rash of systemic lupus erythematosus.
Courtesy Dr. A. S. Hanissian. From Hughes, 1984.

Drooping eyelids, sagging of facial skin, accentuation of the nasolabial folds, appearance of premature aging	Cutis laxa syndrome

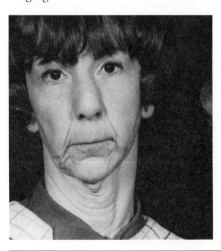

Cutis laxa.
From Goodman and Gorlin, 1977.

Table 5-1—cont'd
Descriptions of Facies and
Their Associated Disorders

Facies	Associated Disorders
Asymmetry of one side of the face, eyelid does not close completely, lower eyelid and corner of mouth droop, loss of nasolabial fold	Bell's palsy, paralysis of facial nerve

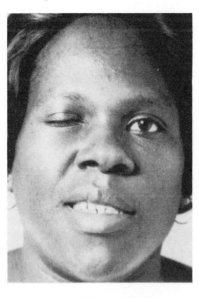

Unilateral facial palsy.
From Dyken and Miller, 1980.

Coarsening of skin and enlargement of bones of face	Acromegaly

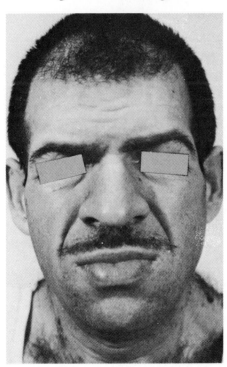

Acromegaly.
From Dyken and Miller, 1980.

Continued.

Table 5-1—cont'd
Descriptions of Facies and
Their Associated Disorders

Facies	Associated Disorders
Multiple osteomas of the facial bones, epidermoid cysts	Gardner's syndrome, osteomatosis–intestinal polyposis syndrome

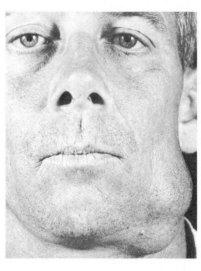

Gardner's syndrome.
From Goodman and Gorlin, 1977.

Coarsening of facial features, thickening and furrowing of face and scalp	Pachydermoperiostosis

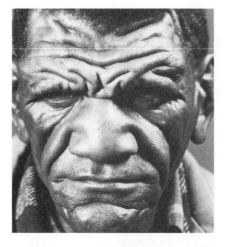

Pachydermoperiostosis.
From Goodman and Gorlin, 1977.

Depressed nasal bridge, epicanthal folds, mongoloid slant of eyes, low set ears, large tongue	Down syndrome

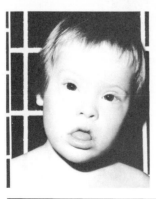

Down syndrome.
From Hughes, 1984.

Table 5-1—cont'd
Descriptions of Facies and
Their Associated Disorders

Facies	Associated Disorders
Pallid, edematous face, especially around the eyes	Nephrotic syndrome

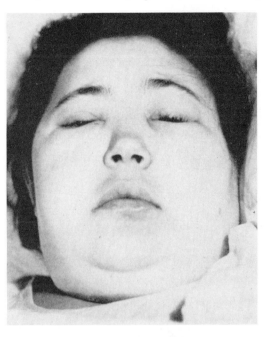

Nephrotic syndrome.
From Kampmeier and Blake, 1970.

Mandibular prognathism, drooping lower lip and short upper lip, parrot beak nose, proptotic eyes	Craniofacial dysostosis

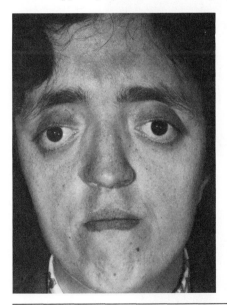

Craniofacial dysostosis.
From Goodman and Gorlin, 1977.

Table 5-1—cont'd
Descriptions of Facies and
Their Associated Disorders

Facies	Associated Disorders
Enlarged skull with low forehead, corneal clouding, short neck	Hurler's syndrome

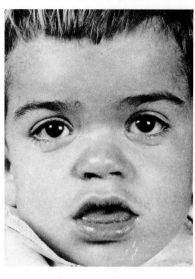

Hurler's syndrome.
From Goodman and Gorlin, 1977.

Enlarged head, bulging fontanel, dilated scalp veins, bossing of the skull, sclerae visible above the iris	Hydrocephalus

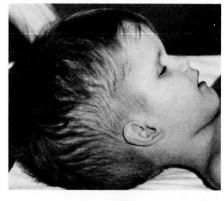

Hydrocephalus.
From Goodman and Gorlin, 1977.

Small palpebral fissures, epicanthal folds, hypoplastic philtrum, thinned upper lip, retrognathia	Fetal alcohol anomaly

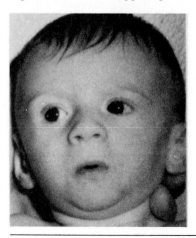

Fetal alcohol anomaly.
Courtesy Dr. Charles Linder, Medical College of Georgia. From Goodman and Gorlin, 1977.

Fig. 5-6
Auscultation for a temporal bruit.

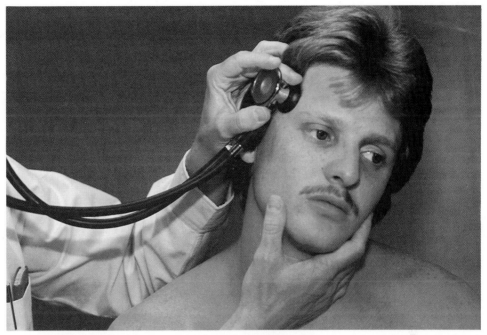

Inspect the skull for size, shape, and symmetry. Examine the scalp by parting the hair in various places, noting any lesions, scabs, tenderness, parasites, nits, or scaliness. Pay special attention to the areas behind the ears, at the hairline, and at the crown of the head. Note any hair loss pattern. In men it is common to see bitemporal recession of hair or balding over the crown of the head.

The skull is palpated in a gentle rotary movement progressing systematically from front to back. The skull should be symmetrical and smooth. The bones should be indistinguishable, because the sites of fusion are not generally palpable after 6 months of age. However, the ridge of the sagittal suture may be felt on some individuals. The scalp should move freely over the skull, and no tenderness, swelling, or depressions on palpation are expected. An indentation or depression of the skull may indicate a skull fracture.

Palpate the patient's hair, noting its texture, color, and distribution. Hair should be smooth, symmetrically distributed, and have no splitting or cracked ends. Coarse, dry, and brittle hair is associated with hypothyroidism. Fine, silky hair is associated with hyperthyroidism.

Palpate the temporal arteries and note their course. Any thickening, hardness, or tenderness over the arteries may be associated with temporal arteritis. If you have any reason to suspect a vascular anomaly of the brain, listen for bruits over the skull and eyes. Place the bell of the stethoscope over the temporal region, the eyes, and below the occiput (Fig. 5-6). A bruit or blowing sound over any of these areas indicates a vascular anomaly.

Neck

Inspect the neck in the usual anatomic position, in slight hyperextension, and as the patient swallows. Look for bilateral symmetry of the sternocleidomastoid and trapezius muscles, alignment of the trachea, the landmarks of the anterior and posterior triangles, and any subtle fullness at the base of the neck. Note any apparent masses, webbing, excess skin folds, unusual shortness, or asymmetry. Observe for any distention of the jugular vein or prominence of the carotid arteries. Carotid artery and jugular vein examination is described in Chapter 9 (Heart and Blood Vessels).

Fig. 5-7
Position of the thumbs to evaluate the midline position of the trachea.

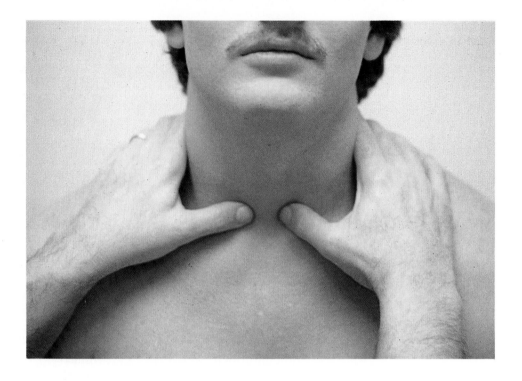

Webbing, excessive posterior cervical skin, and an unusually short neck are associated with chromosomal anomalies. The transverse portion of the omohyoid muscle in the posterior triangle can sometimes be mistaken for a mass. Marked edema of the neck is associated with local infections. A mass filling the base of the neck or visible thyroid tissue that glides upward when the patient swallows may indicate an enlarged thyroid.

Evaluate range of motion by asking the patient to flex, extend, rotate, and laterally bend the head and neck (see Chapter 16, Musculoskeletal System, for details). Movement should be smooth and painless and should not cause dizziness.

The ability to palpate and identify structures in the neck will vary with the patient's habitus. It will be more difficult to examine a short, thick, muscular neck than a long slender one.

Palpate the trachea for midline position. Place a thumb along each side of the trachea in the lower portion of the neck (Fig. 5-7). Compare the space between the trachea and the sternocleidomastoid muscle on each side. An unequal space indicates displacement of the trachea from the midline and is associated with a mass or pathologic condition in the chest.

Identify the hyoid bone and the thyroid and cricoid cartilages. They should be smooth, nontender, and move under your finger when the patient swallows. On palpation, the cartilaginous rings of the trachea in the lower portion of the neck should be distinct and nontender.

With the patient's neck extended, position the index finger and thumb of one hand on each side of the trachea below the thyroid isthmus (Fig. 5-8). A downward tugging sensation, synchronous with the pulse, is evidence of tracheal tugging, suggesting the presence of an aortic aneurysm. Palpation of the lymph nodes is described in Chapter 15, Lymphatic System.

Fig. 5-8
Position of the thumb and finger to detect tracheal tugging.

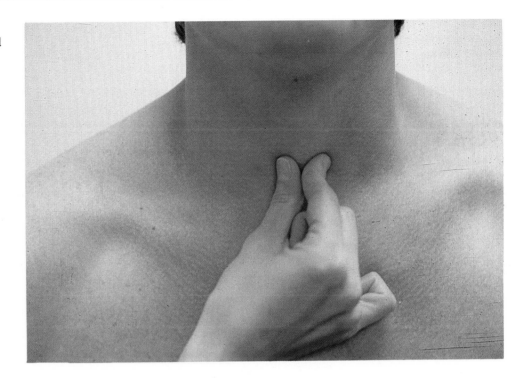

Thyroid Gland

Examination of the thyroid gland mandates a gentle touch. Nodules and asymmetric position will be more difficult to detect if you press too hard. Allow your fingers to almost drift over the gland. Palpate the thyroid for size, shape, configuration, consistency, tenderness, and the presence of any nodules. Use one of two approaches, standing either facing or behind the patient, to palpate the isthmus, main body, and lateral lobes of the thyroid gland. Choose one approach to use consistently.

For both approaches the patient should be positioned to relax the sternocleidomastoid, with the neck flexed slightly forward and laterally toward the side being examined. To facilitate swallowing, give the patient a cup of water. Ask the patient to hold a sip of water in his or her mouth until you have your hands positioned, then instruct the patient to swallow.

To palpate the thyroid using the frontal approach, have the patient sit on the examining table. Using the pads of the first two fingers, palpate the left lobe with your right hand and the right lobe with your left hand. To increase your access to the lobe, gently move the skin medially over the sternocleidomastoid muscle and reach under its anterior borders with your fingers just beneath the cricoid cartilage. Ask the patient to swallow while you palpate the movement of the thyroid isthmus. Slightly displace the trachea to the left to palpate the main body of the right thyroid lobe (Fig. 5-9). The thyroid should move beneath your fingers when the patient swallows. Place your left thumb on the lower left portion of the cricoid cartilage, clasping the right side of the patient's neck, and hook your fingers behind the patient's right sternocleidomastoid. (Make sure your fingernails are well trimmed.) Again ask the patient to swallow. Attempt to palpate the right thyroid lobe between your thumb and fingers, noting its lateral borders. By palpating above the

Fig. 5-9
Palpation of the right
thyroid lobe and lateral
border, facing the patient.

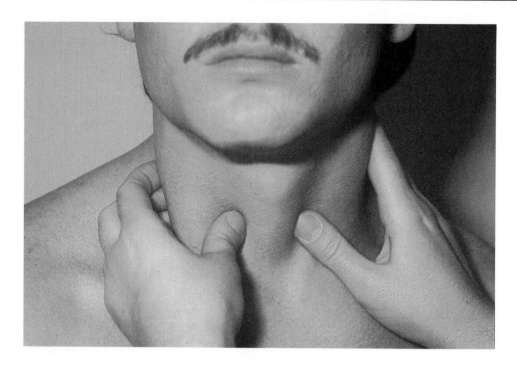

cricoid cartilage, you may be able to feel the pyramidal lobe of the thyroid, if one is present. To examine the left lobe, move your hands to the reverse corresponding positions.

For examining the thyroid from behind, seat the patient on a chair with the neck at a comfortable level. Using both hands, position two fingers of each hand on the sides of the trachea just beneath the cricoid cartilage. Ask the patient to swallow, feeling for movement of the isthmus. Then displace the trachea to the right, ask the patient to swallow, and palpate the main body of the right lobe. To palpate the right lateral border, move the fingers of your left hand between the trachea and the right sternocleidomastoid, placing the fingers of your right hand behind the right sternocleidomastoid. Press your hands together and palpate the right lobe as the patient swallows (Fig. 5-10). Repeat the maneuver for the left lobe with your hands in the reverse corresponding positions.

The thyroid lobes, if felt, should be small, smooth, and free of nodules. The gland should rise freely with swallowing. The thyroid at its broadest dimension is approximately 4 cm, and the right lobe is often 25% larger than the left. The consistency of the thyroid tissue should be firm yet pliable. Coarse tissue or a gritty sensation implies that an inflammatory process has been present. If nodules are present, they need to be characterized by number, whether they are smooth or irregular, and whether they are soft or hard. An enlarged tender thyroid may indicate thyroiditis.

If the thyroid gland is enlarged, auscultate for vascular sounds with the bell of the stethoscope. In a hypermetabolic state, the blood supply is dramatically increased and a vascular bruit or soft, rushing sound will be heard.

Fig. 5-10
Palpation of the right thyroid lobe main body from behind the patient.

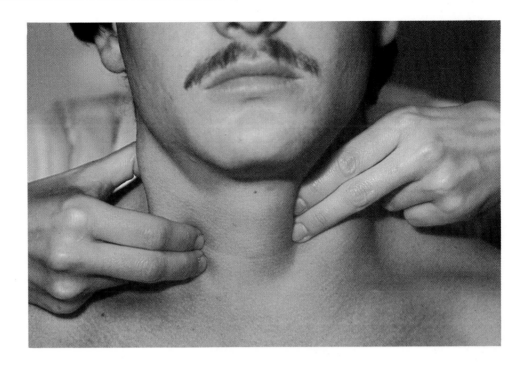

INFANTS

Measure the infant's head circumference and compare it with expected size for age on a growth chart, as detailed in Chapter 3, Growth and Measurement. Inspect the infant's head from all angles for symmetry of shape, noting any prominent bulges or swellings. Inspect the scalp for scaling and crusting, dilated scalp veins, the presence of excessive hair, or an unusual hairline.

You can always tell a pediatric specialist by the first movement in the examination of an infant. The hand goes almost instinctively to palpate the fontanel. Even in a social situation, you will find the pediatric specialist's fingers saying "hello" by drifting over the soft spot.

Birth trauma may cause swelling of the scalp. Caput succedaneum, an edematous swelling of the scalp crossing the suture lines, is a localized response to birth trauma (Fig. 5-11). A subperiosteal hemorrhage along one of the cranial bones, a cephalhematoma, has a soft, fluctuant mass with a well defined outline along the edge of the bone margin. It appears within 24 hours of birth and develops a raised bony margin within 2 to 3 days (Fig. 5-12).

In palpating the edges of a cephalhematoma or a caput succedaneum within 1 or 2 days of delivery, you may feel a sharp depression as if the skull is indented as your fingers move toward the center of the swelling. This is a palpatory illusion, and you should not assume an abnormality is present without additional evidence.

Head shape with an unusual contour may be related to premature or irregular closing of suture lines. Preterm infants often have long narrow heads because their soft cranial bones become flattened with positioning and the weight of their head. Bossing (bulging of the skull) of the frontal areas is associated with prematurity and rickets. Bulging in other areas of the skull may indicate cranial defects or intracranial masses. Dilated scalp veins and a head circumference increasing faster than expected may indicate increased intracranial pressure.

Palpate the infant's head, identifying suture lines and fontanels. Note any tenderness over the scalp. Suture lines feel ridge-like until about 6 months of age, after which they should no longer be palpable. Vaginally delivered newborns may have molding with prominent ridges from overriding sutures. Fontanels may be small or not palpable at birth. Molding of the head at delivery can be very distressing for parents. The football shape disappears relatively quickly, but reassurance is necessary. Drawings can help you explain that the infant's cranial bones overlap and that

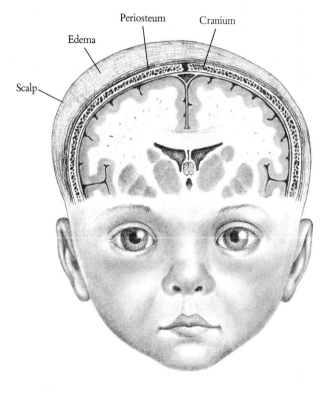

Fig. 5-11
Caput succedaneum.

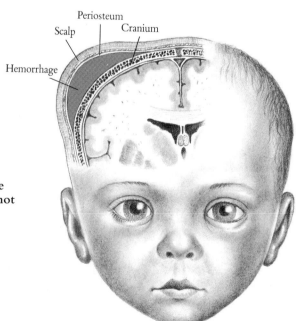

Fig. 5-12
Cephalhematoma. Note that the swelling does not cross suture lines.

their relative lack of development is a protective device for the brain. Assure the parents that symmetry of the head is usually regained within 1 week of birth, with fontanels and suture line resuming their appropriate shape and size. A third fontanel, (the mastoid fontanel), located between the anterior and posterior fontanel, may be a normal variant but is common in infants with Down syndrome. Any palpable ridges in addition to the expected suture lines may indicate fractures.

Measure the size of the anterior and posterior fontanels using two dimensions (anteroposterior and lateral). The anterior fontanel diameter in infants under 6 months of age should not exceed 4 to 5 cm. It should get progressively smaller beyond that age, closing completely by 18 to 24 months of age.

With the infant in a sitting position, palpate the anterior fontanel for bulging or depression. It should feel slightly depressed, and some pulsation is expected. A bulging fontanel feels tense, like the fontanel of an infant during the expiratory phase of crying. A bulging fontanel with marked pulsations may indicate increased intracranial pressure. The infant fontanel gives important clues to what is going on inside the body. If there is infection or increased intracranial pressure, the fontanel will bulge. Interestingly, in the early months of life the fontanel may not be as sensitive an indicator as it becomes later in the first year. You cannot assume that an infant of 3 months whose fontanel is not bulging is free of meningitis.

Palpate the scalp firmly above and behind the ears to detect craniotabes, any softening of the outer table of the skull. A snapping sensation like a ping-pong ball indicates craniotabes, which is associated with rickets and hydrocephalus.

Transilluminate the skull of every newborn and of older infants who have a suspected intracranial lesion or rapidly increasing head circumference. Perform the procedure in a completely darkened room, allowing a few minutes to elapse for your eyes to accommodate. The transilluminator is placed firmly against the infant's scalp so that no light escapes (Fig. 5-13). Begin at the midline frontal region and inch the transilluminator over the entire head. Observe the ring of illumination through the scalp and skull around the light, noting any asymmetry. A ring of 2 cm or less beyond the rim of the transilluminator is expected on all regions of the head except the occiput, where the ring should be 1 cm or less. Illumination beyond these parameters suggests excess fluid or decreased brain tissue in the skull.

Fig. 5-13
Transillumination of the infant's scalp.

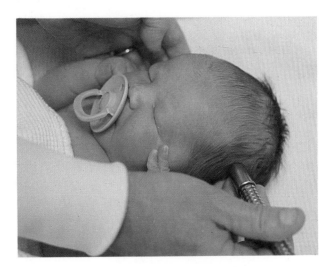

Inspect the face for spacing of the features, symmetry, paralysis, skin color, and texture. Uterine positioning can cause some facial asymmetry.

Observe the infant's head control, position, and movement. Note any jerking, tremors, or inability to move the head in one direction. Chapters 16 (Musculoskeletal System) and 17 (Neurologic System and Mental Status) provide further details.

Inspect the infant's neck for symmetry, size, and shape. Note the presence of edema, distended neck veins, pulsations, masses, webbing, or excess posterior cervical skin. To observe the newborn's neck, which is usually not visible in the supine position, elevate the upper back of the infant and permit the head to fall back into extension. The neck appears short during infancy and lengthens by 3 to 4 years of age. Marked edema may indicate localized infections. A cystic mass high in the neck may be a thyroglossal duct cyst or a branchial cleft cyst. A mass over the clavicle, changing size with crying or respiration, suggests a cystic hygroma. Nuchal rigidity, resistance to flexion of the neck, is associated with meningeal irritation.

Palpate the sternocleidomastoid muscle, noting its tone and the presence of any masses. A mass in the lower third of the muscle may indicate a hematoma. Palpate the trachea. A palpatory thud felt over the trachea suggests the presence of a foreign body. The thyroid is difficult to palpate in infants unless enlarged. The presence of a goiter results from intrauterine deprivation of thyroid hormone.

CHILDREN

Direct percussion of the skull with one finger is useful to detect Macewen's sign, a cracked-pot sound. The sound, which is physiologic when the fontanels are open, may indicate increased intracranial pressure after fontanel closure.

Bruits are common in children up to 5 years of age or in children with anemia. After age 5 years their presence may suggest vascular anomalies or increased intracranial pressure.

The thyroid of the young child may be palpable. Using techniques described for adults, note the size, shape, position, mobility, and any tenderness. No tenderness should be present. An enlarged tender thyroid may indicate thyroiditis.

PREGNANT WOMEN

Beginning after 16 weeks of gestation, many pregnant women develop blotchy, brownish hyperpigmentation of the face, particularly over the malar prominences and the forehead. This "mask of pregnancy" may further darken with sun exposure, and generally fades after delivery.

OLDER ADULTS

The facies of older adults vary with their nutritional status. The eyes may appear sunken with soft bulges underneath and the eyelids may appear wrinkled and hang loose.

Use caution when evaluating range of motion in the older adult's neck. Rather than have the patient perform an entire rotational maneuver, go slowly and evaluate each movement separately. Note any pain, crepitus, dizziness, jerkiness, or limitation of movement.

With aging the thyroid becomes more fibrotic, feeling more nodular or irregular to palpation.

Common Abnormalities

Head

Headaches

Headaches are one of the common complaints and probably one of the most self-medicated. They are not always benign. A history of insistent headache, severe and recurrent, must always be given attention. Sometimes the underlying cause is life threatening, such as a brain tumor. Sometimes it is life intimidating, such as migraines. Sometimes it is easily confronted, such as when it is the result of drinking wine. The patient's history is fully as important as the physical examination in getting at the root of a headache. Various kinds of headaches can be compared as follows*:

Characteristic	Classic Migraine	Common Migraine	Temporal Arteritis	Cluster	Hypertensive	Muscular, Tension
Age at onset	Childhood	Childhood	Older adult	Adult	Adult	Adult
Location	Unilateral	Generalized	Unilateral or bilateral	Unilateral	Bilateral or occipital	Unilateral or bilateral
Prodromal event	Well defined neurologic event, scotoma, aphasia, hemianopia, aura	Vague neurologic changes, change in personality, fluid retention, appetite loss	None	Personality changes, sleep disturbances	None	None
Precipitating event	Menstrual period, missing meals, birth control pills, let down after stress	Menstrual period, missing meals, birth control pills, let down after stress	None	Alcohol consumption	None	Stress, anger, bruxism
Duration	Hours to days	Hours to days	Hours to days	½ to 2 hours	Hours	Hours to days
Time of onset	Morning or night	Morning or night	Anytime	Nocturnal	Morning	Anytime, commonly in afternoon or evening
Quality of pain	Pulsating or throbbing	Pulsating or throbbing	Throbbing	Intense burning, boring, searing, knife-like	Throbbing	Bandlike, constricting
Frequency	< twice a week	< twice a week	Daily	Several times during night for several nights, then none	Daily	Daily
Commonly affects	Females	Females	Males and females	Males	Males and females	Males and females
Other symptoms	Nausea, vomiting	Nausea, vomiting	None	Increased lacrimation, nasal discharge	Generally remits as day progresses	None

*Adapted from Sapar, 1983.

Neck

Thyroglossal Duct Cyst

This freely movable cystic mass lies high in the neck at the midline with the duct at the base of the tongue. It is a remnant of fetal development (Fig. 5-14).

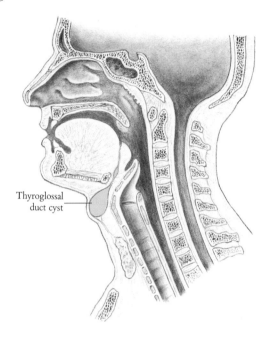

Fig. 5-14
Thyroglossal duct cyst location.

Branchial Cleft Cyst

An oval, moderately movable cystic mass appears near the upper third of the sternocleidomastoid muscle and is a remnant of embryologic development. It may be associated with a fistula (Fig. 5-15).

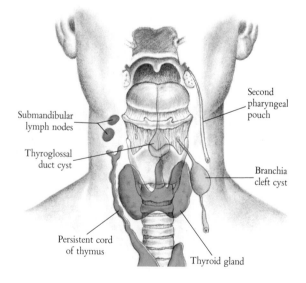

Fig. 5-15
Branchial cleft cyst location in relation to other neck masses.

Torticollis

Torticollis, or wry neck, is often the result of injury during the birth process. The head is tilted and twisted toward the sternocleidomastoid muscle. A hematoma may be palpated shortly after birth, and within 2 to 3 weeks a firm fibrous mass may be felt in the muscle (Fig. 5-16). Torticollis can also occur in older children and adults as a result of trauma or muscle spasms.

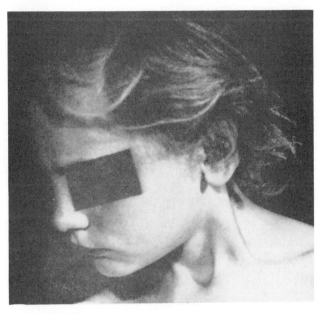

Fig. 5-16
Torticollis, or wry neck.
From Kampmeier and Blake, 1970.

Klippel-Feil Anomaly

Fusion of the cervical vertebrae results in a short neck and painless limitation of head movement. It occurs more commonly in females than in males (Fig. 5-17).

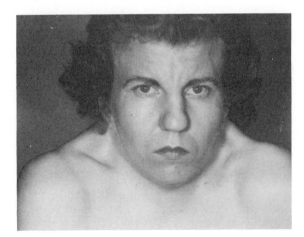

Fig. 5-17
Klippel-Feil anomaly.
From Goodman and Gorlin, 1977.

Thyroid

Myxedema

Adult onset hypothyroidism associated with a decreased metabolic rate produces myxedema. The deposition of glycosaminoglycan in all organ systems leads to the characteristic mucinous edema of facial features (Fig. 5-18). Signs and symptoms of hyperthyroidism and hypothyroidism can be compared as follows:

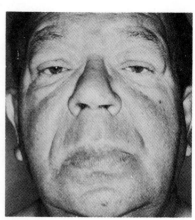

Fig. 5-18
Myxedema.
From Kaye and Rose, 1983.

System or Structure Affected	Signs and Symptoms	
	Hyperthyroidism	**Hypothyroidism**
Constitutional		
Temperature preference	Cool climate	Warm climate
Emotional state	Increased energy, easy irritability, nervousness	Lethargy, complaisance, disinterest
Weight	Loss	Gain
Hair	Fine with hair loss, failure to hold permanent	Coarse, tendency to break
Skin	Warm, fine, hyperpigmentation at pressure points	Coarse, scaling, dry
Fingernails	Thin, tend to break, may become detached from underlying fingers	Thick
Eyes	Increased prominence bilaterally or unilaterally, double or blurred vision	Puffiness in periorbital region
Neck	Swelling in region of thyroid, change in shirt neck size, pain over thyroid	No swelling
Cardiac	Palpitations, rapid pulse rate, irregular heart rhythm	No change noted
Gastrointestinal	Increased frequency of bowel movement, rarely diarrhea	Constipation
Menstrual	Scant flow, amenorrhea	Menorrhagia
Neuromuscular	Increasing weakness especially of proximal muscles	Lethargy, but good muscular strength

Graves' Disease

This thyroid disorder is thought to be autoimmune in origin. It is more common in women during the third and fourth decades of life. Multiple systems are affected, and the disease is often characterized by diffuse thyroid enlargement, hyperthyroidism, and ophthalmologic, dermatologic, and musculoskeletal pathology (Fig. 5-19).

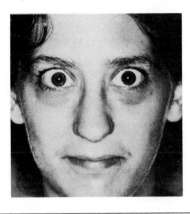

Fig. 5-19
Graves' disease.
From Kaye and Rose, 1983.

Hashimoto's Disease

Hashimoto's disease is a chronic auto-immune disorder that causes symptoms of hypothyroidism. It is common in children and in women between 30 and 50 years of age.

INFANTS

Encephalocele

A protrusion of nervous tissue through a defect in the skull may occur any place on the scalp (Fig. 5-20).

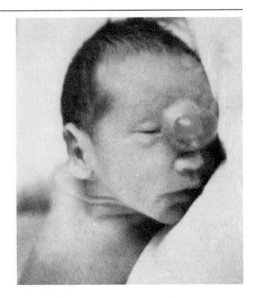

Fig. 5-20
Newborn with frontal, nasal, interocular encephalocele.
Courtesy of Dr. Charles Linder, Medical College of Georgia. From Dyken and Miller, 1980.

Microcephaly

A congenitally small skull caused by cerebral dysgenesis or craniostenosis is usually associated with mental retardation and failure of the brain to develop normally (Fig. 5-21).

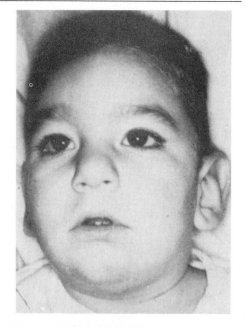

Fig. 5-21
Primary familial microcephaly.
From Dyken and Miller, 1980.

Craniosynostosis

Premature union of cranial sutures leads to a misshapened skull, usually not accompanied by mental retardation. The sutures involved determine the shape of the head (Fig. 5-22).

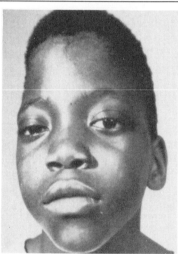

Fig. 5-22
Fourteen-year-old with dolichoscaphocephaly, one of the less threatening of the craniosynostoses.
From Dyken and Miller, 1980.

OLDER ADULTS

Temporal Arteritis (Giant Cell Arteritis)

This inflammatory disorder affects the medium to large arteries, primarily in persons over 60 years of age. It is more common in women and rarely occurs in the black population. Temporal arteritis, a disease of unknown etiology may be accompanied by vision loss if the ophthalmic artery is involved. Headache, fever of unknown origin, and proximal muscle weakness are the usual symptoms, along with a tender, cord-like or tortuous, enlarged temporal artery.

6

Eyes

Anatomy and Physiology

The eye is the sensory organ that transmits visual stimuli to the brain for interpretation (Fig. 6-1). It occupies the orbital cavity with only its anterior aspect exposed. The four rectus and two oblique muscles attached to the eye are innervated by cranial nerves III, IV, and VI (Fig. 6-2). The eye itself is a direct extension of the brain embryologically and is connected to the brain by the optic nerve.

External Eye

The external eye is composed of the eyelid, conjunctiva, lacrimal gland, eye muscles, and the bony skull orbit (Fig. 6-3).

Eyelids. The eyelids are composed of skin, conjunctiva, and both striated and smooth muscle. Their function is (1) to distribute tears over the surface of the eye, (2) to limit the amount of light entering it, and (3) to protect the eye from foreign bodies. Eyelashes extend from the border of each lid.

Conjunctiva. The conjunctiva is a thin membrane covering most of the anterior surface of the eye and the surface of the eyelid in contact with the globe. The conjunctiva protects the eye from foreign bodies and desiccation.

Lacrimal gland. The lacrimal gland (Fig. 6-3) is located in the temporal region of the superior eyelid and produces tears that moisten the eye. Tears flow over the cornea and drain via the lacrimal sac into the nasal meatus.

Internal Eye

The internal structures of the eye are composed of three separate coats, or tunics. The outer fibrous layer is composed of the sclera posteriorly and the cornea anteriorly. The middle tunic, or choroid coat, consists of the choroid posteriorly and the ciliary body and iris anteriorly. The inner nervous tunic is the retina.

Sclera. The sclera is a dense, avascular structure that appears anteriorly as the white of the eye. It physically supports the internal structure of the eye.

Cornea. The cornea comprises the anterior one sixth of the globe and is continuous with the sclera. It has sensory innervation primarily for pain. The cornea separates the watery fluid of the anterior chamber (aqueous humor) from the external environment and permits the transmission of light through the lens to the retina.

Iris. The iris is a circular, contractile muscular disc containing pigment cells that produce the color of the eye. The central aperture of the iris is the pupil through which light travels to the retina. The iris controls the amount of light reaching the retina by dilating and contracting.

Lens. The lens is a cellular structure containing crystalline matter located immediately behind the iris. It is biconvex and transparent. It is supported circumferentially by fibers arising from the ciliary body of the iris. The lens is highly elastic, and contraction or relaxation of the ciliary body changes its thickness, thereby permitting images from varied distances to be focused on the retina.

Retina. The retina is the sensory network of the eye. It transforms light impulses into electrical impulses, which are transmitted through the optic nerve and the optic radiation to consciousness in the cerebral cortex. The optic nerve communicates with the brain, passing through the optic foramen along with the ophthalmic artery, vein, and autonomic nervous system innervation of the eye. Accurate vision

Fig. 6-1
Anatomy of the human eye.

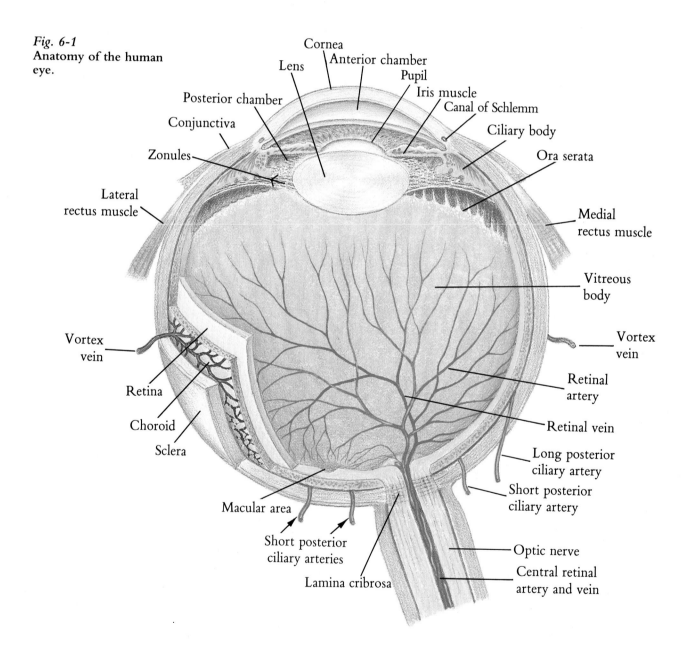

Fig. 6-2
Extraocular muscles of the eye.
From Thompson et. al., 1986.

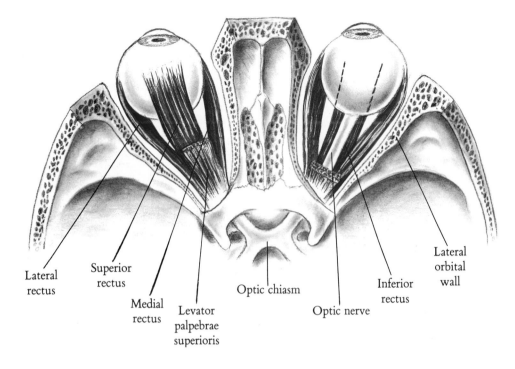

Lateral rectus

Superior rectus

Medial rectus

Levator palpebrae superioris

Optic chiasm

Optic nerve

Inferior rectus

Lateral orbital wall

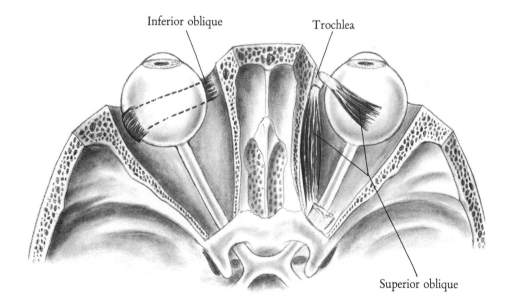

Inferior oblique

Trochlea

Superior oblique

Fig. 6-3
**Important landmarks of the
external eye.**
From Thompson et al., 1986.

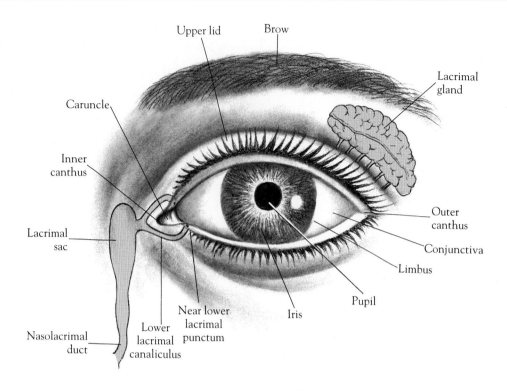

Fig. 6-4
The visual pathway.
From Thompson et al., 1986.

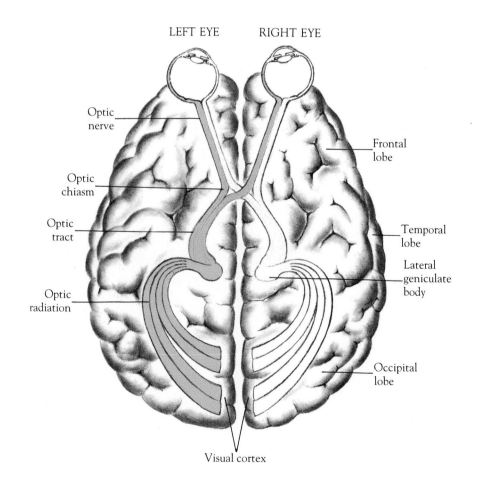

is achieved by focusing an image on the retina through accommodation of the lens. The neural impulses so generated are transmitted along the optic nerve and optic tract, reaching the optic cortex for interpretation. An object may be perceived in each optic cortex even when one eye is covered if the light impulse is cast on the nasal retina. Fibers located there descussate in the optic chiasma (Fig. 6-4). Accurate vision also requires the synchronous functioning of the extraocular muscles.

Major landmarks of the retina include the optic disc from which the optic nerve originates, together with the central retinal artery and vein. The macula densa is the site of central vision and color perception.

INFANTS AND CHILDREN

The eye forms during the first 8 weeks of gestation and may become malformed from the insult of maternal drug ingestion or infection during this time. The development of vision, which is dependent on maturation of the nervous system, occurs over a longer period of time. Term infants are myopic with a visual acuity of 20/200. While peripheral vision is fully developed at birth, central vision develops later. By 2 to 3 months of age the lacrimal ducts begin carrying tears into the nasal meatus, and the infant gains voluntary control of the eye muscles. By 8 months vision has developed sufficiently so the infant can differentiate colors. The eye muscles begin to coordinate, allowing a single image to be perceived by 9 months of age.

Young children have myopic acuity, primarily because the shape of their eyeball is less spherical than adults. The globe of the eye grows as the child's head and brain grow, and adult visual acuity is achieved at about 6 years of age.

OLDER ADULTS

The major physiologic change that occurs with aging is a progressive change in the near point of accommodation. Generally by age 45 the lens becomes more rigid, and the ciliary muscle of the iris becomes weaker. This combination results in presbyopia. The lens also continues to form fibers throughout life. Old fibers are compressed centrally, forming a more dense central region that may cause loss of clarity of the lens and cataract formation.

Review of Related History

General Considerations

1. Employment: exposure to irritating gases, foreign bodies, or high-speed machinery
2. Activities: participation in sporting activities that might endanger the eye (e.g., squash, racquetball, fencing, motorcycle riding)
3. Allergies: type, seasonal, associated symptoms
4. Medications: use of any eyedrops or ointments, and if so, for what reason
5. Lenses: when last changed, how long worn, type (glasses or contact), adequacy of corrected vision; methods of cleaning and storage, insertion and removal procedures of contact lenses; date of last eye examination
6. Use of protective devices during work or activities that might endanger the eye

Present Problem

1. Eyelids: recurrent sties; drooping of the lids so that they interfere with vision (unilateral or bilateral)
2. Difficulty with vision: one or both eyes, corrected by lenses, involving near or distant vision, primarily central or peripheral, transient or sustained; presence of floaters; adequacy of color vision; presence of halos around lights; presence of double vision (when one eye is covered or only with both eyes)
3. Pain: in or around the eye, superficial or deep, insidious or abrupt in onset; burning, itching, or nonspecific uncomfortable sensation
4. Secretions: color (clear or yellow), consistency (watery or foamy), duration, tears that run down the face, decreased tear formation with sensation of gritty eyes; presence of conjunctival redness

Past Medical History

1. Trauma: to the eye as a whole or a specific structure (e.g., cornea) or supporting structures (e.g., the floor of the orbit); events surrounding the trauma; efforts at correction and degree of success
2. Eye surgery: condition requiring surgery, date surgery performed, outcome
3. Chronic illness that may affect vision: hypertension, diabetes, glaucoma

Family History

1. Retinoblastoma or cancer of the retina (often an autosomal dominant disorder)
2. Conditions similar to that of the patient's
3. Color blindness, cataract formation, diabetes, glaucoma, retinitis pigmentosa, macular degeneration, or allergies affecting the eye
4. Nearsightedness, farsightedness, or strabismus

INFANTS AND CHILDREN

1. Preterm: resuscitated, ventilator or oxygen used, given diagnosis of retrolental fibroplasia
2. Failure of infant to gaze at mother's face or other objects, uncertainty of mother that infant looks at her; failure of infant to blink when bright lights or threatening movements are directed at it
3. White area in the pupil on a photograph; inability of one eye to reflect light properly (may indicate retinoblastoma)
4. Excessive tearing over the lower eyelid
5. Crossed eyes some or all of the time
6. Young children: excessive rubbing of the eyes, frequent sties, inability to reach for and pick up small objects, necessity of bringing objects close to examine them
7. Schoolage children: necessity of sitting near the front of the classroom to see the board; poor progress in school not explained by intellectual ability

OLDER ADULT

1. Visual acuity: decrease in central vision, use of dim light to increase visual acuity
2. Production of excess tearing or complaints of blurred vision (caused by loss of contact of the lacrimal duct with the nasal lacrimal lake)
3. Development of arcus senilis, with lipid deposits in the cornea
4. Development of scleral brown spots
5. Difficulty in performing near work without lenses
6. Nocturnal eye pain

Examination and Findings

EQUIPMENT	■ Snellen chart or E chart
	■ Rosenbaum or Jaeger near vision card
	■ Penlight
	■ Cotton wisp
	■ Ophthalmoscope

Visual Testing

Measurement of visual acuity, the discrimination of small details, tests the second cranial nerve and is essentially a measurement of central vision. Position the patient 20 ft away from the Snellen chart (Fig. 2-11, *A*), making sure it is well lighted. Test each eye individually by covering one eye with an opaque card or a gauze, being careful to avoid applying pressure to the eye. Ask the patient to identify all of the letters beginning at any line. Determine the smallest line in which the patient can identify all of the letters and record the visual acuity designated by that line. (If a more precise determination is needed, see pp. 31-32.) When testing the second eye, you may want to ask the patient to read the line from right to left. If you test the patient with and without corrective lenses, record the readings separately. Always test vision without glasses first. The test should be done rapidly enough to prevent the patient from memorizing the chart. However, one of the problems patients confront during the examination of the vision is that the examiner sometimes goes too fast, asking that lines on the chart be read or that other judgments be made more quickly than feels comfortable to the patient. The patient's quick judgment may be helpful. It is wise, however, to pace it a bit more slowly to let the patient be comfortable and to allow time to puzzle out a response. The patient should not have to leave the examination feeling that something had been said too quickly or too uncertainly.

Visual acuity is recorded as a fraction in which the numerator indicates the distance of the patient from the chart (20 ft) and the denominator indicates the distance at which a normal eye can read the line. Thus 20/200 means that the patient can read at 20 ft what the average person can read at 200 ft. The smaller the fraction, the worse the myopia.

Measurement of near vision should be tested in each eye separately, with a hand-held card such as the Rosenbaum near vision card (Fig. 2-12). Have the patient hold the card 15 in from the eyes and read the smallest line possible.

Peripheral vision can be accurately measured with sophisticated instruments, but it is generally estimated by means of the confrontation test. Sit opposite the patient at eye level about 1 m apart. Ask the patient to cover the right eye (Fig. 6-5), while you cover your left eye so the open eyes are directly opposite each other. Both you and the patient should be looking at each other's eye. Fully extend your arm midway between the patient and yourself and then move it centrally with fingers waving. Have the patient tell you when the moving fingers are first seen. Compare the patient's response to the time you first noted the fingers. Test the nasal, temporal, superior, and inferior fields. Remember that the nasal portion of the visual field is interfered with by the nose itself. You can feel comfortable that the fields are full if they correspond with yours. Actually one anticipates that the fields describe an angle of 60 degrees nasally, 90 degrees temporally, 50 degrees superiorly, and 70 degrees inferiorly. The confrontation test is imprecise, however, and can be considered significant only when it is abnormal.

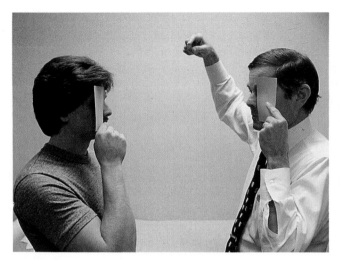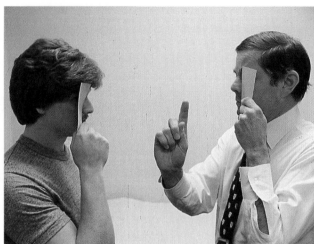

Fig. 6-5
Estimation of peripheral
fields of vision.

Color vision is rarely tested in the routine physical examination. Color plates are available in which numerals are produced in primary colors and surrounded by confusion colors. The tests vary in degree of difficulty. For routine testing check the patient's ability to appreciate primary colors.

Remember that testing of visual acuity involves many complex factors not necessarily related to the ability to see the test object. Motivation and interest as well as intelligence and attention span can modify the results of sensory testing.

External Examination

Examination of the eyes is carried out in a systematic manner beginning with the appendages, i.e., the eyebrows and surrounding tissues, and moving inward.

Inspect the eyebrows for size, extension, and texture of the hair. Note whether the eyebrows extend beyond the eye itself or end short of it. The coarseness of the hair is also important. If the patient's eyebrows are coarse or do not extend beyond the temporal canthus, the patient may have hypothyroidism. If the brows appear unusually thin, ask if the patient waxes or plucks them.

Inspect the orbital area for edema, puffiness, or sagging tissue below the orbit. While puffiness may represent the loss of elastic tissue that occurs with aging, periorbital edema is always abnormal, but the significance varies directly with the amount. It may represent the presence of thyroid hypoactivity, allergies, or (especially in youth) the presence of renal disease. You may see flat, slightly raised, irregularly shaped, yellow tinted lesions on the periorbital tissues that represent depositions of lipids and *may* suggest that the patient has an abnormality of lipid metabolism. These lesions are called xanthelasma (Fig. 6-6), an elevated plaque of cholesterol deposited most commonly in the nasal portion of either the upper or lower lid.

Examine the patient's lightly closed eyes for fasciculations or tremors of the lids, a sign of hyperthyroidism. Inspect the eyelids for their ability to close completely and open widely. Observe for flakiness, redness, or swelling on the eyelid margin. Eyelashes should be present on both lids and turn outward.

When the eye is open, the superior eyelid should cover a portion of the iris but not the pupil itself. If one superior eyelid covers more of the iris than the other or extends over the iris, then ptosis of that lid may be present, indicating a congenital or acquired weakness of the levator muscle or a paresis of a branch of the third cranial nerve (Fig. 6-7). Record the difference between the two lids in millimeters.

If there is drooping of the upper lid with narrowing of the palpebral fissure, blepharoptosis may be present. This condition (Fig. 6-8) may be caused by abnormalities of the musculature of the eyelid or its innervation (cranial nerve III).

You should also note whether the lids evert or invert. When the lower lid is turned away from the eye, ectropion is present and may result in excessive tearing (Fig. 6-9). The inferior punctum, which serves as the tear collecting system, is pulled outward away from the lacrimal lake.

When the lid is turned inward toward the globe, entropion (Fig. 6-10), the lid's eyelashes may cause corneal and conjunctival irritation, increasing the risk of a secondary infection.

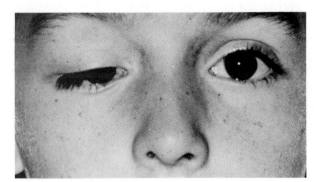

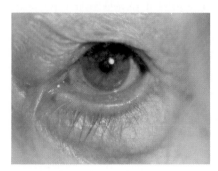

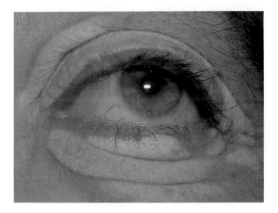

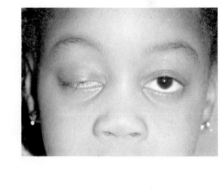

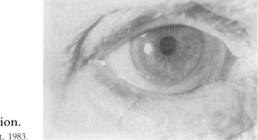

Fig. 6-7
Ptosis, a drooping of the upper eyelid.
From Stein and Slatt, 1983.

Fig. 6-6
Xanthelasma.
From Newell, 1986.

Fig. 6-8
Right blepharoptosis.
From Newell, 1983.

Fig. 6-9
Ectropion.
From Stein and Slatt, 1983.

Fig. 6-10
Spastic entropion.
From Stein and Slatt, 1983.

Fig. 6-11
Acute hordeolum of lower eyelid.
From Newell, 1986.

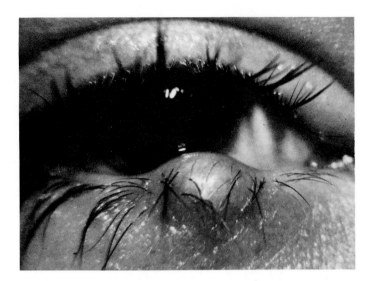

Fig. 6-12
Pulling lower lid down.

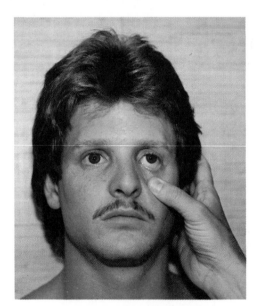

An acute suppurative inflammation of the follicle of an eyelash can cause an erythematous or yellow lump. This hordeolum or sty (Fig. 6-11) is generally caused by staphylococcal organisms.

Palpate the eyelids for nodules. Ask the patient to close his or her eyes and note whether the eyelids meet completely. When the closed lids do not completely cover the globe, a condition called lagophthalmos, the cornea may become dried and be at increased risk of infection.

Next palpate the eye itself. Determine whether it feels hard or can be gently pushed into the orbit without causing discomfort. An eye that feels very firm and resists palpation may indicate hyperthyroidism or a retro-orbital tumor.

The conjunctivae are usually inapparent, clear, and free of erythema. Inspection of the conjunctival covering of the lower lid is easily performed (Fig. 6-12) by having the patient look upward while you draw the lower lid downward.

Inspect the upper tarsal conjunctiva only when there is a suggestion that a foreign body may be present. Ask the patient to look down while you pull the eyelashes gently downward and forward to break the suction between the lid and globe (Fig. 6-13). Next evert the lid on a small cotton covered applicator. After you inspect and remove any foreign body that may be present, return the eyelid to its regular position: ask the patient to look up while you apply forward pressure against the eyelid.

Observe the conjunctivae for increased erythema or exudate. An erythematous or cobblestone appearance may indicate an allergic or infectious conjunctivitis (Fig. 6-14). Bright red blood in a sharply defined area surrounded by normal appearing conjunctiva (Fig. 6-15) indicates subconjunctival hemorrhage. The blood stays red because of direct diffusion of oxygen through the conjunctiva.

Fig. 6-13
Everting upper eyelid.

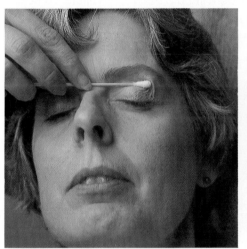
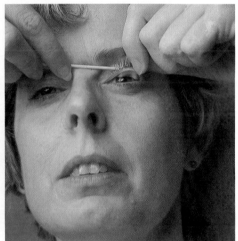

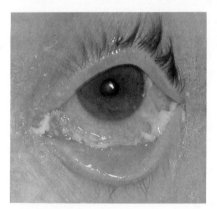

Fig. 6-14
Acute conjunctivitis.
From Newell, 1986.

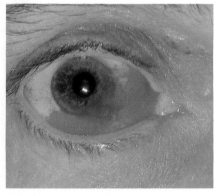

Fig. 6-15
Subconjunctival hemorrhage.
From Newell, 1986.

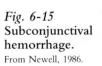

A pterygium is a fold of conjunctiva that progresses over the cornea, usually from the nasal fold (Fig. 6-16). It is most commonly seen in the tropics. It can interfere with vision if it advances over the pupil.

Examine the cornea for clarity by shining a light tangentially on it. Since the cornea is avascular, blood vessels should not be present. Corneal sensitivity, controlled by cranial nerve V, is tested by touching a wisp of cotton to the cornea (Fig. 6-17). The expected response is a blink, which requires intact sensory fibers of cranial nerve V and motor fibers of cranial nerve VII.

You may note a corneal arcus (arcus senilis), which is composed of lipids deposited in the periphery of the cornea (Fig. 6-18). It may in time form a complete circle (circus senilis). An arcus is seen in the majority of individuals over age 60, although it commonly appears in blacks at an earlier age. If present before age 40, arcus senilis may indicate a lipid disorder, most commonly type II hyperlipidemia.

The iris pattern should be clearly visible. Generally the irides are the same color. Note any irregularity in the shape of the pupils. They should be round, regular, and equal in size. Pupil abnormalities are described on pp. 191-192.

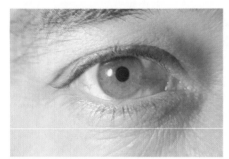

Fig. 6-16
Pterygium.
From Stein and Slatt, 1983.

Fig. 6-17
Testing corneal sensitivity.

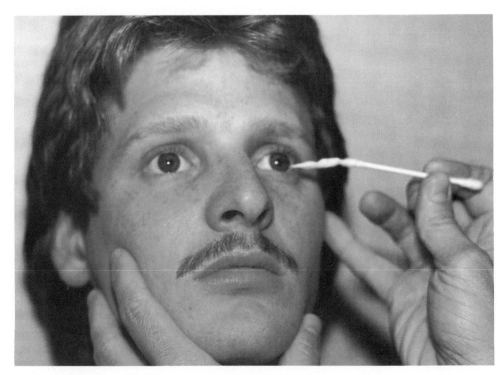

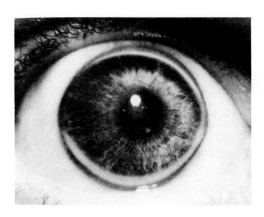

Fig. 6-18
Corneal arcus.
From Newell, 1986.

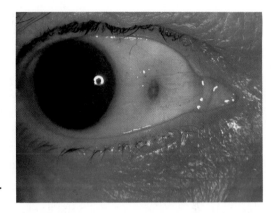

Fig. 6-19
Senile hyaline plaque.
From Newell, 1986.

Test the pupils for response to light both directly and consensually. Dim the lights in the room so the pupils dilate. Shine a penlight directly into one eye and observe the pupil constrict. Note the consensual response of the opposite pupil constricting simultaneously with the tested pupil.

Test the pupils for constriction to accommodation as well. Ask the patient to look at a distant object and then at a test object (either a pencil or your finger) held 10 cm from the bridge of the nose. The pupils should constrict when the eyes focus on the near object. Testing for pupillary response to accommodation is of diagnostic importance only if there is a defect in the pupillary response to light. A failure to respond to direct light but retaining constriction during accommodation is sometimes seen in patients with diabetes or syphilis.

Estimate the pupillary size and compare them for equality. Pupils may show size variation in a number of ways. Miosis is pupillary constriction to less than 2 mm. The miotic pupil fails to dilate in the dark. It is commonly caused by ingestion of drugs such as morphine, but drugs that control glaucoma may cause miosis as well. Mydriasis is pupillary dilation to more than 6 mm, and the pupils fail to constrict with light. Mydriasis is an accompaniment of coma whether caused by diabetes, alcohol, uremia, or epilepsy. Anisocoria, the inequality of pupillary size, is a common normal variation but may also occur in a large variety of disease states.

Inspect the lens, which should be transparent. Shining a light on the lens may cause it to appear grey or yellow, but its ability to transmit light may still be great. Later examination of the lens with the ophthalmoscope will help to judge the clarity.

The sclera should be examined primarily to assure that it is white. The sclera should be visible above the iris only when the eyelids are opened widely. If liver disease is present, the sclera may become pigmented and appear either yellow or green. Senile hyaline plaque (Fig. 6-19) appears as a dark, rust-colored pigment just anterior to the insertion of the medial rectus muscle. Its presence does not imply disease but should be noted.

Extraocular Eye Muscles

Full movement of the eyes is controlled by the integrated function of the third, fourth, and sixth cranial nerves and the six extraocular muscles. Hold the patient's chin to prevent movement of the head and ask him or her to watch your finger as it moves through the six cardinal fields of gaze (Fig. 6-20). Then ask the patient to look to the extreme lateral (temporal) positions. Do not be surprised to observe a few horizontal nystagmic beats.

Occasionally you may note sustained nystagmus, the involuntary rhythmic movements of the eyes that can occur in a horizontal, vertical, rotary, or mixed pattern. Jerking nystagmus, characterized by faster movements in one direction, is defined by its rapid phase. If the eye moves rapidly to the right and then slowly drifts leftward, the patient is said to have nystagmus to the right.

Finally have the patient follow your finger in the vertical plane, going from ceiling to floor. Observe the coordinated movement of the globes and the superior lid. The movement should be accomplished smoothly and without exposure of the sclera. Full movements indicate integrity of muscle strength and cranial nerve action. Lid lag, the exposure of the sclera above the iris when the patient is asked to follow your finger as you direct the eye in a smooth movement from ceiling to floor, may indicate hyperthyroidism.

Fig. 6-20
Testing the six cardinal fields of gaze.

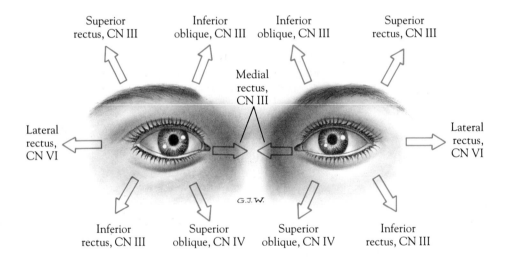

Fig. 6-21
Cover-uncover test.

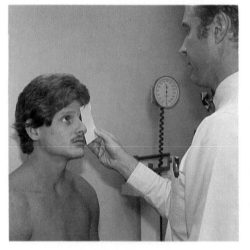
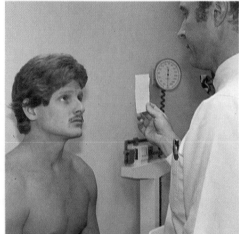

Use the corneal light reflex to test the balance of the extraocular muscles. Direct a light source to the nasal bridge from a distance of about 30 cm. The light should be reflected symmetrically from both eyes.

Muscle balance is also evaluated with the cover-uncover test (Fig. 6-21). Ask the patient to stare straight ahead at a near fixed point. Cover one eye and observe the uncovered eye for movement to focus on the designated point. Remove the cover and watch for movement of this eye as it fixes on the object. Repeat the process, covering the other eye. Movement of the covered or uncovered eye may indicate either esotropia or exotropia.

Inspect the region of the lacrimal gland, and palpate the lower orbital rim near the inner canthus. The puncta should be seen as slight elevations with a central depression on both the upper and lower lid margins. If the temporal aspect of the upper lid feels full, evert the lid and inspect the gland. The lacrimal glands are rarely enlarged but may become so in some conditions such as sarcoid disease and Sjögren's syndrome. Despite the enlargement, the patient may complain of dry eyes because the glands produce inadequate tears.

Ophthalmoscopic Examination

The ophthalmoscopic examination of the eyes is a tiring process. Avoid prolonging it without giving the patient at least brief intervals for rest from the bright light, a respectful consideration that reduces fatigue and improves comfort.

Inspection of the interior of the eye permits visualization of the optic disc, arteries, veins, and retina. Adequate pupillary dilation is necessary and can often be achieved by dimming the lights in the examining room. Instillation of medications that cause mydriasis is used in some cases. Prior to instillation of a mydriatic, inspect the patient's anterior chamber by shining a focused light tangentially at the limbus (the union of the conjunctiva and the sclera). Note the illumination of the iris nasally (Fig. 6-22). This portion of the iris is not lighted when the patient has a shallow anterior chamber, indicating a risk of acute angle glaucoma. Mydriatics should be avoided in these patients.

Fig. 6-22
Evaluation of depth of anterior chambers. A, Normal anterior chamber. B, Shallow anterior chamber.

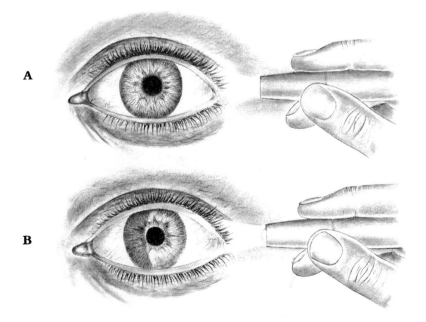

Examine the patient's right eye with your right eye and the patient's left eye with your left. Hold the ophthalmoscope in the hand that corresponds to the examining eye. Change the lens of the ophthalmoscope with your index finger. Start with the lens on the 0 setting and stabilize yourself and the patient by placing your other hand on the patient's shoulder or head (Fig. 6-23).

With the patient looking at a distant fixation point, direct the light of the ophthalmoscope at the pupil from about 30 cm (12 in) away. First visualize a red reflex, which is the light illuminating the retina. Any opacities in the path of the light will stand out as black densities. Absence of the red reflex is often the result of an improperly positioned ophthalmoscope, but it may also indicate total opacity of the pupil by a cataract or by hemorrhage into the vitreous humor. If you locate the red reflex and then lose it as you approach the patient, simply move back and start again.

The fundus, or retina, appears as a yellow or pink background, depending on the amount of melanin in the pigment epithelium. The pigment generally varies with the complexion of the patient (Fig. 6-24). No discrete areas of pigmentation should be seen in the fundus except for crescents or dots at the disc margin, most commonly along the temporal edge.

As you approach the eye gradually, the retinal details should become apparent (Fig. 6-25). A blood vessel will probably be the first structure seen when you are about 3 to 5 cm from the patient. You may have to adjust the ophthalmoscope lens to be able to see the retinal details. If your patient is myopic, you will need to use a

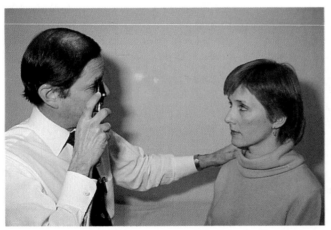
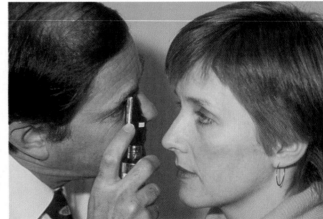

Fig. 6-23
Direct ophthalmoscopy.

Fig. 6-24
A, Normal white adult fundus. **B,** Normal negroid fundus.
From MEDCOM, 1973.

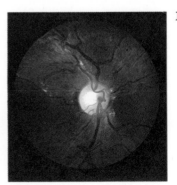

A

B

Fig. 6-25
Retinal structures of left eye.

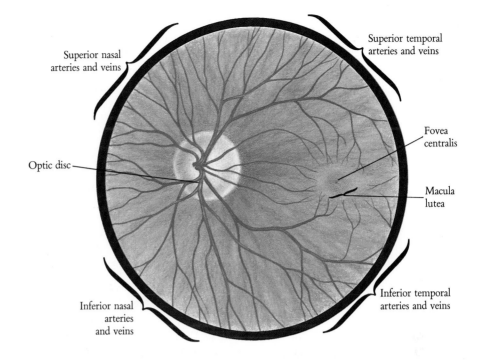

Superior nasal arteries and veins

Superior temporal arteries and veins

Optic disc

Fovea centralis

Macula lutea

Inferior nasal arteries and veins

Inferior temporal arteries and veins

minus (red) lens, and if the patient is hyperopic or lacks a lens (aphakic), you will need a plus (black) reading. When fundus details come into focus, you will note the branching of blood vessels. Since they always branch away from the optic disc, you can use these landmarks to find the optic disc.

Next look at the vascular supply of the retina. The blood vessels divide into superior and inferior branches and then into nasal and temporal ones. Venous pulsations may be seen on the disc and should be noted. Arterioles are smaller than venules, generally at a ratio of 3:5 to 2:3. The light reflected from arterioles is brighter than from venules, and the oxygenated blood is a brighter red. Follow the blood vessels distally as far as you can see them in each of the four quadrants. Note especially the sites of crossing of the arterioles and venules, because their characteristics may change when hypertension is present.

The disc margin should be sharp and well defined, especially in the temporal region. The disc is generally yellow to creamy pink in color, but the color varies with race, being darker in black and Spanish people. It is about 1.5 mm in diameter and is the unit of measurement in describing lesion size and location on the fundus. For example, an abnormality of a blood vessel may occur 2 disc diameters from the optic nerve at 2 o'clock (Fig. 6-26).

Occasionally you may see such unexpected findings as myelinated nerve fibers, papilledema, glaucomatous cupping, drusen bodies, or hemorrhages.

Myelinated nerve fibers appear as a white area with soft, ill-defined peripheral margins (Fig. 6-27). The area is continuous with the optic disc. The absence of pigment, feathery margins, and normal visual fields help distinguish this benign condition from chorioretinitis.

Papilledema is characterized by loss of definition of the optic disc that initially occurs superiorly and inferiorly and then nasally and temporally. It is caused by increased intracranial pressure transmitted along the optic nerve. The central vessels are pushed forward and the veins are markedly dilated. Venous pulsations are not visible and cannot be induced by pressure applied to the globe. Initially vision is not altered (Fig. 6-28).

Fig. 6-26
**Method of giving position
and dimensions of a lesion
in terms of disc diameters
(DD).**

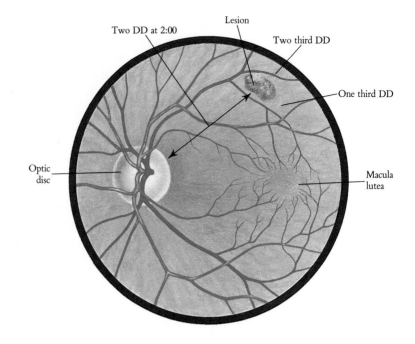

Fig. 6-27
**Myelinated retinal nerve
fibers.**
Courtesy Andrew P. Schachat, M.D.,
The Wilmer Ophthalmological
Institute, The Johns Hopkins
University and Hospital, Baltimore.

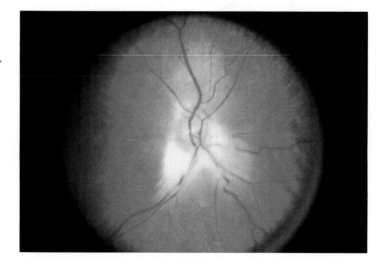

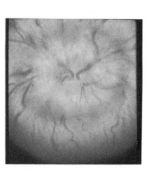

Fig. 6-28
Severe papilledema.
From Stein and Slatt, 1983.

Glaucomatous cupping is a result of increased intraocular pressure and the consequent interruption of the vascular supply to the optic nerve (Fig. 6-29). Blood vessels may disappear over the edge of the physiologic disc and be seen again deep within the disc. Blood vessels may also be displaced nasally. Impairment of the blood supply may lead to optic atrophy, causing the disc to appear much whiter than usual.

Drusen bodies can appear as small, discrete spots slightly pinker than the retina. With time the spots enlarge and become more yellow. They may occur in many conditions that affect the pigment layers of the retina, but most commonly they are a consequence of the aging process (Fig. 6-30).

Hemorrhages in the retina vary in color and shape depending on the cause and location (Fig. 6-31). Preretinal hemorrhages occur between the retina and the vitreous humor. They tend to be large and have a meniscus since the unclotted blood falls. Flame-shaped hemorrhages occur in the nerve fiber layers, and the blood spreads parallel to the nerve fibers. Round hemorrhages tend to occur in the deeper layers and may appear as a dark color instead of the bright red that is characteristic

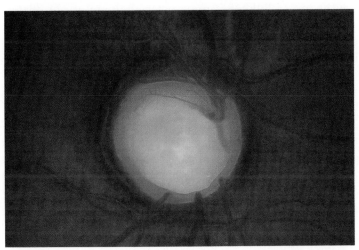

Fig. 6-29
Marked glaucomatous optic nerve head cupping.
Courtesy Andrew P. Schachat, M.D., The Wilmer Ophthalmological Institute, The Johns Hopkins University and Hospital, Baltimore.

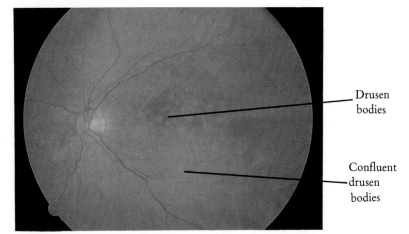

Drusen bodies

Confluent drusen bodies

Fig. 6-30
Drusen bodies in macular area.
Courtesy Andrew P. Schachat, M.D., The Wilmer Ophthalmological Institute, The Johns Hopkins University and Hospital, Baltimore.

Fig. 6-31
A, Preretinal hemorrhages around the disc. B, Flame hemorrhages.
A from MEDCOM, 1973; **B** courtesy Andrew P. Schachat, M.D., The Wilmer Ophthalmological Institute, The Johns Hopkins University and Hospital, Baltimore.

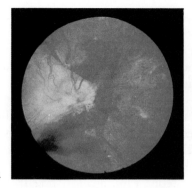

A

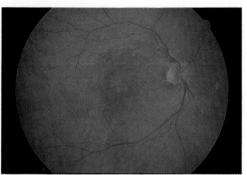

B

of preretinal and flame hemorrhages. Dot hemorrhages may actually represent microaneurysms common in diabetic retinopathy. The direct ophthalmoscope does not permit the distinction between dot hemorrhages and microaneurysms.

Next examine the macula densa, also called the fovea centralis or macula lutea. The site of central vision, it is located approximately two disc diameters temporal to the optic disc. It may be impossible to examine when the pupil is not dilated, because shining light on it induces strong pupillary constriction. To bring it into your field of vision, ask the patient to look directly at the light. No blood vessels enter the fovea, and it appears as a yellow dot surrounded by a deep pink periphery.

INFANTS

Infants often shut their eyes tightly when eye examination is attempted. It is difficult to separate the eyelids, and frequently the lids will evert when too much effort is exerted. Examining the newborn's eyes in a dimly lit room often encourages the baby to open its eyes. Holding the infant upright, suspended under its arms, also encourages the eyes to open. If the parent is present, have him or her hold the infant over a shoulder, and position yourself behind the parent. Even when the infant is crying, there will often be a moment when the eyes open. This gives you an opportunity to learn something about the eyes, their symmetry and extraocular muscular balance, and whether there is a red reflex. The child may then start crying again, but progress has been made.

Begin by inspecting the infant's external eye structures. Note the size of the eyes, paying particular attention to small or different sized eyes. Inspect the eyelids for swelling, epicanthal folds, and position. To detect epicanthal folds, look for a vertical fold of skin nasally that covers the lacrimal caruncle (Fig. 6-32). Prominent epicanthal folds, together with an upward, outer slant of the eyelids is common in Oriental infants, but they may be suggestive of Down syndrome in children of other ethnic groups. Observe the alignment and slant of the palpebral fissures of the infant's eyes. Draw an imaginary line through the medial canthi and extend the line past the outer canthi of the eyes. The medial and lateral canthi should be horizontal. When the outer canthi are above the line, an upward or mongolian slant is present. When the outer canthi are below the line, a downward or antimongolian slant is present (Fig. 6-33).

Inspect the level of the eyelid covering the eye. To detect the setting sun sign rapidly lower the infant from upright to supine position. Look for sclera above the iris. This sign may be a normal variant in newborns; however, it is observed in infants with hydrocephalus and brainstem lesions.

HYPERTENSIVE RETINOPATHY

Retinal changes associated with hypertension are generally classified according to the Keith-Wagner-Barker (KWB) system (Keith, Wagner, and Barker, 1939), which evaluates changes in the vascular supply, the retina itself, and the optic disc. For accurate rating the changes should be present bilaterally.

The arterial-venous size ratio is normally 3:5. As arterioles become smaller because of smooth muscle contraction, hyperplasia, or fibrosis, that ratio decreases. Venules do not have a smooth muscle coat but share the adventitia of the arteriole where the arteriole and venule cross. Thickening of the arteriolar coat results in apparent nicking of the venule where the venule passes beneath the arteriole, or the venule may appear elevated when it passes over the arteriole.

Group I of the KWB classification is characterized by increased light reflex from the arterioles. There is moderate arteriolar attenuation and focal constriction. No arterial-venous changes at crossing are noted.

Group II is marked by the appearance of arteriovenous crossing changes. Arterioles are reduced to about one half normal size, and areas of localized constriction may be observed.

Group III is characterized by a shiny retina and by the appearance of cotton wool spots, which represent ischemic infarcts of the retina. These are yellow areas with poorly defined margins. Hemorrhages may also be present.

Group IV is characterized by the appearance of papilledema.

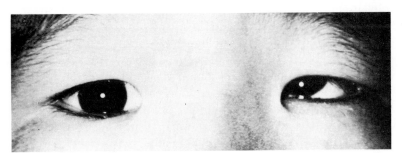

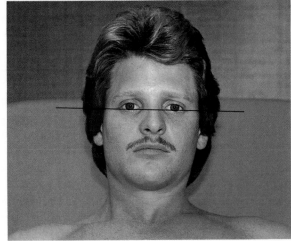

Fig. 6-32
Epicanthal folds.
From Stein and Slatt, 1983.

Fig. 6-33
Drawing a line between medial and lateral canthi to determine if a mongolian or antimongolian slant is present.

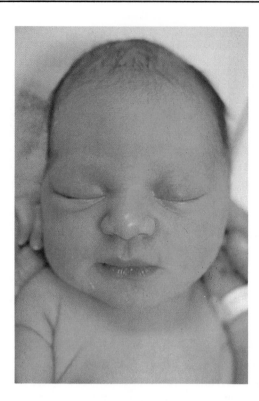

Fig. 6-34
Swollen eyelids in
newborn.

Observe the distance between the eyes, looking for widely spaced eyes or hypertelorism, associated in some instances with mental retardation. Infants often have pseudostrabismus, the false appearance of strabismus because of a flattened nasal bridge or epicanthal fold. Pseudostrabismus generally disappears by about 1 year. Use the corneal light reflex to distinguish pseudostrabismus from strabismus. An asymmetric light reflex may indicate strabismus or hypertelorism.

Inspect the sclera, conjunctiva, pupil, and iris of each eye. The newborn's eyelids may be swollen or edematous, accompanied by conjunctival inflammation and drainage (Fig. 6-34). This may be a consequence of routinely administered antibiotics. Any redness, hemorrhages, discharge, or granular appearance beyond the newborn period may indicate infection, allergy, or trauma. Inspect each iris and pupil for any irregularity in shape. A coloboma or keyhole pupil is associated with other congenital anomalies. White specks scattered in a linear pattern around the entire circumference of the iris, called Brushfield's spots, strongly suggest Down syndrome or mental retardation.

Test the cranial nerves II, III, IV, and VI in the following manner:

• Vision is grossly examined by observing the infant's preference for looking at certain objects. Expect the infant to focus on and track a light or face through 60 degrees.
• Elicit the optical blink reflex by shining a bright light at the infant's eyes, noting the quick closure of the eyes and dorsiflexion of the head.
• The corneal light reflex is performed as in adults, but because of the presence of infantile medial canthi, the reflex may appear asymmetrical until 6 months of age.

A funduscopic examination is very difficult to conduct on a newborn or young infant and is generally deferred until the infant is 2 to 6 months of age unless, as with the visual problems of prematurity, there is a compelling need. Dilation of the eyes for effective visualization of the fundi can be safely achieved in the nursery by using solutions of weak mydriatics. If an infant's irises are blue, very little of a weak solution is necessary; one drop in each eye is generally enough. With darker colored eyes, a second drop a few seconds later is indicated. Caputo drops, a solution that contains Cyclogyl 0.5%, Mydriacyl 0.5%, and Neo-Synephrine 2.5%, may be used (Caputo, Schnitzer, Lindquist, and Sun, 1982).

The red reflex should be elicited bilaterally in every newborn. Observe for any opacities, dark spots, or white spots within the circle of red glow. Opacities or interruption of the red reflex may indicate congenital cataracts or retinoblastoma.

CHILDREN

Perform the inspection of the young child's external eye structures as described for the infant.

Visual acuity is tested when the child is cooperative with the Snellen E game, usually about 3 years of age (Fig. 2-11, B). Have one examiner point to the line on the chart and another assist the child with covering one eye. As with adults, have the child stand 6 m (20 ft) away. Allow the child to practice following the instructions before you administer the test. Instruct the child to point his or her arm or finger in the direction of the legs of the E. If the child has difficulty following these directions, a card with a large E on it can be given the child with instructions to turn the E to match the letter indicated on the chart. Test each eye separately. If the child wears glasses, vision should be tested both with and without corrective lenses.

Examine visual acuity of younger children by observing their activities. Provide an opportunity for the child to play with toys in the examining room. Watch the child's stacking, building, or placing objects inside of others. Children should have no visual difficulties in performing these tasks. The anticipated visual acuity of young children is as follows (Sprague, 1983):

Age	Visual Acuity
3 years	20/50
4 years	20/40
5 years	20/30
6 years	20/20

When you are testing visual acuity in the youngster, any difference in the scores between the eyes should be detected. A two-line difference (e.g., 20/50 and 20/30) may indicate amblyopia.

Examination of extraocular movements and cranial nerves III, IV, and VI are performed as with adults. You may, however, need to hold the child's head still and use an appealing object such as a teddy bear for the child to follow through the six cardinal fields of gaze. Peripheral vision can be tested in cooperative children; the young child may prefer to sit on the parent's lap while these tests are performed.

Patience is very often needed to gain the child's cooperation for the funduscopic examination. The young child is often unable to keep the eyes still and focused on a distant object. Position the young child supine on the examining table, his or her head near one end. Stand at the end of the table and use your right eye to examine the child's left eye and vice versa. Do not hold the child's eyelids open forcibly, because that effort will only lead to some resistance. Remember all retinal findings will appear upside down. Rather than move the ophthalmoscope to visualize all retinal fields, inspect the optic disc, the fovea, and the vessels as they pass by. Often you may do better when the child sits on the parent's lap.

Common Abnormalities

Internal Eye

Band Keratopathy

Band keratopathy is produced by the deposition of calcium in the cornea. It appears as horizontal grayish bands interspersed with dark areas that look like holes. Band keratopathy appears as a line where the eyelids close just below the pupil and passes over the cornea rather than around the iris as arcus senilis does. This finding is most commonly seen in patients with hyperparathyroidism, but it occasionally occurs in individuals with renal failure or syphilis (Fig. 6-35).

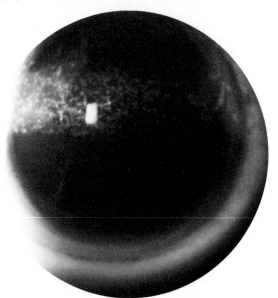

Fig. 6-35
Band keratopathy.
From Apple and Rabb, 1985.

Chorioretinitis

Chorioretinitis is an inflammatory process that involves both the choroid and the retina. It results in a sharply defined lesion that is generally whitish yellow and stippled with dark pigment. The most common cause of these lesions today is laser therapy for diabetic retinopathy, but it may also be seen as a consequence of infectious agents such as cytomegalovirus or toxoplasmosis during fetal life (Fig. 6-36).

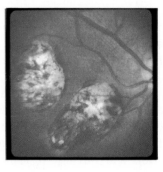

Fig. 6-36
Large patches of chorioretinitis scattered over the fundus.
From Stein and Slatt, 1983.

*Pupil Abnormalities**

Abnormality	Contributing Factors	Appearance
Bilateral		
Miosis (pupillary constriction; usually less than 2 mm in diameter)	Iridocyclitis; miotic eye drops (such as pilocarpine given for glaucoma)	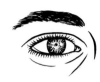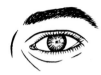
Mydriasis (pupillary dilation; usually more than 6 mm in diameter)	Iridocyclitis; mydriatic or cycloplegic drops (such as atropine); midbrain (reflex arc) lesions or hypoxia; oculomotor (CN III) damage; acute-angle glaucoma (slight dilation)	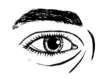
Failure to respond (constrict) with increased light stimulus	Iridocyclitis; corneal or lens opacity (light does not reach retina); retinal degeneration; optic nerve (CN II) destruction; midbrain synapses involving afferent pupillary fibers or oculomotor nerve (CN III) (consensual response is also lost); impairment of efferent fibers (parasympathetic) that innervate sphincter pupillae muscle	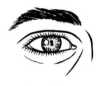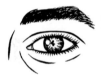
Argyll Robertson pupil	Bilateral, miotic, irregular-shaped pupils that fail to constrict with light but retain constriction with convergence; pupils may or may not be equal in size; commonly caused by neurosyphilis or lesions in midbrain where afferent pupillary fibers synapse	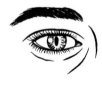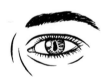
Oval pupil	Sometimes occurs with head injury or intracranial hemorrhage; transitional stage between normal pupil and dilated, fixed pupil with increased intracranial pressure (ICP); in most instances returns to normal when ICP is returned to normal	

*From Thompson et al., 1986.

Pupil Abnormalities	Abnormality	Contributing Factors	Appearance
	Unilateral Anisocoria (unequal size of pupils)	Congenital (approximately 20% of normal people have minor or noticeable differences in pupil size, but reflexes are normal) or caused by local eye medications (constrictors or dilators), amblyopia, or unilateral sympathetic or parasympathetic pupillary pathway destruction (NOTE: Examiner should test whether pupils react equally to light; if response is unequal, examiner should note whether larger or smaller eye reacts more slowly [or not at all], since either pupil could be abnormal size)	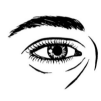
	Iritis constrictive response	Acute uveitis is frequently unilateral; constriction of pupil accompanied by pain and circumcorneal flush (redness)	Normal eye Affected eye 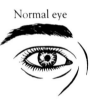
	Oculomotor nerve (CN III) damage	Pupil dilated and fixed; eye deviated laterally and downward; ptosis	Normal eye Affected eye 
	Adie's pupil (tonic pupil)	Affected pupil dilated and reacts slowly or fails to react to light; response to convergence normal; caused by impairment of postganglionic parasympathetic innervation to sphincter pupillae muscle or ciliary malfunction; often accompanied by diminished tendon reflexes (as with diabetic neuropathy or alcoholism)	Normal eye Affected eye 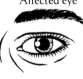

Episcleritis

Episcleritis is an inflammation of the superficial layers of the sclera anterior to the insertion of the rectus muscles. It is generally localized with a purplish elevation of a few millimeters. Often the cause of the inflammation is unknown, but it is a common manifestation of Crohn's disease, rheumatoid arthritis, and other immune disorders (Fig. 6-37).

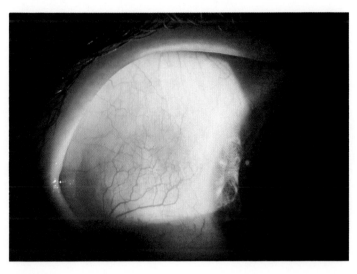

Fig. 6-37
Episcleritis.
Courtesy Andrew P. Schachat, M.D., The Wilmer Ophthalmological Institute, The Johns Hopkins University and Hospital, Baltimore.

Glaucoma

Glaucoma is an abnormal condition of elevated pressure within an eye caused by obstruction of the outflow of aqueous humor. It may occur acutely because the pupil dilates widely and the thickened iris blocks the exit of aqueous humor from the anterior chamber. Acute glaucoma is accompanied by intense ocular pain, blurred vision, a red eye, and a dilated pupil. Glaucoma may also occur chronically in which symptoms are absent except for gradual loss of peripheral vision over a period of years (Fig. 6-38).

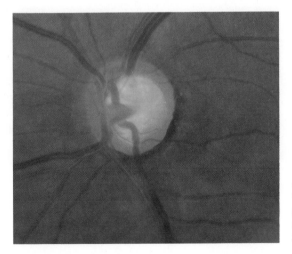

Fig. 6-38
Chronic open-angle glaucoma with optic atrophy.
From Apple and Rabb, 1985.

Horner's Syndrome

Horner's syndrome is caused by the interruption of the sympathetic nerve supply to the eye and results in miosis and ptosis. It is frequently caused by interruption of the cervical sympathetic trunk by mediastinal tumors, bronchogenic carcinoma, metastatic tumors, or operative trauma. Congenital Horner's syndrome has also been described (Fig. 6-39).

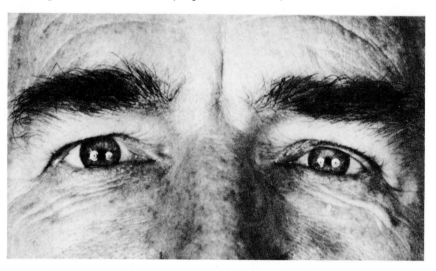

Fig. 6-39
Horner's syndrome, left eye.
From Trevor-Roper, P.D., and Curran, P.V.: The eye and its disorders, ed. 2, Oxford, 1984, Blackwell Scientific Publications, Ltd.

Cataracts

The only common abnormality of the lens is cataract formation. A cataract is an opacity occurring in the lens, most commonly from denaturation of lens protein caused by aging. Almost everyone over the age of 65 has some evidence of lens opacification. With aging the lesion is generally central, but peripheral cataracts occur in conditions such as hypoparathyroidism. Congenital cataracts can result from maternal rubella or other fetal insults during the first trimester of pregnancy (Fig. 6-40).

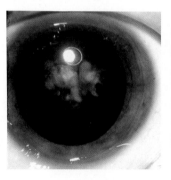 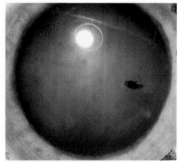

A   **B**

Fig. 6-40
A, Snowflake cataract of diabetes. B, Senile cataract.
From Donaldson, 1976.

Optic Atrophy

Optic atrophy is the result of death of nerve fibers and myelin sheaths. The primary symptom of optic atrophy is loss of central or peripheral vision or both. The disc or a portion of it loses its yellowish hue and becomes stark white (Fig. 6-41).

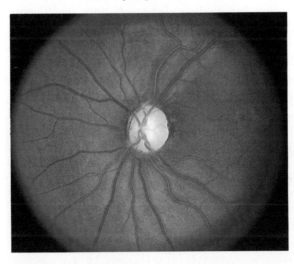

Fig. 6-41
Optic atrophy.
Courtesy Andrew P. Schachat, M.D., The Wilmer Ophthalmological Institute, The Johns Hopkins University and Hospital, Baltimore.

Diabetic Retinopathy (Background)

Diabetic retinopathy is generally divided into background and proliferative retinopathy. Background retinopathy is marked by dot hemorrhages or microaneurysms and the presence of hard and soft exudates. Hard exudates, thought to be the result of lipid transudation through incompetent capillaries, have sharply defined borders and tend to be bright yellow. Soft exudates are caused by infarction of the nerve layer and appear as dull yellow spots with poorly defined margins (Fig. 6-42).

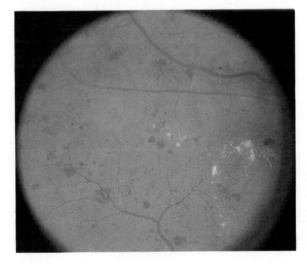

Fig. 6-42
Background diabetic retinopathy.
Courtesy Andrew P. Schachat, M.D., The Wilmer Ophthalmological Institute, The Johns Hopkins University and Hospital, Baltimore.

Diabetic Retinopathy (Proliferative)

Proliferative retinopathy is the development of new vessels as the result of anoxic stimulation. The new vessels lack the supporting structure of normal vessels and are likely to hemorrhage. These vessels grow out of the retina toward the vitreous humor, and visualization may require change in the lens setting of the ophthalmoscope. Bleeding from these vessels is an important cause of blindness in patients with diabetes. The same lesion may be seen in the infant born prematurely who has retrolental fibroplasia as a result of oxygen therapy. Laser therapy for diabetic retinopathy can often control this neovascularization and prevent blindness from occurring. Laser therapy in the premature infant is still experimental (Fig. 6-43).

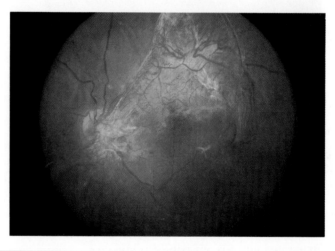

Fig. 6-43
Proliferative diabetic retinopathy.
Courtesy Andrew P. Schachat, M.D., The Wilmer Ophthalmological Institute, The Johns Hopkins University and Hospital, Baltimore.

Lipemia Retinalis

Lipemia retinalis is a dramatic condition that occurs when the serum triglyceride level exceeds 2,000 mg/dl. The blood vessels become progressively pink then white as the triglyceride level rises. This condition may be seen in diabetic ketoacidosis and in some of the hyperlipidemic states (Fig. 6-44).

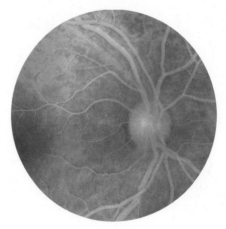

Fig. 6-44
Lipemia retinalis.
From Newell, 1986.

Retinitis Pigmentosa

Retinitis pigmentosa is a congenital condition characterized initially by night blindness that often progresses to loss of peripheral vision circumferentially and to blindness by age 50 or 60 (Fig. 6-45).

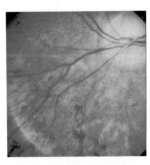

Fig. 6-45
Retinitis pigmentosa.
From Stein and Slatt, 1983.

Visual Fields

Hemianopia

Defective vision or blindness in half the visual field may be a consequence of degenerative changes within the eye itself, such as a cataract, or may stem from a lesion of the optic nerve anterior to its decussation.

Homonymous hemianopia can be caused by a lesion arising in either of two areas of the optic nerve radiation in the brain. The lesion may occur after the optic chiasma and therefore involve nerve fibers arising from the same side of each eye. This disorder is also caused by the complete interruption of the nerve fibers as they progress to the optic cortex (Fig. 6-46, *A*).

Bitemporal hemianopia is caused by a lesion interrupting the optic chiasma, most commonly a pituitary tumor (Fig. 6-46, *B*).

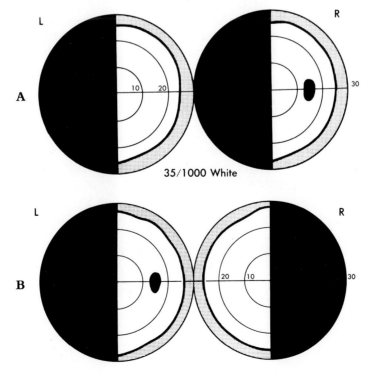

Fig. 6-46
A, Left homonymous hemianopia. B, Bitemporal hemianopia.
From Stein and Slatt, 1983.

Extraocular Muscles

Strabismus (Paralytic and Nonparalytic)

Strabismus is a condition in which both eyes do not focus on an object simultaneously. The condition may be paralytic, caused by impairment of one or more extraocular muscles or their nerve supply, or nonparalytic in which there is no primary muscle weakness. In the nonparalytic form the patient can focus with either eye but not with both simultaneously (Fig. 6-47).

If a nerve supplying an extraocular muscle has been interrupted or the muscle itself has become weakened, the eye will fail to move in the direction of the damaged muscle. For example, if the right sixth nerve is damaged, the right eye does not move temporally. This condition is called paralytic strabismus.

Nonparalytic strabismus implies no muscle weakness or neuronal abnormality. It is detected by having the patient observe a near object. When one eye is covered, the other one will move to focus on the object if the covered eye was the dominant one. (Review cover-uncover testing in the section on examination in this chapter.)

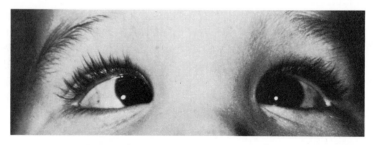

Fig. 6-47
Right convergent strabismus.
From Stein and Slatt, 1983.

External Eye

Exophthalmos

Exophthalmos is an increase in the volume of the orbital content causing a protrusion of the globes forward (Fig. 6-48). It may be bilateral or unilateral. The most common cause is Grave's disease, but when the exophthalmos is unilateral, a retroorbital tumor must be considered. The exophthalmos may be exaggerated by retraction of the upper lid and exposure of the sclera above the iris. Examination for exophthalmos is best conducted with the patient seated and the examiner standing above and looking down over the forehead. Precise quantification of the exophthalmos requires the use of an exophthalmometer. Blacks and whites of Mediterranean descent may have prominent eyes as a normal variant.

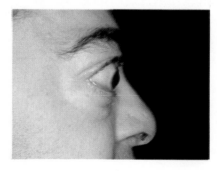

Fig. 6-48
Thyroid exophthalmos.
From Stein and Slatt, 1983.

CHILDREN

Retinoblastoma

Retinoblastoma is a congenital malignant tumor arising from the retina during the first 2 years of life. The retinoblastoma may be transmitted either by an autosomal dominant trait or by a chromosomal mutation. Initial signs are a white reflex, or cat's eye reflex, rather than the usual red reflex. Funduscopic examination reveals an ill-defined mass arising from the retina. Often chalky-white areas of calcification can be seen (Fig. 6-49).

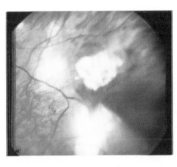

Fig. 6-49
Retinoblastoma, the most common retinal tumor in children.
From Stein and Slatt, 1983.

Retrolental Fibroplasia (Retinopathy of Prematurity)

Retrolental fibroplasia is associated with anoxic episodes and a high oxygen saturation in preterm infants during the first few days of life. The condition may lead to neovascularization, vitreous hemorrhage, retinal detachment, glaucoma, and blindness (Fig. 6-50).

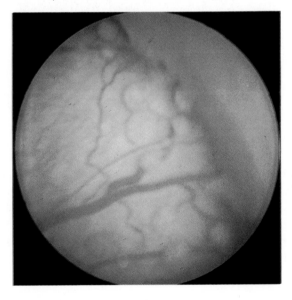

Fig. 6-50
Retrolental fibroplasia (retinopathy of prematurity).
From Garoon, 1980.

Ears, Nose, and Throat

Much information about the function of the respiratory and digestive tracts can be gleaned from their accessible orifices—the ears, nose, mouth, and throat. The special senses of smell, hearing, equilibrium, and taste are also located in the ears, nose, and mouth.

Anatomy and Physiology

Ear

The ear is a sensory organ that functions in the identification, localization, and interpretation of sound as well as in the maintenance of equilibrium. Anatomically, it is divided into the external, middle, and inner ear (Figs. 7-1 and 7-2).

The *external ear,* including the auricle and external auditory canal, is composed of cartilage covered with skin. The auricle, extending slightly outward from the skull, is positioned on a nearly vertical plane. Note its structural landmarks in Fig. 7-3.

The external auditory canal, an S-shaped pathway leading to the middle ear, is approximately 2.5 cm in length in adults. Its skeleton of bone and cartilage is covered with very thin, sensitive skin. This canal lining is protected and lubricated with cerumen, secreted by the sebaceous glands in the distal third of the canal.

The *middle ear* is an air-filled cavity in the temporal bone. It contains the ossicles, three small connected bones (malleus, incus, and stapes) that transmit sound from the tympanic membrane to the oval window of the inner ear. The air-filled cells of the mastoid area of the temporal bone are continuous with the middle ear. The tympanic membrane, surrounded by a dense fibrous ring (annulus), separates the external ear from the middle ear. It is concave, being pulled in at the center (umbo) by the malleus. The tympanic membrane is translucent, permitting visualization of the middle ear cavity, including the malleus. Its oblique position to the auditory canal and conical shape account for the triangular light reflex. Most of the tympanic membrane is tense (the pars tensa), but the superior portion (pars flaccida) is more flaccid (Fig. 7-4).

The middle ear mucosa produces a small amount of mucus, which is rapidly cleared by the ciliary action of the eustachian tube, a cartilaginous and bony passageway between the nasopharynx and the middle ear. This passage opens briefly to equalize the middle ear pressure with that of atmospheric pressure when swallowing, yawning, or sneezing.

The *inner ear* is a membranous curved cavity inside a bony labyrinth consisting of the vestibule, semicircular canals, and cochlea. The cochlea, a coiled structure containing the organ of Corti, transmits sound impulses to the eighth cranial nerve. The semicircular canals contain the end organs for vestibular function.

Fig. 7-1
Cross-section of the external, middle, and inner ear in relationship to other structures of the head and face.

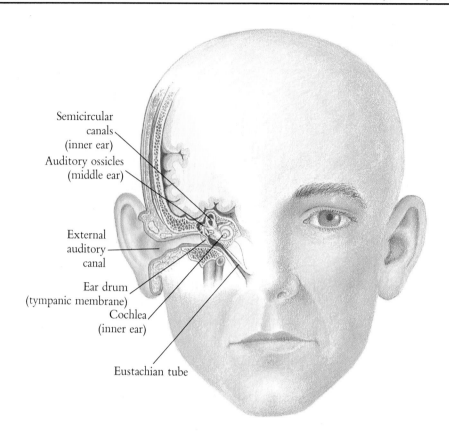

Semicircular canals (inner ear)

Auditory ossicles (middle ear)

External auditory canal

Ear drum (tympanic membrane)

Cochlea (inner ear)

Eustachian tube

Fig. 7-2
Anatomy of the ear.

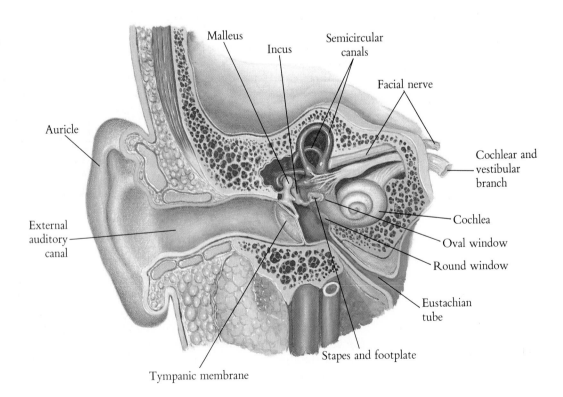

Malleus

Incus

Semicircular canals

Facial nerve

Cochlear and vestibular branch

Auricle

Cochlea

Oval window

Round window

External auditory canal

Eustachian tube

Stapes and footplate

Tympanic membrane

Fig. 7-3
Anatomic structures of the auricle. The helix is the prominent outer rim while the antihelix is the area parallel and anterior to the helix. The concha is the deep cavity containing the auditory canal meatus. The tragus is the protuberance lying anterior to the auditory canal meatus while the antitragus is the protuberance on the antihelix opposite the tragus. The lobule is the soft lobe on the bottom of the auricle.

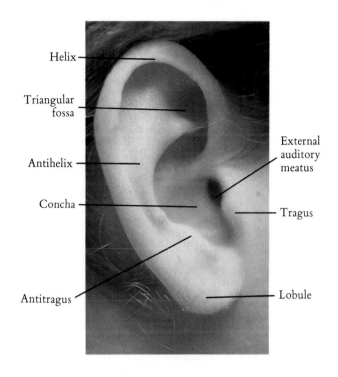

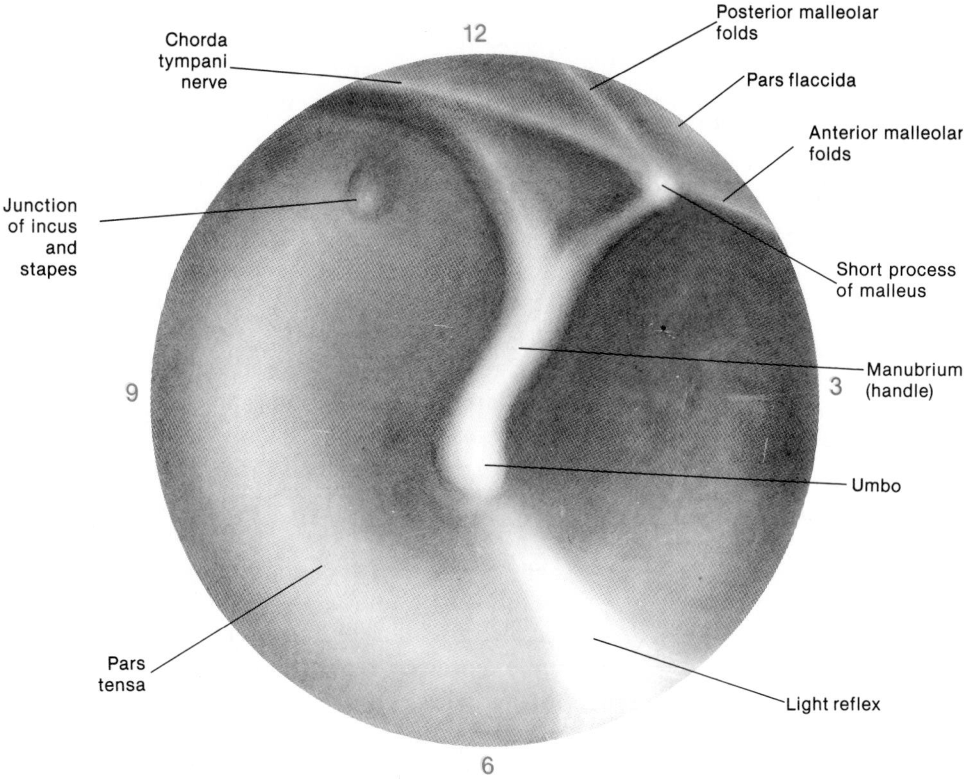

Helix

Triangular fossa

Antihelix

Concha

Antitragus

External auditory meatus

Tragus

Lobule

Fig. 7-4
Structural landmarks of the tympanic membrane.
From Whaley and Wong, 1983.

Chorda tympani nerve

Junction of incus and stapes

Pars tensa

12

9

6

Posterior malleolar folds

Pars flaccida

Anterior malleolar folds

Short process of malleus

Manubrium (handle)

3

Umbo

Light reflex

Fig. 7-5
Ossicles of the right middle
ear.
From Thompson et al., 1986.

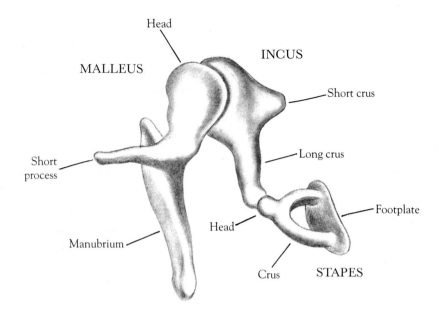

Hearing

Hearing is an interpretation of sound waves by the brain. Sound waves travel through the external auditory canal and strike the tympanic membrane, setting it in vibration. The malleus, attached to the tympanic membrane, begins vibrating as do the incus and stapes, which are attached to the malleus on the other side (Fig. 7-5). The vibrations are passed to the oval window of the inner ear in which the stapes is inserted. From here they travel via the fluid of the cochlea to the round window where they are dissipated. Vibrations in the membrane cause the delicate hair cells of the organ of Corti to impact against the membrane of Corti, stimulating impulses in the sensory endings of the auditory division of the eighth cranial nerve. These impulses are transmitted to the temporal lobe of the brain for interpretation. Sound vibrations may also be transmitted by bone directly to the inner ear.

Nose and Nasopharynx

The nose and nasopharynx have several functions:
- Identification of odors
- Passageway for inspired and expired air
- Humidification, filtration, and warmth of inspired air
- Resonation of laryngeal sound

The external nose is formed by bone and cartilage and covered with skin. The nares, which are the anterior openings of the nose, are surrounded by the cartilaginous ala nasi and columella. The frontal and maxillary bones form the nasal bridge (Fig. 7-6).

The floor of the nose is formed by the hard and soft palate, while the roof is formed by the frontal and sphenoid bone. The internal nose is covered by a vascular mucous membrane thickly lined with small hairs and mucous secretions. This membrane collects and carries debris and bacteria from inspired air to the nasopharynx for swallowing or expectoration.

The internal nose is divided by the septum into two anterior cavities, the vestibules. Inspired air enters the nose through the nares, passes through the vestibules to the choanae, which are posterior openings leading to the nasopharynx. The cribriform plate, housing the sensory endings of the olfactory nerve, lies on the roof of the nose. Kiesselbach's plexus is a convergence of small fragile arteries and veins located superficially on the anterior superior portion of the septum. The adenoids lie on the posterior wall of the nasopharynx (Fig. 7-7).

The lateral walls of the nose are formed by turbinates, curved bony structures covered by vascular mucous membrane, that run horizontally and protrude into the nasal cavity. The inferior, medial, and superior turbinates increase the surface area of the nose to warm, humidify, and filter inspired air. A meatus in the area below each turbinate is named for the turbinate above it. The nasolacrimal duct drains into the inferior meatus, while the paranasal sinuses drain into the medial meatus.

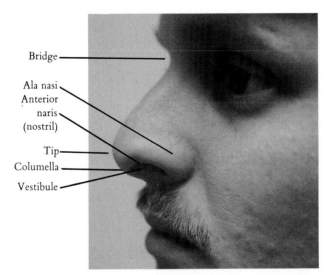

Fig. 7-6
Anatomic structures of the external nose.

Bridge

Ala nasi
Anterior
naris
(nostril)
Tip
Columella
Vestibule

Fig. 7-7
Cross-section view of the anatomic structures of the nose and nasopharynx.

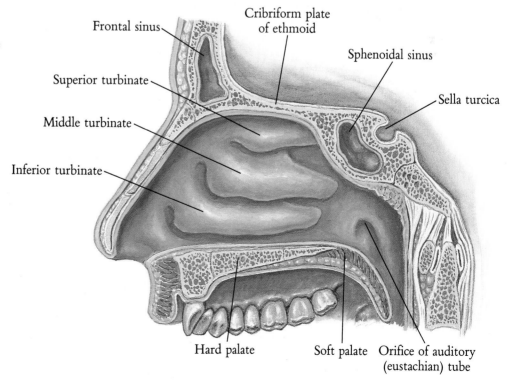

Frontal sinus

Cribriform plate
of ethmoid

Sphenoidal sinus

Superior turbinate

Sella turcica

Middle turbinate

Inferior turbinate

Hard palate

Soft palate

Orifice of auditory
(eustachian) tube

Sinuses

The paranasal sinuses are air-filled, paired extensions of the nasal cavities within the bones of the skull. They are lined with mucous membranes and cilia that move secretions along excretory pathways. Their openings into the medial meatus of the nasal cavity are easily obstructed.

The maxillary sinuses lie along the lateral wall of the nasal cavity in the maxillary bone. The frontal sinuses are in the frontal bone superior to the nasal cavities. Only

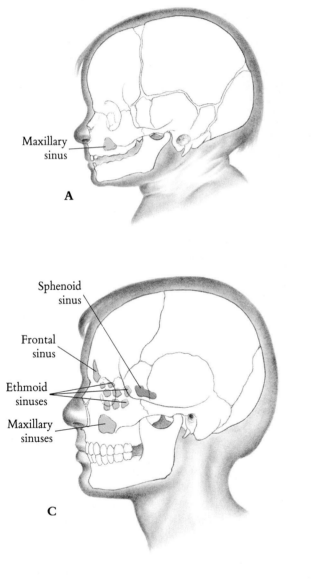

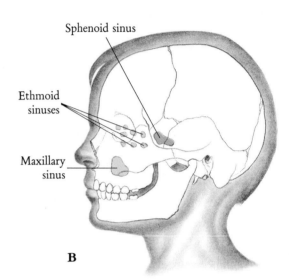

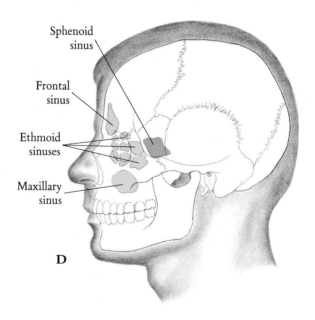

Fig. 7-8
Location of the paranasal sinuses and comparison of their size by age. **A,** Infant, 1 year. **B,** Young child, 6 years. **C,** School-age child, 10 years. **D,** Adult, 21 years.

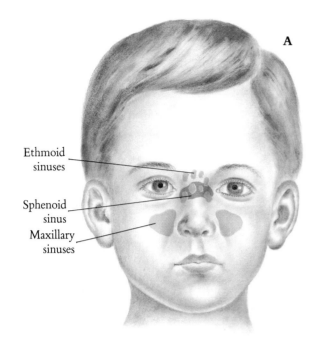

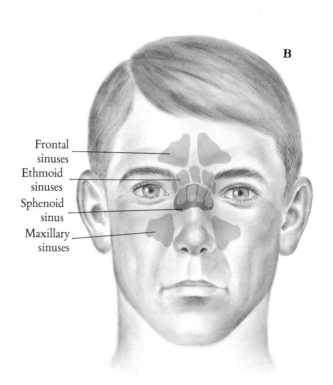

Fig. 7-9
Anterior view of the cranial sinuses. A, Six-year-old child. B, Adult.

the maxillary and frontal sinuses are accessible for physical examination. The ethmoid sinuses lie behind the frontal sinuses and near the superior portion of the nasal cavity. The sphenoid sinuses are deep in the skull behind the ethmoid sinuses (Figs. 7-8 and 7-9).

Mouth and Oropharynx

The mouth and oropharynx have several functions:
- Emission of air for vocalization and non-nasal expiration
- Passageway for food, liquid, and saliva either swallowed or vomited
- Initiation of digestion by masticating solid foods and by salivary secretion
- Identification of taste

The oral cavity is divided into the mouth and the vestibule. The vestibule is the space between the buccal mucosa and the outer surface of the teeth and gums. The mouth, housing the tongue, teeth, and gums, is the anterior opening of the oropharynx. The roof of the mouth is formed by the bony arch of the hard palate and fibrous soft palate. The uvula hangs from the posterior margin of the soft palate (Fig. 7-10).

The floor of the mouth is formed by loose, mobile tissue covering the mandibular bone. The tongue is anchored to the back of the oral cavity at its base and to the floor of the mouth by the frenulum. The dorsal surface of the tongue is covered with thick mucous membrane, supporting the filiform papillae. The ventral surface of the tongue has visible veins and fimbriated folds, thin mucous membrane with ridges (Fig. 7-11).

Fig. 7-10
Anatomic structures of the oral cavity.

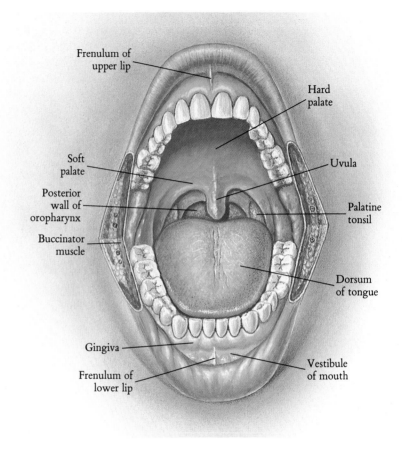

Fig. 7-11
Landmarks of the ventral surface of the tongue.

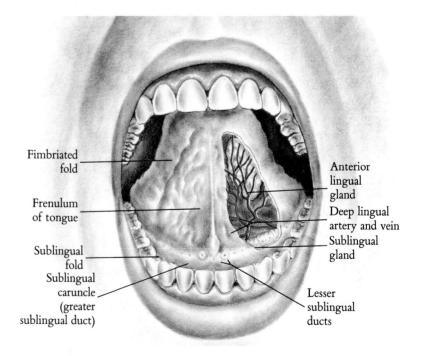

The parotid, submandibular, and sublingual salivary glands are located in tissues surrounding the oral cavity. The secreted saliva initiates digestion and moistens the mucosa. Stenson's ducts are outlets of the parotid gland that open on the buccal mucosa opposite the second molar on each side of the upper jaw. Wharton's ducts, outlets of the submandibular glands, open on each side of the frenulum under the tongue. The sublingual glands have many ducts opening along the sublingual fold.

The gingivae, fibrous tissue covered by mucous membrane, are attached directly to the alveolar surface. The roots of the teeth are anchored to the alveolar ridges, and the gingivae cover the neck and roots of each tooth. Adults have 32 permanent teeth consisting of 4 incisors, 2 canines, 4 premolars, and 6 molars, including wisdom teeth, in each jaw (Fig. 7-12).

The oropharynx, continuous with but inferior to the nasopharynx, is separated from the mouth by the anterior and posterior tonsillar pillars on each side. The tonsils, lying in the cavity between these pillars, have crypts that collect cell debris and food particles.

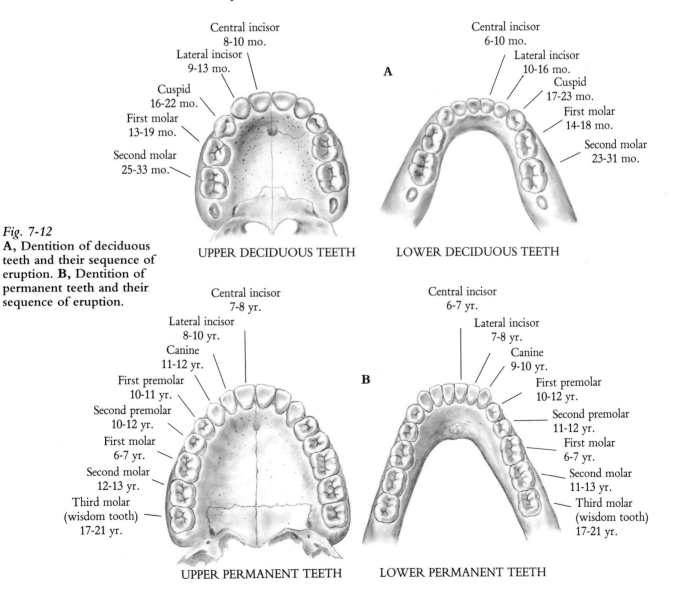

Fig. 7-12
A, Dentition of deciduous teeth and their sequence of eruption. **B,** Dentition of permanent teeth and their sequence of eruption.

Central incisor
8-10 mo.
Lateral incisor
9-13 mo.
Cuspid
16-22 mo.
First molar
13-19 mo.
Second molar
25-33 mo.

Central incisor
6-10 mo.
Lateral incisor
10-16 mo.
Cuspid
17-23 mo.
First molar
14-18 mo.
Second molar
23-31 mo.

A

UPPER DECIDUOUS TEETH   LOWER DECIDUOUS TEETH

Central incisor
7-8 yr.
Lateral incisor
8-10 yr.
Canine
11-12 yr.
First premolar
10-11 yr.
Second premolar
10-12 yr.
First molar
6-7 yr.
Second molar
12-13 yr.
Third molar
(wisdom tooth)
17-21 yr.

Central incisor
6-7 yr.
Lateral incisor
7-8 yr.
Canine
9-10 yr.
First premolar
10-12 yr.
Second premolar
11-12 yr.
First molar
6-7 yr.
Second molar
11-13 yr.
Third molar
(wisdom tooth)
17-21 yr.

B

UPPER PERMANENT TEETH   LOWER PERMANENT TEETH

Fig. 7-13
Positioning of eardrum in A, infant, and B, child over 3 years of age.
From Whaley and Wong, 1983.

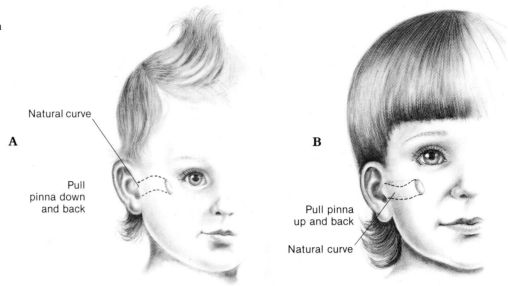

Natural curve

A

Pull
pinna down
and back

B

Pull pinna
up and back

Natural curve

CHILDREN

Because development of the inner ear occurs during the first trimester of pregnancy, an insult to the fetus during that time may impair hearing. The infant's external auditory canal is shorter than the adult's and has an upward curve. The infant's eustachian tube is relatively wider, shorter, and more horizontal than the adult's, which allows easier access for ascending infection from the pharynx. As the child grows, the eustachian tube lengthens and its pharyngeal orifice moves inferiorly (Fig. 7-13). With the growth of lymphatic tissue, specifically the adenoids, the eustachian tube may become occluded, interfering with aeration of the middle ear.

While the maxillary and ethmoid sinuses are present at birth, they are very small. The sphenoid sinus is a tiny cavity at birth that is not fully developed until puberty. The frontal sinus develops by 7 to 8 years of age.

Salivation increases by the time the infant is 3 months old, and the infant drools until it learns to swallow the saliva. Deciduous teeth begin to calcify in the third month of fetal life, each tooth erupting when it has sufficient calcification to withstand chewing. The 20 deciduous teeth usually appear between 6 and 24 months of age. The permanent teeth begin forming in the jaw by 6 months of age. Pressure from these teeth lead to the resorption of the roots of the deciduous teeth until the crown is shed. Eruption of the permanent teeth begins about 6 years of age and continues until about 18 years of age when the third molars (wisdom teeth) usually erupt.

PREGNANT WOMEN

Elevated levels of estrogen cause increased vascularity of the upper respiratory tract. The capillaries of the nose, pharynx, and eustachian tubes become engorged, leading to symptoms of nasal stuffiness, epistaxis, a sense of fullness in the ears, and impaired hearing. Increased vascularity and proliferation of connective tissue of the gums also occurs.

OLDER ADULTS

Hearing tends to deteriorate with degeneration of hair cells in the organ of Corti, usually after age 50. The stria vascularis, a network of capillaries that secrete endolymph and promote the sensitization of hair cells in the cochlea, may atrophy, contributing to hearing loss. Sensorineural hearing loss first occurs with high frequency sounds and then progresses to lower frequency tones.

Hearing deterioration may also result from an excess deposition of bone cells along the ossicle chain, causing fixation of the stapes in the oval window. Fewer sebaceous glands are active, and consequently the cerumen may become very dry. Cerumen may totally obstruct the external auditory canal, interfering with sound transmission. The tympanic membrane becomes more translucent and sclerotic. Conductive hearing loss occurs in each case.

Cartilage formation continues in the ears and nose, making the auricle and nose larger and more prominent. The soft tissues of the mouth change as the granular lining on the lips and cheeks becomes more prominent. The gingival tissue is less elastic and more vulnerable to trauma. The tongue becomes more fissured. The older adult may have altered motor function of the tongue leading to problems with swallowing.

The papillae on the lateral edges of the tongue gradually atrophy after 45 years of age. The decline in number of papillae and taste buds per papillae lead to reduced taste perception, especially sweet and salty tastes.

Gingival recession occurs with increasing age, leaving the root surface of the teeth exposed to caries formation. Teeth darken, losing their translucency, and are worn down from long use.

Review of Related History

General Considerations

1. Environmental hazards: exposure to loud, continuous noises (factory, airport, play in rock band); types of protective hearing devices used
2. Nutrition: excessive sugar intake, foods eaten
3. Oral care patterns: tooth brushing and flossing; last visit to dentist; current condition of the teeth, braces, dentures, bridges, crowns
4. Tobacco use: pipe, cigarettes, cigars, smokeless; amount, number of years (associated with oral cancer)
5. Cocaine use
6. Medications taken
   a. Ototoxic: salicylates, aminoglycosides, furosemide, streptomycin, quinine, ethacrynic acid
   b. Nose drops or sprays: amount, frequency, duration

Present Problem

1. Dizziness or vertigo
   a. Time of onset, duration of attacks
   b. Description (to and fro movement or rotary motion—room moving around patient or patient rotating), change of sensation with position change, associated with head and neck movement
   c. Associated symptoms: nausea, vomiting, presence or absence of tinnitus and hearing loss, visual changes
   d. Unsteadiness, loss of balance, falling

2. Earache
   a. Onset, duration, pain, fever, discharge (serous, mucoid, purulent, sanguinous)
   b. Concurrent upper respiratory infection, frequent swimming, trauma to head; related complaints in the mouth, teeth, sinuses, or throat
   c. Associated symptoms: reduced hearing, ringing in ear, vertigo
   d. Method of ear cleaning
3. Hearing loss: one or both ears
   a. Onset: instant (may indicate vascular disruption), over few hours or days (may indicate viral infection), slow or gradual
   b. Hears best: on telephone, in quiet or noisy environment; all sounds reduced or some sounds garbled
   c. Speech: soft or loud
   d. Management: hearing aid, when worn, battery change frequency; lip reading, sign language
4. Nasal discharge
   a. Character (watery, mucoid, purulent, crusty, bloody), odor, amount, duration, unilateral or bilateral
   b. Associated symptoms: sneezing, nasal congestion, itching nasal mucosa, nasal obstruction, mouth breathing, conjunctival burning or itching
   c. Seasonality of symptoms, concurrent upper respiratory infection, pain and tenderness over sinus
5. Nosebleed
   a. Frequency, amount of bleeding, nasal obstruction, treatment, difficulty stopping bleeding
   b. Predisposing factors: concurrent upper respiratory infection, dry heat, nose picking, forceful nose blowing, trauma, allergies
6. Dental problems
   a. Pain: with chewing, localized to tooth or entire jaw, severity, interference with eating, foods no longer eaten
   b. Dentures or dental appliances: snugness of fit, areas of irritation, length of time dentures worn daily
   c. Malocclusion: difficulty chewing, tooth extractions, previous orthodontic work
7. Mouth lesions
   a. Intermittent or constantly present, duration, pain
   b. Associated with stress, foods, seasons, fatigue, tobacco use, dentures
8. Sore throat
   a. Associated symptoms: painful swallowing or some relief with swallowing, fever, cough, headache, fatigue, decreased appetite, hoarseness, postnasal drip, mouth breathing
   b. Exposure to dry heat, dust, or fumes
   c. Exposure to infection, especially streptococcus

Past Medical History

1. Systemic disease: cardiovascular, diabetes mellitus, nephritis
2. Ear: frequent ear problems during childhood; surgery; antibiotic use, dosage, and duration
3. Nose: trauma, surgery, chronic nosebleeds
4. Sinuses: chronic postnasal drip, repeated sinusitis
5. Throat: frequent documented streptococcal infections, tonsillectomy, adenoidectomy

Family History

1. Hearing problems or hearing loss, Menière's disease
2. Allergies
3. Hereditary renal disease

INFANTS AND CHILDREN

1. Prenatal: maternal infection, irradiation, drug abuse (may indicate risk for congenital defect, hearing loss)
2. Prematurity: birth weight less than 1500 grams, anoxia, ototoxic antibiotic use (risk for hearing loss)
3. Erythroblastosis fetalis, bilirubin greater than 20 mg/100 ml serum (risk of hearing loss)
4. Infection: meningitis, encephalitis, recurrent otitis media, unilateral mumps, congenital syphilis (risk of hearing loss)
5. Congenital defect: cleft palate (risk of hearing loss and chronic otitis media)
6. Playing with small objects (risk of foreign body in nose, ear, throat)
7. Behaviors indicating hearing loss: no reaction to loud or strange noises, no babbling after 6 months of age, no communicative speech and reliance on gestures after 15 months of age, inattention to children the same age
8. Dental care: fluoride supplementation or fluoridated water; goes to sleep with bottle of milk or juice; when first tooth erupted, number of teeth present; thumbsucking, pacifier use

OLDER ADULTS

1. Hearing loss causing any interference with daily life
2. Any physical disability: interference with oral care, problems operating hearing aid
3. Deterioration of teeth, extractions, difficulty chewing
4. Medications decreasing salivation: anticholinergics, diuretics, antihypertensives, antihistamines, antispasmodics, antidepressants, tranquilizers

Examination and Findings

EQUIPMENT

- Otoscope with pneumatic attachment
- Nasal speculum
- Tongue blades
- Tuning fork (500 to 1000 Hz, approximates vocal frequencies)
- Gauze
- Gloves
- Penlight, sinus transilluminator, or light from otoscope

Ear

External Ear

Inspect the auricles for size, shape, symmetry, landmarks, color, and position on the head. Examine the lateral and medial surfaces and surrounding tissue, noting color, presence of deformities, lesions, and nodules. The auricle should have the same color as the facial skin, without moles, cysts or other lesions, deformities, or nodules. No openings or discharge should be present in the preauricular area. Darwin's tubercle, a thickening along the upper ridge of the helix, is a normal variation.

The color of the auricles may vary with certain conditions. Blueness may indicate some degree of cyanosis. Pallor or excessive redness may be the result of vasomotor instability. Frostbite can cause extreme pallor.

An unusual size or shape of the auricle may be a familial trait or indicate abnormality. A cauliflower ear is the result of blunt trauma and necrosis of the underlying cartilage. Tophi—small, whitish uric acid crystals along the peripheral margins of the auricles—may indicate gout. Sebaceous cysts, which are elevations in the skin with a punctum indicating a blocked sebaceous gland, are common (Fig. 7-14).

To determine the position of the auricle, draw an imaginary line between the outer canthus of the eye and the most prominent protuberance of the occiput. The top of the auricle should touch or be above this line. Then draw another imaginary line perpendicular to the previous line just anterior to the auricle. The auricle's position should be almost vertical, with no more than a 10 degree lateral posterior angle (Fig. 7-15). An auricle with a low-set or unusual angle may indicate chromosomal aberrations or renal disorders.

Palpate the auricles and mastoid area for tenderness, swelling, or nodules. The consistency of the auricle should be firm, mobile, and without nodules. If folded forward it should readily recoil to its usual position. Pulling gently on the lobule should cause no pain. If pain is present, inflammation of the external auditory canal may be present. Tenderness or swelling in the mastoid area may indicate mastoiditis.

Fig. 7-14
A, Preauricular skin tag and sinus. **B,** Darwin's tubercle. **C,** Cauliflower ear. **D,** Tophi. **E,** Sebaceous cysts. **F,** Malformation of the auricle.

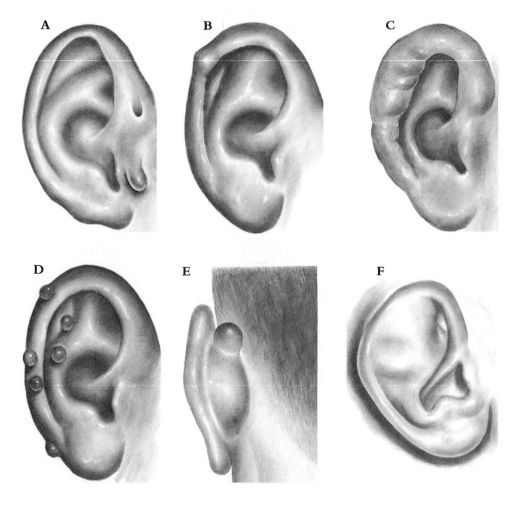

Fig. 7-15
Assessment of auricle alignment, showing expected position.

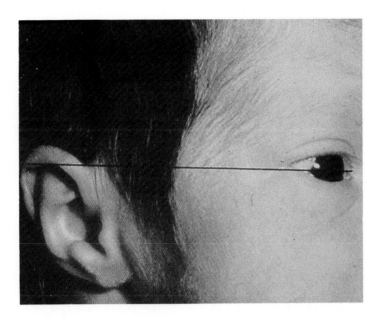

Otoscopic Examination

The otoscope is used to inspect the external auditory canal and middle ear. Select the largest size speculum that will fit comfortably in the patient's ear. Hold the handle of the otoscope in the space between your thumb and index finger, supported on the middle finger (right hand for the right ear and left hand for the left ear). This leaves the ulnar side of your hand to rest against the patient's head, stabilizing the otoscope as it is inserted into the canal. The handle of the otoscope can be held facing either up or down. Tilt the patient's head toward the opposite shoulder and simultaneously pull the patient's auricle upward and back as the speculum is inserted, thereby straightening the auditory canal to give you the best view (Fig. 7-16).

Examination of the tympanic membrane with the otoscope requires that you manipulate the auricle. This is one of innumerable times when the admonition to be gentle is underscored. A vise-like grip is not necessary; a firm, gentle grasp is. The entire procedure need not be at all uncomfortable for the patient.

As you slowly insert the speculum to a depth of 1.0 or 1.5 cm (0.5 in), inspect the auditory canal from the meatus to the tympanic membrane, noting discharge, scaling, excessive redness, lesions, foreign bodies, and cerumen. Touching the bony walls of the auditory canal (the inner two thirds) with the speculum will be painful for the patient. Expect to see minimal cerumen, a uniformly pink color, and hairs in the outer third of the canal. Cerumen may vary in color and texture but should have no odor. No lesions, discharge, or foreign body should be present.

Inspect the tympanic membrane for landmarks, color, contour, and perforations. Vary the direction of the light to see the entire tympanic membrane and the annulus. The landmarks (umbo, handle of malleus, and light reflex) should be visible (Fig. 7-17). The tympanic membrane should have no perforations and be a translucent pearly gray color. Its contour should be slightly conical with a concavity at the umbo. A bulging tympanic membrane is more conical, usually with a loss of bony landmarks and a distorted light reflex. A retracted tympanic membrane is more concave, usually with accentuated bony landmarks and a distorted light reflex (Fig. 7-18).

Fig. 7-16
Straightening the external auditory canal by pulling the helix up and out to examine the ear with the otoscope.

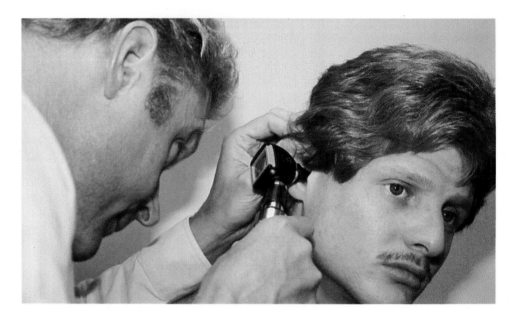

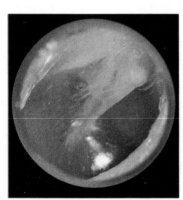

Fig. 7-17
Normal tympanic membrane.
Courtesy Dr. Richard A. Buckingham, Abraham Lincoln School of Medicine, University of Illinois, Chicago; from Malasanos et al., 1986.

A   B

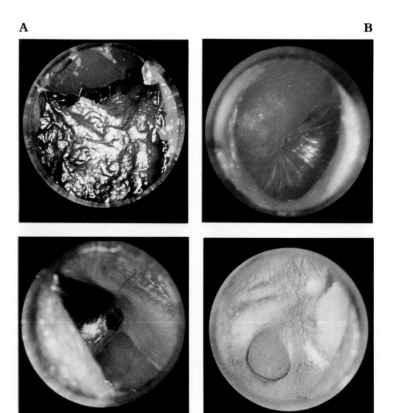

Fig. 7-18
A, Tympanic membrane partially obscured by cerumen. **B,** Bulging tympanic membrane with loss of bony landmarks. **C,** Perforated tympanic membrane. **D,** Perforated tympanic membrane that has healed.
Courtesy Dr. Richard A. Buckingham, Abraham Lincoln School of Medicine, University of Illinois, Chicago; from Malasanos et al., 1986.

C   D

CLEANING AN OBSTRUCTED AUDITORY CANAL

If the tympanic membrane is obscured by cerumen, the canal can be cleaned by warm water irrigation or by a cerumen spoon. Although a cerumen spoon is an acceptable tool for clearing out ear wax, you must remember that the auditory canal is easily abraded and bleeds readily, and when this happens, you cause pain. Water irrigation is the preferable approach, particularly with the young. If you suspect perforation of the tympanic membrane or if the auditory canal is filled with blood or discharge, it should never be irrigated.

The pneumatic attachment of the otoscope is used to evaluate the mobility of the tympanic membrane. Make sure the speculum inserted into the canal seals it from the outside air. Gently apply positive and negative pressure into the canal, either by alternately puffing and sucking on the tube or by using the squeeze bulb attachment. Observe the membrane moving in and out, indicated by a change in the appearance of the cone of light.

Tympanic membrane characteristics are associated with different conditions. A bulging tympanic membrane with no mobility is associated with pus or fluid behind the membrane. A retracted tympanic membrane with no mobility or mobility only with negative pressure is associated with obstruction of the eustachian tube resulting in a vacuum in the middle ear. Excess mobility in small areas of the tympanic membrane is associated with healed perforations.

A change in the color of the tympanic membrane is usually related to middle ear or tympanic membrane disorders. White flecks or dense white plaques indicate a healed inflammation. An amber color, fluid, or air bubbles are caused by serous fluid in the middle ear. Blue or deep red color indicates blood behind the membrane. A chalky white appearance behind the membrane or redness of the membrane may result from infection. Dullness of the membrane indicates fibrosis.

While pneumatic otoscopy has made it easier to assess the mobility of the tympanic membrane and the pressures within the middle ear, improper technique may produce misleading results. Dilation of the vessels overlying the malleus can result from applying negative pressure too slowly. The consequent redness, described as a mallear blush, may be the result of the otoscopy and can occur in the absence of infection (Bluestone and Shurin, 1974).

Hearing Evaluation

The auditory nerve (cranial nerve VIII) is tested by evaluating hearing. Screening of auditory function begins when the patient responds to your questions and directions. The patient should respond without excessive requests for repetition. Speech with a monotonous tone and erratic volume may indicate hearing loss.

WHISPERED VOICE. Check the patient's response to your whispered voice, one ear at a time. Mask the hearing in the other ear by placing your finger in the patient's ear canal, gently moving it rapidly up and down. Stand to the side of the patient, about 30 to 60 cm (1 to 2 ft) away from the ear being tested. Whisper one and two syllable words very softly and ask the patient to repeat the words heard. If the patient has difficulty, increase the loudness of the whisper gradually until the patient responds appropriately. Repeat the procedure with the other ear. The patient should hear softly whispered words in each ear at a distance of 1 to 2 ft, responding correctly at least 50% of the time.

TICKING WATCH TEST. Use a nonelectric ticking watch to test high frequency hearing. Because of the variable loudness of ticking between watches, determine the average distance from the ear at which the ticking of your watch is heard by several persons. Use this distance as the criteria to judge the patient's hearing. Mask the hearing in one ear, as described previously, and position the watch about 5 in from the other ear, slowly moving it toward the ear. Ask the patient to tell you when the ticking is heard. Repeat the procedure with the other ear.

WEBER, RINNE, AND SCHWABACH TESTS. The tuning fork is used to compare hearing by bone conduction with that by air conduction. Hold the base of the tuning fork with one hand without touching the tines, and tap the tines gently against your other hand, setting the tuning fork in vibration.

Perform the Weber test by placing the base of the vibrating tuning fork on the midline vertex of the patient's head (Fig. 7-19). Ask the patient if the sound is heard equally in both ears or is better in one ear (lateralization of sound). Avoid giving the patient a cue as to the best response. The patient should hear the sound equally in both ears. If the sound is lateralized, have the patient identify which ear hears the sound better. To test the reliability of the patient's response, repeat the procedure while occluding one ear, asking the patient in which ear the sound is best heard. It should be heard best in the occluded ear.

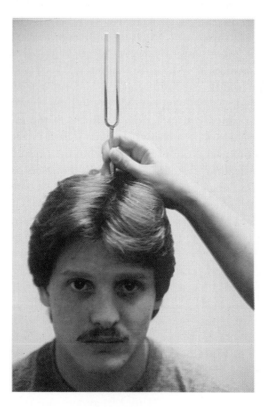

Fig. 7-19
Weber test. Place the tuning fork on the midline of the skull.

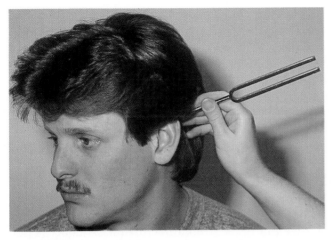
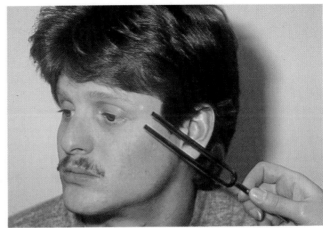

A   **B**

Fig. 7-20
Rinne test. A, Place the tuning fork on the mastoid bone for bone conduction. B, Place the tuning fork in front of the ear for air conduction.

The Rinne test is performed by placing the base of the vibrating tuning fork against the patient's mastoid bone. Begin counting or timing the interval with your watch. Ask the patient to tell you when the sound is no longer heard, noting the number of seconds. Quickly position the still vibrating tines 1 to 2 cm (0.5 to 1 in) from the auditory canal, and ask the patient to tell you when the sound is no longer heard. Continue counting or timing the interval to determine the length of time the sound is heard by air conduction (Fig. 7-20). Compare the number of seconds sound is heard by bone conduction versus air conduction. Air-conducted sound should be heard twice as long as bone-conducted sound after bone conduction stops. For example, if bone conduction is heard for 15 seconds, air conduction should be heard for an additional 30 seconds.

The Schwabach test is a comparison of the patient's and examiner's hearing by bone conduction. Alternately place the vibrating tuning fork against the patient's mastoid bone and your mastoid bone, until one of you no longer hears the sound. You should both hear the sound an equal length of time.

Determining the type of hearing loss is accomplished by integrating findings from all tuning fork techniques (Table 7-1).

Table 7-1
Interpretation of Tuning Fork Tests

Test	*Conductive Hearing Loss*	*Sensorineural Hearing Loss*
Weber	Lateralization of sound to deaf ear	Lateralization of sound to better ear
Rinne	Bone conduction heard longer than or equal to air conduction	Air conduction heard longer but not twice as long as bone conduction
Schwabach	Patient hears longer than examiner	Examiner hears longer than patient

Adapted from Prior et al., 1981.

Nose and Nasopharynx

External Nose

The nose is inspected for deviations in shape, size, or color. Observe the nares for discharge and for flaring or narrowing. The skin should be smooth without swelling and conform to the color of the face. The columella should be directly midline, and its width should not exceed the diameter of a naris. The nares are usually oval in shape and symmetrically positioned.

If discharge is present describe its character (watery, mucoid, purulent, crusty, or bloody), amount, odor, and whether unilateral or bilateral. The characteristics of nasal discharge are associated with various conditions. Bloody discharge occurs from epistaxis or trauma. Mucoid discharge is typical of rhinitis, and bilateral purulent discharge can occur with an upper respiratory infection. Unilateral, purulent, thick, greenish, and extremely malodorous discharge may indicate a foreign body.

A depression of the nasal bridge can result from a fractured nasal bone. Nasal flaring is associated with respiratory distress, while narrowing of the nares on inspiration may be indicative of chronic nasal obstruction and mouth breathing. A transverse crease at the juncture between the cartilage and bone of the nose may indicate chronic nasal itching and allergies (Fig. 7-21).

Palpate the ridge and soft tissues of the nose. Note any displacement of bone and cartilage, tenderness, or masses. Place one finger on each side of the nasal arch and gently palpate, moving the fingers from the nasal bridge to the tip. The nasal structures should feel firm and stable to palpation. No tenderness or masses should be present.

Evaluate the patency of the nares. Occlude one naris by placing a finger on the side of the nose, and ask the patient to breathe in and out with mouth closed. Repeat the procedure with the other naris. Nasal breathing should be noiseless and easy through the open naris.

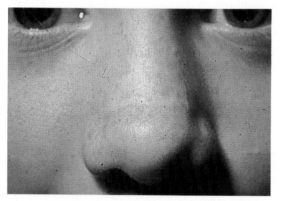

Fig. 7-21
Transverse nasal crease.

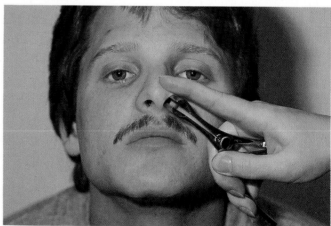

Fig. 7-22
Use of the nasal speculum.

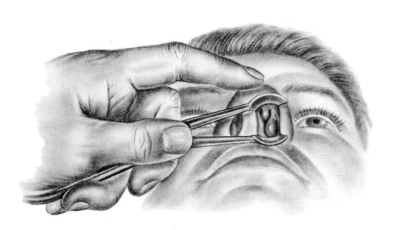

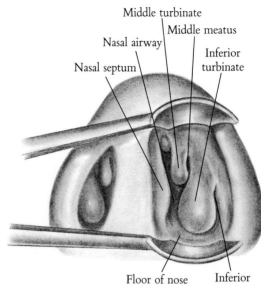

Middle turbinate

Middle meatus

Nasal airway

Inferior turbinate

Nasal septum

Floor of nose

Inferior meatus

Fig. 7-23
View of the nasal mucosa through the nasal speculum.

Nasal Cavity

Use a nasal speculum and good light source to inspect the nasal cavity. Hold the speculum in the palm of the hand and keep the index finger free for stabilization on the patient's nose. Use your other hand to change the patient's head position and to direct the light source. The speculum should be inserted slowly and cautiously. Make sure you do not overdilate the naris or touch the nasal septum, which causes pain (Fig. 7-22). Inspect the nasal mucosa for color, discharge, masses, lesions, and swelling of the turbinates. Inspect the nasal septum for alignment, perforation, bleeding, and crusting.

Only the inferior and middle turbinates will be visible. Keep the patient's head erect to examine the vestibule and inferior nasal turbinate. Tilt the patient's head back to visualize the middle meatus and middle turbinate. Then cautiously move the speculum tip toward the midline to examine the septum. Repeat the procedure in the other naris (Fig. 7-23).

The nasal mucosa should appear deep pink (pinker than the buccal mucosa) and glistening. A film of clear discharge is often apparent on the nasal septum. Hairs may be present in the vestibule. Increased redness of the mucosa may occur with an infection, whereas localized redness and swelling in the vestibule may indicate a furuncle. Unilateral purulent discharge results from the presence of a foreign body.

The turbinates should be the same color as the surrounding area and have a firm consistency. Turbinates that appear bluish gray or pale pink with a swollen, boggy consistency may indicate allergies. A rounded, elongated mass projecting into the nasal cavity from boggy mucosa may be a polyp.

The nasal septum should be close to midline and fairly straight, appearing thicker anteriorly than posteriorly. Asymmetric size of the posterior nasal cavities may indicate deviation of the nasal septum. No perforations, bleeding, or crusting should be apparent. Crusting over the anterior portion of the nasal septum may occur at the site of epistaxis (Fig. 7-24).

Fig. 7-24
Unexpected findings on
nasal examination.
A, Nasal polyp (allergic).
B, Purulent discharge.
C, Deviation of the nasal
septum.
C from Bull, 1974.

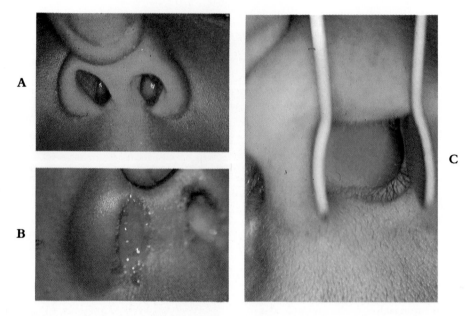

Fig. 7-25
A, Palpation of frontal
sinuses. **B,** Palpation of
maxillary sinuses.

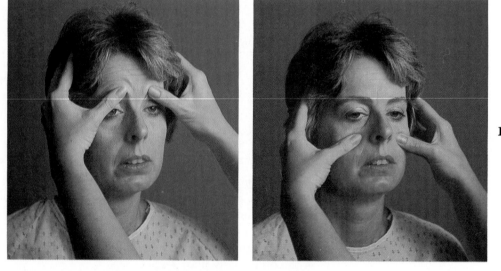

The sense of smell (olfactory nerve) is often tested. This procedure is described in Chapter 17 (Neurologic System and Mental Status) in the examination of cranial nerves.

Sinuses

Inspect the frontal and maxillary sinus areas for swelling. To palpate the frontal sinuses, use your thumbs to press up under the bony brow on each side of the nose. Then press up under the zygomatic processes, using either your thumbs or index and middle fingers to palpate the maxillary sinuses (Fig. 7-25). No tenderness or swelling over the soft tissue should be present.

Percuss the sinus areas to detect tenderness. Lightly tap directly over each sinus area with your index finger, using your wrist to produce the force behind the finger. Swelling, tenderness, and pain over the sinuses may indicate infection or obstruction.

Mouth and Oropharynx

Lips

With the patient's mouth closed, inspect and palpate the lips for symmetry, color, edema, and surface abnormalities. Make sure the female patient removes her lipstick. The lips should be pink and have vertical and horizontal symmetry, both at rest and with movement. The distinct border between the lips and the facial skin should not be interrupted by lesions. The surface characteristics of the lips should be smooth and free of lesions.

Dry, cracked lips (cheilitis) may be caused by dehydration from wind chapping. Deep fissures at the corners of the mouth (cheilosis) may indicate riboflavin deficiency or overclosure of the mouth, allowing saliva to macerate the tissue. Swelling of the lips may be caused by infection, while edema may indicate allergy. Lesions, plaques, vesicles, nodules, and ulcerations may be signs of infections, irritations, or skin cancer (Fig. 7-26).

Fig. 7-26
Unexpected findings on the lips. **A,** Angular cheilitis. **B,** Actinic cheilitis. **C,** Angioedema. **D,** Herpes labialis. **E,** Squamous cell carcinoma of the lip.
A to **C** from Habif, 1985; **D** courtesy Antoinette Hood, M.D., The Johns Hopkins University School of Medicine, Baltimore; **E** from Stewart et al., 1978.

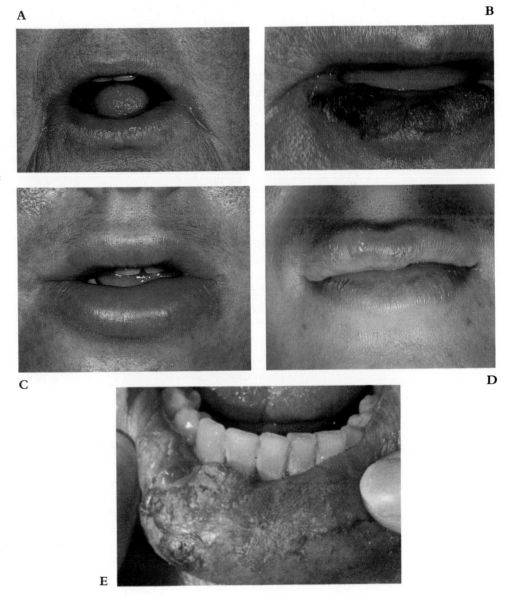

The color of the lips is influenced by various conditions. Pallor of the lips is associated with anemia, while circumoral pallor is associated with scarlet fever. Cyanosis from a respiratory or cardiovascular problem produces bluish-purple lips. A cherry red color is associated with acidosis and carbon monoxide poisoning. Round, oval, or irregular bluish gray macules of various intensity on the lips and buccal mucosa are associated with Peutz-Jeghers syndrome.

Buccal Mucosa, Teeth, and Gums

Ask the patient to clench his or her teeth and smile so you can observe the occlusion of the teeth. The facial nerve (cranial nerve VII) is also tested with this maneuver. Proper tooth occlusion is apparent when the upper molars rest directly on lower molars and the upper incisors slightly override the lower incisors. Protrusion of the upper or lower incisors, failure of the upper incisors to overlap with the lower incisors, and back teeth that do not meet are indications of malocclusion (Fig. 7-27).

Have the patient remove any dental appliances and open the mouth partially. Using a tongue blade and bright light, inspect the buccal mucosa, gums, and teeth. The mucous membrane should be pinkish red, smooth, and moist. Stenson's duct should appear as a whitish yellow or whitish pink protrusion in approximate alignment with the second upper molar.

Fordyce spots are ectopic sebaceous glands that appear on the buccal mucosa and lips as numerous small, yellow-white raised lesions and are a normal variant. Deeply pigmented buccal mucosa may indicate endocrine pathology. Whitish or pinkish scars are a common result of trauma from poor tooth alignment. Inflammation of Stenson's duct indicates parotitis (mumps). Aphthous ulcers on the buccal mucosa appear as white, round, or oval ulcerative lesions with a red halo (Fig. 7-28).

The gums should have a slightly stippled, pink appearance with a clearly defined, tight margin at each tooth. Patchy dark pigmentation may be noted in dark skinned patients. The gum surface beneath dentures should be free of inflammation, swelling, or bleeding.

Using gloves, palpate the gums for any lesions, induration, thickening, or masses. No tenderness on palpation should be elicited. Epulis, a localized gingival enlargement or granuloma, is usually an inflammatory rather than neoplastic change. Enlargement of the gums occurs with pregnancy, dilantin therapy, puberty, and leukemia. A blue-black line about 1 mm from the gum margin may indicate chronic lead or bismuth poisoning. Easily bleeding, swollen gums that have enlarged crevices between the teeth and gum margins or pockets containing debris at tooth margins are associated with gingivitis or periodontal disease (Fig. 7-29).

Inspect and count the teeth, noting wear, notches, caries, and missing teeth. Make sure teeth are firmly anchored, probing each with a tongue blade. The teeth generally have an ivory color but may be stained yellow from tobacco or brown from coffee or tea. Loose teeth can be the result of periodontal disease or trauma. Discolorations on the crown of a tooth should raise the suspicion of caries.

Oral Cavity

Inspect the dorsum of the tongue, noting any swelling, variation in size or color, coating, or ulcerations. Ask the patient to extend the tongue while you inspect for deviation, tremor, and limitation of movement. The procedure also tests the hypoglossal nerve (cranial nerve XII). The protruded tongue should not be atrophied and should be maintained at the midline without fasciculations. Deviation to one side indicates tongue atrophy and hypoglossal nerve impairment.

Fig. 7-27
A, Normal occlusion.
B, Malocclusion.
From Bowers and Thompson, 1984.

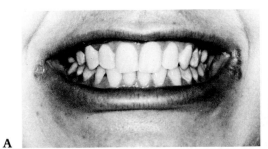

A

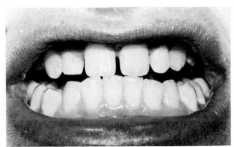

B

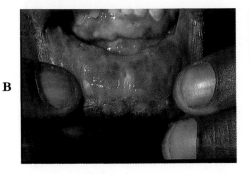

A

B

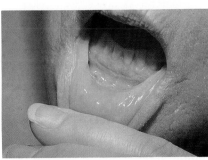

C

Fig. 7-28
Findings on the buccal mucosa. A, Fordyce spots.
B, Aphthous ulcer.
C, Pemphigus.

A from Wood and Goaz, 1985; **B** and C courtesy Antoinette Hood, M.D., The Johns Hopkins University School of Medicine, Baltimore.

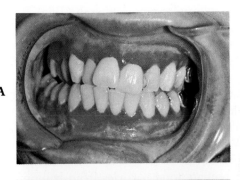

A

B

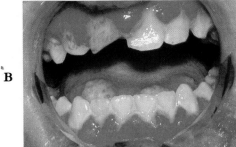

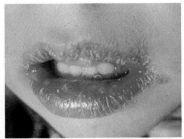

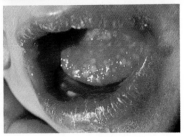

C

Fig. 7-29
Unexpected findings of the gingiva. A, Plasma cell gingivitis. **B,** Primary herpetic gingivostomatitis.
C, Primary gingivostomatitis showing lesions on the lips, tongue, and gums.

A and **B** from Wood and Goaz, P.W.: 1985; C reproduced with kind permission of the Wellcome Foundation Ltd.

Fig. 7-30
Findings on the tongue.
A, Geographic tongue.
B, Smooth tongue
resulting from vitamin
deficiency. **C,** Glossitis.
D, Dome-shaped varicosity
resembling a ranula.
E, Black hairy tongue.

A to **C** courtesy Antoinette Hood,
M.D., The Johns Hopkins University
School of Medicine, Baltimore; **D**
from Wood and Goaz, 1985; **E** from
Bull, 1974.

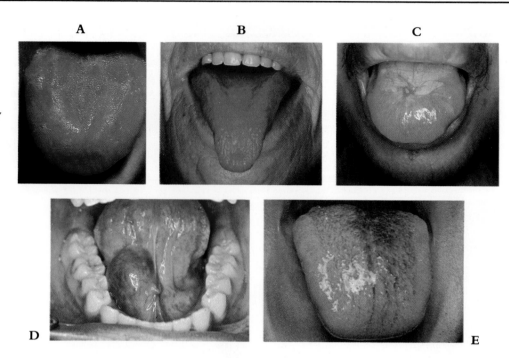

The tongue should appear dull red, moist, and glistening. Its anterior portion should have a smooth, yet roughened surface with papillae and small fissures. The posterior portion should have a smooth, slightly uneven or rugated surface with a thinner mucosa than the anterior portion. The geographic tongue, a normal variant, has superficial denuded circles or irregular areas exposing the tips of papillae. A smooth red tongue with a slick appearance may indicate niacin deficiency. The hairy tongue with yellow-brown to black elongated papillae on the dorsum sometimes follows antibiotic therapy (Fig. 7-30).

Ask the patient to touch the tongue tip to the palate area directly behind the upper incisors. Inspect the floor of the mouth and the ventral surface of the tongue for swelling and varicosities, also observing the frenulum, sublingual ridge, and Wharton's ducts. The tip of the tongue should have no difficulty touching the hard palate behind the upper central incisors. The ventral surface of the tongue should be pink and smooth with large veins between the frenulum and fimbriated folds. Wharton's ducts should be apparent on each side of the frenulum.

Wrapping the tongue with a piece of gauze, pull the tongue to each side, inspecting its lateral borders (Fig. 7-31). Any white or red margins should be scraped to differentiate food particles from leukoplakia or another fixed abnormality. Then palpate the tongue and the floor of the mouth for lumps, nodules, or ulcerations. The tongue should have a smooth, even texture without nodules, ulcerations, or areas of induration. Any ulcer, nodule, or thickened white patch on the lateral or ventral surface of the tongue should be suspect of malignancy.

Ask the patient to tilt his or her head back for you to inspect the palate and uvula. The whitish hard palate should be dome-shaped with transverse rugae. The pinker soft palate should be contiguous with the hard palate. The uvula, a midline continuation of the soft palate, varies in length and thickness. The hard palate may have a bony protuberance at the midline, called torus palatinus, which has no clinical consequence (Fig. 7-32). A nodule on the palate that is not at the midline may indicate a tumor.

Movement of the soft palate is evaluated by asking the patient to say "ah." Depressing the tongue may be necessary for this maneuver. As the patient vocalizes, observe the soft palate rise symmetrically with the uvula remaining in the midline. This maneuver also tests the glossopharyngeal and vagus nerves (cranial nerves IX and X). Failure of the soft palate to rise bilaterally with vocalization may result from paralysis of the vagus nerve. The uvula will deviate to the unaffected side (Fig. 7-33). A bifid uvula may indicate a submucous cleft of the soft palate.

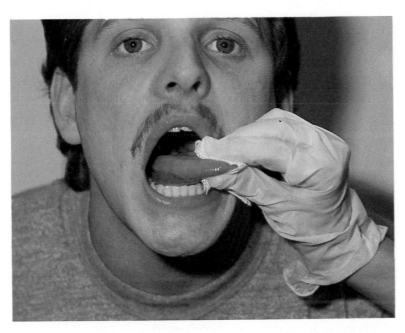

Fig. 7-31
Inspection of the lateral borders of the tongue.

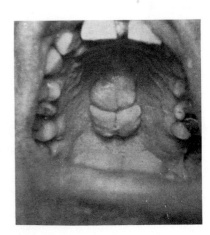

Fig. 7-32
Torus palatinus.
From DeWeese and Saunders, 1982.

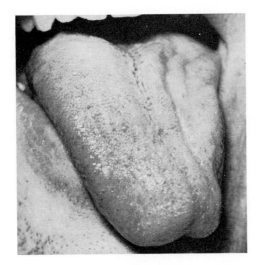

Fig. 7-33
Left hypoglossal paralysis. The tongue deviates toward the weak side.
From Saunders et al., 1979.

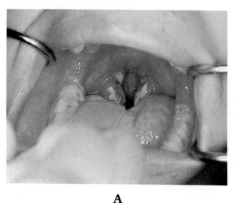

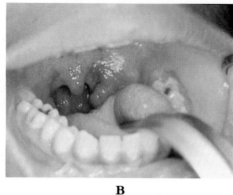

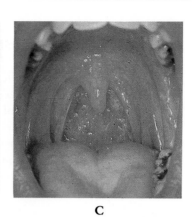

A

B

C

Fig. 7-34
Findings of the oropharynx. **A,** Tonsillitis and pharyngitis. **B,** Acute viral pharyngitis. **C,** Postnasal drip.

A and B courtesy Dr. Edward L. Applebaum, University of Illinois Medical Center, Chicago; from Malasanos et al., 1986.

Oropharynx

Inspect the oropharynx using a tongue blade to depress the tongue. A patient of any age will possibly anticipate the use of the tongue blade with some degree of anxiety. If the patient is an easy gagger, there probably is little you can do to avoid setting off this reflex. Moistening the tongue blade with warm water helps, since a warm, wet blade will not trigger the gag as frequently as a dry one. Observe the tonsillar pillars, noting the size of tonsils, if present, and the integrity of the retropharyngeal wall. The tonsils usually blend into the pink color of the pharynx and should not project beyond the limits of the tonsillar pillars. Tonsils may have crypts where cellular debris and food particles collect. If reddened, hypertrophied, and covered with exudate, an infection may be present.

The posterior wall of the pharynx should be smooth, glistening pink mucosa with some small irregular spots of lymphatic tissue and small blood vessels. A red bulge adjacent to the tonsil and extending beyond the midline may indicate a peritonsillar abscess. A yellowish mucoid film in the pharynx is typical of postnasal drip. A grayish membrane is associated with diphtheria (Fig. 7-34).

Touch the posterior wall of the pharynx on each side to elicit the gag reflex, testing the glossopharyngeal and vagus nerves (cranial nerves IX and X). This should produce a bilateral response.

Additional Procedures

Equilibrium

The Romberg test, described in Chapter 17 (Neurologic System and Mental Status) is used to screen for equilibrium in most patients. When a vestibular function disorder is suspected, as indicated by a loss of balance by the Romberg test, further evaluation of the vestibular branch of the auditory nerve (cranial nerve VIII) is indicated. In most cases, the patient is referred to a specialist for the cold caloric test or Nylen-Barany test.

For the cold caloric test have the patient sit and hyperextend the head to 60 degrees. Irrigate one auditory canal with cold water (32 to 50° F) for 20 seconds. (Caution! Do not perform this test if the patient has an acute middle ear infection or a perforated tympanic membrane.) The patient should feel nausea, dizziness, and nystagmus, appearing in about 30 seconds and lasting about 90 seconds. Normal response is horizontal nystagmus, with conjugate eye movement, turning slowly toward the ear being irrigated and then quickly to the other side. Repeat the procedure in the other auditory canal. The response should be bilaterally equal.

To perform the Nylen-Barany test, the patient should be supine with the head hyperextended about 45 degrees over the end of the examining table. When the patient turns his or her head to one side, observe for nystagmus. Repeat the procedure with the patient's head turned to the other side. Nystagmus is an unexpected finding, and if present, note the duration and the direction of eye movement (horizontal or vertical).

Transillumination

Transillumination of the frontal and maxillary sinuses is performed if sinus tenderness is present or infection is suspected. The examination must be performed in a completely darkened room. A sinus transilluminator or small bright light is used.

To transilluminate the maxillary sinuses, place the light source lateral to the nose, just beneath the medial aspect of the eye. Look through the patient's open mouth for illumination of the hard palate. To transilluminate the frontal sinuses, place the light source against the medial aspect of each supraorbital rim. Look for a dim red glow as light is transmitted just above the eyebrow. The sinuses will usually show differing degrees of illumination. The absence of a glow indicates either the sinus is filled with secretions or it never developed (Fig. 7-35).

Fig. 7-35
Transillumination of the sinuses: Placement of the light source and expected area of transillumination. A, For the maxillary sinus. **B,** For the frontal sinus.

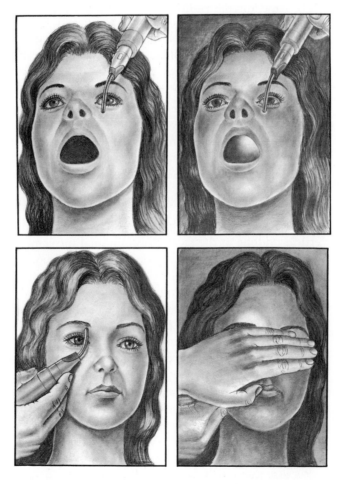

INFANTS

Because the ears, nose, mouth, and throat are frequent sites of congenital malformations in the newborn, thorough examination is important.

Ears

The auricle should be well formed with all landmarks present on inspection. The tip of the auricle should cross the imaginary line between the outer canthus of the eye and the prominent portion of the occiput, varying no more than 10 degrees from vertical. Auricles either poorly shaped or positioned below the imaginary line are associated with renal disorders or congenital anomalies.

The newborn's auricle is very flexible but should have instant recoil after bending. The premature infant's auricles may appear flattened with limited incurving of the upper auricle, and ear recoil is slower.

No skin tags or small openings in the preauricular area should be present. A small preauricular skin tag or pit is sometimes found just anterior to the tragus, indicating a remnant of the first branchial cleft.

The newborn's auditory canals are often obstructed with vernix, but they should be examined within the first few weeks of life. The infant is placed in either supine or prone position so the head can be turned side to side. Hold the otoscope so the ulnar surface of your hand rests against the infant's head, alternating the hand used (right hand for the right ear and left hand for the left ear). As the infant's head moves, the otoscope moves, preventing trauma to the auditory canal. Use your other hand to stabilize the infant's head as the thumb and index finger pull the auricle down to straighten the upward curvature of the canal. Because the tympanic membrane does not become conical for several months, the light reflex may appear diffuse.

Knowledge of the sequence of hearing development is necessary to evaluate the infant's hearing (Table 7-2). Use a noise maker, your voice, or clap your hands as a sound stimulus, taking care that the infant does not respond to the air movement generated by any of these maneuvers. Remember that responses to repeated sound stimuli will diminish as the infant tunes out the stimulus.

Nose and Sinuses

The external nose should have a symmetrical appearance and be positioned in the vertical midline of the face. Only minimal movement of the nares with breathing should be apparent. A deviation of the nose may be related to fetal position. A saddle-shaped nose with a low bridge and broad base, a short small nose, or a large nose may suggest a congenital anomaly.

Inspect the internal nose by shining a light inside after gently tilting the nose tip upward with your thumb. Infants may discharge small amounts of clear fluid with crying.

Newborns are obligatory nose breathers, so nasal patency must be determined at the time of birth. With the infant's mouth closed, occlude one naris and then the other, observing the respiratory pattern. With total obstruction, the infant will not be able to inspire or expire through the noncompressed naris. With any breathing difficulty, pass a small catheter through each naris to the choana, the posterior nasal opening. An obstruction may indicate choanal atresia or septal deviation from delivery trauma.

Because the maxillary and ethmoid sinuses are small during infancy, few problems arise in these areas, and examination is generally unnecessary.

Table 7-2
The Sequence of Expected
Hearing Response by Age

Age	Response
Birth to 3 months	Startle reflex, crying, cessation of breathing or movement in response to sudden noise; quiets to parent's voice
4 to 6 months	Turns head toward source of sound but may not always recognize location of sound; responds to parent's voice; enjoys sound-producing toys
6 to 10 months	Responds to own name, telephone ringing, and person's voice, even if not loud; begins localizing sounds above and below, turns head 45 degrees toward sound
10 to 12 months	Recognizes and localizes source of sound; imitates simple words and sounds

Adapted from Caufield, 1978.

Mouth

The lips should be well formed with no cleft. The newborn may have sucking calluses on the upper lips appearing as plaques or crusts for the first few weeks of life. Healthy newborns may have circumoral cyanosis at birth and for a short while afterwards.

The crying infant provides the opportune time to examine the mouth. Avoid depressing the tongue as this stimulates a strong reflex protrusion making visualization of the mouth difficult (Fig. 7-36).

The buccal mucosa should be pink and moist with sucking pads but have no other lesions. Scrape any white patches on the tongue or buccal mucosa with a tongue blade. Nonadherent patches are usually milk deposits, while adherent patches may indicate candidiasis (thrush). Secretions that accumulate in the newborn's mouth requiring frequent suctioning may indicate esophageal atresia.

The newborn's gums should be edentulous, smooth with a serrated edge of tissue along the buccal margins. Occasionally you will find a tooth or tooth buds in a newborn. Determine if natal teeth are loose and their potential for aspiration. The question is whether to leave them there or remove them. Such teeth are not usually firmly fixed and it is probably wisest, in most instances, to remove them. Never do this without consulting the parents first, however. In older infants, count the deciduous teeth, noting any unusual sequence of eruption. Pearl-like retention cysts that sometimes appear along the buccal margin disappear in 1 to 2 months.

The tongue should fit well in the floor of the mouth. The frenulum of the tongue usually attaches at a point midway between the ventral surface of the tongue and its tip. If the tongue protrudes beyond the alveolar ridge, no feeding difficulties should occur. Macroglossia is associated with congenital anomalies—another reminder that external clues to pathophysiologically severe problems abound. A large tongue protruding from the mouth so that it does not close should make you think of congenital hypothyroidism, for example.

The palatal arch should be dome-shaped with no clefts in either the hard or soft palate. A narrow flat palate roof or a high arched palate (associated with congenital anomalies) will affect the tongue's placement, leading to feeding and speech problems. The soft palate should rise symmetrically when the infant cries. Petechiae are often seen on the newborn's soft palate. Epstein's pearls, small whitish yellow

Fig. 7-36
Findings in the infant's mouth. A, Thrush. B, Natal teeth. C, Short frenulum. D, Macroglossia. E, Epstein's pearls.
Courtesy Mead Johnson and Co., Evansville, Indiana.

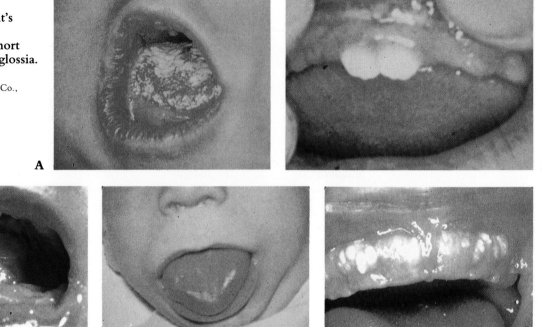

masses at the juncture between the hard and soft palate, are common and disappear within a few weeks of birth.

Insert your index finger into the infant's mouth, with the fingerpad to the roof of the mouth. Simultaneously evaluate the infant's suck and palpate the hard and soft palates. (This maneuver may be performed when quieting the infant to auscultate the heart and lungs.) The infant should have a strong suck, the tongue pushing vigorously upward against the finger. Neither the hard nor soft palate should have palpable clefts. Stimulate the gag reflex by touching the tonsillar pillars. A bilateral gag reflex should be present.

CHILDREN

Because the young child often resists otoscopic and oral examination, it is often wise to postpone these procedures until the end. Be prepared to use restraint if encouraging the child to cooperate fails. Another person, usually the parent, is needed to effectively restrain the child.

Children of any age who are not too big to sit on their parent's lap are better examined there than in a prone or supine position on the examining table. If the baby or toddler is comfortably seated in the parent's lap, back to the parent and legs between the adult's legs, the parent can then reach comfortably around to restrain the child's arms with one arm and control the child's head with the other. This can usually be accomplished without forcing, which avoids extra grief for the child, the parent, and you.

For the otoscopic examination, face the child sideways with one arm placed around th parent's waist. The parent holds the child firmly against his or her trunk, using one arm to restrain the child's head and the other arm to restrain the child's body. You further stabilize the child's head as you insert the otoscope. For the oral examination, face the child forward (Fig. 7-37).

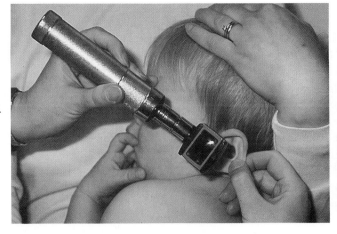

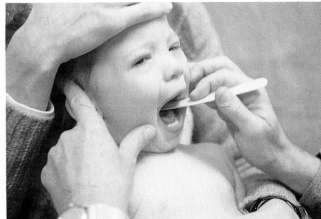

Fig. 7-37
Sitting position of toddlers and young children.
A, Otoscopic examination.
B, Oral examination.

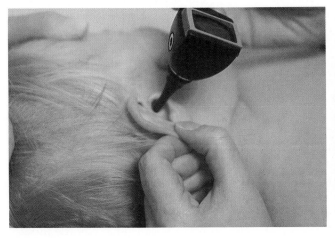

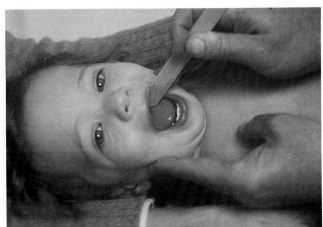

Fig. 7-38
Supine positioning of toddlers and young children. A, Otoscopic examination. **B,** Oral examination.

When the child actively resists your efforts to examine the ears and mouth, place him or her in supine position on the examining table. The parent holds the child's arms extended above the head and assists in restraining the head. You lie across the child's trunk and stabilize the child's head with your hands as you insert the otoscope or tongue blade. A third person may hold the child's legs, if necessary (Fig. 7-38).

Ears

When performing the otoscopic examination, pull the auricle either downward and back or upward and back to gain the best view of the tympanic membrane. As the child grows, the shape of the auditory canal changes to the **S**-shaped curve of the adult. If the child is crying or has recently cried vigorously, dilation of blood vessels in the tympanic membrane can cause redness. Thus you cannot assume that redness of the membrane alone is a hallmark of middle ear infection. The pneumatic otoscope is especially important to differentiate a red tympanic membrane caused by crying (the membrane is mobile) from that resulting from disease (no mobility).

Evaluate the toddler's hearing by observing the response to a whispered voice and various noisemakers (e.g., rattle, bell, tissue paper). Position yourself behind the child while the parent distracts the child. Whisper or use noisemakers outside the child's field of vision. The child should turn toward the sound consistently. Development of speech provides another indication of hearing acuity. When whispering, particularly to children, use words that will have more meaning for them, such as the name of a popular television personality or a comic strip character—Big Bird or Mickey Mouse, for example.

In addition to these procedures, evaluate the young child's hearing by asking the child to perform tasks, using a soft voice. Avoid giving visual cues. The Weber, Rinne, and Schwabach tests are used when the child understands directions and can cooperate with the examiner, usually between 3 and 4 years of age. Audiometric evaluation should be performed in all young children.

Nose and Sinuses

As with infants, when inspecting the internal nose, it is usually adequate to tilt the nose tip upward with your thumb. However, if visualization of a larger area is needed, the largest otoscopic speculum may be used.

The transverse crease at the juncture between the cartilage and the bone of the nose is often the result of the "adenoidal salute." Children are particularly prone to wipe their noses with an upward sweep of the palm of the hand, which if repeated often enough causes the crease.

The maxillary sinuses may be palpated, but few sinus problems occur in this age group since it takes many years for the sinuses to develop in children. However, there is a wide variation in the development of sinuses, so you cannot assume that the very young will not have sinusitis simply on the basis of age.

Mouth

Encourage the child to cooperate with the oral examination. Letting the child hold and manipulate the tongue blade and light may reduce the fear of the procedure. Begin by asking the child to show you his or her teeth, usually not a threatening request. Flattened edges on the teeth may indicate bruxism, unconscious grinding of the teeth. Multiple brown areas or caries on the upper and lower incisors may be the result of a bedtime bottle of juice or milk, commonly called baby bottle mouth syndrome (Fig. 7-39). Teeth with a black or gray color may indicate pulp decay or

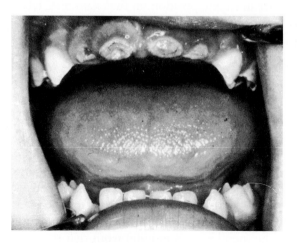

Fig. 7-39
Baby bottle syndrome.
From McDonald and Avery, 1983.

CAUTION! SPECIAL PROCEDURE IF EPIGLOTTITIS IS SUSPECTED

Suspect epiglottitis when the child has a croupy cough, sudden high fever, signs of upper respiratory obstruction, and is drooling, having difficulty swallowing, and looks as if he or she is holding a piece of hot potato in the mouth. One examination by a skilled examiner with intubation equipment available is generally performed, often in the operating room. A markedly swollen and cherry red epiglottis is diagnostic. Repeated oral examinations are not performed because of the potential for complete laryngeal obstruction.

oral iron therapy. Mottled or pitted teeth are often the result of tetracycline treatment during tooth development or enamel dysplasia.

If the child will protrude the tongue and say "ah," the tongue blade is often unnecessary for the oral examination. When the child refuses to open the mouth, insert a tongue blade through the lips to the back molars. Gently but firmly insert the tongue blade between the back molars and press the tongue blade to the tongue. This maneuver should stimulate the gag reflex and give you a brief view of the mouth and oropharynx.

Koplik spots, white specks with a red base on the buccal mucosa opposite the first and second molars, occur with rubeola in a child with fever, coryza, and cough. A highly arched palate may be observed in children who are chronic mouth breathers.

The tonsils, lying deep in the oral cavity, should blend into the color of the pharynx. They gradually enlarge to their peak size between 2 and 6 years of age, but the oropharynx should retain an unobstructed passage. If the tonsils appear pushed backward or forward, possibly displacing the uvula, consider a peritonsillar abscess.

When the tongue is depressed, the epiglottis is visible as a glistening pink structure behind the base of the tongue.

PREGNANT WOMEN

Edema and erythema in the nose and pharynx of the pregnant woman results from the increased vascularization of the respiratory tract. Tympanic membranes may have increased vascularity and be retracted or bulging with serous fluid. The gums will appear reddened, swollen, and spongy, with the hypertrophy resolving within 2 months of delivery.

OLDER ADULTS

Ears and Hearing

Inspect the auditory canal of the patient who wears a hearing aid for areas of irritation from the ear mold. Coarse, wirelike hairs are often present along the periphery of the auricle. On otoscopic examination, the tympanic membrane landmarks may appear slightly more pronounced from sclerotic changes.

Some degree of sensorineural hearing deterioration with advancing age (presbycusis) may be noted. This is marked by greater difficulty understanding sounds rather than a reduction in all sounds heard. Problems will be most prominent when the patient is in a room with considerable background noise. Conductive hearing loss from otosclerosis may also occur.

Nose

The nasal mucosa may appear dryer, less glistening. An increased number of bristly hairs in the vestibule are common, especially in men.

Mouth

The lips will have increased vertical markings and appear dryer when salivary flow is reduced. The buccal mucosa is thinner, less vascular and shiny than that of the younger adult. Dark skinned patients will have increased pigmentation on the buccal mucosa and gums. The tongue may appear more fissured, and veins on its ventral surface may appear varicose (Fig. 7-40).

Many adults over 65 years of age are edentulous. Natural teeth may be worn down, and dental restorations may have deteriorated. The teeth often appear longer as resorption of the gum and bone progresses. Dental malocclusion are commonly caused by the migration of remaining teeth after extractions. The lower jaw may protrude in patients with a stooping and head thrusting posture.

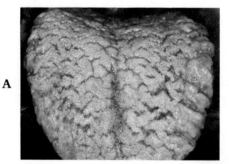

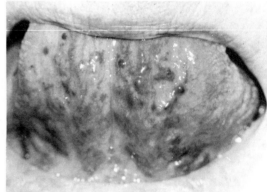

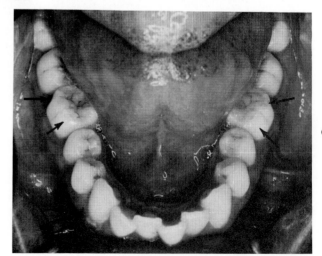

Fig. 7-40
Common findings in the older adult's mouth.
A, Fissured tongue.
B, Varicose veins on tongue. **C,** Attrition of teeth.
A from Wood and Goaz, 1985; **B** from Bowers and Thompson, 1984; C from Halstead et al., 1982.

Common Abnormalities

Ear

Acute Otitis Media

An infection of the middle ear often follows or accompanies an upper respiratory infection. Symptoms include pain, fever, and a red tympanic membrane without mobility. Occasionally, purulent discharge will be found in the auditory canal when the tympanic membrane perforates (Fig. 7-41).

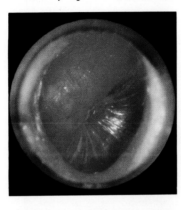

Fig. 7-41
Acute otitis media.
Courtesy Dr. Richard A. Buckingham, Clinical Professor, Otolaryngology, Abraham Lincoln School of Medicine, University of Illinois, Chicago; from Malasanos et al., 1986.

Serous Otitis Media (Secretory Otitis Media)

Serous fluid in the middle ear results from an obstructed or dysfunctional eustachian tube. This can be caused by allergies, residual otitis media, or enlarged lymphoid tissue in the nasopharynx that block the middle ear. Once blocked, the middle ear space absorbs the air creating a vacuum, and a transudate from the mucosa fills the middle ear. The tympanic membrane appears to be yellow, either retracted or bulging, and may have a fluid level or air bubbles. The patient rarely has pain but may experience pressure sensation. Conductive hearing loss occurs (Fig. 7-42).

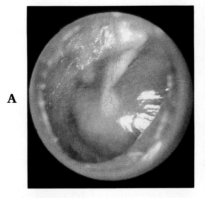
A

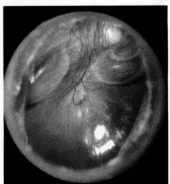
B

Fig. 7-42
Serous otitis media. A, Middle ear filled with serous fluid. B, Air fluid levels in upper middle ear.
Courtesy Dr. Richard A. Buckingham, Clinical Professor, Otolaryngology, Abraham Lincoln School of Medicine, University of Illinois, Chicago; from Malasanos et al., 1986.

Otitis Externa (Swimmer's Ear)

Otitis externa is an infection of the auditory canal resulting when trauma or a moist environment favors bacterial or fungal growth. The auditory canal mucosa is edematous and filled with foul smelling, thick gray or white exudate. The patient experiences pain when the auricle is touched or tugged. One of the ways to tell otitis media from otitis externa is to tug *very gently* on the patient's auricle. Otitis externa responds with pain or tenderness that is accentuated by the tug, whereas otitis media does not. Swimmer's ear really hurts when you do this, so perform this maneuver gently.

Cholesteatoma

A growth of keratinizing squamous epithelium and cholesterol in the middle ear is termed cholesteatoma. It may be a congenital defect or result from chronic infection. Signs include a reddened color behind the tympanic membrane and sometimes a perforated tympanic membrane with persistent, foul smelling discharge (Fig. 7-43).

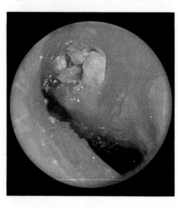

Fig. 7-43
Cholesteatoma.
Courtesy Dr. Richard A. Buckingham, Clinical Professor, Otolaryngology, Abraham Lincoln School of Medicine, University of Illinois, Chicago; from Malasanos et al., 1986.

Acute Mastoiditis

Infection of the air spaces of the mastoid process is the result of an untreated or incompletely treated otitis media. Signs include fever, a red bulging tympanic membrane, and erythema and swelling over the mastoid process. The auricle on the involved side may be pushed forward and stick out from the head. Happily, it is unlikely that you will see acute mastoiditis during your career. It was a frequent and a devastating complication of otitis media before the advent of antibiotics and chemotherapeutic agents, but now it is a rarity.

Otosclerosis

Otosclerosis is a hereditary condition that is more common in women. Irregular ossification occurs within the labyrinthine capsule, resulting in fixation of the stapes. Symptoms include tinnitus and conductive hearing loss, usually noticed between 11 and 30 years of age.

Menière's Disease

Menière's disease affects the vestibular labyrinth, leading to profound sensorineural hearing loss. Symptoms include a sensation of fullness in one ear with some degree of hearing loss, tinnitus, and later disabling vertigo, all occurring episodically. Hearing improves after the attack but deteriorates over time.

Conductive Hearing Loss

Transmission of sound through the external or middle ear to the sensorineural apparatus of the inner ear is impaired. The patient experiences reduction of all sounds heard, rather than difficulty interpreting sounds (Fig. 7-44).

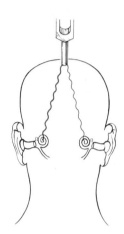
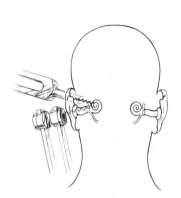

Fig. 7-44
Conductive hearing loss.
From Malasanos et al., 1986.

Sensorineural Hearing Loss (perceptual)

Transmission of sound through the external and middle ear to the inner ear is unimpaired. A defect in the inner ear leads to a distortion of sound, so the patient has difficulty interpreting sounds heard (Fig. 7-45).

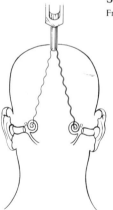
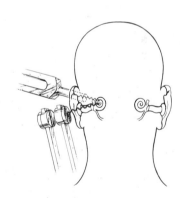

Fig. 7-45
Sensorineural hearing loss.
From Malasanos et al., 1986.

Labyrinthitis

Inflammation of the labyrinthine canal of the inner ear occurs as a complication of an acute upper respiratory infection. Symptoms of vertigo, associated with nystagmus, increase in severity with head movement.

Nose and Sinuses

Rhinitis

Rhinitis is an inflammatory response of the nose to infection or allergy. With an allergy the patient has watery discharge, sneezing, and stuffiness. With an infec-tion the patient has either mucoid or purulent discharge and other symptoms of sore throat, coughing, and general malaise (Fig. 7-46).

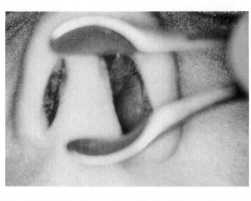

Fig. 7-46
Allergic rhinitis.
From Malasanos et al., 1986.

Sinusitis

An infection of one or more of the para-nasal sinuses may be a complication of an upper respiratory infection, dental infection, allergies, or a structural defect of the nose. Symptoms include fever, headache, local tenderness, and pain. There may be swelling of the skin over-lying the involved sinus and copious purulent nasal discharge (Fig. 7-47).

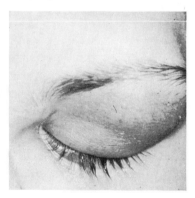

Fig. 7-47
Acute frontal sinusitis with orbital edema.
From Saunders et al., 1979.

Mouth and Oropharynx

Peutz-Jegher's Syndrome

This is an autosomal dominant genetic disorder characterized by round to oval areas of bluish-gray pigmentation over the lips and buccal mucosa. The syndrome is associated with intestinal polyposis, sometimes causing partial intestinal obstruction, intussusception, and malignant degeneration (Fig. 7-48).

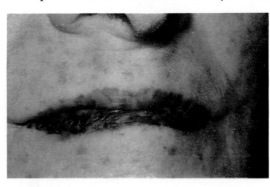

Fig. 7-48
Peutz-Jegher's syndrome.
From Diagnostic picture tests in clinical medicine, 1984.

Tonsillitis

Inflammation or infection of the tonsils is frequently caused by streptococcus. Symptoms include sore throat, dysphagia, fever, fetid breath, and malaise. The tonsils appear red and swollen, and tonsillar crypts are filled with purulent exudate (Fig. 7-49).

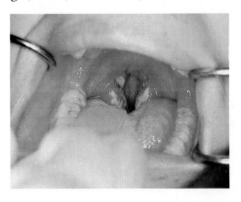

Fig. 7-49
Tonsillitis and pharyngitis.
Courtesy Dr. Edward L. Applebaum, Head, Department of Otolaryngology, University of Illinois Medical Center, Chicago; from Malasanos et al., 1986.

Peritonsillar Abscess

Infection of the tissue between the tonsil and pharynx occurs as a complication of tonsillitis. Symptoms include dysphagia, pain radiating to the ear, and fever. The tonsil, tonsillar pillar, and adjacent soft palate become red and swollen. The tonsil may appear pushed forward or backward, possibly displacing the uvula.

Retropharyngeal Abscess   Infection of the retropharyngeal space lymph nodes, followed by abscess formation, occurs after an upper respiratory infection. Symptoms include fever, difficulty swallowing, and pain. Respiratory distress can occur if the airway becomes obstructed. The fullness of the posterior pharyngeal wall can be seen and palpated (Fig. 7-50).

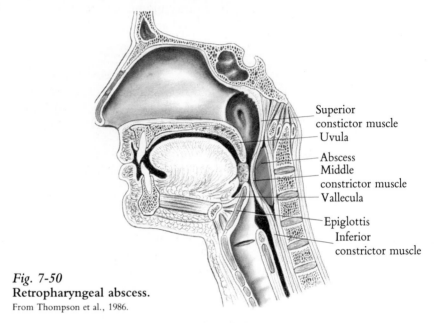

Fig. 7-50
Retropharyngeal abscess.
From Thompson et al., 1986.

INFANTS AND CHILDREN

Choanal Atresia   Choanal atresia is a congenital nasal obstruction of the posterior nares at the junction between the nasal cavity and nasopharynx. Newborns who have this anomaly experience respiratory distress without prompt intervention, because they are obligatory nose breathers.

Cleft Lip and Palate

This congenital malformation of the face appears as a fissure of the upper lip or palate. Each may occur without the other; however, they often occur together. There may be a complete cleft extending through the lip and hard and soft palates to the nasal cavity, or there may be a partial cleft in any of these tissues. Long term problems for the affected child include hearing loss, chronic otitis media, speech difficulties, and improper tooth development and alignment (Fig. 7-51).

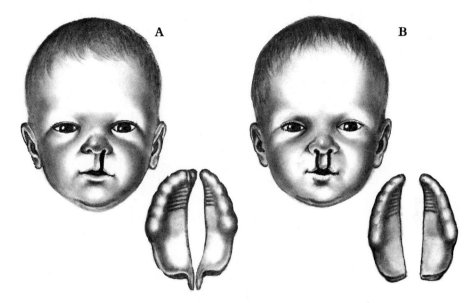

Fig. 7-51
A, Unilateral cleft lip and palate. **B,** Bilateral cleft lip and palate.
From Whaley and Wong, 1983.

OLDER ADULTS

Presbycusis

Presbycusis is a common auditory disorder in which there is bilateral sensorineural hearing loss associated with aging. It is caused by degenerative changes in the inner ear or auditory nerve. There is a loss in the perception of auditory stimuli, initially of high frequency sounds. Speech may be poorly understood when spoken quickly or when background noise is present.

Xerostomia

A dry mouth caused by the ingestion of anticholinergic drugs interferes with the production of saliva. Xerostomia is also caused by systemic diseases (rheumatoid arthritis, SLE, scleroderma, polymyositis) and is seen in Sjögren's syndrome. This occurs most often in women over age 50.

Chest and Lungs

Anatomy and Physiology

The chest, or thorax, is a cage of bone, cartilage, and muscle that is capable of movement as the lungs expand (Fig. 8-1). The anterior portion consists of the sternum, manubrium, xiphoid process, and costal cartilages. The lateral portions are formed by the 12 pairs of ribs, and the posterior part consists of the 12 thoracic vertebrae (Fig. 8-2). All the ribs are connected to the thoracic vertebrae; the upper 7 are attached anteriorly to the sternum by the costal cartilages. The transverse diameter of the chest normally exceeds the anteroposterior diameter in adults.

The primary muscles of respiration are the diaphragm and the intercostal muscles. The diaphragm contracts and moves downward during inspiration, lowering the abdominal contents to increase the intrathoracic space. The external intercostal muscles increase the anteroposterior chest diameter during inspiration, and the internal intercostals decrease the transverse diameter during expiration. The sternocleidomastoid and trapezius muscles also contribute to respiratory movements (Fig. 8-3).

The interior of the chest is divided into three major spaces: the right and left pleural cavities and the mediastinum (Fig. 8-1). The mediastinum, situated between the lungs, contains all of the thoracic viscera except the lungs. The pleural cavities are lined with the parietal and visceral pleurae, serous membranes that enclose the lungs.

The spongy and highly elastic lungs are paired but not symmetric, the right having three lobes and the left two. Each lobe consists of blood vessels, lymphatics, nerves, and an alveolar duct connecting with the alveoli (as many as 300 million in an adult). The entire lung parenchyma is shaped by an elastic subpleural tissue that limits its expansion. Each lung is conical; the apex is rounded and extends anteriorly about 4 cm above the first rib into the base of the neck in adults. Posteriorly, the apices of the lungs rise to about the level of T1. The lower borders descend on deep inspiration to about T12 and rise on forced expiration to about T10. The base of each lung is broad and concave, resting on the convex surface of the diaphragm. The medial surfaces of the lung are to some extent concave, providing a cradle for the heart.

The tracheobronchial tree is a tubular system that provides a pathway for air to move from the upper airway to the farthest alveolar reaches. The trachea is 10 to 11 cm long and about 2 cm in diameter. It lies anterior to the esophagus and posterior to the isthmus of the thyroid. The trachea divides into the right and left main bronchi at about the level of T4 or T5 vertebra and just below the manubriosternal joint.

The right bronchus is wider, shorter, and more vertically placed than the left bronchus (and therefore more susceptible to aspiration of foreign bodies). The main bronchi are divided into three branches on the right and two on the left, each branch supplying one lobe of the lungs. The branches then begin to subdivide into terminal bronchioles and ultimately into respiratory bronchioles so small that each is associated with one acinus, or terminal respiratory unit. The acini consist of the respiratory bronchioles, alveolar ducts, alveolar sacs, and alveoli. The bronchi transport air and, to some extent, trap noxious foreign particles in the mucus of their cavities and sweep them toward the pharynx with their cilia.

The bronchial arteries branch from the anterior thoracic aorta and the intercostal arteries, supplying blood to the lung parenchyma and stroma. The bronchial vein is formed at the hilum of the lung, but most of the blood supplied by the bronchial arteries is returned by the pulmonary veins.

Chemical and Neurologic Control of Respiration

The purpose of respiration is to keep the body adequately supplied with oxygen and protected from excess accumulation of carbon dioxide. Control of this complex process is not yet fully understood. Chemoreceptors in the medulla oblongata are exquisitely sensitive and respond quickly to changes in hydrogen ion concentration in the blood and spinal fluid. Peripherally, chemoreceptors in the carotid body at the bifurcation of the common carotid arteries also respond to changes in arterial oxygen and carbon dioxide levels. Both types of chemoreceptors respond by sending signals to the respiratory center in the medulla oblongata. Nerve impulses from

Fig. 8-1
Chest cavity and related anatomic structures.

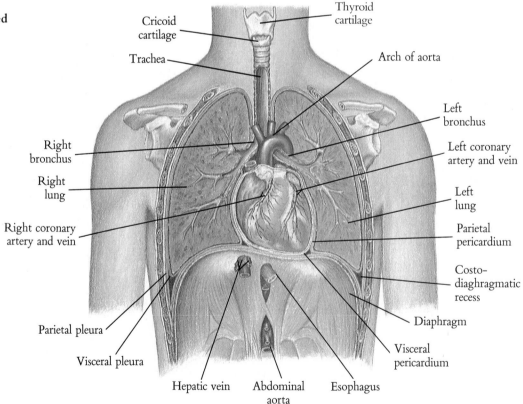

Thyroid cartilage

Cricoid cartilage

Trachea

Arch of aorta

Left bronchus

Left coronary artery and vein

Right bronchus

Right lung

Left lung

Parietal pericardium

Right coronary artery and vein

Costo-diaghragmatic recess

Diaphragm

Parietal pleura

Visceral pleura

Visceral pericardium

Hepatic vein

Abdominal aorta

Esophagus

Fig. 8-2
Ventilatory structures of the thorax. A, Anterior view. **B,** Posterior view.
From Thompson et al., 1986.

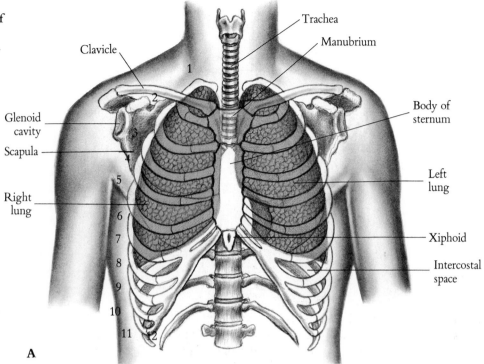

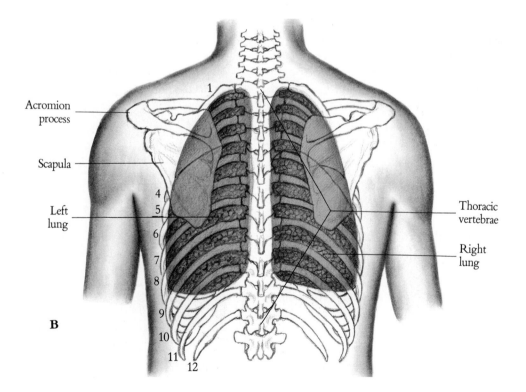

Fig. 8-3
**Muscles of ventilation. A,
Anterior view. B, Posterior
view.**

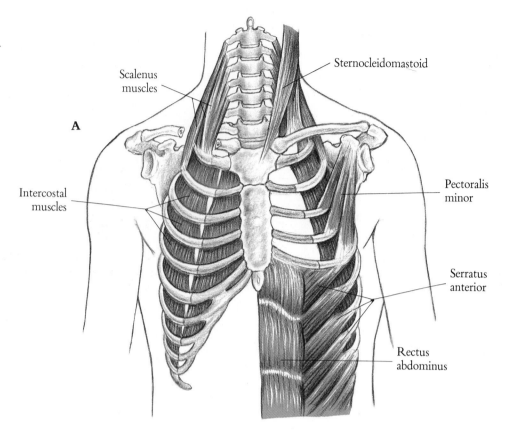

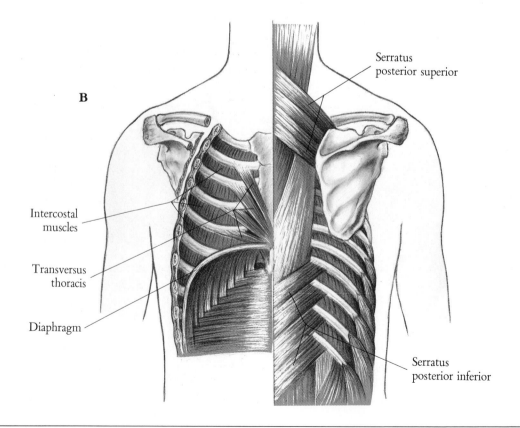

here are transmitted to two subcenters in the pons, which regulate the respiratory muscles. Excess levels of carbon dioxide stimulate the rate and depth of respiration.

Anatomic Landmarks

The following topographic markers on the chest are used to describe findings:
1. The nipples.
2. The manubriosternal junction (angle of Louis): a visible and palpable angulation of the sternum and the point at which the second rib articulates with the sternum. One can count the ribs and intercostal spaces from this point. The number of each intercostal space corresponds to that of the rib immediately above it.
3. The suprasternal notch: a depression, easily palpable and most often visible at the base of the ventral aspect of the neck, just superior to the manubriosternal junction.
4. Costal angle: the angle formed by the blending together of the costal margins at the sternum. It is usually no more than 90 degrees, with the ribs inserted at approximately 45-degree angles.
5. Vertebra prominens: the spinous process of C7. It can be more readily seen and felt with the patient's head bent forward. If two prominences are felt, the upper is that of the spinous process of C7, and the lower is that of T1. It is difficult to use this as a guide to counting ribs posteriorly, because the spinous processes from T4 down project obliquely, thus overlying the rib *below* the number of its vertebra.
6. The clavicles.

INFANTS AND CHILDREN

At about 4 weeks gestation the lung is a groove on the ventral wall of the gut. It evolves ultimately from a simple sac to an involuted structure of tubules and spaces. The lungs contain no air and the alveoli are collapsed. Relatively passive respiratory movements occur throughout much of gestation; they do not open the alveoli or move the lung fluids. Rather they prepare the term infant to respond to postnatal chemical and neurologic respiratory stimuli. Fetal gas exchange is supplied by the placenta.

At birth the change in respiratory function is rapid and intense. After the cord is cut, the lungs fill with air for the first time only with great respiratory effort. Blood, no longer coursing through the placenta, flows through the lungs more vigorously. The pulmonary arteries expand and relax, offering much less resistance than the systemic circulation. This relative decrease in pulmonary pressure leads to closure of the foramen ovale within minutes after birth, and the increased oxygen tension in the arterial blood stimulates contraction and closure of the ductus arteriosus. The pulmonary and systemic circulations adopt their mature configurations, and the lungs are fully integrated for postnatal function.

The chest of the newborn is generally round, the anteroposterior diameter approximating the transverse, and the circumference is roughly equal to that of the head until the child is about 2 years old (Fig. 8-4). With growth, the chest assumes adult proportions with the lateral diameter exceeding the anteroposterior diameter (see Table 3-4, p. 59).

The relatively thin chest wall of the infant and young child makes the bony structure more prominent than in the adult. It is more cartilaginous and yielding, and the xiphoid process is often more prominent and a bit more movable.

Fig. 8-4
Chest of healthy infant.
Note that AP diameter is
approximately the same as
transverse diameter.

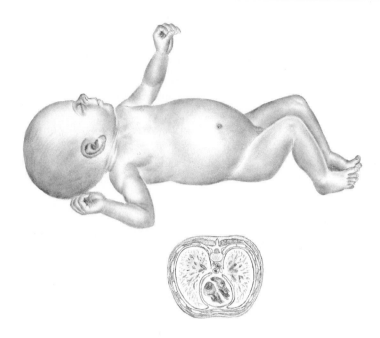

PREGNANT WOMEN

Elevated levels of estrogen cause the ligaments of the rib cage to relax, permitting increased chest expansion. In preparation for the enlarging uterus, the length of the lungs decrease and the diaphragm rises as much as 4 cm. The anteroposterior chest diameter increases by about 2 cm, and the circumference increases by 5 to 7 cm. Ventilation is increased by deeper breathing accompanied by only a slight increase in respiratory rate.

OLDER ADULTS

The barrel chest characteristic of many older adults results from loss of muscle strength in the thorax and diaphragm, coupled with the loss of lung resiliency. In addition, skeletal changes of aging tend to emphasize the dorsal curve of the thoracic spine, resulting in an increased anteroposterior chest diameter. There may also be stiffening and decreased expansion of the chest wall.

The alveoli become less elastic and relatively more fibrous. The associated loss of some of the interalveolar folds decreases the alveolar surface available for gas exchange. This and the loss of some tensile strength in the muscles of respiration result in underventilation of the alveoli in the lower lung fields and a decreased tolerance for exertion. Dyspnea can occur when older persons exceed their accustomed light or moderate exertional demands.

Aging mucous membranes tend to become drier and less able to rid themselves of mucus. Retained mucus encourages bacterial growth and predisposes the older adult to respiratory infection.

Review of Related History

General Considerations

1. Employment: nature of work, environmental hazards, exposure to chemicals, vapors, dust, pulmonary irritants, allergens, use of protective devices
2. Home environment: location, possible allergens, type of heating, use of air conditioning, humidifier, ventilation

3. Tobacco use: type of tobacco (cigarettes, cigars, pipe, smokeless), duration and amount, age started
4. Exposure to respiratory infections, influenza, tuberculosis
5. Nutritional status: weight loss or obesity

Present Problem

1. Coughing
   a. Onset: sudden, gradual; duration
   b. Nature of cough: dry, moist, wet, hacking, hoarse, barking, whooping, bubbling, productive, nonproductive
      1. Sputum production: duration, frequency, with activity, at certain times of day
      2. Sputum characteristics: amount, color (clear, mucoid, purulent, blood-tinged, mostly blood), foul odor
   c. Pattern: occasional, regular, paroxysmal; related to time of day, weather, activities, talking, deep breaths; change over time
   d. Severity: severe enough to tire patient, disrupt sleep or conversation, cause chest pain
   e. Associated symptoms: shortness of breath, chest pain or tightness with breathing, fever, upper respiratory signs, noisy respirations, hoarseness, gagging, choking, stress
   f. Efforts to treat: prescription or nonprescription drugs, vaporizers, effectiveness
2. Shortness of breath
   a. Onset: sudden or gradual; duration; gagging or choking event few days before onset
   b. Pattern
      1. Position most comfortable, number of pillows used
      2. Related to extent of exercise, certain activities, time of day, eating
      3. Harder to inhale or exhale
   c. Severity: extent of activity limitation, tiring or fatigue with breathing, anxiety about getting air
   d. Associated symptoms: pain or discomfort (relationship to specific point in respiratory exertion, location), cough, diaphoresis, swelling of ankles
3. Chest pain
   a. Onset and duration; associated with trauma, coughing, lower respiratory infection
   b. Associated symptoms: shallow breathing, fever, uneven chest expansion, coughing, anxiety about getting air, radiation of pain to neck or arms
   c. Efforts to treat: heat, splinting, pain medication

Past Medical History

1. Thoracic trauma or surgery, hospitalizations for pulmonary disorders, dates
2. Use of oxygen or ventilation-assisting devices
3. Chronic pulmonary diseases: tuberculosis (date, treatment, compliance), bronchitis, emphysema, bronchiectasis, asthma, cystic fibrosis
4. Other chronic disorders: cardiac, cancer
5. Testing: allergy, pulmonary function tests, tuberculin and fungal skin tests, chest x-rays

Family History

1. Tuberculosis
2. Cystic fibrosis
3. Emphysema
4. Allergy, asthma, atopic dermatitis
5. Smoking by household family members
6. Malignancy

INFANTS AND CHILDREN

1. Low birth weight: premature, duration of ventilation assistance if any, respiratory distress syndrome, bronchopulmonary dysplasia
2. Coughing or difficulty breathing of sudden onset
   a. Possible aspiration of small object, toy, or food
   b. Possible ingestion of kerosene or other hydrocarbon
3. Difficulty feeding: increased perspiration, cyanosis, tiring quickly, disinterest in feeding, inappropriate weight gain
4. Apnea episodes: use of apnea monitor, sudden infant death in sibling
5. Recurrent spitting up and choking, recurrent pneumonia (possible gastroesophageal reflux)

OLDER ADULTS

1. Exposure to and frequency of respiratory infections, history of annual influenza immunization
2. Effects of weather on respiratory efforts and occurrence of infections
3. Immobilization or marked sedentary habits
4. Difficulty swallowing
5. Alteration in daily living habits or activities as a result of respiratory symptoms
6. Since older adults are at risk for chronic respiratory diseases (lung cancer, chronic bronchitis, emphysema, and tuberculosis), specifically inquire about:
   a. Smoking history
   b. Cough, dyspnea on exertion, or breathlessness
   c. Fatigue
   d. Significant weight changes
   e. Fever, night sweats

RISK FACTORS FOR RESPIRATORY DISABILITY IN OLDER ADULTS

History of smoking
History of frequent respiratory infections
Immobilization or marked sedentary habits
History of chronic exposure to environmental pollutants or
   toxic inhalants
Difficulty swallowing
Weakened chest muscles
Family history of respiratory disability

Examination and Findings

- Marking pencil
- Centimeter ruler and tape measure
- Stethoscope with bell and diaphragm (for children, the diaphragm may have a smaller diameter)

Inspection

Have the patient sit upright, if possible without support, naked to the waist. A drape should be available to cover the patient when full exposure is not necessary. The room and stethoscope should be comfortably warm, and a bright tangential light is needed to highlight chest movement.

Note the shape and symmetry of the chest from both the back and front. The bony framework is obvious, the clavicles prominent superiorly, the sternum usually rather flat and free of an abundance of overlying tissue. The chest will not be absolutely symmetric, but one side can be used as a measure of comparison for the other. The anteroposterior (AP) diameter of the chest is normally less than that of the transverse diameter, often by as much as half (Fig. 8-5).

"Barrel chest" results from compromised respiration as, for example, in chronic asthma, emphysema, or cystic fibrosis. The ribs are more horizontal, the spine at least somewhat kyphotic, and the sternal angle more prominent (Fig. 8-6).

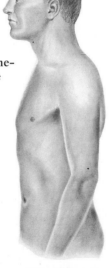

Fig. 8-5
Thorax of healthy adult male. Note that AP diameter is less than transverse diameter.

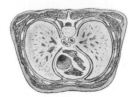

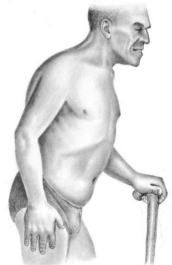

Fig. 8-6
Barrel chest. Note increase in AP diameter.

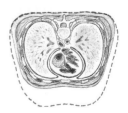

THORACIC LANDMARKS

In conjunction with the anatomic landmarks of the chest, the following imaginary lines on the surface will help localize the findings on physical examination (Fig. 8-7):

1. Midsternal line: vertically down the midline of the sternum
2. Right and left midclavicular lines: parallel to the midsternal line, beginning at midclavicle; the inferior borders of the lungs generally cross the sixth rib at the midclavicular line
3. Right and left anterior axillary lines: parallel to midsternal line, beginning at the anterior axillary folds
4. Right and left midaxillary lines: parallel to the midsternal line, beginning at the midaxilla
5. Right and left posterior axillary lines: parallel to the midsternal line, beginning at the posterior axillary folds
6. Midspinal line: vertically down the spinal processes
7. Right and left scapular lines: parallel to the midspinal line, through the inferior angle of the scapula when the patient is erect

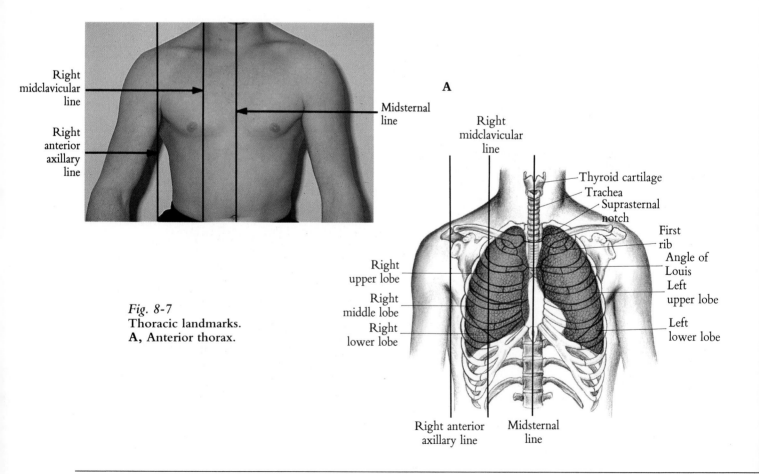

Fig. 8-7
Thoracic landmarks.
A, Anterior thorax.

A

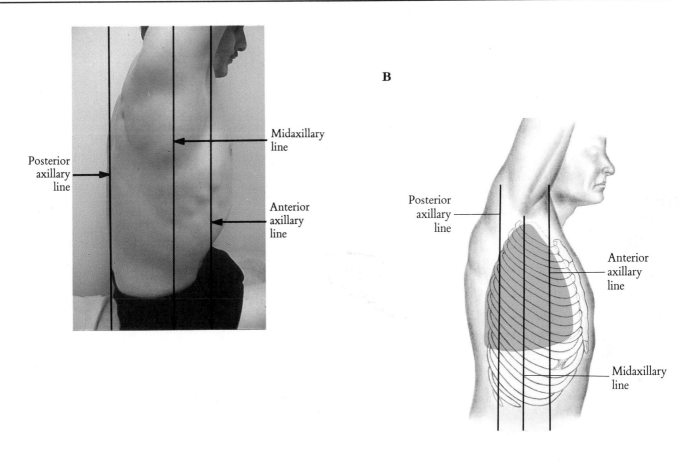

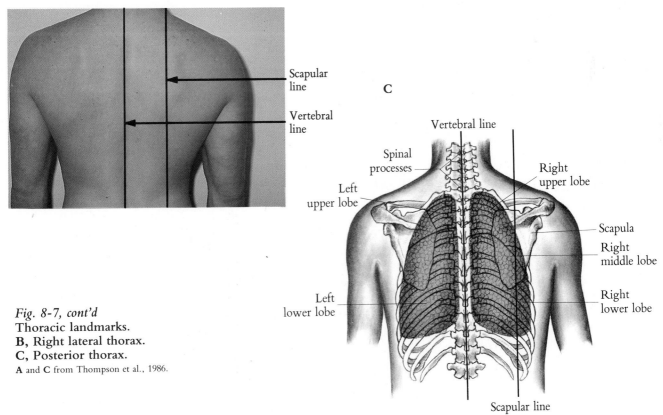

Fig. 8-7, cont'd
Thoracic landmarks.
B, Right lateral thorax.
C, Posterior thorax.
A and C from Thompson et al., 1986.

Fig. 8-8
A, Pectus carinatum (pigeon chest). **B,** Pectus excavatum (funnel chest). Dotted lines indicate structural deviations.

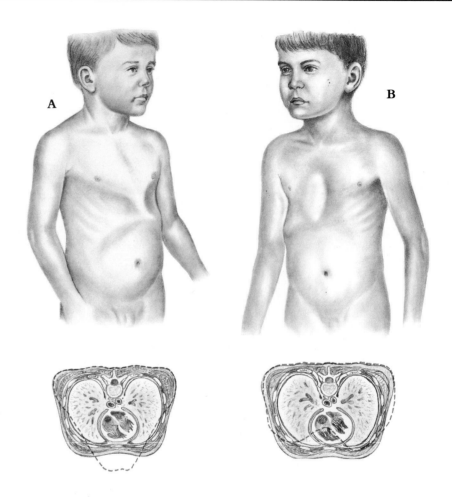

Other changes in the chest wall contour may be the result of structural problems in the spine, rib cage, or sternum. Two common structural problems are pigeon chest (pectus carinatum), a prominent sternal protrusion, and funnel chest (pectus excavatum), an indentation of the lower sternum above the xiphoid process (Fig. 8-8).

Inspect the skin and nipples, noting whether there is any cyanosis or pallor. Look for any superficial venous patterns over the chest, which could be a sign of heart disorders or vascular obstruction or disease. The underlying fat and relative prominence of the ribs give some clue to general nutrition.

Respiration

Count the respiratory rate for 60 seconds, or count for 30 seconds and double the count. The rate should be 12 to 20 per minute; the ratio of respirations to heartbeats is approximately 1:4.

Note the pattern (or rhythm) of respiration and the way in which the chest moves (Fig. 8-9). Expansion of the chest should be bilaterally symmetric. Expect the patient to breathe easily, regularly, and without apparent distress. The pattern of breathing should be even, neither too shallow nor too deep. Note any variations in respiratory rate.

Tachypnea is a persistent respiratory rate faster than 20 per minute. Doublecheck to be sure that it is persistent. Rapid shallow breathing is often a symptom of protective splinting from pain of a broken rib or pleurisy. Massive liver enlargement or abdominal ascites may prevent descent of the diaphragm and produce a similar pattern. Bradypnea, a rate slower than 12 respirations per minute, may indicate neurologic or electrolyte disturbance, infection, or a sensible response to protect against the pain of pleurisy or other irritative phenomena.

Note any variations in respiratory rhythm. If the patient is breathing rapidly and deeply (hyperpnea), hyperventilation results. Exercise and anxiety can cause hyperpnea, but so can central nervous system and metabolic disease.

A regular periodic pattern of breathing, with intervals of apnea followed by a crescendo/decrescendo sequence of respiration, is called periodic breathing or Cheyne-Stokes respirations. Children and older adults may breathe in this pattern during sleep, but otherwise it occurs only in patients who are seriously ill.

An occasional deep, audible sigh that punctuates an otherwise regular respiration is associated with emotional distress or an incipient episode of more severe hyperventilation. Sighs are significant only if they exceed the infrequent and inconsequential sighs of daily life.

If the pulmonary tree is seriously obstructed for any reason, inspired air has difficulty overcoming the resistance and getting out. Air-trapping is the result of a prolonged but inefficient expiratory effort. The rate of respiration increases in order to compensate; as this happens, the effort becomes more shallow, the amount of trapped air increases, and the lungs inflate.

Biot's respiration consists of irregular respirations varying in depth and interrupted by intervals of apnea, but lacking the repetitive pattern of periodic respiration. On occasion, the respirations may be regular, but the apneic periods may occur in an irregular pattern. Biot's respiration usually is associated with severe and persistent increased intracranial pressure. Changes in breathing pattern are usually significant. When breathing is labored or respirations are deeper than usual, the accessory muscles of respiration, the sternocleidomastoids and trapezii, may be used.

Inspect the chest wall movement during respiration. Expansion should be symmetric without apparent use of accessory muscles. Chest asymmetry can be asso-

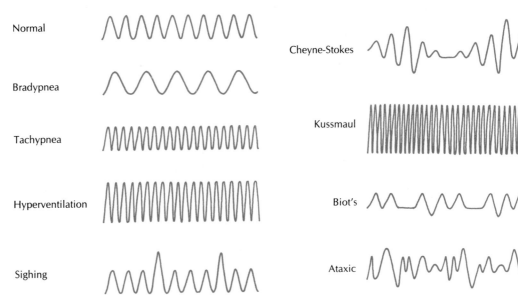

Fig. 8-9
Patterns of respiration.
From Abels, 1986.

Normal

Bradypnea

Tachypnea

Hyperventilation

Sighing

Cheyne-Stokes

Kussmaul

Biot's

Ataxic

ciated with unequal expansion and respiratory compromise caused by a collapsed lung or limitation of expansion by extrapleural air, fluid, or a mass. Unilateral or bilateral bulging can be a reaction of the ribs and interspaces to respiratory obstruction. A prolonged expiration and bulging on expiration are probably caused by outflow obstruction or the valve-like action of compression by a tumor, aneurysm, or enlarged heart. The costal angle widens beyond 90 degrees.

Retractions suggest an obstruction to inspiration at any point in the respiratory tract. The musculature "pulls back" in the effort to overcome blockage. Any significant obstruction makes the retraction observable with each inspiratory effort. The degree and level of retraction depend on the extent and level of obstruction. When the obstruction is high in the respiratory tree (e.g., with tracheal or laryngeal involvement), breathing is characterized by stridor, and the chest wall seems to cave in at the sternum, between the ribs, in the suprasternal notch, above the clavicles, and at the lowest costal margins.

A foreign body in one or the other of the bronchi (usually the right because of its broader bore and more vertical placement) causes unilateral retraction, but the suprasternal notch is not involved. Retraction of the lower chest occurs with asthma and bronchiolitis.

Observe the lips and nails for cyanosis, the lips for pursing, the fingers for clubbing, and the ala nasi for flaring. Any of these peripheral clues suggest pulmonary or cardiac difficulty. Pursing of the lips is an accompaniment of increased expiratory effort. Clubbing of the fingers is associated with chronic fibrotic changes within the lung, the chronic cyanosis of congenital heart disease, or cystic fibrosis. (Oddly, other chronic problems involving the lungs, for example, asthma and emphysema, are not associated with clubbing.) Flaring of the ala nasi during inspiration is a common sign of air hunger, particularly when the alveoli are considerably involved.

Palpation

Palpate the thoracic muscles and skeleton, feeling for pulsations, tenderness, bulges, depressions, unusual movement, and unusual positions. There should be bilateral symmetry and some elasticity of the rib cage, but the sternum and xiphoid should be relatively inflexible and the thoracic spine rigid.

Crepitus, a crackly or crinkly sensation, can be both palpated and heard. It indicates air in the subcutaneous tissue from a rupture somewhere in the respiratory system. It may be localized (for example, over the suprasternal notch and base of the neck) or cover a wider area of the thorax, usually anteriorly and toward the axilla. Crepitus is always a matter for attention.

A palpable coarse, grating vibration, usually on inspiration, suggests a pleural friction rub caused by inflammation of the pleural surfaces.

To evaluate thoracic expansion during respiration, stand behind the patient and place your thumbs along the spinal processes at the level of the tenth rib, with your palms lightly in contact with the posterolateral surfaces (Fig. 8-10). Watch your thumbs diverge during quiet and deep breathing. A loss of symmetry in the movement of the thumbs suggests a problem on one or both sides. Then face the patient and place your thumbs along the costal margin and the xiphoid process, with your palms touching the anterolateral chest. Again, watch your thumbs diverge as the patient breathes.

Note the quality of the tactile fremitus, the palpable vibration of the chest wall that results from speech or other verbalizations. Fremitus is best felt parasternally at the second intercostal space, at the level of the bifurcation of the bronchi. There is great variability depending on the intensity and pitch of the voice and the structure and thickness of the chest wall.

Ask the patient to recite a few numbers or say a few words while you systematically palpate the chest with the palmar surfaces of the fingers or with the ulnar aspects of a clenched fist. Use a firm, light touch, establishing even contact. For comparison palpate both sides simultaneously and symmetrically, or use one hand, quickly alternating between the two sides. Move about the patient, palpating each area carefully: front to back, right side to left side, the lung apices (Fig. 8–11).

Decreased or absent fremitus is caused by excess air in the lungs and may indicate emphysema, pleural thickening or effusion, massive pulmonary edema, or bronchial obstruction. Increased fremitus, often coarser or rougher in feel, occurs in the presence of fluids or a solid mass within the lungs and may be caused by lung consolidation, heavy but nonobstructive bronchial secretions, compressed lung, or tumor. Gentle, more tremulous fremitus than expected occurs with some lung consolidations and inflammatory and infectious processes.

Note the position of the trachea. Place an index finger in the suprasternal notch and move it gently, side to side, along the upper edges of each clavicle and in the spaces above to the inner borders of the sternocleidomastoid muscles. These spaces should be equal on both sides, and the trachea should be in the midline directly above the suprasternal notch (Fig. 8-12).

Fig. 8-10
Palpating thoracic expansion. The thumbs are at the level of the tenth rib.

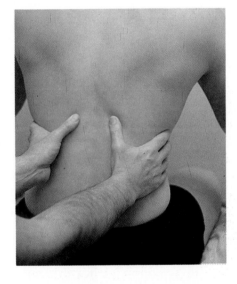

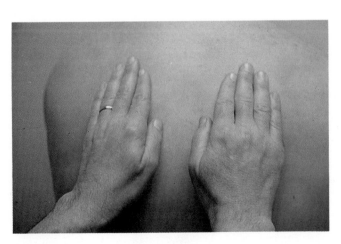

Fig. 8-11
Evaluating tactile fremitus with palmar surface of both hands.

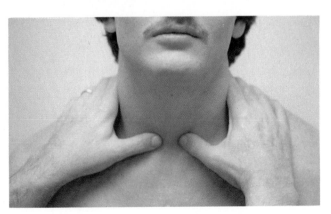

Fig. 8-12
Palpating to evaluate midline position of the trachea.

Fig. 8-13
Percussion tones through-out chest. A, Anterior view. B, Posterior view.
From Thompson et al., 1986.

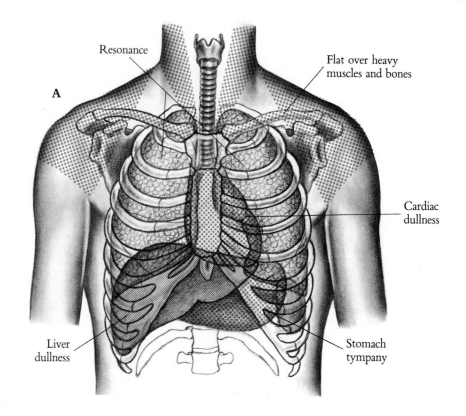

A

Resonance

Flat over heavy muscles and bones

Cardiac dullness

Liver dullness

Stomach tympany

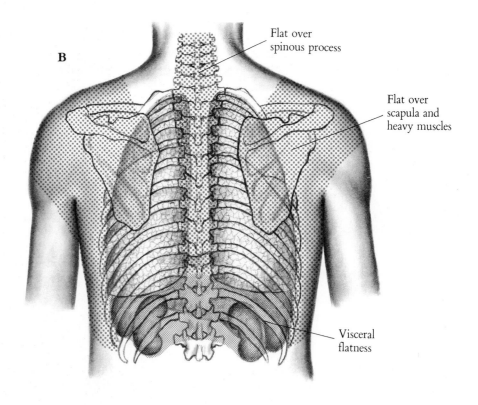

B

Flat over spinous process

Flat over scapula and heavy muscles

Visceral flatness

The trachea may be deviated because of problems within the chest and may, on occasion, seem to pulsate. The trachea may be pulled to the right or left by atelectasis, thyroid enlargement, or pleural effusion. It may be pushed to one side by tension pneumothorax, a tumor, or nodal enlargements on the contralateral side or by a tumor on the side to which it deviates. A palpable pull out of the midline with respiration is called a tug.

Percussion

Percussion tones heard over the chest, as elsewhere, are described in Chapter 2 (Examination Techniques and Equipment) and summarized in Table 8-1 and Fig. 8-13). You can percuss directly or indirectly, as described in Chapter 2 (Fig. 8-14).

Compare all areas bilaterally, using one side as a control for the other. The following sequence serves as a model; however, the examiner may vary the approach. First, examine the back with the patient sitting with head bent forward and arms folded in front. This moves the scapulae laterally, exposing more of the lung. Then ask the patient to raise his or her arms overhead while you percuss the lateral and anterior chest. For all positions percuss at 4- to 5-cm intervals, over the intercostal spaces, moving systematically from superior to inferior and medial to lateral (Fig. 8-15). Resonance is usually heard over all areas of the lungs. Hyperresonance associated with hyperinflation may indicate emphysema, pneumothorax, or asthma. Dullness or flatness suggests atelectasis, pleural effusion, or lung consolidation.

Measure the diaphragmatic excursion. Remember that the diaphragm is usually higher on the right than on the left because it sits over the bulk of the liver.

1. Ask the patient to breathe deeply and hold.
2. Percuss along the scapular line until you locate the lower border, the point marked by a change in note from resonance to dullness.
3. Mark the point with a skin pencil at the scapular line. Allow the patient to breathe, and then repeat the procedure on the other side.
4. Ask the patient to take several breaths and then to exhale as much as possible and hold.
5. On each side, percuss up from the marked point and make a mark at the change from dullness to resonance. Remind the patient to start breathing.
6. Measure and record the distance in centimeters between the marks on each side. The excursion distance is usually 3 to 5 cm (Fig. 8-16).

Fig. 8-14
A, Direct percussion using ulnar aspect of fist. **B,** Indirect percussion.

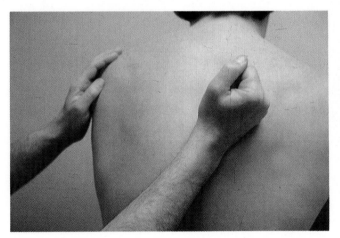

A

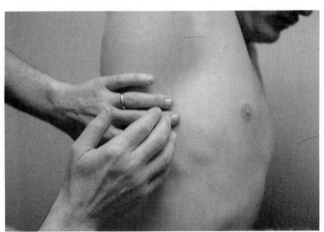

B

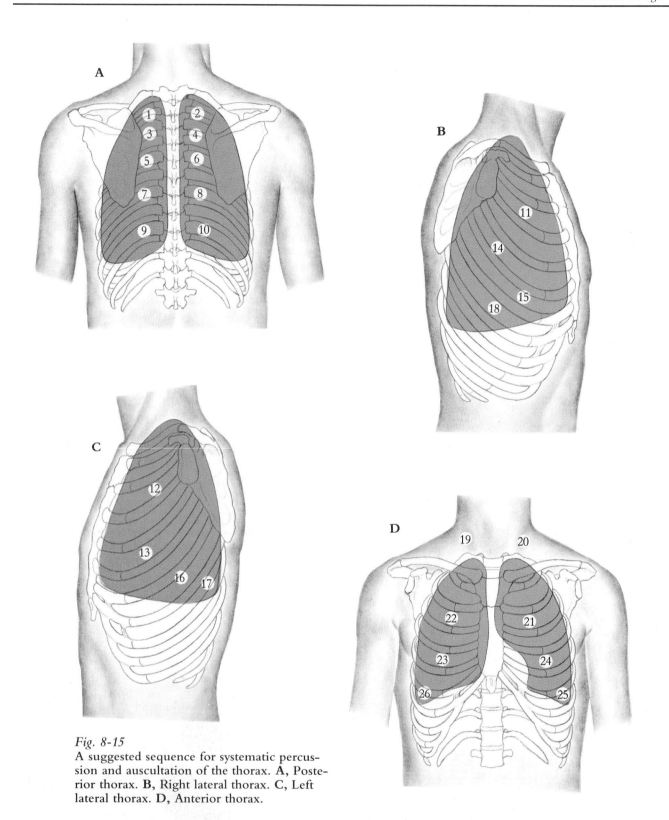

Fig. 8-15
A suggested sequence for systematic percussion and auscultation of the thorax. **A,** Posterior thorax. **B,** Right lateral thorax. **C,** Left lateral thorax. **D,** Anterior thorax.

Fig. 8-16
Measuring diaphragmatic excursion. Excursion distance is usually 3-5 cm.

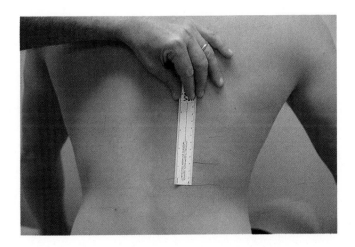

Table 8-1
Percussion Tones Heard over the Chest

Type of Tone	Intensity	Pitch	Duration	Quality
Resonant	Loud	Low	Long	Hollow
Flat	Soft	High	Short	Extremely dull
Dull	Medium	Medium-high	Medium	Thud-like
Tympanic	Loud	High	Medium	Drum-like
Hyperresonant*	Very loud	Very low	Longer	Booming

From Thompson et al., 1986.
*Hyperresonance is abnormal sound in adults. It represents air trapping such as occurs in obstructive lung diseases.

Auscultation

Auscultation with a stethoscope provides important clues to the condition of the lungs and pleura. (On relatively rare occasions, a sound is apparent to the ear directly that might be lost via the stethoscope, for example, the click of an aspirated foreign body.) All sounds can be characterized in the same manner as the percussion notes: intensity, pitch, quality, and duration (Table 8-2).

Have the patient sit upright, if possible, and breathe slowly and deeply through the mouth, exaggerating normal respiration. Demonstrate it yourself. Caution the patient to keep a pace consistent with comfort; hyperventilation is easier to achieve than one might think and causes faintness. Remember that exaggerated breathing can be tiring, especially for the aged or the ill.

The diaphragm of the stethoscope is usually preferable to the bell for listening to the lungs, because it transmits the ordinarily high-pitched sounds better, and it provides a broader area of sounds. Place the stethoscope firmly on the skin. When the individual breath sound is being evaluated, there should be *no* movement of patient or stethoscope except for the respiratory excursion.

To auscultate the back, ask the patient to sit as for percussion, with head bent forward and arms folded in front to enlarge the listening area. Then have the patient sit more erect with arms overhead for auscultating the lateral chest. Finally, ask the patient to sit erect with the shoulders back, and auscultate the anterior chest. As with so much else, the exact sequence you use is not as important as using the same sequence each time to ensure that the examination is thorough.

Listen systematically for each position, moving from side to side for comparison as you move downward from apex to base at intervals of several centimeters (Fig. 8-15).

Breath sounds are made by the flow of air through the respiratory tree. They can be characterized by their pitch, intensity, and quality and the relative duration of their inspiratory and expiratory phases. Breath sounds are classified as vesicular, bronchovesicular, and bronchial (tubular) (Table 8-2 and Fig. 8-17).

Vesicular breath sounds are low-pitched, low-intensity sounds heard over normal lung tissue. Bronchovesicular sounds are heard over the major bronchi and are normally moderate in pitch and intensity. The sounds highest in pitch and intensity are the bronchial breath sounds, which are normally heard only over the trachea. Both bronchovesicular and bronchial breath sounds are abnormal if they are heard over the peripheral lung tissue.

Breath Sounds

Breath sounds are relatively more difficult to hear or are absent if fluid or pus has accumulated in the pleural space, secretions or a foreign body obstructs the bronchi, the lungs are hyperinflated, or breathing is shallow from splinting for pain. Breath sounds are easier to hear when the lungs are consolidated; the mass surrounding the tube of the respiratory tree promotes sound transmission better than do air-filled alveoli.

Most of the unexpected sounds heard during lung auscultation are superimposed on the breath sounds. Extraneous sounds such as the crinkling of hair must be carefully distinguished from far more significant adventitious sounds. The common terms used to describe adventitious sounds are rales, rhonchi, wheezes, and friction rub (Fig. 8-18).

A rale, or crackle, is an abnormal respiratory sound heard most often during inspiration and characterized by discrete noncontinuous sounds. The individual noise tends to be brief and the interval to the next one similarly brief.

Table 8-2
Characteristics of Normal Breath Sounds

Sound	Characteristics	Findings
Vesicular	Heard over most of lung fields; low pitch; soft and short expirations (Fig. 8-18)	
Bronchovesicular	Heard over main bronchus area and over upper right posterior lung field; medium pitch; expiration equals inspiration	
Bronchial	Heard only over trachea; high pitch; loud and long expirations	

From Thompson et al., 1986.

Fig. 8-17
**Normal auscultatory
sounds. A, Anterior view.
B, Posterior view.**
From Thompson et al., 1986.

A

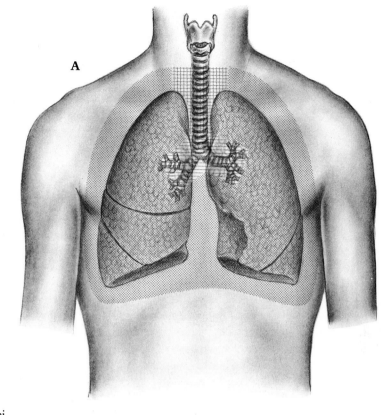

KEY:

Bronchovesicular
over main bronchi

Vesicular over lesser
bronchi, bronchioles, and lobes

Bronchial over trachea

B

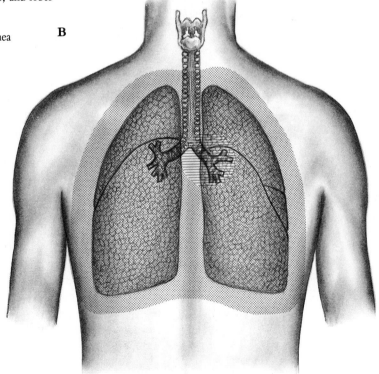

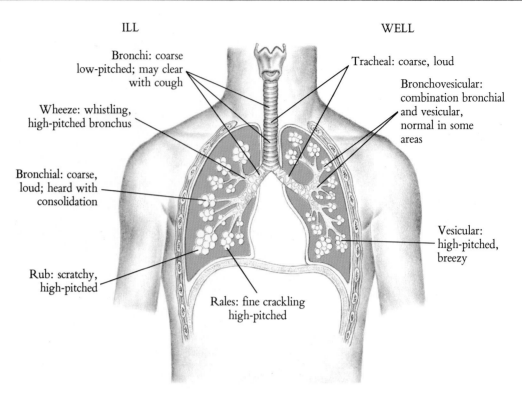

Fig. 8-18
Schema of breath sounds in the well and ill patient.

ILL — WELL

Bronchi: coarse low-pitched; may clear with cough

Wheeze: whistling, high-pitched bronchus

Bronchial: coarse, loud; heard with consolidation

Rub: scratchy, high-pitched

Rales: fine crackling high-pitched

Tracheal: coarse, loud

Bronchovesicular: combination bronchial and vesicular, normal in some areas

Vesicular: high-pitched, breezy

Rales are caused by the passage of air through the small airways in the lung that have become sticky and adherent due to the presence of fluid, mucus, or pus. The coarser and lower-pitched the rales sound, the higher their origin in the respiratory tree. High-pitched rales are described as sibilant; the more low-pitched are termed sonorous. Rales with a dry quality, more crisp than gurgling, are apt to occur higher in the respiratory tree.

Rhonchi are deeper, more rumbling, more pronounced during expiration, more likely to be continuous, and less discrete than rales. They are caused by the passage of air through an airway obstructed by thick secretions, muscular spasm, new growth, or external pressure. The more sibilant higher-pitched rhonchi arise from the smaller bronchi, as in asthma; the more sonorous lower-pitched rhonchi arise from larger bronchi, as in tracheobronchitis.

It may be difficult at times to distinguish between rales and rhonchi. In general, rhonchi tend to disappear after coughing, whereas rales do not. If such sounds are present, listen to several respiratory excursions, a few with the patient's accustomed effort, a few with deeper breathing, a few before coughing, a few after.

A wheeze is sometimes thought of as a form of rhonchus. It is a continuous, high-pitched, musical sound, almost a whistle, heard during inspiration or expiration. It is caused by a relatively high-velocity air flow through a narrowed airway. Wheezes may be composed of complex combinations of a variety of pitches or of a single pitch, and they may vary from area to area and minute to minute. If a wheeze is heard bilaterally, it may be caused by the bronchospasm of asthma or acute or chronic bronchitis. Unilateral or more sharply localized wheezing may occur with a foreign body. A tumor compressing a part of the bronchial tree can create a consistent wheeze or whistle of single pitch at the site of compression.

A friction rub occurs outside the respiratory tree. It has a dry, crackly, grating, low-pitched sound and is heard in both expiration and inspiration. It may have a machine-like quality. It may have no significance if heard over the liver or spleen. However, a friction rub heard over the heart or lungs is caused by inflamed, roughened surfaces rubbing together. Over the pericardium, this sound suggests pericarditis; over the lungs, pleurisy.

Vocal Resonance

The spoken voice vibrates and transmits sounds through the lung fields that may be judged with reasonable ease. Ask the patient to recite numbers, names, or other words. These transmitted sounds are usually muffled and indistinct and best heard medially. Pay particular attention to vocal resonance if there are other unexpected

ADVENTITIOUS BREATH SOUNDS

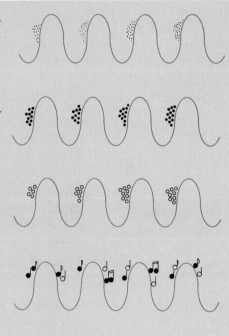

Fine rales: high-pitched, discrete, non-continuous crackling sounds heard during the end of inspiration

Medium rales: lower, more moist sound heard during the midstage of inspiration; not cleared by a cough

Coarse rales: loud, bubbly noise heard during inspiration; not cleared by a cough

Rhonchi: loud, low, coarse sounds like a snore heard at any point of inspiration or expiration; coughing may clear sound (usually means mucus accumulation in trachea or large bronchi)

Wheeze: musical noise sounding like a squeak; may be heard during inspiration or expiration; usually louder during expiration

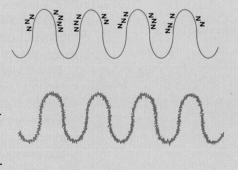

Pleural friction rub: dry, rubbing, or grating sound, usually caused by inflammation of pleural surfaces; heard during inspiration or expiration; loudest over lower lateral anterior surface

Modified from Thompson et al., 1986.

SUMMARY OF EXPECTED FINDINGS OF CHEST AND LUNGS

When the lungs are healthy, the respiratory tree clear, the pleurae unaffected by disease, and the chest wall symmetrically and appropriately structured and mobile, there will be
  Symmetry of movement on expansion
  Midline trachea without a "tug"
  Range of 3 to 5 cm in the descent of the diaphragm on inspiration
  Resonant percussion note
  Moderate tactile fremitus and muffled vocal resonance
  Absence of adventitious sounds
  Vesicular breath sounds, except for bronchovesicular sounds beside the
    sternum and more prominent bronchial components in the area of the
    larger bronchi

findings during any part of the examination of the lungs, such as dullness on percussion or changes in tactile fremitus. The factors that influence tactile fremitus similarly influence vocal resonance.

Greater clarity and increased loudness of spoken sounds are defined as bronchophony. If bronchophony is extreme, even a whisper can be heard clearly through the stethoscope (whispered pectoriloquy). When the intensity of the spoken voice is increased and there is a nasal quality (*e*'s become stuffy broad *a*'s), the auditory quality is called egophony. These auditory changes may be present in any condition that consolidates lung tissue. Conversely, vocal resonance diminishes and loses intensity when there is blockage of the respiratory tree for any reason, such as emphysema.

Cough

Coughs are a common symptom of a respiratory problem. The causes may be related to localized or more general insults at any point in the respiratory tract. Coughs are reflexive responses to an irritant such as a foreign body (microscopic or larger), an infectious agent, or a mass of any sort compressing the respiratory tree.

Describe a cough according to its moisture, frequency, regularity, pitch and loudness, and quality. The type of cough may offer some clue to the cause. While a cough may not have a serious cause, do not ignore it.

Dry or moist. A moist cough may be caused by infection and can be accompanied by sputum production. A dry cough can have a variety of causes, which may be indicated by the quality of its sound.

Frequency of occurrence. Note whether the cough is seldom or often present. An infrequent cough may result from allergens or environmental insults.

Regularity. A regular, paroxysmal cough is seen in pertussis. An irregularly occurring cough may have a variety of causes, such as smoking, early congestive heart failure, an inspired foreign body or irritant, or a tumor within or compressing the bronchial tree.

Pitch and loudness. A cough may be loud and high-pitched or quiet and relatively low-pitched.

Quality. A dry cough may sound brassy if it is caused by compression of the respiratory tree (as by a tumor) or hoarse if it is caused by croup. Pertussis produces an inspiratory whoop at the end of a paroxysm of cough.

INFANTS

The approach to examination of the chest and lungs of the newborn follows a similar sequence as for adults. Inspection, before you disturb the baby, is key. Percussion, however, is usually unreliable. The examiner's fingers are too large for the baby's chest, particularly the premature infant.

A newborn's Apgar scores at 1 and 5 minutes after birth tell you a great deal about the infant's respiratory efforts. An infant whose respirations are inadequate but who is otherwise normal may initially score 1 or even 0 on heart rate, muscle tone, response to a catheter, or color. Depressed respiration often has its origins in the maternal environment during labor, such as sedatives or compromised blood supply to the child, or it may result from mechanical obstruction by mucus. Table 8-3 explains the Apgar scoring system.

Inspect the thoracic cage, noting its size and shape; measure the chest circumference, which in the healthy full-term infant is usually in the range of 30 to 36 cm, generally 2 to 3 cm smaller than the head circumference. The difference between the two increases with prematurity. As a rough measure, the distance between the nipples is about one quarter the circumference of the chest.

Observe the nipples for symmetry in size and for the presence of swelling and discharge, as detailed in Chapter 10 (Breasts and Axillae). On occasion you will see supernumerary nipples, ordinarily not fully developed, in a line drawn caudad from the primary nipple. In white children, but not in blacks, they may be associated with congenital abnormalities.

The newborn's lung function is particularly susceptible to a number of environmental factors. The pattern of respirations will vary with room temperature, feeding, and sleep. In the first few hours after birth, the respiratory effort can be depressed by the passive transfer of drugs given the mother before delivery.

Look for cyanosis, and note its extent and distribution. Cyanosis of the hands and feet is common in the newborn and can persist for several days in a cool environment.

Count the respiratory rate for 1 minute. The normal rate varies from 40 to 60, although 80 respirations per minute is not uncommon. Babies delivered by cesarean section generally have a more rapid rate than babies delivered vaginally. If the room temperature is very warm or cool, a noticeable variation in the rate occurs, most often tachypnea but sometimes bradypnea.

Table 8-3
Infant Evaluation at Birth—Apgar Scoring System

	0	1	2
Heart rate	Absent	Slow (below 100 beats/minute)	Over 100 beats/minute
Respiratory effort	Absent	Slow or irregular	Good crying
Muscle tone	Limp	Some flexion of extremities	Active motion
Response to catheter in nostril (tested after oropharynx is clear)	No response	Grimace	Cough or sneeze
Color	Blue or pale	Body pink, extremities blue	Completely pink

Note the regularity of respiration. The more preterm an infant at birth, the more likely some irregularity in the respiratory pattern will be present. Periodic breathing, a sequence of relatively vigorous respiratory efforts followed by apnea of as much as 10 to 15 seconds, is common. It is cause for concern if the apneic episodes tend to be prolonged and the baby becomes cyanotic. The persistence of periodic breathing episodes in preterm infants is relative to the gestational age of the baby, the apneic period diminishing in frequency as the baby approaches term status. In the term infant, periodic breathing should wane a few hours after birth.

Newborns rely primarily on the diaphragm for their respiratory effort, only gradually adding the intercostal muscles. Infants quite commonly also use the abdominal muscles.

If the chest expansion is asymmetric, suspect some compromise of the baby's ability to fill one of the lungs, as can occur in pneumothorax or diaphragmatic hernia.

Palpate the rib cage and sternum, noting loss of symmetry, unusual masses, or crepitus. Crepitus around a fractured clavicle (with no evidence of pain) is common after a difficult forcep delivery. The newborn's xiphoid process is more mobile and prominent than that of the older child or adult. It has a sharp inferior tip that moves slightly back and forth under your finger.

Listen to the chest. If the baby is crying and restless, it pays to wait for a more quiet moment. Localization of breath sounds is difficult, particularly in the very small chest of the preterm infant. Breath sounds are easily transmitted from one segment of the auscultatory area to another, and therefore the absence of sounds in any given area may be difficult to detect. Sometimes it helps to listen to both sides of the chest simultaneously. Some neonatologists use a double-belled stethoscope for this purpose.

It is not uncommon to hear rales and rhonchi immediately after birth since fetal fluid has not been completely cleared. Whenever auscultatory findings are asymmetric, a problem should be suspected. Adventitious sounds, gurgling from the intestinal tract, slight movement, and mucus in the upper airway may all contribute to adventitious sounds, making evaluation difficult. If gastrointestinal gurgling sounds are persistently heard in the chest, one must suspect diaphragmatic hernia, but wide transmission of these sounds can sometimes be deceptive.

Stridor is a high-pitched, piercing sound, most often heard during inspiration. It is the result of an obstruction high in the respiratory tree. A compelling sound, it

ASSESSMENT OF RESPIRATION IN THE INFANT

There are several important observations that should be made of an infant's respiratory effort (Silverman and Anderson, 1956):
1. Does a loss of synchrony between left and right occur during the respiratory effort? Is there a lag in movement of the chest on one side?
2. Is there retraction at the suprasternal notch, intercostally, or at the xiphoid process?
3. Do the nares dilate with respiratory effort?
4. Is there an audible expiratory grunt? Is it audible with the stethoscope only or without the stethoscope?

Table 8-4
Normal Respiratory Rates in Children

Age	Rate per Minute
Newborn	30–80
1 year	20–40
3 years	20–30
6 years	16–22
10 years	16–20
17 years	12–20

cannot be dismissed as inconsequential. If it is accompanied by a cough, hoarseness, and retraction, it signifies a serious problem in the trachea or larynx: a floppy epiglottis, congenital defects, croup, or an edematous response to an infection, allergen, smoke, chemicals, or aspirated foreign body. Infants who have a narrow tracheal lumen readily respond with stridor to its compression by a tumor, abscess, or double aortic arch.

Respiratory grunting is a mechanism by which the infant tries to expel trapped air or fetal lung fluid while trying to retain air and increase oxygen levels.

CHILDREN

Children use the thoracic (intercostal) musculature for respiration by the age of 6 or 7 years. In young children obvious intercostal exertion (retractions) on breathing suggests some pulmonary or airway problem. Normal respiratory rates for children are shown in Table 8-4.

If the "roundness" of the young infant's chest persists past the second year of life, be concerned about the possibility of a chronic obstructive pulmonary problem such as cystic fibrosis. The persistence of a barrel chest at the age of 5 or 6 years can be ominous.

Seize the opportunity a crying child presents. A sob is frequently followed by a deep breath. The sob itself allows the evaluation of vocal resonance and the feel for tactile fremitus; use the whole hand, palm and fingers, gently. The crying child may pause occasionally and the heart sounds may be heard. These pauses may be a bit prolonged as the breath is held, giving the chance to distinguish a murmur from a breath sound.

Children's chests are thinner and ordinarily more resonant than adults, the intrathoracic sounds are easier to hear, and hyperresonance is common in young children. With either direct or indirect percussion, it is easy to miss the dullness of an underlying consolidation. If you sense some loss of resonance, give it as much importance as you would give frank dullness in the adolescent or adult.

Because of the thin chest wall, the breath sounds of the young may sound louder, harsher, and more bronchial than those of the adult. Bronchovesicular breath sounds may be heard throughout the chest.

PREGNANT WOMEN

Pregnant women experience both structural and ventilatory changes. The costal angle of approximately 68 degrees before pregnancy increases to about 103 degrees in the third trimester. The lower rib cage appears to flare out. Breathing becomes more thoracic than abdominal as a result of the enlarging uterus. The respiratory rate may increase slightly, by about 2 breaths per minute, and each breath will be deeper. After delivery, the chest may not return to its prepregnant state.

The examination procedure for older adults is the same as that for younger adults although there may be variation in some expected findings. Chest expansion is often decreased. The patient may be less able to use the respiratory muscles because of muscle weakness, general physical disability, or a sedentary life-style. Calcification of rib articulations may also interfere with chest expansion, requiring use of accessory muscles. Bony prominences are marked and there is loss of subcutaneous tissue. The dorsal curve of the thoracic spine is pronounced with flattening of the lumbar curve (kyphosis) (Fig. 8-19). The anteroposterior diameter of the chest is increased in relation to the lateral diameter.

Older patients may have more difficulty breathing deeply and holding their breath than younger patients.

Some older patients may display hyperresonance as a result of increased distensibility of the lungs. This finding must be evaluated in the context of the presence or absence of other symptoms.

Fig. 8-19
Pronounced dorsal curvature in older adult. **A,** Kyphosis. **B,** Gibbus (extreme kyphosis).

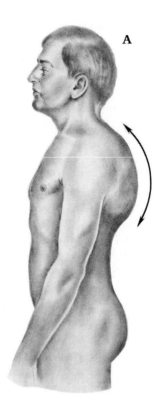
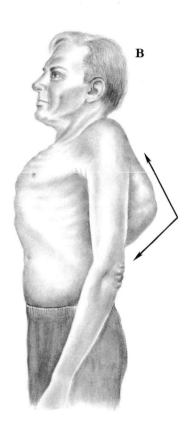

Common Abnormalities

Asthma	Asthma consists of episodes of dyspnea, tachypnea, cough, and prolonged expirations that last minutes, hours, or days. The episodes are accompanied by wheezing, cough, and a feeling of chest tightening. It may be triggered by a response to allergans, anxiety, upper respiratory infections, or exercise. The bronchial tree is narrowed in spasm, and there may be secretion and edema of the bronchial mucosa. Asthma can be variable and can change in intensity, sometimes from moment to moment and often from area to area, but it is always acutely anxiety provoking to the patient. It is a common disorder that often begins in childhood.
Atelectasis	Atelectasis is the incomplete expansion of the lung at birth or the collapse of the lung at any age. Collapse can be caused by compression by pressure from without (exudates, tumors) or resorption of gas from one alveolus in the presence of complete internal obstruction (loss of elastic recoil of the lung for any reason—thoracic or abdominal surgery, plugging, exudates, foreign body). The affected area of the lung is airless. The overall effect is to dampen or mute the sounds in the involved area.
Bronchiectasis	Chronic dilation of the bronchi or bronchioles is caused by repeated pulmonary infections and bronchial obstruction. The dilations may involve the tube uniformly (cylindric) or irregularly (saccular); at the terminal ends, the enlargement may be bulbous. Bronchiectasis may lead to malfunction of bronchial muscle tone and loss of elasticity. The extent of findings on physical examination is governed by the degree of "wetness." The cough and expectoration are most often the major clues.
Bronchitis	Bronchitis is an inflammation of the mucous membranes of the bronchial tubes. Acute bronchitis may be more or less severe than chronic bronchitis, and it may be accompanied by fever and chest pain. Chronic bronchitis has a wide variety of causes and physical manifestations, including excessive secretion of mucus in the bronchial tree. In either type the initial stimulus is irritation by an internal or external noxious influence. Either an acute or chronic condition can show varying degrees of involvement, with the possibility of obstructive phenomena and even atelectasis, but bronchitis is most often quite mild.
Emphysema	Emphysema is a chronic obstructive pulmonary disorder in which air may take over and dominate a space in a way that disrupts function. When the lung is involved, the air spaces beyond the terminal bronchioles dilate, rupturing alveolar walls, permanently destroying them, reducing their number, and permanently hyperinflating the lung. Alveolar gas is trapped, essentially in expiration, and gas exchange is seriously compromised. Chronic bronchitis is the frequent precursor. The overinflated lungs tend to hyperresonant on percussion. Further expansion on inspiration is limited; occasionally there is a prolonged expiratory effort to expel air.

Pleural Effusion	Excessive nonpurulant fluid in the pleural space can result in permanent fibrotic thickening. The sources of fluid vary; infection, neoplasm, and trauma are all possible causes. The extent of embarrassment varies with the amount of fluid, and the degree of fibrosis varies with	the chronicity of the condition. The findings vary with severity and also with the position of the patient. Fluid is mobile; it will gravitate to the most dependent position. In the affected areas the sounds are muted.
Pneumonia	Pneumonia is an inflammatory response of the bronchioles and alveolar spaces to an infective agent (bacterial, fungal, or viral). Exudates lead to lung consolida-	tion, resulting in dyspnea, tachypnea, and rales. Diminished breath sounds and dullness to percussion occur over the area of consolidation.
Pneumothorax	The presence of air or gas in the pleural cavity may be the result of trauma or may occur spontaneously without discoverable cause. The air in the pleural space may not communicate with that in the lung, but in tension pneumothorax air continues to leak from the lung into the pleural space. Air enters the pleural space on inspiration in tension pneumothorax but becomes trapped on	expiration, resulting in increasing pressure in the pleural space. Minimal collections of air without the presence of associated inflammatory lesions may easily escape detection at first. Larger collections cause varying degrees of the possible findings. Overall, the breath sounds are distant but the percussion note may boom.
Lung Cancer	Lung cancer generally refers to bronchogenic carcinoma, a malignant tumor that evolves from bronchial epithelial structures. Etiologic agents include tobacco smoke, asbestos, ionizing radiation, and other inhaled chemicals and noxious agents. It may cause cough,	wheezing, a variety of patterns of emphysema and atelectasis, pneumonitis, and hemoptysis. The extent of the tumor and the patterns of its invasion and metastasis are often determined by its histologic nature.
Cor Pulmonale	Cor pulmonale is an acute or chronic condition involving right-sided heart failure. In the acute phase, the right side of the heart is dilated and fails, most often as a direct result of pulmonary embolism. In chronic cor pulmonale a chronic, massive disease of the lungs causes gradual obstruction that	produces a more gradual hypertrophy of the right ventricle, increasing stress, and ultimate heart failure. An isolated failure of the right side of the heart is rare except in the circumstance of pulmonary obstruction caused by emboli or extensive infection and noxious involvement of the lung.
Pulmonary Hypertension	Pulmonary hypertension is defined as a pulmonary artery pressure greater than 30/15 mm Hg. Elevation must always be recognized as indicative of a disease process, such as pulmonary artery embolism or thrombosis, pulmonic stenosis, failure of the left heart, or extensive parenchymal disease of the lung. When pulmonary hypertension is chronic, it	clearly adds to the stress imposed on the heart and the coronary vasculature, compounding the initial problem. The patient with pulmonary hypertension may have only vague complaints of weakness, dyspnea, or fatigue. However, severe disease produces intense fatigue, precordial pain and, occasionally, fainting.

INFANTS AND CHILDREN

Cystic Fibrosis

Cystic fibrosis is an autosomal recessive disorder of exocrine glands involving the lungs, pancreas, and sweat glands. Heavy secretions of abnormally thick mucus cause progressive clogging of the bronchi and bronchioles, leading to frequent and progressive pulmonary infections. Initially areas of hyperinflation and atelectasis are evident. As pulmonary dysfunction progresses, pulmonary hypertension and cor pulmonale often occur. Recent advancements in treatment have extended life expectancy into adulthood.

Croup

Croup is a syndrome that generally results from infection with a variety of viral agents, particularly the parainfluenza viruses. It occurs most often in very young children, generally from about age 1½ to 3 years old. Boys are more frequently affected than girls, and for reasons unknown, some children are prone to recurrent episodes. It is not unusual to have an episode begin in the evening, often after the child has gone to sleep. The child awakens suddenly, often very frightened, with a harsh rough stridorous cough, somewhat like the bark of a seal. Labored breathing, retraction, and inspiratory stridor are characteristic. Fever does not always accompany croup. The inflammation is subglottic.

Epiglottitis

Epiglottitis is an acute, life-threatening disease almost always caused by *Haemophilus influenzae* type B. It begins suddenly and progresses rapidly, often to full obstruction of the airway resulting in a fatal outcome. It occurs most often in children between the ages of 3 and 7. The child appears very anxious and ill, unable to swallow, drooling from an open mouth; cough is not common. The fever may be high. The epiglottis appears beefy red. It is vital to note that there should be no vigorous attempt to visualize the epiglottis and that any suspicion of epiglottitis should be treated as a medical emergency. Immediate attention is required with the help of an otolaryngologist and radiologist in an emergency department. The tentative diagnosis should be based on the history and clinical appearance of the child before physical examination. Any attempt to visualize the epiglottis without skilled assistance and appropriate equipment for establishing an artificial airway is not justified.

Bronchiolitis

Bronchiolitis occurs most frequently in young infants less than 6 months old. The principle characteristic is hyperinflation of the lungs. The cause is viral, usually the respiratory syncytial virus. Expiration becomes difficult, and the infant appears anxious and tachypneic. Generalized retraction and perioral cyanosis are common. Because of lung hyperinflation, the anteroposterior diameter of the thoracic cage may be increased and the percussion not hyperresonant. Wheezing may or may not be apparent. In the presence of severe tachypnea, air exchange is poor and the breaths are rapid and short, with the expiratory phase prolonged. Rales may or may not be heard. The abdomen appears distended from swallowed air.

CHAPTER

9

Heart and Blood Vessels

Anatomy and Physiology

Heart

The heart lies in the thoracic cavity toward the middle of the mediastinum, left of the midline, just above the diaphragm, and cradled between the medial and lower borders of the lungs. It is positioned behind the sternum and the contiguous parts of the third to the sixth costal cartilages. The area of the chest overlying the heart is the precordium. Paradoxically, because of its conelike shape, the broader upper portion of the heart is called the base and the narrower lower tip of the heart the apex (Fig. 9-1).

The position of the heart can vary considerably, depending on body build, configuration of the chest, and level of the diaphragm. In the tall, slender person, the heart tends to hang more vertically and to be positioned more centrally. With increasing stockiness and shortness, it tends to lie more to the left and more horizontally (Fig. 9-2). In some rare cases the heart lies on the right side instead of the left, a condition known as dextrocardia.

Fig. 9-1
Frontal section of heart.

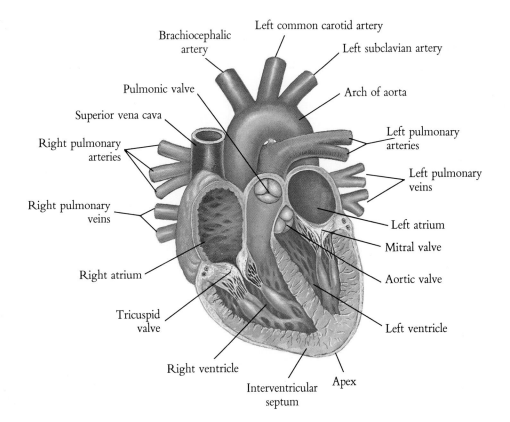

Fig. 9-2
Position of heart in the chest. A, Average person. **B,** Tall, thin person. **C,** Short, stocky person.

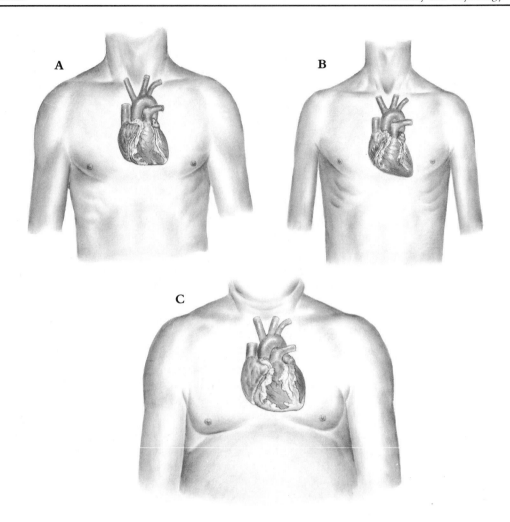

Structure

The pericardium is a tough, double-walled, fibrous sac encasing and protecting the heart. Several cubic centimeters of fluid are present between the inner and outer layers of the pericardium, providing for easy, low friction movement.

The epicardium, the thin outermost muscle layer, covers the surface of the heart and extends to the great vessels. The myocardium, the thick muscular middle layer, is responsible for the major pumping action of the ventricles. The endocardium, the innermost layer, lines the inner chambers of the heart and covers the heart valves and the small muscles associated with the opening and closing of these valves (Fig. 9-3).

The heart is divided into four chambers. The two top chambers are the right and left atria (or auricles, because of their earlike shape), and the two bottom chambers are the right and left ventricles. The left atrium and left ventricle together are referred to as the left heart; the right atrium and right ventricle together are referred to as the right heart. The left heart and right heart are divided by a blood-tight partition called the cardiac septum.

The atria are small, thin-walled structures that act primarily as a reservoir for the blood returning to the heart from the veins throughout the body. The ventricles are large, thick-walled chambers that pump blood to the lungs and throughout the body. The right and left ventricles together form the primary muscle mass of the heart.

Most of the anterior surface of the heart is formed by the right ventricle. The left ventricle is set behind the right and extends more to the left, forming the left border of the heart. (Its contraction and thrust are responsible for the apical impulse usually felt in the fifth left intercostal space along the midclavicular line.) The right atrium lies above and slightly to the right of the right ventricle, forming the right border of the heart. The left atrium is above the left ventricle, forming the more posterior aspect of the heart. The heart is, in effect, turned ventrally on its axis, putting its right side more forward. The adult heart is about 12 cm long, 8 cm wide at the widest point, and 6 cm thick (Fig. 9-4).

The four chambers of the heart are connected by two sets of valves: the atrioventricular and semilunar valves. In the fully formed heart that is free of defect, these are the only intracardiac pathways. They permit the flow of blood in only one direction (Fig. 9-5).

The atrioventricular valves, which are situated between the atria and the ventricles, include the tricuspid and mitral valves. The tricuspid valve, which has three cusps or leaflets, leads from the right atrium into the right ventricle. The mitral valve, which has two cusps, leads from the left atrium into the left ventricle. When the atria contract, the atrioventricular valves swing open, allowing the blood to flow down into the ventricles. When the ventricles contract, these valves shap shut, preventing any blood from flowing back up into the atria.

The two semilunar valves each have three cusps. The pulmonic valve separates the right venticle from the pulmonary artery. The aortic valve lies between the left ventricle and the aorta. Contraction of the ventricles opens the semilunar valves, causing blood to rush into the pulmonary artery and aorta. When the ventricles relax, the valves close, shutting off any backward flow into the ventricles.

Fig. 9-3
Cross section of cardiac muscle showing its three layers and pericardium.
From Thompson et al., 1986.

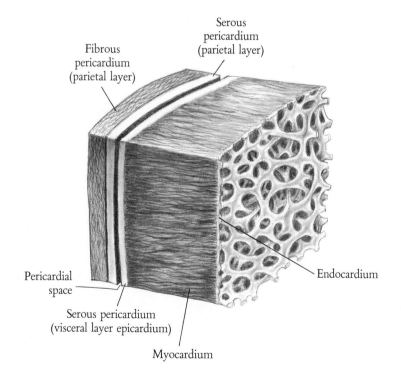

Fig. 9-4
A, Anterior. **B,** Posterior
views of heart.

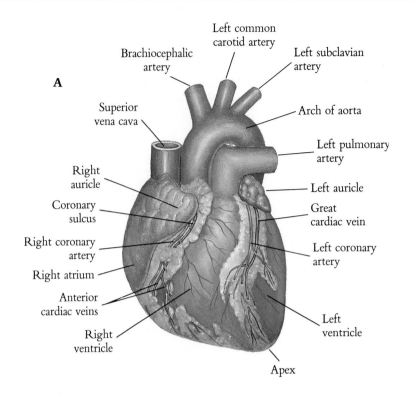

A

Left common
carotid artery

Brachiocephalic
artery

Left subclavian
artery

Superior
vena cava

Arch of aorta

Left pulmonary
artery

Right
auricle

Left auricle

Coronary
sulcus

Great
cardiac vein

Right coronary
artery

Left coronary
artery

Right atrium

Anterior
cardiac veins

Left
ventricle

Right
ventricle

Apex

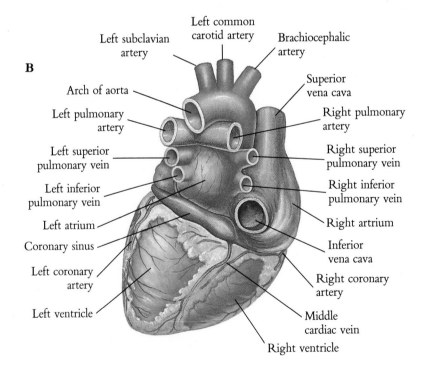

B

Left subclavian
artery

Left common
carotid artery

Brachiocephalic
artery

Arch of aorta

Superior
vena cava

Left pulmonary
artery

Right pulmonary
artery

Left superior
pulmonary vein

Right superior
pulmonary vein

Left inferior
pulmonary vein

Right inferior
pulmonary vein

Left atrium

Right artrium

Coronary sinus

Inferior
vena cava

Left coronary
artery

Right coronary
artery

Left ventricle

Middle
cardiac vein

Right ventricle

Fig. 9-5
Anterior cross section showing the valves and chambers of the heart.

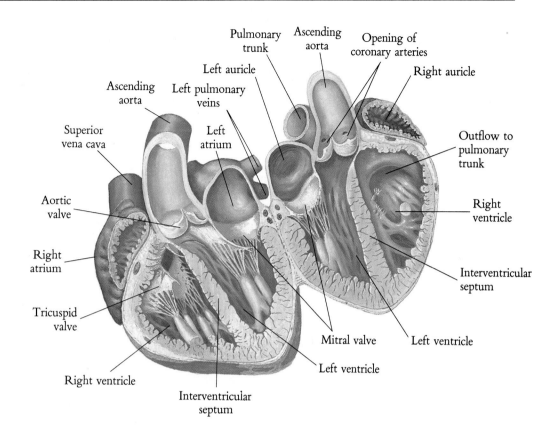

Fig. 9-6
Anatomic location of the heart valves and their relationship to the great vessels.

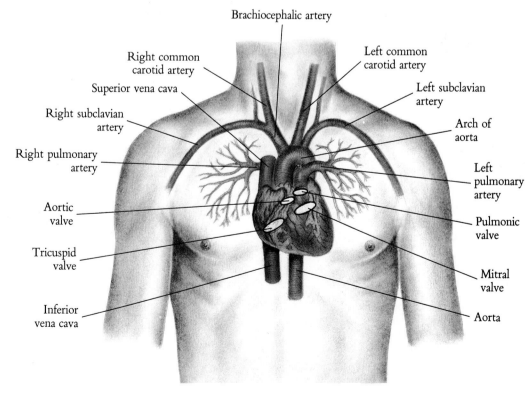

The arteries and veins attached to the heart are called the great vessels. They circulate blood to and from the body and the lungs. The great vessels, located in a cluster at the base of the heart, include the aorta, superior and inferior vena cavae, pulmonary arteries, and pulmonary veins (Fig. 9-6). The aorta carries oxygenated blood out of the left ventricle to the body. The superior and inferior vena cavae carry blood from the upper and lower body, respectively, to the right atrium. The pulmonary artery, which leaves the right ventricle and bifurcates almost immediately into the right and left bronchial arteries, carries blood to the lungs. The pulmonary veins branch right and left and return oxygenated blood from the lungs to the left atrium.

Cardiac Cycle

The muscular heart contracts and relaxes rhythmically to assure proper circulation, a process that creates two phases in the cardiac cycle. During systole the ventricles contract, ejecting blood from the left ventricle into the aorta and from the right ventricle into the pulmonary artery. During diastole the ventricles relax and the atria contract, moving blood from the atria to the ventricles (Figs. 9-7 and 9-8).

As systole begins, ventricular contraction raises the pressure in the ventricles and forces the mitral and tricuspid valves closed, preventing backflow. This valve closure produces the first heart sound (S_1), the characteristic "lubb." The intraventricular pressure rises until it exceeds that in the aorta and pulmonary artery. Then the aortic and pulmonic valves are forced open and ejection of blood into the arteries begins. Valve opening is normally a silent event.

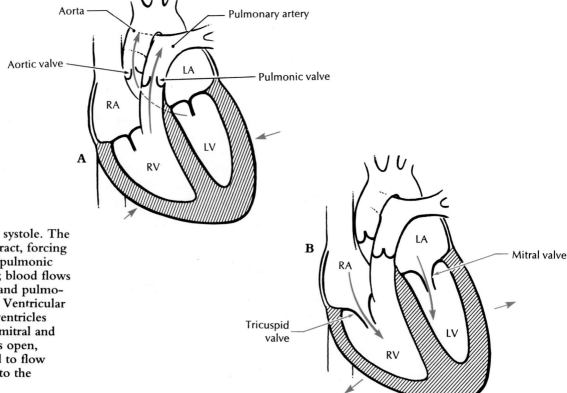

Fig. 9-7
A, Ventricular systole. The ventricles contract, forcing the aortic and pulmonic valves to open; blood flows into the aorta and pulmonary artery. B, Ventricular diastole. The ventricles relax, and the mitral and tricuspid valves open, allowing blood to flow from the atria to the ventricles.

From Malasanos et al., 1986.

Fig. 9-8
Events of cardiac cycle, showing venous pressure waves, ECG, and heart sounds in systole and diastole.
From Guzzetta and Dossey, 1984.

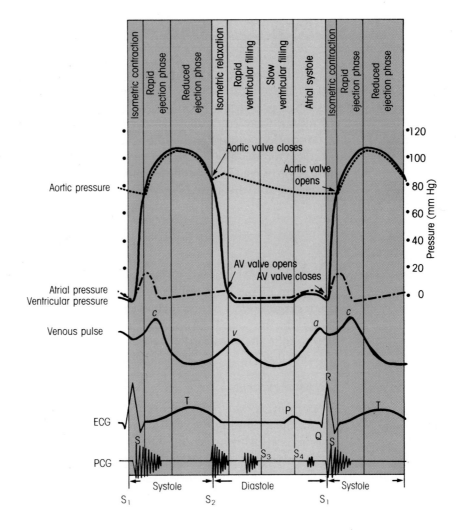

When the ventricles are almost empty, the pressure in the ventricles falls below that in the aorta and pulmonary artery, allowing the aortic and pulmonic valves to close. Closure of these valves causes the second heart sound (S_2), "dubb," which has two components—A_2 is produced by aortic valve closure and P_2 is produced by pulmonic valve closure. As ventricular pressure falls below atrial pressure, the mitral and tricuspid valves open to allow the blood collected in the atria to refill the relaxed ventricles. Diastole is a relatively passive interval until ventricular filling is almost complete. This filling sometimes produces a third heart sound (S_3). Then the atria contract to ensure the ejection of any remaining blood. This can sometimes be heard as a fourth heart sound (S_4). The cycle begins anew with ventricular contraction and atrial refilling occurring at about the same time.

For the sake of simplicity this discussion describes the events of the cardiac cycle as identical on both sides of the heart. Actually, however, the pressures in the right ventricle, right atrium, and pulmonary artery are lower than those on the left side of the heart, and the same events occur slightly later on the right side than on the left. The effect is that heart sounds sometimes have two distinct components, the first produced by the left side and the second by the right side. For example, the aortic valve closes slightly before the pulmonic, so that S_2 is often heard as two distinct components, referred to as "split S_2."

VALVULAR CONTROL OF BLOOD FLOW

Systole: Systole is the time period during which the ventricles contract and eject blood into their respective arteries. The mitral and tricuspid valves close (S_1), preventing backflow, and the aortic and pulmonic valves open, permitting forward flow.

Diastole: During diastole the ventricles are in a relaxed state and the atria contract, forcing blood into the ventricles. The aortic and pulmonic valves close (S_2), preventing backflow, and the mitral and tricuspid valves open, permitting forward flow.

Closure of the heart valves during the cardiac cycle produces heart sounds in rapid succession. The simultaneous muscular tension and flow of blood give "body" to the sounds. Although the valves are anatomically close to each other, their sounds are best heard in an area away from the anatomic site (in the direction of blood flow).

Electrical Activity

An electrical conduction system coordinates the sequence of muscular contractions that take place during the cardiac cycle. An electrical current or impulse stimulates each myocardial contraction. The impulse originates in and is paced by the sino-atrial node (SA node), located in the wall of the right atrium. The impulse then travels through both atria to the atrioventricular node (AV node), located in the atrial septum. The AV node stimulates atrial contraction. Before its passage down the bundle of His and its branches, the impulse is slightly delayed; it then travels to the Purkinje fibers in the ventricular myocarium, where it stimulates ventricular contraction (Fig. 9-9).

An electrocardiogram (ECG) is a graphic recording of electrical activity during the cardiac cycle. The ECG records electrical current generated by movement of ions in and out of the myocardial cell membrane. The ECG records two basic events: depolarization, which is the spread of a stimulus through the heart muscle, and repolarization, which is the return of the stimulated heart muscle to a resting state. The ECG records electrical activity as specific waves (Fig. 9-10):

P wave—the spread of a stimulus through the atria (atrial depolarization)

PR interval—the time from initial stimulation of the atria to initial stimulation of the ventricles

QRS complex—the spread of a stimulus through the ventricles (ventricular depolarization)

ST segment and T wave—the return of stimulated ventricular muscle to a resting state (ventricular repolarization)

U wave—a small deflection sometimes seen just after the T wave, representing the final phase of ventricular repolarization

Since the electrical stimulus starts the cycle, it must precede the mechanical response by a brief moment; the sequence of myocardial depolarization is the cause of events on the left of the heart occurring slightly before those on the right. When the heart is beating at a rate of 68 to 72 beats per minute, ventricular systole is

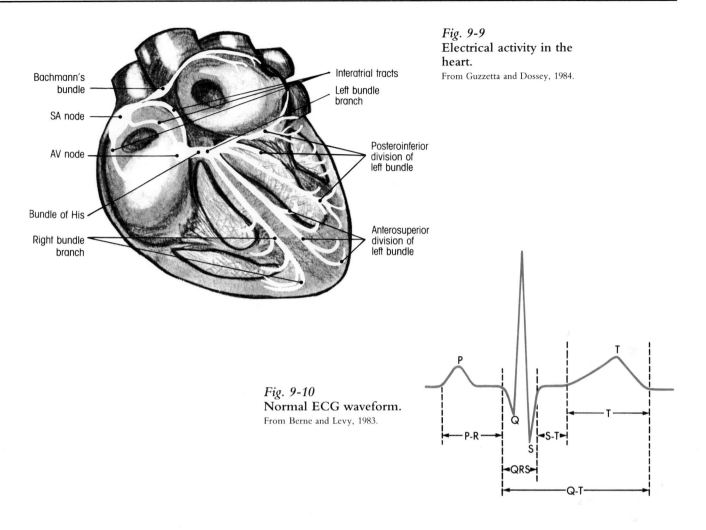

Fig. 9-9
Electrical activity in the heart.
From Guzzetta and Dossey, 1984.

Fig. 9-10
Normal ECG waveform.
From Berne and Levy, 1983.

shorter than diastole; but as the rate increases to about 120 because of stress or pathology, the two phases of the cardiac cycle tend to approximate each other in length.

Blood Circulation

Once it leaves the heart, the blood flows through two circulatory systems: the pulmonary and the systemic. The heart and these two systems create a closed system that distributes oxygen to all parts of the body.

The pulmonary circulation routes blood through the lungs, where it is reoxygenated before being dispatched to the rest of the body. Venous blood arrives at the right atrium via the superior and inferior vena cavae and moves through the tricuspid valve to the right ventricle. During systole, unoxygenated blood is ejected through the pulmonic valve into the pulmonary artery; it travels through increasingly smaller and more numerous arteries, arterioles, and capillaries of the lungs until it reaches the alveoli, where gas exchange occurs.

Oxygenated blood returns to the heart through the pulmonary veins into the left atrium, then through the mitral valve into the left ventricle. The left ventricle contracts, forcing a volume of blood (stroke volume) through the aortic valve into the aorta, through the arterial system and capillaries, where the deoxygenated blood passes into the venous system and returns to the heart (Fig. 9-11).

Fig. 9-11
Systemic circulation.
A, Arteries.

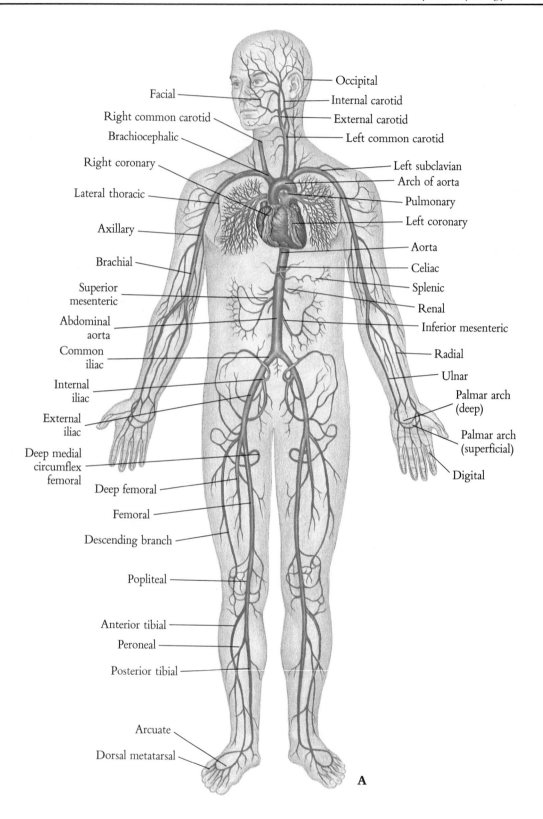

Occipital
Internal carotid
External carotid
Left common carotid

Facial
Right common carotid
Brachiocephalic

Right coronary

Lateral thoracic

Axillary

Brachial

Superior
mesenteric

Abdominal
aorta

Common
iliac

Internal
iliac

External
iliac

Deep medial
circumflex
femoral

Deep femoral

Femoral

Descending branch

Popliteal

Anterior tibial

Peroneal

Posterior tibial

Arcuate

Dorsal metatarsal

Left subclavian
Arch of aorta
Pulmonary
Left coronary

Aorta
Celiac
Splenic
Renal
Inferior mesenteric

Radial

Ulnar

Palmar arch
(deep)

Palmar arch
(superficial)

Digital

A

Fig. 9-11, cont'd
Systemic circulation.
B, Veins.

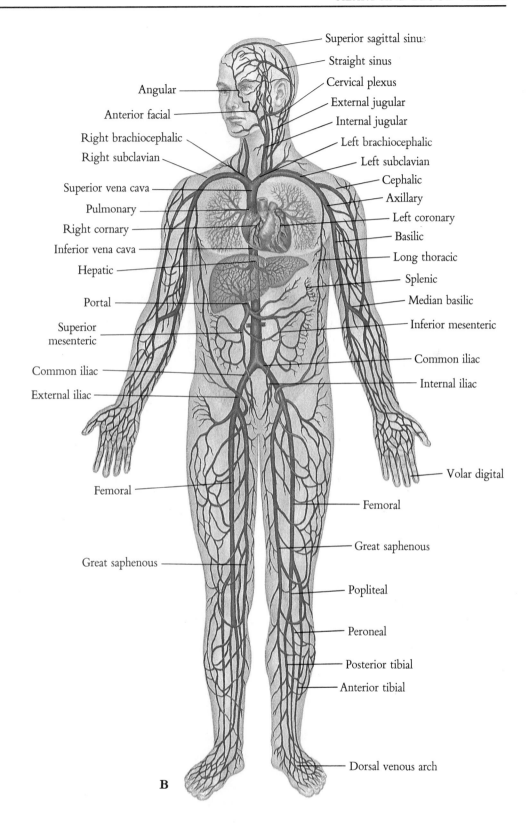

Superior sagittal sinus
Straight sinus
Cervical plexus
External jugular
Internal jugular
Left brachiocephalic
Left subclavian
Cephalic
Axillary
Left coronary
Basilic
Long thoracic
Splenic
Median basilic
Inferior mesenteric
Common iliac
Internal iliac
Volar digital
Femoral
Great saphenous
Popliteal
Peroneal
Posterior tibial
Anterior tibial
Dorsal venous arch

Angular
Anterior facial
Right brachiocephalic
Right subclavian
Superior vena cava
Pulmonary
Right cornary
Inferior vena cava
Hepatic
Portal
Superior
mesenteric
Common iliac
External iliac
Femoral
Great saphenous

B

Fig. 9-12
Structure of arteries and veins. Note thickness of venous walls.
From Thompson et al., 1986.

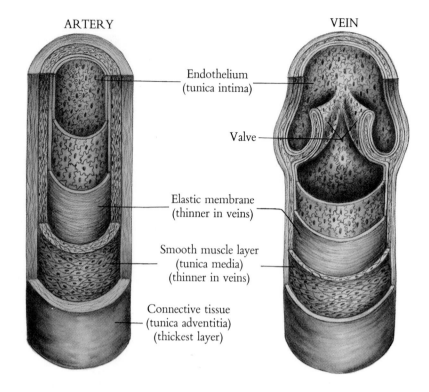

The structure of the arteries and veins reflects their function. The arteries are tougher, more tensile, and less distensible. They are subjected to much more pressure than the veins. The veins are less sturdy and more passive than the arteries (Fig. 9-12). Since venous return is less forceful than blood flow through the arteries, veins contain valves to keep blood flowing in one direction. If blood volume increases significantly, the veins can expand and act as a repository for extra blood. This compensatory mechanism diminishes stress on the heart up to a point.

Arterial Pulse and Pressure

The palpable and sometimes visible arterial pulses are the result of ventricular systole, which produces a pressure wave throughout the arterial system (arterial pulse). The arterial blood pressure is the force exerted by the blood against the wall of an artery as the ventricles of the heart contract and relax.

A normal pulse is felt as a forceful wave that is smooth and more rapid on the ascending part of the wave, becoming domed, less steep, and slower on the descending part. Since the carotid arteries are the most accessible arteries closest to the heart, they have the most suitable pulse for evaluation of cardiac function (Fig. 9-13).

Arterial blood pressure has both systolic and diastolic components. Systolic pressure is the force exerted against the wall of the artery when the ventricles contract and is largely the result of cardiac output and blood volume. Blood pressure is highest in systole. Diastolic pressure is the force exerted against the wall of the artery when the heart is in the filling or relaxed state and is primarily the function of peripheral vascular resistance. During diastole, pressure falls to its lowest point. Pulse pressure is the difference between systolic and diastolic pressure.

Fig. 9-13
Diagram of normal pulse.
From Malasanos et al., 1986.

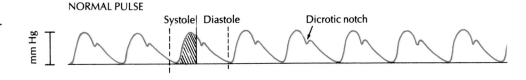

NORMAL PULSE

Systole | Diastole   Dicrotic notch

mm Hg

Fig. 9-14
Jugular venous pressure.
From Malasanos et al., 1986.

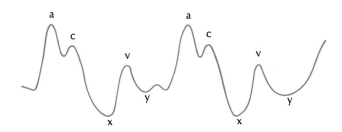

Variables that contribute to the characteristics of the pulses are:
• Volume of the blood ejected (stroke volume)
• Distensibility of the aorta and large arteries
• Viscosity of the blood
• Rate of ejection (cardiac output)
• Peripheral arteriolar resistance

Jugular Venous Pulse and Pressure

The jugular veins, which empty directly into the superior vena cava, reflect the activity of the right side of the heart and offer clues to its competency. The level at which the jugular venous pulse is visible gives an indication of right atrial pressure (Fig. 9-14).

The external jugulars are more superficial and are more visible bilaterally above the clavicle, close to the insertion of the sternocleidomastoid muscles. The larger internal jugulars run deep to the sternocleidomastoids, near the carotid arteries, and are less accessible to inspection. (See Fig. 9-33.)

The activity of the right side of the heart is transmitted back through the jugular veins as a pulse* that has five identifiable components—three peaks and two descending slopes:

a wave	The a wave, the first and highest component, is the result of a brief backflow of blood to the vena cava during right atrial contraction.
c wave	The c wave is a transmitted impulse from the nearby carotid artery and from the vigorous backward push produced by closure of the tricuspid valve during ventricular systole.
v wave	The v wave is caused by the increasing volume and concomitant increasing pressure in the right atrium. It occurs a split moment after the c wave, late in ventricular systole.
x slope	The downward x slope is evident during the displacement of the base of the ventricles during ventricular systole and atrial diastole.
y slope	The y slope following the v wave reflects the open tricuspid valve and the relatively passive filling of the ventricle.

*Although often referred to as a pulse, this is not the same as an arterial pulse, since it is reflected back from the right heart rather than pushed forward by the left heart.

INFANTS AND CHILDREN

The heart becomes very much like its adult self early in fetal life. The fetal circulation, including the umbilical vessels, compensates for the nonfunctional fetal lung. The left ventricle pumps blood through the patent ductus arteriosus rather than into the lungs. The right and left ventricles are equal in weight and muscle mass because they both pump blood into the systemic circulation (Figs. 9-15 and 9-16).

The changes at birth include closure of the ductus arteriosus, usually within 24 to 48 hours, and the functional closure of the interatrial foramen ovale as the pressure in the left atrium rises. The changing demand on the right ventricle as the pulmonary circulation is established and on the left ventricle as it assumes total responsibility for the systemic circulation results in a relative increase in the mass of the left ventricle. By 1 year of age, the relative sizes of the left and right ventricles approximates the adult ratio of 2:1.

In infants and young children, the heart lies more horizontally in the chest than in the adult, and as a result the apex of the heart rides higher, sometimes well out into the fourth left intercostal space. Usually, by the age of 7 years the adult heart position is reached (Fig. 9-17).

Fig. 9-15
Anatomy of fetal heart.
From Thompson et al., 1986.

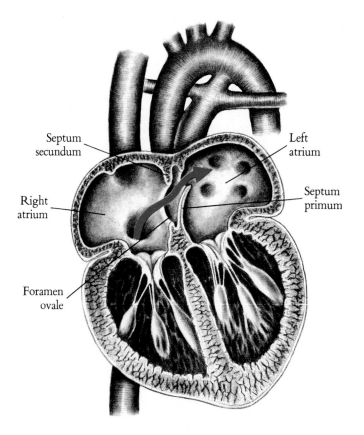

Fig. 9-16
Fetal circulation.
From Thompson et al., 1986.

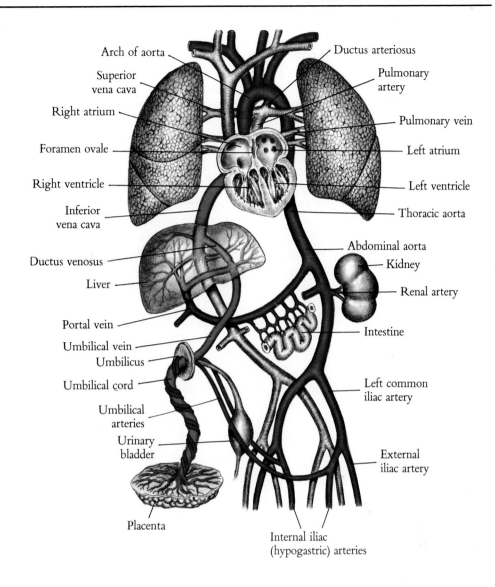

Arch of aorta
Superior vena cava
Right atrium
Foramen ovale
Right ventricle
Inferior vena cava
Ductus venosus
Liver
Portal vein
Umbilical vein
Umbilicus
Umbilical cord
Umbilical arteries
Urinary bladder
Placenta

Ductus arteriosus
Pulmonary artery
Pulmonary vein
Left atrium
Left ventricle
Thoracic aorta
Abdominal aorta
Kidney
Renal artery
Intestine
Left common iliac artery
External iliac artery
Internal iliac (hypogastric) arteries

Fig. 9-17
Position of heart at various ages.

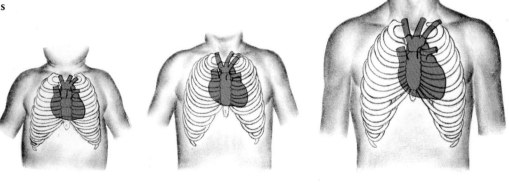

Early infancy   Early childhood   Adulthood

PREGNANT WOMEN

The maternal blood volume begins to increase by 10 to 12 weeks gestation and reaches its maximum by 32 to 34 weeks, with an increase in total blood volume of approximately 30% to 40% over the prepregnant state. The heart works harder and may dilate to accommodate the increased heart rate and stroke volume required for this expanded blood volume. By 6 weeks postpartum, the blood volume returns to its prepregnant level. With the enlarging uterus and movement of the diaphragm upward, the position of the heart is shifted upward and to the left and rotated forward.

Peripheral vascular changes include vasodilation of the blood vessels, resulting from hormonal changes. As a result, blood pressure drops during early pregnancy and varies with position, slowly rising during the third trimester. The capacity of the venous system is increased during pregnancy, leading to venous pooling. Increased venous pressure results from obstruction of the iliac veins and inferior vena cava by the uterus, causing edema of the lower extremities and varicosities.

OLDER ADULTS

Heart size may decrease with age unless there is enlargement associated with hypertension or heart disease. The heart rate slows, stroke volume decreases, and cardiac output declines by 30% to 40%. The endocardium thickens. The myocardium becomes less elastic and more rigid so that recovery of myocardial contractility and irritability is delayed. Thus the response to stress and increased oxygen demand is less efficient, tachycardia is poorly tolerated, and after stress for any reason, the return to a normal heart rate takes longer.

Calcification of the walls of the arteries causes dilation and tortuosity of the aorta, aortic branches, and the carotid arteries. The superficial vessels of the forehead, neck, and extremities also become tortuous and more prominent. The arterial walls lose elasticity and vasomotor tone, thus increasing peripheral vascular resistance, which elevates systolic blood pressure. Increased vasopressor lability tends to increase both systolic and diastolic pressures. Cardiac function is further compromised by fibrosis and sclerosis in the region of the SA node and in the heart valves (particularly the mitral valve and aortic cusps), increased vagal tone, and decreased baroreceptor sensitivity.

Electrocardiographic changes occur secondary to cellular alteration, fibrosis within the conduction system, and neurogenic changes. Common ECG changes in older patients include first degree atrioventricular block, bundle branch block, ST-T wave abnormalities, premature systole (atrial and ventricular), left anterior hemiblock, left ventricular hypertrophy, and atrial fibrillation.

Review of Related History

General Considerations

1. Employment: physical demands, environmental hazards such as heat, chemicals, dust
2. Tobacco: type (cigarettes, cigars, pipe, chewing tobacco, snuff), duration, amount, age started
3. Nutritional status
   a. Usual diet: proportion of fat, food preferences, history of dieting
   b. Weight: loss or gain, amount and speed
   c. Alcohol consumption: amount, frequency, duration of current intake

Table 9-1
Exercise Intensity

Intensity	Sample Activities
Light	Walking 10-15 steps Preparing simple meal for one Retrieving newspaper from just outside door Pulling down bedspread Brushing teeth
Moderate	Making bed Dusting and sweeping Walking a level, short block Office filing
Moderately heavy	Climbing 1-2 flights of stairs Lifting full cartons Long walks Sexual intercourse
Heavy	Jogging Vigorous athletics of any kind Cleaning entire house in less than a day Raking large number of leaves Mowing large lawn Shoveling deep snow

4. Relaxation
   a. Hobbies
   b. Exercise: type, amount, frequency, intensity (Table 9-1)
   c. Sexual activity: frequency of intercourse
5. Drug use: nitroglycerin, digoxin, diuretics, beta blockers, antihypertensives, prophylactic penicillin, aspirin, over-the-counter agents

Present Problem

Chest Pain

1. Onset and duration: sudden or gradual, time episode lasted; cyclic nature; related to physical exertion, rest, emotional experience, eating, coughing, cold temperatures
2. Character: aching, sharp, tingling, burning, pressure, stabbing, crushing, or clenched fist sign; location; radiation down arms, to neck, jaws, teeth, scapula; relief with rest or position change
3. Severity: interference with activity, need to stop all activity until subsiding, disrupts sleep
4. Associated symptoms: anxiety, dyspnea, diaphoresis, dizziness, nausea and vomiting, faintness, cold clammy skin, cyanosis, pallor, swelling or edema (noted anywhere, constant or certain times during day)
5. Treatment: rest, position change, exercise, nitroglycerin

Fatigue

1. Unusual or persistent, unable to keep up with contemporaries, inability to maintain usual activities, bedtime earlier
2. Associated symptoms: dyspnea on exertion, chest pain, palpitations, orthopnea, anorexia, nausea, vomiting

Leg Pain or Cramps

1. Onset and duration: with activity or rest, with elevation of legs, recent injury or immobilization
2. Character
   a. Continuous burning in toes, pain when pointing toes, pain in thighs or buttocks, charley horses, aching, pain over specific location
   b. Skin changes: cold skin, pallor, hair loss, sores, redness or warmth over vein, visible veins
   c. Fatigue or limping: occurs with walking, improves with walking
   d. Wake up at night

Past Medical History

1. Cardiac surgery or hospitalization for cardiac evaluation or disorder
2. Acute rheumatic fever, unexplained fever, swollen joints, inflammatory rheumatism, St. Vitus' dance (Sydenham's chorea)
3. Chronic illness: hypertension, bleeding disorder, hyperlipidemia, diabetes, coronary artery disease, congenital heart defect

Family History

1. Diabetes
2. Heart disease
3. Hyperlipidemia
4. Hypertension
5. Congenital heart defects, ventricular septal defects
6. Sudden death, particularly in young and middle-aged relatives

INFANTS

1. Tiring easily during feeding
2. Breathing changes: more heavily or more rapidly than expected during feeding or defecation
3. Cyanosis: perioral during eating, more widespread and more persistent, related to crying
4. Weight gain as expected
5. Knee-chest position or other position favored for rest
6. Mother's health during pregnancy: rubella in first trimester, unexplained fever, drug use

CHILDREN

1. Tiring during play: amount of time before tiring, activities that are tiring, inability to keep up with other children, reluctance to go out to play
2. Naps: longer than expected, usual length
3. Positions: squatting instead of sitting when at play or watching television
4. Leg pains during exercise
5. Headaches
6. Nosebleeds
7. Unexplained joint pain
8. Unexplained fever
9. Expected height and weight gain (and any substantiating records)
10. Expected physical and cognitive development (and any substantiating records)

<table>
<tr><td>

PREGNANT WOMEN

</td><td>

1. Blood pressure: prepregnancy levels, elevation during pregnancy; associated with headaches, edema of face and hands
2. Legs: edema, varicosities, pain or discomfort
3. Dizziness or faintness on standing

</td></tr>
<tr><td>

OLDER ADULTS

</td><td>

1. Common symptoms of cardiovascular disorders
   a. Confusion, dizziness, blackouts, syncope
   b. Palpitations
   c. Coughs and wheezes
   d. Hemoptysis
   e. Shortness of breath
   f. Chest pains or chest tightness
   g. Fatigue
   h. Leg edema: pattern, frequency, time of day most pronounced
2. If heart disease has been diagnosed
   a. Drug reactions: potassium excess (weakness, bradycardia, hypotension, confusion); potassium depletion (weakness, fatigue, muscle cramps, dysrhythmias); digitalis toxicity (anorexia, nausea, vomiting, diarrhea, headache, confusion, dysrhythmias, yellow vision)
   b. Interference with activities of daily living
   c. Ability of the patient and family to cope with the condition

</td></tr>
</table>

Examination and Findings

<table>
<tr><td>

EQUIPMENT

</td><td>

- **Marking pencil**
- **Centimeter rule**
- **Stethoscope, with bell and diaphragm (for children, the diaphragm may have a smaller diameter)**
- **Sphygmomanometer with appropriately sized cuff**

</td></tr>
</table>

A complete examination of the cardiovascular system includes the following: (1) observing and palpating the pulses, comparing each with the contralateral pulse and comparing pulses of the upper extremity with those of the lower; (2) inspecting the veins, particularly the jugular veins; (3) measuring blood pressure in both lower and upper extremities and, when there is clinical indication, with the patient sitting, standing, and supine; and (4) auscultating the heart.

Observations may be integrated with other parts of the physical examination in a sequence that is comfortable for you. Performing a successful examination requires both a mastery of the mechanics of each procedure and the ability to interpret findings in relation to the cardiac events they reflect.

Heart

In assessing cardiac function, it is a common error to listen to the heart first. However, it is important to follow the proper sequence, beginning with inspection, palpation, percussion, and then auscultation. Be sure that lighting includes a tangential source to allow shadows to accent the surface flicker of underlying cardiac movement. The room should be quiet, because subtle, low-pitched sounds are hard to hear. Stand to the patient's right, at least at the start. A thorough examination of the heart requires the patient to assume a variety of positions: sitting erect and leaning forward, supine, and left lateral recumbent. These necessary changes in position mandate a comfortable examining table on which movement is easy. Large breasts can make examination difficult. Either you or the patient can move the left breast up or to the left.

Inspection

Look first at the precordium with the patient supine and the light source tangential. Visible pulsations and more exaggerated lifts and heaves of the chest can provide clues to the size and symmetry of the heart. The apical impulse is the visible, palpable, pushing force against the chest caused by left ventricular contraction. It is generally synchronous with the carotid impulse and the first heart sound. Since it usually appears near the apex of the heart, its location offers a clue to cardiac size.

In about half of all adults the apical impulse is visible 5 to 7 cm from the midsternal line (at the midclavicular line) in the fifth left intercostal space, but it is easily obscured by obesity, large breasts, and great muscularity. However, the apical impulse may become visible only when the patient sits up and the heart is brought closer to the anterior wall. This is an expected finding.

Readily visible and palpable findings when the patient is supine suggest an intensity that may be the result of a problem. The absence of an apical impulse and faint heart sounds, particularly when the patient is in the left lateral recumbent position, suggest some intervening extracardiac problem, such as pleural or pericardial fluid. In any event, what is seen is affected by the shape and thickness of the chest wall and the amount of tissue, air, and fluid through which the impulses are transmitted.

Palpation

Make sure that your hands are warm, and with the patient supine, feel the precordium. Use the proximal halves of the four fingers held gently together or the whole hand. Touch gently and let the movements rise to your hand, because sensation will decrease as you increase pressure.

Fig. 9-18
Sequence for palpation of precordium. A, Apex. B, Left sternal border. C, Base.

As always, be methodical. One suggested sequence is to begin at the apex, move to the left sternal border and then to the base, going down to the right sternal border and into the epigastrium or axillae if the circumstance dictates (Fig. 9-18).

A   B   C

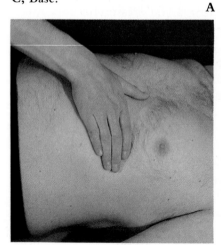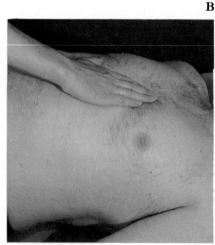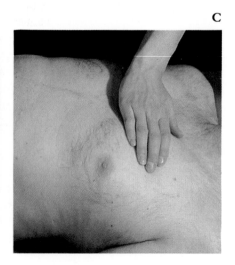

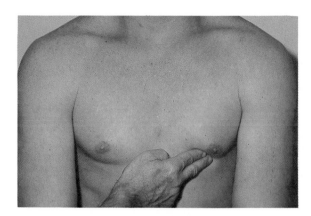

Fig. 9-19
Palpation of apical
impulse.

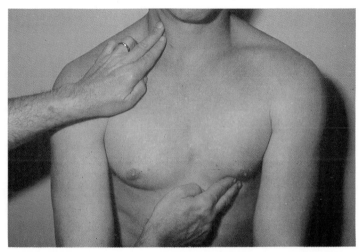

Fig. 9-20
Palpation of carotid artery
to time events felt over
precordium.

Feel for the apical impulse and identify its location by the intercostal space and the distance from the midsternal line. Determine the width of the arc in which it is felt. Usually it is palpable within a small radius—no more than 1 cm. The impulse is usually gentle and brief, not lasting as long as systole. If it is more vigorous than expected, characterize it as a heave or lift. In many adults, you may not be able to feel the apical impulse because of the thickness of the chest wall (Fig. 9-19).

An apical impulse that is more forceful and widely distributed, fills systole, or is displaced laterally and downward may indicate increased cardiac output or left ventricular hypertrophy. A lift along the left sternal border may be caused by right ventricular hypertrophy. A loss of thrust may be related to overlying fluid or air or to displacement beneath the sternum. Displacement to the right or left without a loss or gain in thrust suggests dextrocardia, diaphragmatic hernia, distended stomach, or pulmonary abnormality.

Feel for a thrill—a fine, palpable, rushing vibration over the base of the heart in the area of the right or left second intercostal space. It indicates a disruption of the expected blood flow related to some defect in the closure of one of the semilunar valves (generally aortic or pulmonic stenosis), pulmonary hypertension, or atrial septal defect.

While palpating the precordium, use your other hand to palpate the carotid artery so that you can describe the carotid pulse in relation to the cardiac cycle. The carotid pulse and S_1 are practically synchronous. The carotid pulse is located just medial to and below the angle of the jaw. Locate each sensation in terms of its intercostal space and relationship to the midsternal, midclavicular, and axillary lines (Fig. 9-20). Chapter 8 (Chest and Lungs) describes the method for counting ribs and intercostal spaces.

Percussion

Percussion is of limited value in defining the borders of the heart or determining its size, since the shape of the chest is relatively rigid and can to some extent make the more malleable heart conform. Left ventricular size is better judged by the location of the apical impulse. The right ventricle tends to enlarge in the anteroposterior diameter rather than laterally, thus diminishing the value of percussion of the left heart border. A chest roentgenogram is far more useful for defining the heart borders.

Should you wish to estimate the size of the heart by percussion, begin tapping at the anterior axillary line, moving medially along the intercostal spaces toward the sternal borders. The change from a resonant to a dull note marks the cardiac border. Ordinarily no change in note is expected before the right sternal border is encountered. On the left, the loss of resonance will generally be close to the point of maximal impulse at the apex of the heart. Measure this point from the midsternal line at each intercostal space. Obesity, unusual muscular development, and some pathologic events (such as air or fluids) can easily distort the findings.

Auscultation

Since all heart sounds are of relatively low frequency, in a range somewhat difficult for the human ear to detect, you must be compulsive about obtaining ambient quiet. Because shivering and movement increase adventitious sound, make certain the patient is warm and relaxed before beginning.

It is a common error to try to hear *all* of the sounds in the cardiac cycle at one time. Take the time to isolate each sound and each pause in the cycle, listening separately and selectively for as many beats as necessary to evaluate the sounds. It takes time to tune in, so you must not rush. Avoid "jumping" the stethoscope from one site to another; instead, "inch" the endpiece along the route. This maneuver helps prevent missing important sounds.

Fig. 9-21
Areas for auscultation of heart.

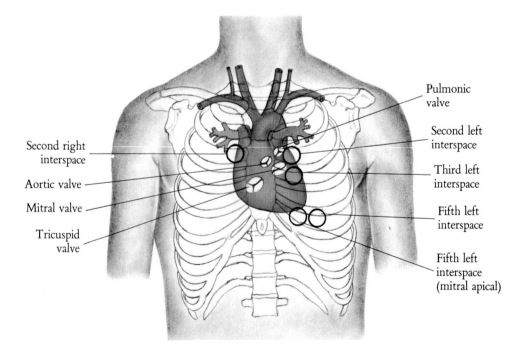

Since sound is transmitted in the direction of blood flow, specific heart sounds are best heard over areas where the blood flows after it passes through a valve. Approach each of the precordial areas systematically in a sequence that is comfortable for you.

Auscultation should be performed in each of the five cardiac areas using first the diaphragm and then the bell of the stethoscope. Use firm pressure with the diaphragm and light pressure with the bell.

There are five auscultatory areas, located as follows (Fig. 9-21):

- Aortic valve area: second right intercostal space at the right sternal border
- Pulmonic valve area: second left intercostal space at the left sternal border
- Second pulmonic area: third left intercostal space at the left sternal border
- Tricuspid area: fourth left intercostal space along the lower left sternal border
- Mitral (or apical) area: at the apex of the heart in the fifth left intercostal space at the midclavicular line

PROCEDURE FOR AUSCULTATING THE HEART

Adopt a routine for the various positions the patient is asked to assume, although you should be prepared to alter the sequence if the patient's condition requires it. Instruct the patient when to breathe normally and when to hold the breath in expiration and inspiration. Listen carefully for each heart sound, especially while the respirations are momentarily suspended. The following sequence is suggested:

1. Patient sitting up and leaning slightly forward: listen in all five areas (Fig. 9-22, *A*). This is the best position to hear relatively high-pitched murmurs with the stethoscope diaphragm.
2. Patient supine: listen in all five areas (Fig. 9-22, *B*).
3. Patient left lateral recumbent: listen in all five areas. This is the best position to hear the low-pitched filling sounds in diastole with the stethoscope bell (Fig. 9-22, *C*).
4. Other positions depend on your findings. Patient right lateral recumbent: listen in all five areas. This is best position for evaluating right rotated heart or dextrocardia.

Fig. 9-22
Sequence of patient positions for auscultation. A, Sitting up, leaning slightly forward. B, Supine. C, Left lateral recumbent.

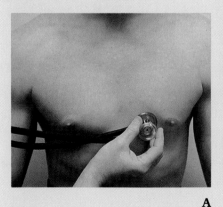
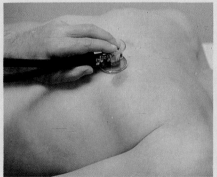
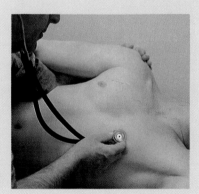

A   B   C

As you examine each of the five auscultatory areas, listen selectively for each component:

1. Assess the overall rate and rhythm of the heart, noting the auscultatory area in which you are listening each time.
2. Instruct the patient to breathe normally and then hold the breath in expiration. Listen for S_1 while you palpate the carotid pulse. S_1 coincides with the rise (upswing) of the carotid pulse. Note the intensity, any variations, the effect of respirations, and any splitting of S_1.
3. Concentrate on systole, listening for any extra sounds or murmurs. S_1 marks the beginning of systole.
4. Concentrate on diastole, which is a longer interval than systole, listening for any extra sounds or murmurs. (Note, however, that systole and diastole are equal in duration when the heart rate is rapid.) S_1 immediately follows diastole.
5. Instruct the patient to breathe normally, listening closely for S_2 to become two components (split S_2) during inspiration.
6. Instruct the patient to exhale and hold the breath, then inhale and hold the breath. Listen for S_2 to become a single sound in both instances.

BASIC HEART SOUNDS. Heart sounds are characterized in much the same way as respiratory and other body sounds: by frequency (pitch), intensity (loudness), duration, and timing in the cardiac cycle. Heart sounds are relatively low in pitch, except in the presence of significant pathologic events. Table 9-2 summarizes their relative differences according to auscultatory area. (Also see Fig. 9-27.)

There are four basic heart sounds: S_1, S_2, S_3, and S_4. S_1 and S_2 are the most distinct heart sounds and should be characterized separately, since variations can offer important clues to cardiac function. S_3 and S_4 may or may not be present; their absence is not an unusual finding, but their presence does not necessarily indicate a pathologic condition. Thus S_3 and S_4 must be evaluated in relation to other sounds and events in the cardiac cycle.

S_1 and S_2. S_1 is best heard toward the apex where it is louder than S_2. At the base, S_1 is louder on the left than on the right but softer than S_2 in both areas. It is lower in pitch and a bit longer than S_2, and it occurs immediately after diastole (Fig. 9-23).

Table 9-2
Relative Differences of Heart Sounds According to Auscultatory Area

	Aortic	Pulmonic	Second Pulmonic	Mitral	Tricuspid
Pitch	$S_1<S_2$	$S_1<S_2$	$S_1<S_2$	$S_1<S_2$	$S_1<S_2$
Loudness	$S_1<S_2$	$S_1<S_2$	$S_1<S_2$*	$S_1>S_2$†	$S_1>S_2$
Duration	$S_1>S_2$	$S_1>S_2$	$S_1>S_2$	$S_1>S_2$	$S_1>S_2$
S_2 split	>inhale	>inhale	>inhale	>inhale‡	>inhale
	<exhale	<exhale	<exhale	<exhale	<exhale
A_2	Loudest	Loud	Decreased		
P_2	Decreased	Louder	Loudest		

*S_1 is relatively louder in second pulmonic area than in aortic area.
†S_1 may be louder in mitral area than in tricuspid area.
‡S_2 split may not be audible in mitral area if P_2 is inaudible.

S₁ INTENSITY: DIAGNOSTIC CLUES

When systole begins with the mitral valve wide open, the valve snaps shut more vigorously, producing a louder S₁. This occurs in the following situations:

- Blood velocity is increased, such as occurs in anemia, fever, hyperthyroidism, anxiety, and during exercise.
- The mitral valve is stenotic.

If the mitral valve is not completely open, ventricular contraction forces it shut. The loudness produced by valve closure depends on the degree of opening, so the intensity of S₁ varies in the following situations:

- Complete heart block is present.
- Gross disruption of rhythm occurs, such as during fibrillation.

The intensity of S₁ is decreased in the following situations:

- Increased overlying tissue, fat, or fluid (as occurs in emphysema, obesity, or pericardial fluid) obscures sounds.
- Systemic or pulmonary hypertension is present, which contributes to more forceful atrial contraction. If the ventricle is noncompliant, the contraction may be delayed or diminished, especially if valve is partially closed when contraction begins.
- Fibrosis and calcification of a diseased mitral valve can result from rheumatic heart disease. Calcification diminishes valve flexibility so that it closes with less force.

Although there is some asynchrony between closure of the mitral and tricuspid valves, S₁ is usually heard as one sound. If the asynchrony is more marked than usual, the sound may be split and is then best heard in the tricuspid area. Other variations in S₁ depend on the competency of the pulmonary and systemic circulations, the structure of the heart valves, their position when ventricular contraction begins, and the force of the contraction.

S₂ is best heard in the aortic and pulmonic areas. It is of lower pitch and shorter duration than S₁ and occurs at the end of systole. S₂ is louder than S₁ at the base of the heart but softer than S₁ at the apex.

Fig. 9-23
First and second heart sounds.
From Malasanos et al., 1986.

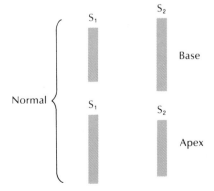

S₂ INTENSITY: DIAGNOSTIC CLUES

The intensity of S_2 increases in the following conditions:
- Systemic hypertension (S_2 in toto may ring or boom), syphilis of the aortic valve, exercise, or excitement accentuate A_2.
- Pulmonary hypertension, mitral stenosis, and congestive heart failure accentuate P_2.
- The valves are diseased but still fully mobile; the component of S_2 affected depends on which valve is compromised.

The intensity of S_2 decreases in the following conditions:
- A shock-like state with arterial hypotension causes loss of valvular vigor.
- The valves are immobile, thickened, or calcified; the component of S_2 affected depends on which valve is compromised.
- Aortic stenosis affects A_2.
- Pulmonic stenosis affects P_2.
- Overlying tissue, fat, or fluid mutes S_2.

S_2 is actually two sounds that merge during expiration. The closure of the aortic valve (A_2) contributes to most of the sound of S_2 when it is heard in the aortic and pulmonic areas. A_2 tends to mask the sound of pulmonic valve closure (P_2). During inspiration P_2 occurs slightly later, giving S_2 two distinct components—split S_2.

Splitting. Splitting of S_1 is not usually heard because the sound of the tricuspid valve closing is too faint to hear. Occasionally, however, it may be audible in the tricuspid area.

Splitting of S_2 is a normal event, because pressures are higher and depolarization occurs earlier on the left side of the heart. Ejection times on the right are longer, and the pulmonic valve closes a bit later than the aortic valve. Consequently, the normal S_2 often has two audible components.

Splitting is greatest at the peak of inspiration (Fig. 9-24). During expiration the disparity in ejection times tends to diminish, and the split may disappear. Ejection times tend to equalize when the breath is held in inspiration, so this maneuver also tends to eliminate the split. Thus, the degree of S_2 splitting varies widely from very explicit to nondetectable, from inspiration to expiration. The respiratory cycle is not always the dominant factor in the variation, however, and the interval between the components tends to remain easily discernible, if variable, throughout.

Fig. 9-24
Normal splitting of S_2.
From Malasanos et al., 1986.

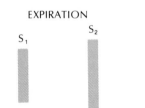

EXPIRATION

S_1 S_2

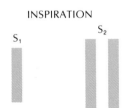

INSPIRATION

S_1 S_2

UNEXPECTED SPLITTING OF HEART SOUNDS

Wide Splitting: The split becomes wider when there is delayed activation of contraction or emptying of the right ventricle resulting in delay in pulmonic closure. This occurs, for example, in right bundle branch block, which splits both S_1 and S_2. Wide splitting of S_2 also occurs when stenosis delays closure of the pulmonic valve or when mitral regurgitation induces early closure of the aortic valve. The split becomes narrower and is even eliminated when closure of the aortic valve is delayed, such as in left bundle branch block.

Fixed Splitting: Splitting is said to be fixed when it is unaffected by respiration. This occurs with delayed closure of the pulmonic valve when output of the right ventricle is greater than that of the left (such as occurs in large atrial septal defects or right ventricular failure).

Paradoxical Splitting: Paradoxical splitting occurs when closure of the aortic valve is delayed (such as in left bundle branch block) so that P_2 occurs first, followed by A_2. In this case, the interval between P_2 and A_2 is heard during expiration and disappears during inspiration.

Variations in splitting of S_2.

From Malasanos et al., 1986.

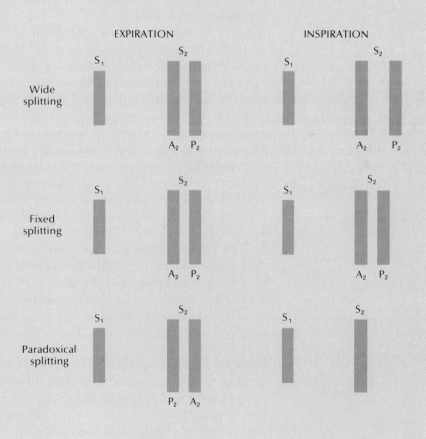

Fig. 9-25
S₃, an early diastolic sound.
From Malasanos et al., 1986.

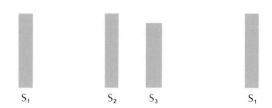

Fig. 9-26
S₄, a late diastolic sound.
From Malasanos et al., 1986.

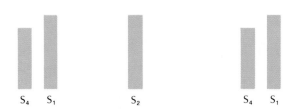

S₃ and S₄. During diastole, the ventricles fill in two steps: an early, passive flow of blood from the atria is followed by a more vigorous, muscular ejection. The passive phase occurs quickly relatively early in diastole, distending the ventricular walls and causing vibration. The resultant sound, S₃, is quiet and somewhat difficult to hear (Fig. 9-25).

In the second phase of ventricular filling, vibration in the valves, papillae, and ventricular walls produces S₄ (Fig. 9-26). Because it occurs so late in diastole (presystole), S₄ may be confused with a split S₁.

S₃ and S₄ should be quiet and somewhat difficult to hear. Increased intensity of either sound is suspect.

When S₃ becomes intense and easy to hear, the resultant sequence of sounds simulates a gallop—the protodiastolic gallop rhythm. S₄ may also become more intense, producing a readily discernible presystolic gallop rhythm. This is most frequent in older patients, but it may happen at any age where there is increased resistance to filling because of loss of compliance of the ventricular walls (such as in hypertensive disease and coronary artery disease) or the increased stroke volume of high output states (such as in profound anemia and thyrotoxicosis).

EXTRA HEART SOUNDS. The cardiac valves generally open noiselessly unless thickened, roughened, or otherwise altered as a result of disease. Valvular stenosis may produce an opening snap (mitral valve), ejection clicks (semilunar valves), or mid-to-late systolic clicks (mitral prolapse). Extra heart sounds often accompany murmurs and should always be viewed as possibly representing a pathologic process.

Pericardial friction rub can be easily mistaken for cardiac-generated sounds. Inflammation of the pericardial sac causes a roughening of the parietal and visceral surfaces, which produces a rubbing sound audible through the stethoscope. It occupies both systole and diastole and overlays the intracardiac sounds. Pericardial friction rub may have three components that are associated in sequence with the atrial component of systole, ventricular systole, and ventricular diastole. It is usually heard widely but is more distinct toward the apex. A three-component friction rub is a grating sound that may be intense enough to obscure the heart sounds. However, if there are only one or two components, the sound may not be particularly intense or machine-like and may then be more difficult to distinguish from an

Table 9-3
Extra Heart Sounds

Sound	Detection	Description
Increased S_3	Bell at apex; patient left lateral recumbent	Early diastole, low pitch
Increased S_4	Bell at apex; patient supine or semilateral	Late diastole or early systole, low pitch
Gallops	Bell at apex; patient supine or left lateral recumbent	Presystole, intense, easily heard
Mitral valve opening snap	Diaphragm medial to apex, may radiate to base; any position, second left intercostal space	Early diastole briefly, before S_3; high pitch, sharp snap or click; not affected by respiration; easily confused with S_2
Ejection clicks	Diaphragm; patient sitting or supine	
Aortic valve	Apex, base in second right intercostal space	Early systole, intense, high pitch; radiates; not affected by respirations
Pulmonary valve	Second left intercostal space at sternal border	Early systole, less intense than aortic click; intensifies on expiration, decreases on inspiration
Pericardial friction rub	Widely heard, sound clearest toward apex	May occupy all of systole and diastole; intense, grating, machine-like; may have 3 components and obliterate heart sounds; if only 1 or 2 components, may sound like murmur

Heart sounds	Events	Cause	End-piece	Location	Pitch	Respirations	Position	Variables
First heart sound = S_1 (M_1T_1)		Closure of tricuspid and mitral valves	Diaphragm	Entire precordium (apex)	High	Softer on inspiration	Any position	Increased with excitement, exercise, amyl nitrate, epinephrine, and atropine
Second heart sound = S_2 (A_2P_2)		Closure of pulmonary and aortic valves	Diaphragm	A_2 at 2nd RICS; P_2 at 2nd LICS	High	Fusion of A_2P_2 on expiration; physiologic split on inspiration	Sitting or supine	Increased in thin chest walls and with exercise
Third heart sound = S_3 (ventricular gallop)		Rapid ventricular filling	Bell	Apex	Low	Increased on inspiration	Supine or left lateral	Increased with exercise, fast heart rate, elevation of legs, and increased venous return
Fourth heart sound = S_4 (atrial gallop)		Forceful atrial ejection into distended ventricle	Bell	Apex	Low	Increased on forced inspiration	Supine or left semilateral	Same as for S_3
Quadruple rhythm		S_1, S_2, S_3, and S_4 all heard separately	Bell	Apex	Low	Increased on inspiration	Supine or left lateral	Same as for S_3
Summation gallop = triple gallop		S_3 and S_4 fuse with fast heart rates	Bell	Apex	Low	Increased on inspiration	Supine or left lateral	Same as for S_3
Ejection sounds		Opening of deformed semilunar valves	Diaphragm	2nd RICS, 2nd LICS, or apex	High	Increases on expiration with pulmonary stenosis	Sitting or supine	Aortic ejection sound same as S_1 and S_2; pulmonary ejection sound increased on expiration
Systolic click		Prolapse of mitral valve leaflet	Diaphragm	Apex	High	Increased on expiration	Sitting or supine	Occurs later in systole with increased venous return (e.g.) with elevated legs or supine position
Opening snap		Abrupt recoil of stenotic mitral or tricuspid valve	Diaphragm	Apex	High	No effect	Any position	May be confused with S_3

Fig. 9-27
Heart sounds. *RICS,* **Right intercostal space;** *LICS,* **left intercostal space.**
From Guzzetta and Dossey, 1984.

intracardiac murmur. The detection of extra heart sounds are detailed in Table 9-3, along with associated disorders (Fig. 9-27).

HEART MURMURS. Heart murmurs are relatively prolonged extra sounds heard during systole or diastole; they frequently indicate a problem. Murmurs are caused by some disruption in the flow of blood into, through, or out of the heart. The characteristics of a murmur depend on the adequacy of valve function, the size of the opening, the rate of blood flow, the vigor of the myocardium, and the thickness and consistency of the overlying tissues through which the murmur must be heard.

Table 9-4
Characterization of Heart Murmurs

	Classification	*Description*
Timing and duration*	Early systolic	Begins with S_1, decrescendos, ends well before S_2
	Midsystolic	Begins after S_1, ends before S_2
	Late systolic	Begins mid-to-late systole, crescendos, ends at S_2; often introduced by mid-to-late systolic clicks
	Early diastolic	Begins with S_2
	Mid-diastolic	Begins at clear interval after S_2
	Late diastolic (presystolic)	Begins immediately before S_1
	Holosystolic	Begins with S_1, occupies all of systole, ends at S_2
	Holodiastolic	Begins with S_2, occupies all of diastole, ends at S_1
	Continuous	Starts in systole, continues without interruption through S_2 into all or part of diastole; does not necessarily persist throughout entire cardiac cycle
Pitch	High, medium, low	Depends on pressure and rate of blood flow
Intensity	Grade I	Barely audible in quiet room
	Grade II	Quiet but clearly audible
	Grade III	Moderately loud
	Grade IV	Loud, associated with thrill
	Grade V	Very loud, thrill easily palpable
	Grade VI	Very loud, audible with stethoscope not in contact with chest, thrill palpable and visible
Pattern	Crescendo	Increasing intensity caused by increased blood velocity
	Decrescendo	Decreasing intensity caused by decreased blood velocity
Quality	Harsh, raspy, machine-like, vibratory, musical, blowing	Quality depends on several factors including degree of valve compromise, force of contractions, blood volume
Location	Anatomic landmarks (e.g., 2nd left intercostal space on sternal border)	Area of greatest intensity, usually area to which valve sounds are normally transmitted
Radiation	Anatomic landmarks (e.g., to axilla)	Site farthest from location of greatest intensity at which sound is still heard; sound usually transmitted in direction of blood flow
Respiratory phase variations	Intensity, quality, and timing may vary	Venous return increases on inspiration and decreases on expiration

*Systolic murmurs are best described according to time of onset and termination; diastolic murmurs are best classified according to time of onset only.

ARE SOME MURMURS INNOCENT?

Many murmurs, particularly in children and adolescents, have no apparent cause. They are presumably a result of vigorous myocardial contraction and the consequent stronger blood flow in early or midsystole. The thinner chests of the young make these sounds easier to hear, particularly with a lightly held bell. They are usually grade I or II, without radiation, of medium pitch, blowing, and brief. They are often located in the second left intercostal space near the left sternal border. Such murmurs heard in a recumbent position may disappear when the patient sits or stands because of the tendency of the blood to pool.

Diseased valves, a common cause of murmurs, do not close well. When the leaflets are thickened and the passage narrowed, forward blood flow is restricted (stenosis). When valve leaflets, which are intended to fit together snugly, lose competency, the slack openings allow backwards flow of blood (regurgitation). Table 9-4 summarizes the characteristics of heart murmurs.

The discovery of a heart murmur requires careful assessment and diagnosis. Although some murmurs are benign, others represent a lethal process at work. Therefore, solid evidence from ECG testing is mandatory before a murmur is dismissed as "functional."

Not all murmurs are the result of valvular defects, however. Other causes include:

- High output demands that increase speed of blood flow
- Structural defects, either congenital or acquired, that allow blood to flow through inappropriate pathways (such as the myocardial septa)
- Diminished strength of myocardial contraction
- Altered blood flow in the major vessels near the heart

Arteries

Arterial Pulses

The pulses are best palpated over arteries that are close to the surface of the body and lie over bones. These include the carotid, brachial, radial, femoral, popliteal, dorsalis pedis, and posterior tibial (Table 9-5 and Fig. 9-28).

An arterial pulsation is essentially a bounding wave of blood with varying vigor that diminishes with increasing distance from the heart. Of all the arterial pulses, the carotids are easily accessible and closest to the cardiac source and thus most useful in evaluating heart activity. The arterial pulses in the extremities are examined to determine the sufficiency of the entire arterial circulation. At least one pulse point is palpated in each extremity, usually at the most distal point.

Examine the arterial pulses with the distal pads of the second, third, and fourth fingers. Do not use your thumb, because your own pulse may be more readily felt than the patient's. Palpate firmly but not so hard that the artery is occluded.

If you have difficulty finding a pulse, try varying your pressure, feeling carefully throughout the area. Make sure when you locate it that you are not feeling your own pulse. In some areas, particularly the ankle, fat or edema may make the pulse difficult to feel.

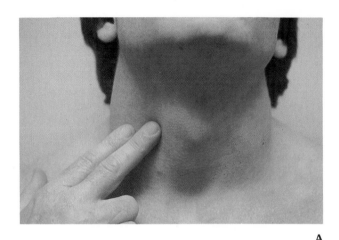

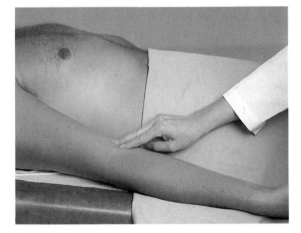

Fig. 9-28
Palpation of arterial pulses.
A, Carotid. **B,** Brachial.

B

A

Table 9-5
Locations of Palpable Pulses

Pulse	Location
Carotid	In the neck, just medial to and below angle of the jaw (do not palpate both sides simultaneously)
Brachial	Just medial to biceps tendon
Radial	Medial and ventral side of wrist (gentle pressure)
Femoral	Inferior to inguinal ligament; if patient is obese, midway between anterior superior iliac spine and pubic tubercle (press harder here than in most areas)
Popliteal	Popliteal fossae (press firmly)
Dorsalis pedis	Medial side of dorsum of foot with foot slightly dorsiflexed (pulse may be hard to feel and may be absent in some well persons)
Posterior tibial	Behind and slightly inferior to medial malleolus of ankle

CAUTION: CAROTID SINUS MASSAGE

When palpating the carotid arteries, *never palpate both sides simultaneously*. Excessive carotid massage can cause slowing of the pulse or a drop in blood pressure. The result could be possible circulatory embarrassment, particularly in older adults who may already have compromised cardiovascular function. If you have difficulty feeling the pulse, rotate the patient's head to the side being examined to relax the sternocleidomastoid muscle.

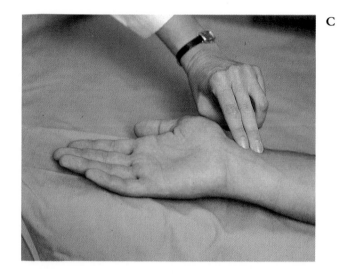

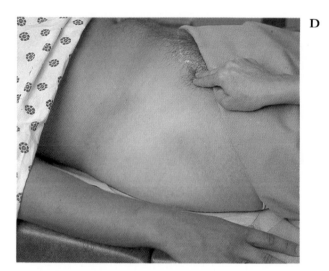

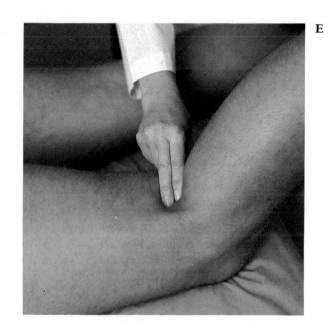

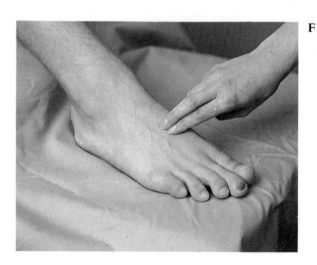

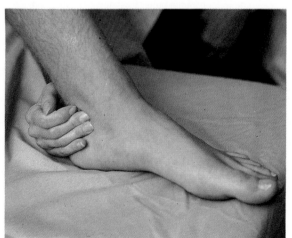

C

D

E

F

G

Fig. 9-28, cont'd
**Palpation of arterial pulses.
C, Radial. D, Femoral. E,
Popliteal. F, Dorsalis pedis.
G, Posterial tibial.**
E and **F** from Potter and Perry, 1987.

CHARACTERISTICS. Palpation of arterial pulses can indicate heart rate and rhythm, pulse contour (wave form), amplitude (strength), symmetry, and sometimes obstructions to blood flow. Variations from the expected findings are described in Table 9-6 and Fig. 9-29.

The pulse rate (heart rate) is determined by counting the pulsations for 60 seconds (or counting for 30 seconds and doubling the count). The resting pulse rate should range between 60 and 90 per minute.

Determine the steadiness of the heart rhythm, which should be regular. A heart rate that is irregular but occurs in a repeated pattern may indicate a cyclical variation of the heart rate, increasing on inspiration and decreasing on expiration. A patternless, unpredictably irregular rate suggests heart disease or conduction system impairment.

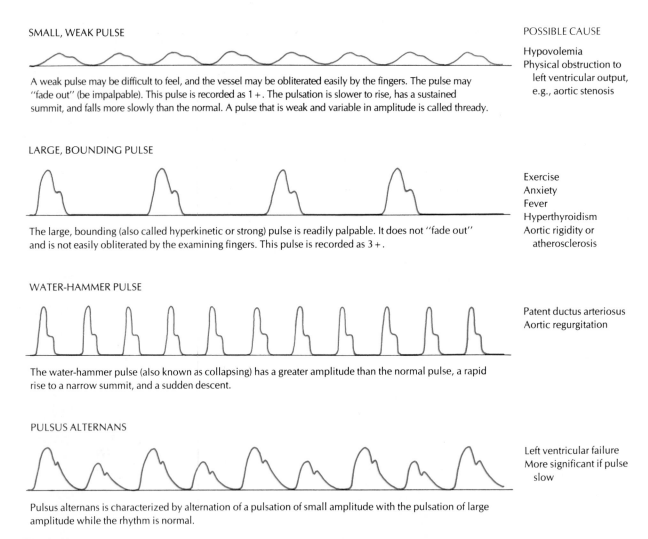

SMALL, WEAK PULSE

A weak pulse may be difficult to feel, and the vessel may be obliterated easily by the fingers. The pulse may "fade out" (be impalpable). This pulse is recorded as 1 +. The pulsation is slower to rise, has a sustained summit, and falls more slowly than the normal. A pulse that is weak and variable in amplitude is called thready.

POSSIBLE CAUSE

Hypovolemia
Physical obstruction to
 left ventricular output,
 e.g., aortic stenosis

LARGE, BOUNDING PULSE

The large, bounding (also called hyperkinetic or strong) pulse is readily palpable. It does not "fade out" and is not easily obliterated by the examining fingers. This pulse is recorded as 3 +.

Exercise
Anxiety
Fever
Hyperthyroidism
Aortic rigidity or
 atherosclerosis

WATER-HAMMER PULSE

The water-hammer pulse (also known as collapsing) has a greater amplitude than the normal pulse, a rapid rise to a narrow summit, and a sudden descent.

Patent ductus arteriosus
Aortic regurgitation

PULSUS ALTERNANS

Pulsus alternans is characterized by alternation of a pulsation of small amplitude with the pulsation of large amplitude while the rhythm is normal.

Left ventricular failure
More significant if pulse
 slow

Fig. 9-29
Pulse abnormalities.
From Malasanos et al., 1986.

The contour of the pulse wave normally has a smooth, rounded, or domed shape. Attention should be paid to the ascending portion, the peak, and the descending portion. Each wave crest should be compared with the next to detect cyclic differences.

The amplitude of the pulse is described on a scale of 0 to 4:

4 = bounding
3 = full, increased
2 = expected
1 = diminished, barely palpable
0 = absent, not palpable

Lack of symmetry between the left and right extremities suggests impaired circulation. Compare the strength of the upper extremity pulses with those of the lower extremities and the left with the right. Ordinarily, the femoral is as strong as or stronger than the radial pulse. If this is reversed or if the femoral pulsation is absent, coarctation of the aorta must be suspected.

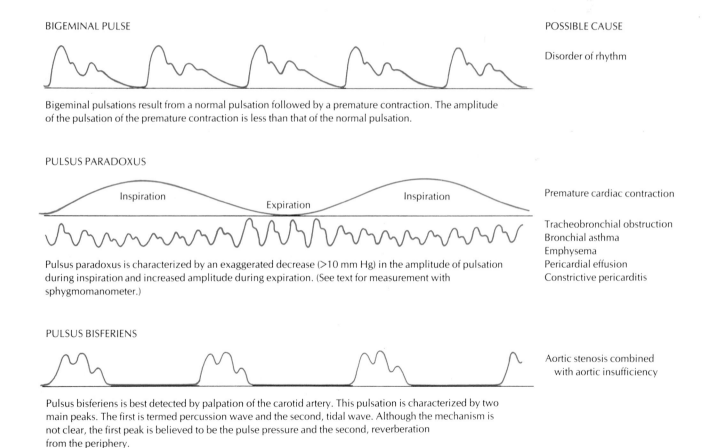

BIGEMINAL PULSE

POSSIBLE CAUSE

Disorder of rhythm

Bigeminal pulsations result from a normal pulsation followed by a premature contraction. The amplitude of the pulsation of the premature contraction is less than that of the normal pulsation.

PULSUS PARADOXUS

Inspiration   Expiration   Inspiration

Premature cardiac contraction

Tracheobronchial obstruction
Bronchial asthma
Emphysema
Pericardial effusion
Constrictive pericarditis

Pulsus paradoxus is characterized by an exaggerated decrease (>10 mm Hg) in the amplitude of pulsation during inspiration and increased amplitude during expiration. (See text for measurement with sphygmomanometer.)

PULSUS BISFERIENS

Aortic stenosis combined
with aortic insufficiency

Pulsus bisferiens is best detected by palpation of the carotid artery. This pulsation is characterized by two main peaks. The first is termed percussion wave and the second, tidal wave. Although the mechanism is not clear, the first peak is believed to be the pulse pressure and the second, reverberation from the periphery.

Fig. 9-29, cont'd
Pulse abnormalities.
From Malasanos et al., 1986.

Table 9-6
Arterial Pulse Abnormalities

Type	Description	Associated Disorders
Alternating pulse (pulsus alternans)	Regular rate; amplitude varies from beat to beat with weak and strong beats	Left ventricular failure
Biferious pulse (pulsus biferiens)	Two strong systolic peaks separated by a midsystolic dip	Aortic regurgitation alone or with stenosis
Bigeminal pulse (pulsus bigeminus)	Two beats in rapid succession followed by longer interval; easily confused with alternating pulse	Regularly occurring ventricular premature beats
Bounding pulse	Increased pulse pressure; contour may have rapid rise, brief peak, rapid fall	Atherosclerosis, aortic regurgitation, patent ductus arteriosus, fever, anemia, hyperthyroidism, anxiety, exercise
Bradycardia	Rate less than 60	Hypothermia, hypothyroidism, drug intoxication, impaired cardiac conduction, excellent physical conditioning
Labile pulse	Normal when patient is resting but increases on standing or sitting	Not necessarily associated with disease; not a specific indicator of a problem
Paradoxical pulse (pulsus paradoxus)	Amplitude decreases on inspiration	Chronic obstructive pulmonary disease, constrictive pericarditis
Pulsus differens	Inequal pulses between left and right extremities	Impaired circulation, usually from local obstruction
Tachycardia	Rate over 100	Fever, hyperthyroidism, anemia, shock, heart disease, anxiety, exercise
Trigeminal pulse (pulsus trigeminus)	Three beats followed by a pause	Often benign, such as after exercise; cardiomyopathy, severe ventricular hypertrophy, severe aortic stenosis, dysfunctional right ventricle
Water-hammer pulse (Corrigan's pulse)	Jerky pulse with full expansion followed by sudden collapse	Aortic regurgitation

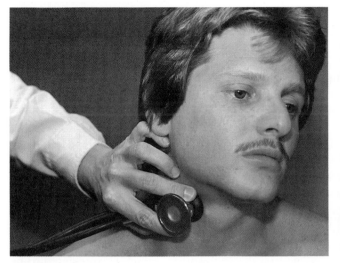

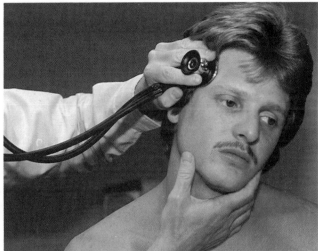

A

B

Fig. 9-30
Auscultation for bruits. A, Carotid artery. B, Temporal artery.

Auscultation over an artery for a bruit (murmur or unexpected sound) is indicated when you are following the radiation of murmurs or looking for evidence of local obstruction. These sounds are usually low pitched and relatively hard to hear. Using the bell of your stethoscope and asking the patient to hold the breath for a few heart beats will help. Sites at which to auscultate for a bruit are the carotid, jugular, temporal, abdominal, aortic, renal, and femoral arteries (Fig. 9-30).

Peripheral Arteries

Arteries in any location can become occluded, resulting in insufficient circulation to the tissues. As a result, a variety of changes occur in the area distal to the occlusion. Examine each arm and leg, noting any evidence of the following:

- Diminished pulse (weak and thready or even absent)
- Audible systolic bruits over the artery that may extend through diastole
- Loss of expected body warmth
- Localized pallor cyanosis
- Collapsed superficial veins with delay in venous filling
- Thin, atrophied skin, muscle atrophy, and loss of hair (long-term insufficiency accentuates skin mottling and increases the likelihood of ulceration, localized anesthesia, and tenderness)
- Pain, often severe, particularly if there is an acute occlusion

Blood Pressure

Blood pressure is usually measured in the patient's arm and should be measured in both arms at least once. The patient's arm should be slightly flexed and comfortably supported on a table, pillow, or your hand. Be sure that the arm is free of clothing. Center the deflated bladder over the brachial artery, just medial to the biceps tendon, with the lower edge 2 to 3 cm above the antecubital crease. Apply the cuff snugly and securely, because a loose cuff will give an inaccurate measurement.

Checking the palpable systolic blood pressure first will help you avoid being misled by an auscultatory gap when you listen with the stethoscope. Place the fingers of one hand over the brachial artery. Rapidly inflate the cuff with the hand bulb 20 to 30 mm Hg above the point at which you no longer feel the brachial pulse. Deflate the cuff slowly at a rate of 2 to 3 mm Hg per second until you again feel the brachial pulse. This point is the palpable systolic blood pressure. Immediately deflate the cuff completely (Fig. 9-31, *A*).

Now place the bell of the stethoscope over the brachial artery, and again inflate the cuff until it is 20 to 30 mm Hg above the palpable systolic blood pressure (Fig. 9-31, *B*). The bell of the stethoscope is more effective than the diaphragm in transmitting the low-pitched sound produced by the turbulence of blood flow in the artery (Korotkoff sounds). Deflate the cuff slowly as previously described, listening for the following sounds (Fig. 9-32):

1. Two consecutive beats indicate the systolic pressure and also the beginning of phase 1 of the Korotkoff sounds.
2. Occasionally, the Korotkoff sounds will be heard, disappear, and reappear 10 to 15 mm Hg later (phase 2). The period of silence is the auscultatory gap.
3. Note the point at which the sounds, which are first crisp (phase 3), become muffled (phase 4). This is the first diastolic sound, which is considered to be the closest approximation of direct diastolic arterial pressure. It signals imminent disappearance of the Korotkoff sounds.
4. Note the point at which the sounds disappear (phase 5). This is the second diastolic sound. Now deflate the cuff completely.

The American Heart Association recommends recording three values for the blood pressure: the systolic and both diastolic measures (for example, 110/76/68). If only two values are recorded, they are the systolic and the second diastolic pressures (for example, 100/68). The difference between the systolic and diastolic pressures is the pulse pressure. The normal range is approximately 100 to 140 mm Hg for the systolic pressure and 60 to 90 for the (second) diastolic. The pulse pressure should be 30 to 40 mm Hg.

Repeat the process in the other arm. Readings between the arms may vary by as much as 10 mm Hg and tend to be higher in the right arm; the higher reading should be accepted as closest to the patient's blood pressure. Record both sets of measurements.

Since the systolic pressure is more labile and more readily responsive to a wide range of physical and emotional stimuli, hypertension is usually defined on the basis of the generally more stable diastolic pressure. A patient may be considered to

Fig. 9-31
Blood pressure measurement. **A,** Checking palpable systolic pressure. **B,** Using bell of stethoscope.

A   **B**

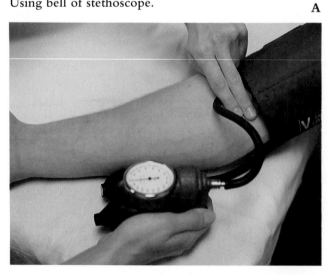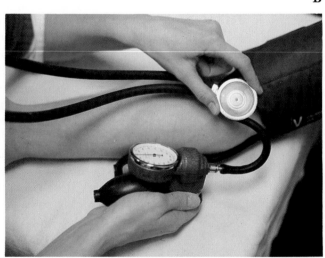

315

Examination and Findings   HEART AND BLOOD VESSELS

Fig. 9-32
Phases of Korotkoff sounds.

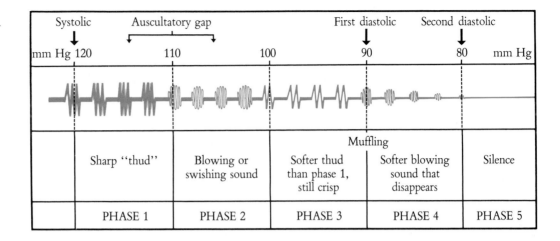

have high blood pressure if three consecutive diastolic pressures are found to be equal to or above 90 mm Hg. It may be considered mild at that level, moderate when it reaches 105 mm Hg, and severe above 115 mm Hg. Most cases of hypertension have no discoverable cause. Since the elevation of blood pressure may, for a time, be the only significant clinical finding, persons with hypertension are unsymptomatic.

If the diastolic pressure in the arms is above 90 mm Hg or you suspect coarctation of the aorta or aortic insufficiency, measure the blood pressure in the legs. The patient should be prone, if possible; if supine, the leg should be flexed as little as possible. Center the bladder over the posterior surface and wrap the cuff securely on the distal third of the femur. Measure the pressure over the popliteal artery using the same procedure as for the brachial artery. Leg pressures, which are usually higher than arm pressures, will be lower with coarctation of the aorta or aortic insufficiency.

If the patient is taking antihypertensive medications, has a depleted blood volume, or complains of fainting or postural dizziness, blood pressure in the arm should be measured with the patient standing. Normally, as a patient changes position from supine to standing, there is a slight or no drop in systolic pressure and a slight rise in diastolic pressure. However, if postural hypotension is present, expect to see a significant drop in systolic pressure (greater than 15 mm Hg) and a drop in diastolic pressure. Even a mild blood loss (such as from blood donation), drugs, autonomic nervous system disease, or prolonged stay in a recumbent position can all contribute to postural hypotension.

With even impeccable technique the accuracy of the blood pressure reading may be undermined by some conditions:

- Cardiac arrhythmias: An infrequent odd beat may be ignored, but if the irregularity is sustained, it is a good idea to take the average of several pressures and to note the uncertainty.
- Aortic regurgitation: The sounds of aortic regurgitation do not disappear, thus obscuring the diastolic pressure.
- Venous congestion: Sluggish venous flow from a pathologic event can cause the systolic pressure to be heard lower than it actually is and the diastolic pressure higher. Repeated, slow inflations of the cuff can also cause venous congestion.

Veins

Jugular Venous Pressure

After evaluating the carotid pulses, look for the jugular venous pulse with the patient reclining at a 45-degree angle. This position achieves the maximum excursion of the internal jugular veins. Because the internal jugular veins lie close to the carotid arteries, their pulsations are easily confused with the carotid pulse. However, the internal jugular pulse is not palpable (Fig. 9-33). Table 9-7 provides instructions on differentiating between the jugular and carotid pulses.

The light should be tangential to illuminate highlights and shadows. Clothing should not obstruct flow (as a tight necktie might). A pillow may be used for the patient's comfort, but the neck should not be sharply flexed. A pulse more rapid than 90 beats per minute will cause enough turbulence and distortion to minimize the value of the observation.

Observation of both jugular veins can provide a reliable indication of the volume and pressure in the right side of the heart, since internal jugular veins pulsate in response to phasic changes in right atrial pressure. Usually pulsations are not evident when the patient is sitting. As the patient slowly leans back into a supine position, the level of venous pulsations begins to rise above the level of the manubrium as much as 1 or 2 cm when the patient reaches a 45-degree angle. Finally, when the patient is supine, the effect of gravity diminishes and the veins fill. The jugular venous pressure is determined as follows (Fig. 9-34):

1. Using a centimeter ruler, measure the vertical distance between the angle of Louis (manubriosternal joint) and the highest level of jugular vein pulsation on both sides. A straight edge intersecting the ruler at a right angle assists in accurate measurement.
2. Record this measurement as the jugular venous pressure; 2 cm or less is considered normal.

Table 9-7
Differentiation of the Jugular and Carotid Pulse Waves

	Jugular	Carotid
Quality and Character Palpate the carotid artery on one side of the neck and look at the jugular vein on other to tell the difference	Three positive waves in normal sinus rhythm More undulating	One wave More brisk
Effect of Respiration	Level of pulse wave decreased on inspiration and increased on expiration	No effect
Effect of Changing Position	More prominent when recumbent; less prominent when sitting	No effect
Venous Compression Apply gentle pressure over vein at base of neck above clavicle	Easily eliminates pulse wave	No effect
Abdominal Pressure Place the palm moderately firmly over the right upper quadrant of the abdomen for half a minute	May cause some increased prominence even in well persons; with right-sided failure, jugular vein may be more visible	No effect

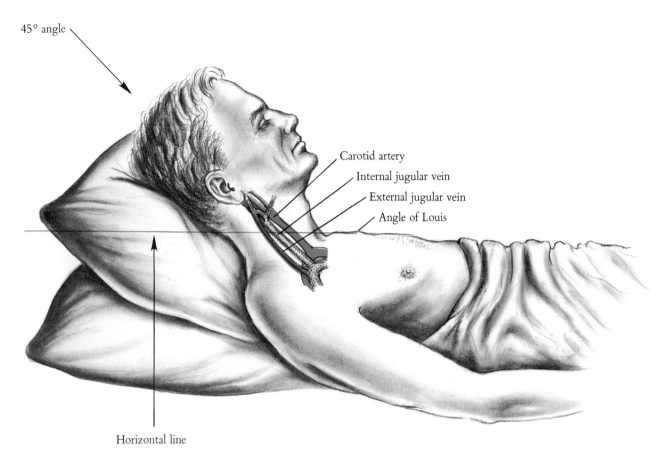

45° angle

Carotid artery

Internal jugular vein

External jugular vein

Angle of Louis

Horizontal line

Fig. 9-33
Inspection of jugular venous pressure.
From Thompson et al., 1986.

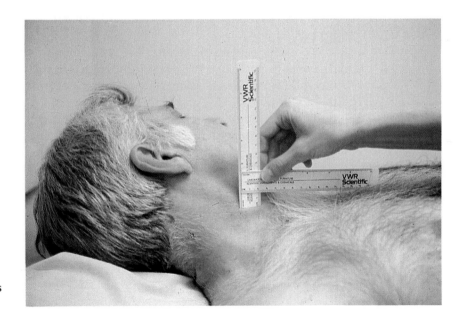

Fig. 9-34
Measuring jugular venous pressure.

ALTERED WAVES OF JUGULAR VENOUS PULSE

The a wave is accentuated when the contracting right atrium cannot empty into the right ventricle and, in the effort to achieve this, contracts more forcibly. This can be the result of reduced right ventricular compliance or tricuspid valve obstruction.

The x descent and c and v waves can be distorted and accentuated in a jugular pulse wave that simulates an exaggerated arterial pulsation. The cause may be insufficiency of the tricuspid valve from either organic change or generalized cardiac failure. The resultant regurgitation into the right atrium during ventricular systole may obliterate the x descent with a force that also blends the usually discernible c and v waves.

The y descent depends on intravascular and intracardiac pressures and volumes and on resistance to flow across the tricuspid valve. Delay in the y descent suggests tricuspid stenosis.

While the patient is positioned at a 45-degree angle, observe the left and right jugular veins for symmetry. Distension on one side only suggests a localized abnormality. When the venous pressure is increased because of intracardiac events, the veins are distended bilaterally. (In general, the internal jugulars provide more reliable information in this regard than the external veins, but both are generally observed.) Abnormal distention is caused by increasing pressure in the right heart when the right ventricle fails because of left ventricular failure, in constrictive pericarditis, or in superior vena cava obstruction. The pattern of the jugular venous pulse waves can be disrupted as the various components respond.

Peripheral Veins

Inspect the extremities for signs of venous insufficiency (thrombosis, varicose veins, and edema). Further tests are performed if evidence of peripheral vein compromise is present.

Note any redness, thickening, and tenderness along a superficial vein, a combination of findings that suggest thrombophlebitis of a superficial vein. A deep vein thrombosis cannot be confirmed on physical examination alone, but suspect it if there is swelling, pain, and tenderness over a vein. (An occluded artery does not result in swelling.) Acutely dorsiflex the foot to test for Homans' sign. The complaint of calf pain with this procedure is a positive sign and usually indicates thrombosis. Be certain you do not mistake calf pain with Achilles tendon pain, a common finding in athletes who frequently stress the Achilles tendon and in women who wear high heels. Avoid this confusion by keeping the knee slightly flexed when you dorsiflex the foot.

Inspect the extremities for edema, noted as a change in the usual contour of the leg. Press your index finger over the bony prominence of the tibia or medial malleolus for several seconds. A depression that does not rapidly refill and resume its original contour indicates orthostatic (pitting) edema. Pitting edema is not usually accompanied by thickening or pigmentation of the overlying skin (Fig. 9-35).

Edema caused by deep venous obstruction or valvular incompetence may be accompanied by some thickening and ulceration of the skin. Right-sided heart failure leads to an increased fluid volume, which in turn elevates the hydrostatic pressure in the vascular space, causing edema in dependent parts of the body. Edema related to valvular incompetence or an obstruction of a deep vein (usually in the legs) is caused by mechanical pressure of blood volume to the area served by the affected vein. Nonpitting edema caused by circulatory disorders must be distinguished from lymphedema (see Chapter 15, Lymphatic System).

Varicose veins are dilated and swollen veins that have a diminished rate of blood flow and an increased intravenous pressure. This may be the result of imcompetence of the vessel wall or valves or an obstruction in a more proximal vein (Fig. 9-36).

Superficial varicosities are easy to detect on inspection. The veins appear dilated and often tortuous when the extremities are dependent. When varicosities are present, Trendelenburg's test is used to evaluate venous incompetence. With the patient supine, lift the leg above the level of the heart until the veins empty. Then lower the leg quickly. An incompetent system will allow rapid filling of the veins.

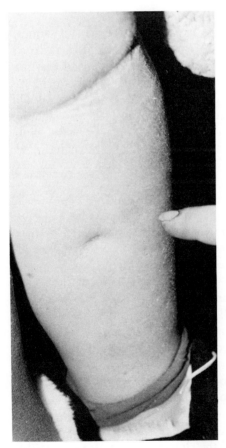

Fig. 9-35
Testing for pitting edema.
From Bowers and Thompson, 1984.

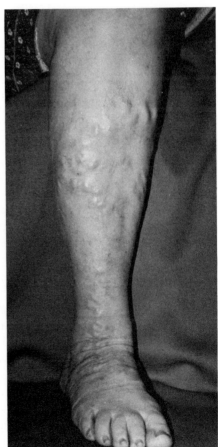

Fig. 9-36
**Varicose veins on lower
leg with nodular bulges.**
From Bowers and Thompson, 1984.

Perthes' test is used to evaluate the patency of deep veins. Occlude the subcutaneous veins with a tourniquet just above the knee to prevent filling of superficial varicosities from above. As the patient walks around, muscular tension will act on the deep veins and empty the dilated superficial varicosities. When these superficial veins fail to empty, suspect that the deep veins are also somewhat incompetent.

In the event of arteriovenous fistulae or venous obstruction, evaluate the direction of blood flow and the possible presence of a compensatory circulation. Distend visible veins by putting the affected limb in a dependent position. Then empty or "strip" a vein by first compressing it with two fingers held closely together (generally the second and third fingers on one hand) and then pushing one finger with pressure along the course of the vessel. If the stripped vessel fills before pressure is released, there is collateral circulation. Releasing the pressure of one finger should permit the blood to flow in the direction from whence the pressure is released. If the vein does not fill, try releasing the pressure in the other direction. Sometimes the vein does not fill from the second direction, an indication that the circulation is poor indeed (Fig. 9-43).

INFANTS

The newborn presents a challenge because of the immediate change from fetal to systemic and pulmonary circulation. Examine the heart within the first 24 hours and again at about 2 to 3 days of age.

Complete evaluation of heart function includes examination of the skin, lungs, and liver. Infants with right-sided congestive heart failure have large, firm livers with the inferior edge distended up to 5 to 6 cm below the right costal margin. Unlike adults, this finding may precede that of moisture in the lungs.

Inspect the color of the skin and mucous membranes. The well newborn should be reassuringly pink. A purplish plethora is associated with polycythemia, an ashy white color indicates shock, and cyanosis indicates congenital heart disease. Note the distribution and intensity of discoloration as well as the extent of change after vigorous exertion.

Cyanosis distinguishes the problems that lead to admixture of arterial and venous blood or prevent the expected oxygenation of blood. Severe cyanosis evident at birth or shortly thereafter suggests transposition of the great vessels, tetralogy of Fallot, tricuspid atresia, a severe septal defect, or severe pulmonic stenosis. Cyanosis that may not appear until after the neonatal period suggests a pure pulmonic stenosis, Eisenmenger's complex, tetralogy of Fallot, or large septal defects.

The apical impulse in the newborn is usually seen and felt at the fourth to fifth left intercostal space just medial to the midclavicular line. The smaller the baby, the thinner the chest, and the more obvious it will be. It may be somewhat farther to the right in the first few hours of life, sometimes even substernal.

Note any enlargement of the heart. It is especially important to note the position of the heart if a baby is having trouble breathing. A pneumothorax shifts the apical impulse away from the area of the pneumothorax. A diaphragmatic hernia, more commonly found on the left, shifts the heart to the right. A dextrocardia results in an apical impulse on the right.

The right ventricle is relatively more vigorous in a well, full-term newborn. If the baby is thin, you might even be able to feel the closure of the pulmonary valve in the second left intercostal space.

S_2 in infants is somewhat higher in pitch and more discrete than S_1. The vigor and quality of the heart sounds of the newborn (and throughout infancy and early childhood) are major indicators of the function of the heart. Diminished vigor may be the only apparent change when an infant is already in heart failure. Splitting of the heart sounds is common. S_2 is usually heard without a split at birth, then often splits within a few hours.

Murmurs are relatively frequent in the newborn until about 48 hours of age. Most are innocent, caused by the transition from fetal to pulmonic circulation rather than a significant congenital abnormality. These murmurs are usually grade I or II intensity, systolic, and unaccompanied by other signs and symptoms; they usually disappear within 2 to 3 days. Paradoxically, a significant congenital abnormality may be unaccompanied by a murmur.

If you cannot tell a murmur from respiration, pinch the nares briefly, listen while the baby is feeding, or time the sound with the carotid pulsation. Because of the rapid heart rate in infants, the heart sounds must be evaluated with great care. A murmur heard immediately at birth is apt to be less significant than one detected after the first few hours of life. If a murmur persists beyond the second or third day of life, is intense, fills systole, occupies diastole to any extent, or radiates widely, it must be investigated. If you push up on the liver, thereby increasing right atrial pressure, the murmur of a left-to-right shunt through a septal opening or patent ductus will disappear briefly, whereas the murmur of a right-to-left shunt will intensify.

Murmurs that extend beyond S_2 and occupy diastole are said to have a machine-like quality; they may be associated with a patent ductus arteriosus. The murmur should disappear when the patent ductus closes in the first 2 or 3 days of life.

In the newborn suspected of having cardiovascular difficulty, auscultate the head and the abdomen for bruits to detect arteriovenous malformations.

Infant's heart rates are more variable than those of older children. Eating, sleeping, and waking can change the rate considerably. The variation is greatest at birth or shortly after and is even more marked in premature infants. Rates close to 200 per minute are not uncommon, but they may also indicate paroxysmal atrial tachycardia. Ordinarily, the decrease in rate is relatively rapid, and at a few hours of age the rate may be much closer to 120. A relatively fixed tachycardia is a clue to some difficulty.

The brachial, radial, and femoral pulses of the newborn are easily palpable. When the pulse is weaker or thinner than expected, the cardiac output may be diminished or peripheral vasoconstriction may be present. A bounding pulse is associated with a large left-to-right shunt produced by a patent ductus arteriosus. Difference in pulse amplitude between the upper extremities or between the femoral and radial pulses suggests a coarctation of the aorta, as does absence of the femoral pulses.

Electronic sphygmomanometers sense vibrations, convert them to electrical impulses, and transmit them to a device that produces a digital readout. It is relatively sensitive and is also capable of simultaneously measuring the pulse rate. The normal newborn blood pressure ranges from 60 to 96 systolic and 30 to 62 diastolic. A sustained increase in blood pressure is almost always significant.

CHILDREN

The precordium of a child tends to bulge over an enlarged heart if the enlargement is of long standing. A child's thoracic cage, being more cartilaginous and yielding than that of an adult, responds more to the thrust of cardiac enlargement.

Sinus arrhythmia is a physiologic event during childhood. The heart rate varies in a cyclic pattern, usually faster on inspiration and slower on expiration.

The heart rates of children are more variable than those of adults, reacting with wider swings to stress of any sort (exercise, fever, tension). It is not uncommon to discover an increase of 10 to 20 beats in the heart rate for each degree of temperature elevation. The expected heart rates in children vary with age:

Age	Rate
Newborn	120-170
1 year	80-160
3 years	80-120
6 years	75-115
10 years	70-110

A venous hum, which is common in children, has no pathologic significance; it is caused by the turbulence of blood flow in the internal jugular veins. To detect a venous hum, ask the child to sit with the head turned to the left and tilted slightly upward. Auscultate over the right supraclavicular space with the stethoscope bell (Fig. 9-37). When present the hum is a continuous low-pitched sound that is louder during diastole. It may be interrupted by gentle pressure over the vein in the space between the trachea and the sternocleidomastoid muscle at about the level of the thyroid cartilage.

Most organic murmurs in infants and children are now the result of congenital heart disease. However, acute rheumatic fever still accounts for most acquired murmurs.

When examining a child with known heart disease, take careful note of weight gain (or loss), developmental delay, cyanosis, and clubbing of fingers and toes. Cyanosis is a major key to congenital heart defects that impede oxygenation of blood.

Blood pressure is easy to measure in children past the age of 2 or 3. Children like to explore the sphygmomanometer, and a moment of playing with the instrument can facilitate examination. If a child seems anxious, wait until later in the examination. If your ability to hear is compromised by crying or a deeply placed brachial

Fig. 9-37
Auscultation for venous hum.

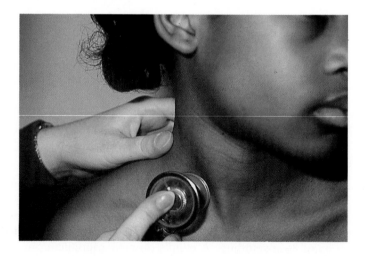

artery, palpate the radial artery if a digital sphygmomanometer is not available. This will yield a systolic pressure about 10 mm Hg less than that at the brachial artery.

Do not make the diagnosis of hypertension on the basis of one reading. Many readings should be taken over time. If the systolic pressure is elevated and the diastolic not, transient anxiety may be responsible. Take time to reassure the child to alleviate his or her anxiety. Children with pressures consistently above the 95th percentile must be carefully studied and followed. It is unlikely for a child to have essential hypertension (the possibility is greater in the adolescent). Most often hypertension in children is caused by kidney disease, renal arterial disease, coarctation of the aorta, or pheochromocytoma.

PREGNANT WOMEN

The heart rate gradually increases throughout pregnancy until it is 15 to 20 beats per minute higher by the end of the third trimester. Blood pressure varies with the woman's position, being highest when sitting, lowest when in the left lateral recumbent position, and in between when supine. Blood pressure readings above those recorded before pregnancy in the same position should make you suspect hypertension.

The heart position is shifted during pregnancy, but the position varies with the size and position of the uterus. The apical impulse is upward and more lateral by 1 to 1.5 cm. Some changes in auscultated heart sounds are expected because of the increased blood volume and extra effort of the heart. There is more audible splitting of S_1 and S_2, and S_3 may be readily heard after 20 weeks of gestation. Additionally, grade II systolic ejection murmurs may be heard over the pulmonic area.

OLDER ADULTS

You may need to slow the pace of your examination when asking some older patients to assume positions that may be uncomfortable or perhaps too difficult. Some may not be able to lie flat for an extended time, and some may not be able to control their breathing pattern at your request.

The heart rate may be slower because of increased vagal tone, or more rapid, with a wide range from the low 40s to more than 100. Occasional ectopic beats are fairly common and may or may not be significant.

The apical impulse may be harder to find in many persons because of the increased anteroposterior diameter of the chest. In obese older adults, the diaphragm is raised and the heart is more transverse.

S_4 is more common in older adults and may indicate decreased left ventricular compliance. Early, soft, physiologic murmurs may be heard, caused by aortic lengthening, tortuosity, and sclerotic changes.

The dorsalis pedis and posterior tibial pulses may be more difficult to find, and the superficial vessels are more apt to appear tortuous and distended.

The blood pressure tends to be higher; hypertension in this age group is usually defined by 170/95 on repeated measurement. Kinking of the left innominate artery may interfere with measurement of the jugular venous pressure. Trying a number of different positions (more or less erect, moving from side to side) may make it possible to get a more reliable reading.

Common Abnormalities

Acquired Cardiac Disorders

Heart Murmurs *(Figs. 9-38 and 9-39)*	Type and Detection	Findings on Examination	Description
	Mitral Stenosis Heard with bell at apex, patient in left lateral decubitus	Low frequency diastolic rumble, more intense in early and late diastole, does not radiate; systole usually quiet; palpable thrill at apex in late diastole common; S_1 increased and often palpable at left sternal border; S_2 split often with accented P_2; opening snap follows P_2 closely Visible lift in right parasternal area if right ventricle hypertrophied Arterial pulse amplitude decreased	Narrowed valve restricts forward flow; forceful ejection into ventricles Often occurs with mitral regurgitation Caused by rheumatic fever or cardiac infection
	Aortic Stenosis Heard over aortic area; ejection sound at 2nd right intercostal border	Midsystolic murmur, medium pitch, coarse, diamond-shaped,* crescendo-decrescendo; radiates down left sternal border (sometimes to apex) and to carotid with palpable thrill; S_1 normal often followed by ejection click; S_2 soft or absent and may not be split; S_4 palpable Apical thrust shifts down and left and is prolonged in left ventricle hypertrophy	Calcification of valve cusps restricts forward flow; forceful ejection from ventricle into systemic circulation Caused by congenital bicuspid valves, rheumatic heart disease
	Subaortic Stenosis Heard at apex and along left sternal border	Murmur fills systole, diamond shaped, medium pitch, coarse; thrill often palpable during systole at apex and right sternal border; multiple waves in apical impulses; S_2 usually split; S_3 and S_4 often present Arterial pulse brisk, double wave in carotid common; jugular venous pulse prominent	Fibrous ring, usually 1 to 4 mm below aortic valve; most pronounced on ventricular septal side; may become progressively severe with time
	Pulmonic Stenosis Heard over pulmonic area radiating to left and into neck; thrill in 2nd and 3rd left intercostal space	Systolic murmur, diamond shaped, medium pitch, coarse; usually with thrill; S_1 often followed quickly by ejection click; S_2 often diminished, usually wide split; P_2 soft or absent; S_4 common in right ventricular hypertrophy	Valve restricts forward flow; forceful ejection from ventricle into pulmonary circulation Cause is almost always congenital

*Diamond-shaped murmur is named for its recorded shape on phonocardiogram (a crescendo-decrescendo sound).

Type and Detection	Findings on Examination	Description
Tricuspid Stenosis Heard with bell over tricuspid area	Diastolic rumble accentuated early and late in diastole, resembling mitral stenosis but louder on inspiration; diastolic thrill palpable over right ventricle; S_2 may be split during inspiration Arterial pulse amplitude decreased; jugular venous pulse prominent, especially A wave; slow fall of V wave	Calcification of valve cusps restricts forward flow; forceful ejection into ventricles Usually seen with mitral stenosis, rarely occurs alone Caused by rheumatic heart disease, endocardial fibroelastosis, right atrial myxoma, congenital defect
Mitral Regurgitation Heard best at apex; loudest there, transmitted into left axilla	Holosystolic, plateau-shaped intensity, high pitch, harsh blowing quality, often quite loud; radiates from apex to base or to left axilla; thrill may be palpable at apex during systole; S_1 intensity diminished; S_2 more intense with P_2 often accented; S_3 often present; S_3-S_4 gallop common in late disease; If mild, late systolic murmur crescendos; if severe, early systolic intensity decrescendos; apical thrust more to left and down in ventricular hypertrophy	Valve incompetence allows backflow from ventricle to atrium Caused by rheumatic fever, myocardial infarction, myxoma
Aortic Regurgitation Heard with diaphragm, patient sitting and leaning forward; Austin-Flint murmur heard with bell; ejection click heard in 2nd intercostal space	Early diastolic, high pitch, blowing, often with diamond-shaped midsystolic murmur, sounds often not prominent; duration varies with blood pressure; low-pitched rumbling murmur at apex common (Austin-Flint); early ejection click sometimes present; S_1 soft; S_2 split may have tambour-like quality; M_1 and A_2 often intensified; S_3-S_4 gallop common In left ventricular hypertrophy, prominent prolonged apical impulse down and to left Pulse pressure wide; water-hammer or biferiens pulse common in carotid, brachial, and femoral arteries	Valve incompetence allows backflow from aorta to ventricle Caused by rheumatic heart disease, endocarditis, aortic diseases (Marfan's syndrome, medial necrosis), syphilis, ankylosing spondylitis, dissection, cardiac trauma
Pulmonic Regurgitation	Difficult to distinguish from aortic regurgitation on physical examination	Valve incompetence allows backflow from pulmonary artery to ventricle Cause secondary to pulmonary hypertension or bacterial endocarditis

Text continued on p. 330.

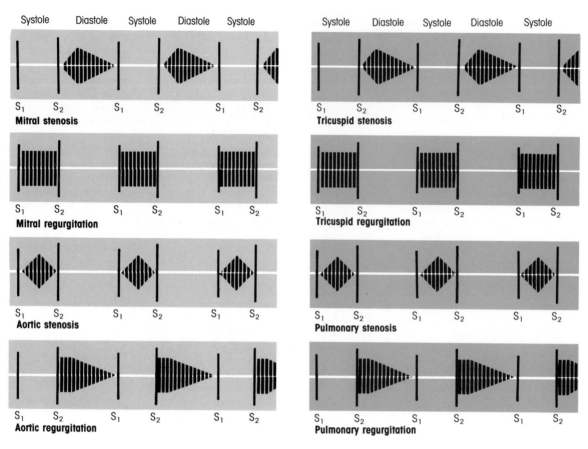

Fig. 9-38
Valvular heart disease murmurs.
From Guzzetta and Dossey, 1984.

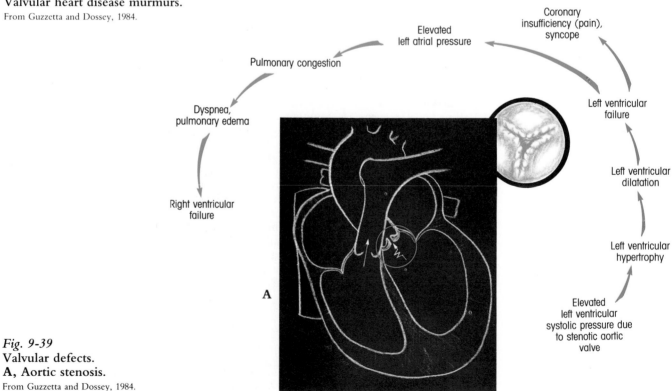

Fig. 9-39
Valvular defects.
A, Aortic stenosis.
From Guzzetta and Dossey, 1984.

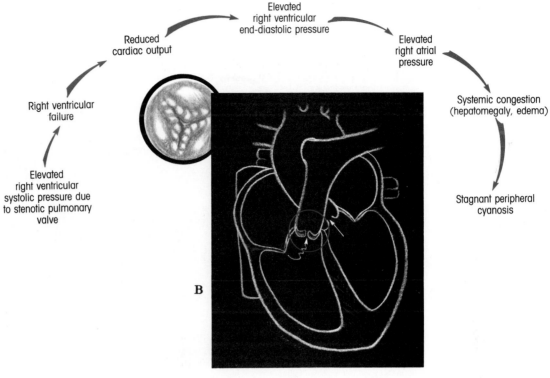

Fig. 9-39, cont'd
Valvular defects.
B, Pulmonic stenosis.
C, Mitral regurgitation.
From Guzzetta and Dossey, 1984.

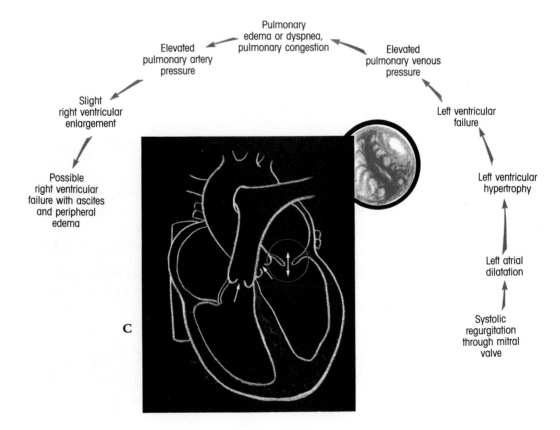

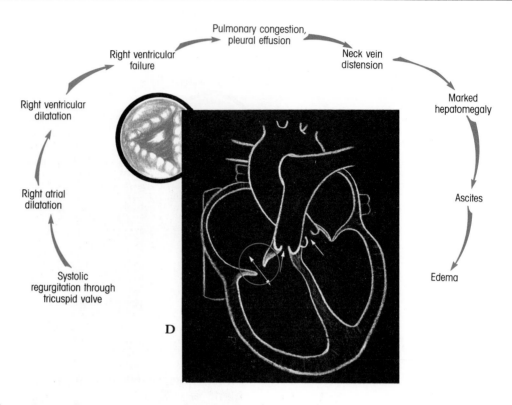

Fig. 9-39, cont'd
Valvular defects.
D, Tricuspid regurgitation.
E, Aortic regurgitation.
From Guzzetta and Dossey, 1984.

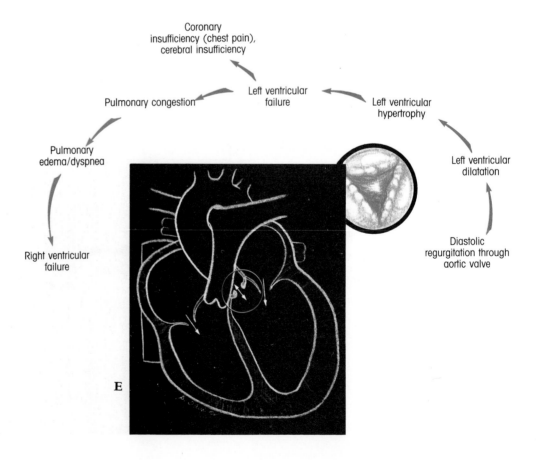

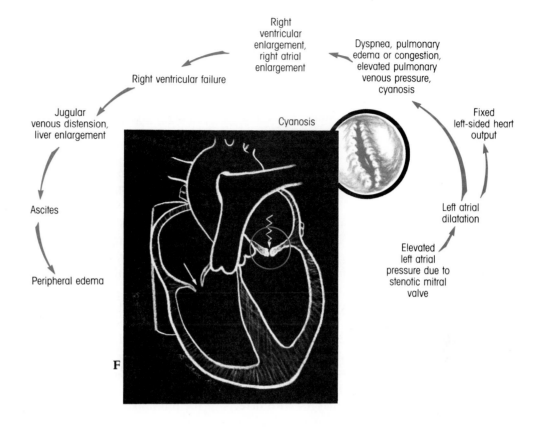

Right
ventricular
enlargement,
right atrial
enlargement

Right ventricular failure

Dyspnea, pulmonary
edema or congestion,
elevated pulmonary
venous pressure,
cyanosis

Jugular
venous distension,
liver enlargement

Cyanosis

Fixed
left-sided heart
output

Ascites

Left atrial
dilatation

Peripheral edema

Elevated
left atrial
pressure due to
stenotic mitral
valve

F

Fig. 9-39, cont'd
Valvular defects.
F, Mitral stenosis.
G, Triscuspid stenosis.
From Guzzetta and Dossey, 1984.

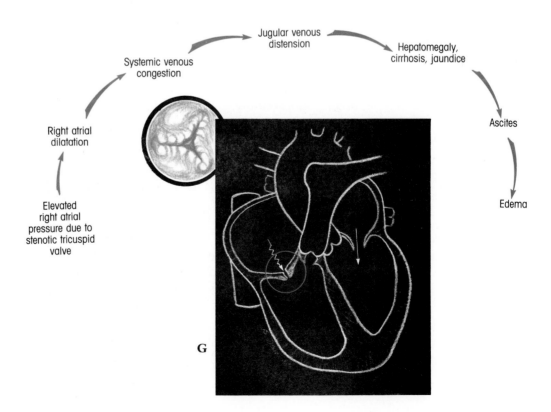

Jugular venous
distension

Systemic venous
congestion

Hepatomegaly,
cirrhosis, jaundice

Right atrial
dilatation

Ascites

Elevated
right atrial
pressure due to
stenotic tricuspid
valve

Edema

G

	Type and Detection	Findings on Examination	Description
	Tricuspid Regurgitation Heard at left lower sternum, occasionally radiating a few centimeters to left	Holosystolic murmur over right ventricle, blowing, increased on inspiration; S_3 and thrill over tricuspid area frequent In pulmonary hypertension, pulmonary artery impulse palpable over second left intercostal space and P_2 accented; in right ventricular hypertrophy, visible lift to right of sternum Jugular venous pulse has large v waves	Valve incompetence allows backflow from ventricle to strium Caused by pulmonary hypertension, cardiac trauma, congenital defects, bacterial endocarditis
Left Ventricular Hypertrophy	The left ventricle works harder and longer with each beat when it meets increased resistance to the emptying of blood into the systemic circulation, as with aortic stenosis, volume overload, and systemic hypertension. It hypertrophies because of the extra exercise and, sometimes, becomes displaced laterally.	A vigorous sustained lift is palpable during ventricular systole, sometimes over a broader area than usual, as much as 2 cm or more. The displacement of the apical impulse can be most impressive, well beyond the midclavicular line and downward.	
Right Ventricular Hypertrophy	The right ventricle works harder and enlarges with defects of the pulmonary vascular bed and pulmonary hypertension. This is less common than left ventricular hypertrophy. It can cause a lift along the left sternal border in the third	and fourth left intercostal spaces accompanied by occasional systolic retraction at the apex. The left ventricle is not itself particularly affected, but it is displaced and turned posteriorly by the enlarged right ventricle.	
Sick Sinus Syndrome	In sick sinus syndrome, sinoatrial dysfunction occurs secondary to hypertension, arteriosclerotic heart disease, or rheumatic heart disease; it may also occur idiopathically. The condition	causes fainting, transient dizzy spells, light headedness, seizures, palpitations, and symptoms of angina and congestive heart failure.	
Bacterial Endocarditis	A bacterial infection of the endothelial layer of the heart and valves should be suspected with prolonged fever, signs of neurologic dysfunctions, and sudden onset of congestive heart failure. A	murmur may or may not be present. Individuals with valvular defects, congenital or acquired, are particularly susceptible.	
Congestive Heart Failure	Congestive heart failure is a syndrome in which the heart fails to propel blood forward normally, resulting in congestion in the pulmonary or systemic circulation. Decreased cardiac output causes	decreased blood flow to the tissues. Congestive heart failure may be predominantly left- or right-sided. It can develop gradually or suddenly with acute pulmonary edema.	

Cor Pulmonale	Cor pulmonale is the enlargement of the right ventricle secondary to pulmonary malfunction. Usually chronic but occasionally acute, cor pulmonale results from chronic obstructive pulmonary disease. The alterations in the pulmonary	circulation lead to pulmonary arterial hypertension, which imposes a mechanical load on right ventricular emptying. Signs include left parasternal systolic lift and a loud S_2.
Myocardial Infarction	Ischemic myocardial necrosis is caused by abrupt decrease in coronary blood flow to a segment of the myocardium. It predominantly affects the left ventricle, but damage may extend into the right ventricle or atria. Symptoms commonly include deep substernal or visceral pain that often radiates to the jaw, neck, and left arm, although discomfort	may be mild, especially in older adults. Arrhythmias are common and S_4 is usually present. Heart sounds are typically distant, with a soft systolic blowing apical murmur. Pulse may be thready, and blood pressure varies, although hypertension is usual in the early phases. Atherosclerosis is the underlying cause.
Myocarditis	Focal or diffuse inflammation of the myocardium can result from infectious agents or toxins. Initial symptoms are typically vague and include fatigue, dyspnea, fever, and palpitations. As the	disease process advances, cardiac enlargement, murmur, gallop rhythms, tachycardia, arrhythmias, and pulsus alternans develop.
Temporal Arteritis (giant cell arteritis)	Chronic generalized inflammatory disease of the branches of the aortic arch principally affect arteries of the carotid system and the temporal and occipital arteries. Temporal arteritis usually affects persons over 50. Flu-like symptoms (low-grade fever, malaise, anorexia) are accompanied by polymyalgia involving the trunk and proximal mus-	cles. Headache is severe, there is throbbing in the temporal region on one or both sides, and the area over the temporal artery becomes red, swollen, tender, and nodulated. The temporal pulse may be variously strong, weak, or absent. Ocular symptoms, including loss of vision, are common. (Also see p. 161.)

Abnormalities in Heart Rates and Rhythms

	Finding on Examination	Description
Atrial (auricular) flutter	Atrial rate far in excess of ventricular rate; heart sounds not necessarily weak	Regular uniform atrial contractions occur in excess of 200/min as a result of heart block. The conduction system cannot respond to the rapidity of the atrial rate, causing variance from the ventricle rate. The ECG may look like a saw-tooth cog.

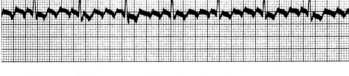

Atrial flutter with a constant 4:1 conduction ratio.
From Guzzetta and Dossey, 1984.

| Sinus bradycardia | Slow rate, sometimes below 50 or 60/min | No disruption in origin or conduction, which may not indicate illness. |

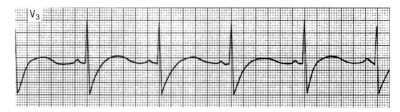

Sinus bradycardia.
From Guzzetta and Dossey, 1984.

| Atrial fibrillation | Arrhythmic contraction of the atria gives way to rapid series of irregular spasms of the muscle wall; no discernible regularity in rhythm or pattern | The conduction system is malfunctioning and is in an anarchic state. Any contraction of the atria that gets through to the ventricle is irregular. The sounds are best described as chaotic. |

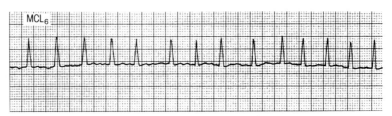

Atrial fibrillation with rapid ventricular response.
From Guzzetta and Dossey, 1984.

| Heart block | Heart rate slower than expected, often 25-45/min at rest | Conduction from atria to ventricles partially or completely disrupted. If conduction is completely disrupted, the ventricle may be left to beat on its own and the heart rate slows considerably. ECG is necessary to determine the nature and extent of heart block in conduction. |

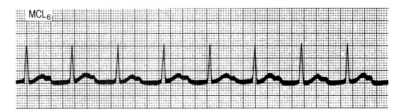

Normal sinus rhythm with first-degree AV block.
From Guzzetta and Dossey, 1984.

| Atrial tachycardia | Rapid, regular heart rate (≅200/min) without disruption of the rhythm; may be heard only on occasion (in paroxysms) and without loss of vigor in heart sounds | This is the result of electrical stimulus originating in a focus in the atrium separate from the SA. Conduction through to the ventricle is usually complete. Often there is no other evidence of disease, and the patient is usually a young adult. The rate will occasionally respond to vagal stimulation, holding a deep breath, or gentle massage of a carotid sinus. (Remember that massage must always be done with care.) |

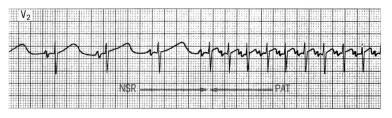

Paroxysmal atrial tachycardia (PAT).
From Guzzetta and Dossey, 1984.

| Ventricular tachycardia | Rapid, relatively regular heart beat (often nearly 200/min) without loss in apparent strength | The electrical source of the beat is in an unusual focus somewhere in the ventricles. This usually arises in serious heart disease and is a grave prognostic sign. |

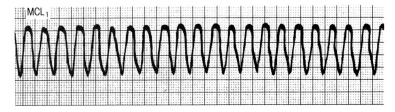

Ventricular tachycardia.
From Guzzetta and Dossey, 1984.

| Ventricular fibrillation | Complete loss of regular heart rhythm with expected conduction pattern absent; if weakened and rapid, ventricular contraction is irregular | The ventricle has lost the rhythm of its expected response, and all evidence of vigorous contraction is gone. It calls for immediate action and may immediately precede sudden death. |

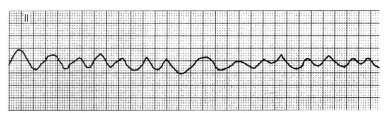

Ventricular fibrillation.
From Guzzetta and Dossey, 1984.

Congenital Defects

Tetralogy of Fallot

Four cardiac defects make up the tetralogy of Fallot: ventricular septal defect, pulmonic stenosis, dextroposition of the aorta, and right ventricular hypertrophy. Infants with tetralogy of Fallot have paroxysmal dyspnea with loss of consciousness; older children have cyanosis with clubbing of fingers and toes. There is a parasternal heave and precordial prominence. A systolic ejection murmur is heard over the third intercostal space, sometimes radiating to the left side of the neck. A single S_2 is heard (Fig. 9-40).

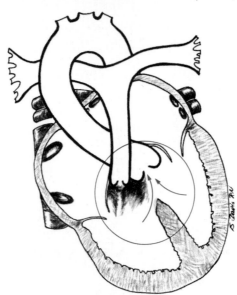

Fig. 9-40
Tetralogy of Fallot.
From Guzzetta and Dossey, 1984.

Ventricular Septal Defect

Ventricular septal defect is an opening between the left and right ventricles. The arterial pulse is small and the jugular venous pulse is unaffected. Regurgitation occurs through the septal defect; as a result, the murmur tends to be holosystolic. It is frequently loud, coarse, high-pitched, and best heard along the left sternal border in the third to fifth intercostal spaces. A distinct lift is often discernible along the left sternal border and the apical area. A smaller defect causes a more easily felt thrill than a large one (Fig. 9-41).

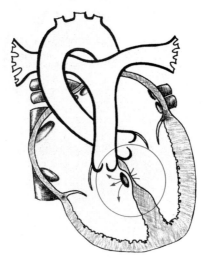

Fig. 9-41
Ventricular septal defect.
From Guzzetta and Dossey, 1984.

Patent Ductus Arteriosus

Sometimes the ductus arteriosus, which is patent in the fetal circulation, fails to close after birth. Blood flows through the ductus during systole and diastole, increasing the pressure in the pulmonary circulation and consequently the work load of the right ventricle. A small shunt can be asymptomatic; a larger one causes dyspnea on exertion. The neck vessels are dilated and pulsate, and the pulse pressure is wide. A harsh, loud, continuous murmur is heard at the first to third intercostal spaces and the lower sternal border. It has a machine-like quality (Fig. 9-42).

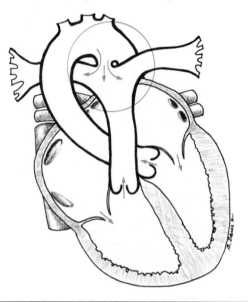

Fig. 9-42
Patent ductus arteriosus.
From Guzzetta and Dossey, 1984.

Atrial Septal Defect

A congenital defect in the septum dividing the left and right atria causes a systolic ejection murmur that is diamond-shaped, often loud, high in pitch, and harsh. It is heard best over the pulmonic area and may be accompanied by a brief, rumbling early diastolic murmur. It does not usually radiate beyond the precordium. A systolic thrill may be felt over the area of the murmur along with a palpable parasternal thrust. S$_2$ may be split fairly widely (Fig. 9-43).

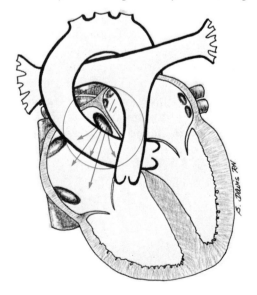

Fig. 9-43
Atrial septal defect.
From Guzzetta and Dossey, 1984.

Vessel Disorders

Arterial Aneurysm	An aneurysm is a localized dilation of an artery caused by a weakness in the arterial wall. It is noticed as a pulsatile swelling along the course of an artery. Aneurysms occur most commonly in the	aorta, although abdominal, renal, femoral, and popliteal arteries are also common sites. A thrill or bruit may be evident over the aneurysm.
Arteriovenous Fistula	An arteriovenous fistula is a pathologic communication between an artery and a vein; it may result in an aneurysmal	dilation. A continuous bruit or thrill over the area of a fistula suggests its presence.
Venous Thrombosis	Thrombosis can occur suddenly or gradually with varying severity of symptoms. It can be the result of trauma or prolonged immobilization. Clinical findings of thrombosis in a superficial vein include redness, thickening, and tenderness along the involved segment. Deep vein thrombosis in the femoral and pelvic circulations may have no symptoms, and pulmonary embolism, sometimes fatal, may occur without warning. Signs and symptoms sugges-	tive of deep vein thrombosis include tenderness along the iliac vessels and the femoral canal, in the popliteal space, and over the deep calf veins, as well as slight swelling that may be distinguished only by measuring and comparing the upper and lower legs bilaterally, minimal ankle edema, low grade fever, and tachycardia. Homans' sign can be helpful but not absolutely reliable in suggesting deep vein thrombosis.
Peripheral Atherosclerotic Disease (Arteriosclerosis Obliterans)	Occlusion of the blood supply to the extremities by atherosclerotic plaques causes symptoms that vary in severity. Intermittent claudication produces pain, ache, or cramp in the exercising muscle that receives a deficient blood supply. The amount of exercise necessary to cause the discomfort is predictable, occurring after the same distance walked each time. A brief rest relieves	the pain. The limb appears healthy, but pulses are weak or absent. Progressive occlusion results in severe ischemia in which the foot or leg is painful at rest, cold, numb, and skin changes occur (dry and scaling, with poor hair and nail growth). Edema seldom accompanies this disorder, but ulceration is common in severe disease, and the muscles may atrophy.
Raynaud's Disease	Idiopathic spasm of the arterioles in the digits (occasionally in the nose and tongue) causes intermittent skin pallor or cyanosis. The vasospasm may last from minutes to hours. It occurs bilaterally, and the skin over the digits eventually appear smooth, shiny, and tight from loss of subcutaneous tissue. Ulcers	may appear on tips of the digits. Raynaud's disease occurs most frequently in young, otherwise healthy women. Raynaud's phenomenon is secondary to connective tissue diseases, neurogenic lesions, drug intoxication, primary pulmonary hypertension, and trauma.

OLDER ADULTS

Atherosclerotic Heart Disease	Atherosclerotic heart disease may cause myocardial insufficiency, angina pectoris, dysrhythmias, and congestive heart failure.	
Mitral Insufficiency	Mitral insufficiency is usually silent and painless until it produces sudden heart failure, stroke, or dysrhythmias. It also occurs after infarction, along with	tachycardia, pallor, a variety of alterations in the heart sounds, occasional pericardial friction rub, various murmurs, and arrhythmias.
Angina	Angina produces retrosternal pain radiating to neck, jaws, arms, and back. It is often accompanied by symptoms of	shortness of breath, fatigue, faintness, and syncope.
Senile Cardiac Amyloidosis	Amyloid deposits in the heart cause heart failure. Electrocardiography shows a small, thickened left ventricle,	and the right ventricle may also be thickened. The contractility of the heart may be normal or reduced.
Conduction Disturbances	Conduction disturbances occur either proximal to the bundle of His or diffusely throughout the conduction system. They produce symptoms of transient weakness, fainting spells, or	stroke-like episodes (Adams-Stokes attacks).

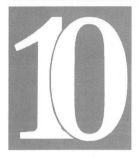

CHAPTER

10

Breasts and Axillae

Anatomy and Physiology

The breasts are paired mammary glands located on the anterior chest wall, superficial to the pectoralis major and serratus anterior muscles (Fig. 10-1). In women the breast extends from the second or third rib to the sixth or seventh rib, and from the sternal margin to the midaxillary line. The nipple is located centrally, surrounded by the areola. The male breast consists of a small nipple and areola overlying a thin layer of breast tissue that is indistinguishable by palpation from surrounding tissue.

The female breast is composed of glandular and fibrous tissue and subcutaneous and retromammary fat. The glandular tissue is arranged into 15 to 20 lobes per breast that radiate about the nipple. Each lobe is composed of 20 to 40 lobules, which consist of the milk-producing acini cells that empty into lactiferous ducts. These cells are small and inconspicuous in the nonpregnant, nonlactating woman. A lactiferous duct drains milk from each lobe onto the surface of the nipple.

The layer of subcutaneous fibrous tissue provides support for the breast. Suspensory ligaments (Cooper's ligaments) extend from the connective tissue layer, through the breast, and attach to the underlying muscle fascia, providing further support for the breast. The muscles forming the floor of the breast are the pectoralis major, pectoralis minor, serratus anterior, latissimus dorsi, subscapularis, external oblique, and rectus abdominus.

Vascular supply to the breast is primarily through branches of the internal mammary artery and the lateral thoracic artery. This network provides most of the blood supply to the deeper tissues of the breast and to the nipple. The intercostal arteries assist in supplying the more superficial tissues.

The subcutaneous and retromammary fat that surround the glandular tissue compose most of the bulk of the breast. The proportions of each of the component tissues vary with age, nutritional status, pregnancy, lactation, and genetic predisposition.

For the purposes of examination the breast is divided into 5 segments: four quadrants and a tail (Fig. 10-2). The greatest amount of glandular tissue lies in the upper outer quadrant. Breast tissue extends from this quadrant into the axilla, forming the tail of Spence. In the axillae the mammary tissue is in direct contact with the axillary lymph nodes.

The nipple, onto which the lactiferous ducts empty, is located centrally on the breast and is surrounded by the pigmented areola. The nipple is composed of epithelium that is infiltrated with circular and longitudinal smooth muscle fibers. Contraction of the smooth muscle, induced by tactile, sensory, or autonomic stimuli,

Fig. 10-1
**Anatomy of the breast
showing position and
major structures.**

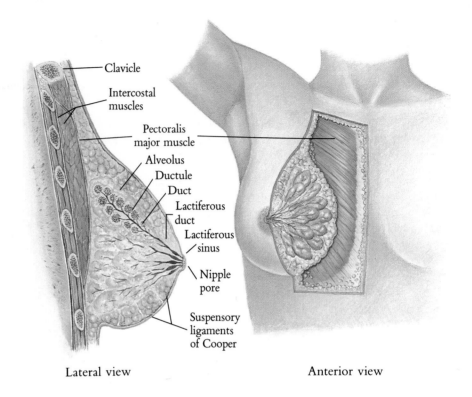

Lateral view   Anterior view

Fig. 10-2
**Quadrants of left breast
and axillary tail of Spence.**

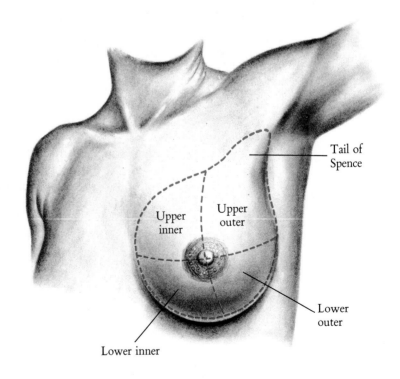

Table 10-1
Patterns of Lymph Drainage

Area of Breast	Drainage
Superficial	
Upper outer quadrant	Scapular, brachial, intermediate nodes toward axillary nodes
Medial portion	Internal mammary chain toward opposite breast and abdomen
Deep	
Posterior chest wall and portion of the arm	Posterior axillary nodes (subscapular)
Anterior chest wall	Anterior axillary nodes (pectoral)
Upper arm	Lateral axillary nodes (brachial)
Retroareolar area	Interpectoral (Rotter's) nodes into the axillary chain
Areola and nipple	Midaxillary, subclavicular, and supraclavicular nodes

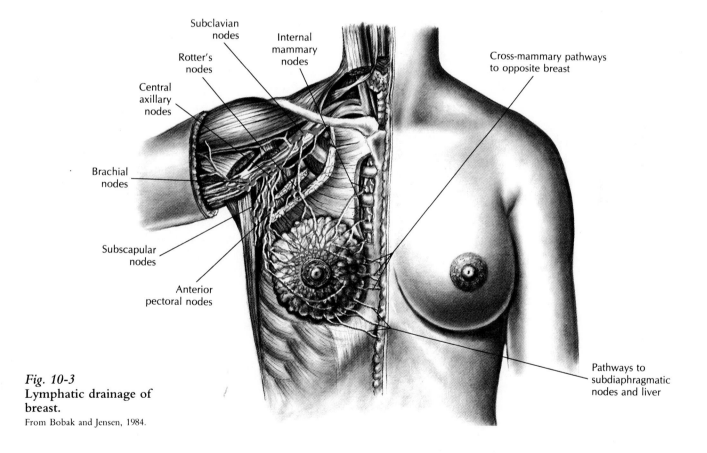

Fig. 10-3
Lymphatic drainage of breast.
From Bobak and Jensen, 1984.

produces erection of the nipple and causes the lactiferous ducts to empty. The process of erection is supported by venous stasis in the erectile vascular tissue. Tiny sebaceous glands may be apparent on the areolar surface (Montgomery tubercles or follicles). Some hair follicles may be found about the circumference of the areola. Supernumerary nipples or breast tissue is sometimes present along the mammary ridge that extends from the axilla during embryonic development.

Each breast contains a lymphatic network that drains the breast radially and deeply to underlying lymphatics. Superficial lymphatics drain the skin, and deep lymphatics drain the mammary lobules. Table 10-1 summarizes the patterns of lymph drainage.

The complex of lymph nodes, their locations, and direction of drainage are illustrated in Fig. 10-3. The axillary nodes are more superficial and are therefore more accessible and relatively easily palpable. The anterior axillary (pectoral) nodes are located along the lower border of the pectoralis major inside the lateral axillary fold. The mid axillary (central) nodes are high in the axilla close to the ribs. The posterior axillary (subscapular) nodes lie along the lateral border of the scapula and deep in the posterior axillary fold, while the lateral axillary (brachial) nodes can be felt along the upper humerus.

CHILDREN AND ADOLESCENTS

The breast evolves in structure and function throughout life. Childhood and pre-adolescence represent a latent phase of breast development during which only minimal branching of primary ducts occurs. Thelarche (breast development) represents an early sign of puberty in adolescent girls. The developmental process has been classified and described a number of ways. Tanner's five stages of developing sexual maturity, discussed in Chapter 3 (Growth and Measurement), is the classification most commonly used.

In using the Tanner charts to stage breast development, it is important to note certain temporal relationships. It is unusual for the onset of menses to occur before stage III. About 25% of females begin menstruation at stage III. Seventy five percent are menstruating at stage IV and are beginning a reasonably regular menstrual cycle. Some 10% of young women do not begin to menstruate until stage V. The average interval from the appearance of the breast bud (stage II) to menarche is 2 years. Stage IV may not occur in as many as 25% of all adolescents and may be only minimal in another 25%. It is also important to remember that breasts develop at different rates, which can result in asymmetry.

PREGNANT WOMEN

Striking changes occur in the breasts during pregnancy. In response to luteal and placental hormones, the lactiferous ducts proliferate and the alveoli increase extensively in size and number, causing the breasts to enlarge two to three times their prepregnancy size. The increase in glandular tissue displaces connective tissue and, as a result, the tissue becomes softer and looser. Toward the end of pregnancy as epithelial secretory activity increases, colostrum is produced and accumulates in the acini cells (alveoli).

The areolae become more deeply pigmented and their diameter increases. The nipples become more prominant, darker, and more erectile. Montgomery tubercles often develop as sebaceous glands hypertrophy.

Mammary vascularization increases, causing veins to engorge and become visible as a blue network beneath the surface of the skin.

LACTATING WOMEN

In the first few days following delivery, small amounts of colostrum are secreted from the breasts. Milk production to replace colostrum begins 3 to 5 days after delivery in response to surging prolactin levels, declining estrogen levels, and the stimulation of sucking. Between the third and sixth days colostrum changes to transitional milk with a high protein content. By about day 10 the protein content decreases and the lactose content increases, stabilizing by the end of the first month. As the alveoli and lactiferous ducts fill, the breasts become full and tense. This, combined with tissue edema, produces breast engorgement.

At the termination of lactation, involution occurs over a period of about 3 months. Decrease in breast size is accomplished without loss of lobular and alveolar components. The breasts rarely return to their prelactation size.

OLDER ADULTS

Before menopause there is a moderate decrease in glandular tissue and some decomposition of alveolar and lobular tissue. After menopause glandular tissue continues to gradually atrophy and is replaced by fat deposited in the breasts. The inframammary ridge at the lower edge of the breast thickens. The breasts tend to hang more loosely from the chest wall because of these tissue changes and the relaxation of the suspensory ligaments. The nipples become smaller, flatter, and lose some erectile ability.

The skin may take on a relatively dry, thin texture. Loss of hair in the axillae may also occur.

Review of Related History

General Considerations

1. Age
2. Any changes in breast characteristics: pain, tenderness, lumps, discharge, skin changes, size or shape changes
3. Changes in the breast that occur with the menstrual cycle: tenderness, swelling, pain, enlarged nodes
4. Date of first day of last menstrual period
5. Menopause: onset, course, associated problems, residual problems
6. Breast support used with strenuous exercise or sports activities
7. Medications, particularly oral contraceptives or other hormones: name, dosage, length of time taking
8. Breast self-examination: frequency; at what time in the menstrual cycle; have woman describe her procedure
9. Risk factors for breast cancer: see top of p. 344

Present Problem

1. Breast discomfort
   a. Temporal sequence: onset gradual or sudden; length of time symptom has been present; does symptom come and go or is it always present
   b. Relationship to menses: timing, severity
   c. Character: stinging, pulling, burning, drawing, stabbing, aching, throbbing; unilateral or bilateral; localization; radiation
   d. Associated symptoms: lump or mass, discharge from nipple
   e. Contributory factors: skin irritation under breasts from tissue-to-tissue contact or from rubbing of brassiere; strenuous activity; recent injury to breast

FACTORS ASSOCIATED WITH INCREASED RISK OF BREAST CANCER IN THE UNITED STATES

Age (risk rises steadily with age then peaks at 45-49)
Early age at menarche (under age 12)
Rapid establishment of regular cycles after menarche (within a year)
Later age at menopause (over age 55)
Nulliparity
Later age at first full-term pregnancy (over age 30)
Postmenopausal weight gain
Benign breast disease (fibrocystic, fibroadenoma)
Family history of breast cancer

Adapted from Henderson et al., 1984.

2. Breast mass or lump
   a. Temporal sequence: length of time since lump first noted; does lump come and go or is it always present; relationship to menses
   b. Symptoms: tenderness or pain (characterize as described previously), dimpling or change in contour
   c. Changes in lump: size, character, relationship to menses (timing or severity)
   d. Associated symptoms: nipple discharge or retraction, tender lymph nodes
3. Nipple discharge
   a. Character: onset gradual or sudden, duration, color, consistency, odor, amount
   b. Associated symptoms: nipple retraction, breast lump or discomfort
   c. Associated factors: relationship to menses or other activity; medications (contraceptives, phenothiazines, digitalis, diuretics, steroids); recent injury to breast

Past Medical History

1. Previous breast disease: cancer, fibroadenomas, fibrocystic disease
2. Surgeries: breast biopsies, aspirations, implants, reduction plasties; oophorectomy
3. Menstrual history: age of menarche or menopause; cycle length, duration and amount of flow, regularity; associated breast symptoms (nipple discharge; pain or discomfort)
4. Pregnancy: age at each pregnancy, length of each pregnancy, date of delivery or termination
5. Lactation: number of children breast-fed; duration of time for breast-feeding; date of termination of last breast-feeding; medications used to suppress lactation
6. Past use of hormonal medications: name and dosage, reason for use (contraception, menstrual control, menopausal symptom relief), length of time on hormones, date of termination

Family History

1. Breast cancer: which relative (particularly mother or sister); type of cancer; age at time of occurrence; treatment and results
2. Other breast disease in female and male relatives: type of disease; age at time of occurrence; treatment and results

PREGNANT WOMEN

1. Sensations: fullness, tingling, tenderness
2. Use of supportive brassiere
3. Preparation procedures for breast-feeding

LACTATING WOMEN

1. Cleaning procedures for breasts: daily washing or after each feeding, if dried milk is present; soap or solution used for cleaning; lubrication of nipples
2. Use of nursing brassiere
3. Nipples: tenderness, pain, cracking, bleeding; retracted; related problems with feeding
4. Associated problems: engorgement, leaking breasts, plugged duct (localized tenderness and lump), fever, infection; treatment and results; infant with oral candidal infection
5. Nursing routine: number of minutes for each breast, rotation of breast used first

OLDER ADULTS

1. Skin irritation under pendulous breasts from tissue-to-tissue contact or from rubbing of brassiere; treatment
2. Hormone therapy during or since menopause: name and dosage of medication; duration of therapy

Examination and Findings

EQUIPMENT

- **Flashlight with transilluminator**
- **Ruler**
- **Small pillow or folded towel**
- **Glass slide and cytologic fixative, if nipple discharge is present**

Adequate lighting is essential for revealing shadows and subtle variations in skin color and texture. Adequate exposure is also essential, requiring that the patient be disrobed to the waist. Draping one breast while examining the other to protect the patient's modesty is more a disservice than a consideration, because simultaneous observation of both breasts is necessary in order to detect minor differences between them that may be significant. Modesty is a concern, however, and you or the patient may be uncomfortable at first. A matter-of-fact and composed approach with attention to the patient as a person will go a long way in reassuring the patient of your regard and sensitivity.

Take a few extra minutes during this examination to have the patient demonstrate how she does her breast self-exam. This gives you an opportunity to review the process and rationale for self-examination with her, and to instruct her in the correct techniques if necessary.

BREAST SELF-EXAMINATION

A, Steps in breast self-examination. Inspect and palpate breasts (1) in the shower, (2) before a mirror, and (3) lying down. In all positions use the palmar surface of the examining fingers to inch along the breast tissue. Examine each breast using a circular movement until you are confident that the tail of the breast and all four quadrants have been evaluated. Gently express each nipple. Observe for discharge and bleeding. During inspection and palpation look for the following: swelling or elevated area **(B),** redness or inflammation **(C),** puckering or dimpling **(D),** nipple pulled inward **(E),** depression or sunken area **(F),** and nipple pulled askew compared with the other nipple **(G).**

A

Step 1

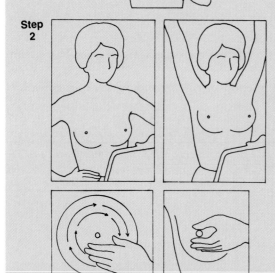

Step 2

Step 3

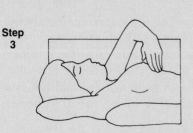

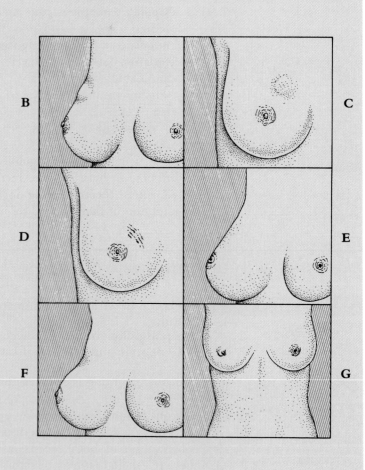

B   C

D   E

F   G

Courtesy American Cancer Society: Teaching breast self-examination, Instructional material no. 77-1R-50M, no. 2015-LE, June 1977.

Inspection

With the patient in a sitting position and arms hanging loosely at the sides, inspect each breast and compare them for size, symmetry, contour, skin color and texture, venous patterns, and lesions. Perform this portion of the examination for both women and men. With female patients lift the breasts with your fingertips, inspecting the lower and lateral aspects to determine if there are any changes in the color or texture of the skin.

Women's breasts are rather convex in shape, frequently with one breast somewhat smaller in size than the other. Men's breasts are generally even with the chest wall, although some men, particularly when overweight, have breasts with a convex shape.

The skin texture should appear smooth and the contour should be uninterrupted. Retractions and dimpling signify the contraction of fibrotic tissue that occurs with carcinoma. Alterations in contour are best seen on bilateral comparison of one breast with another. A peau d'orange appearance of the skin indicates edema of the breast caused by blocked lymph drainage in advanced carcinoma (Fig. 10-4). The skin appears thickened with enlarged pores and accentuated skin markings. Healthy skin may look similar if the pores of the skin are large.

Venous patterns should be bilaterally similar. Venous networks may be visible, although these are usually pronounced only in the breasts of pregnant or obese women. If these are bilateral, there is no cause for concern. However, unilateral venous patterns can be produced by dilated superficial veins from increased blood flow to a malignancy. This finding should alert you to the need for further investigation.

Other markings and nevi that are long standing, unchanging, or nontender are of little concern. Changes or the recent appearance of any lesions always signal the need for closer investigation. A mammogram, xerogram, or biopsy is indicated.

Inspect the areola and nipples in both men and women. The areola should be round or oval and bilaterally equal or nearly equal. The color ranges from pink to brown. In light skinned women the areola usually turns brown with the first pregnancy and remains dark. In women with dark skin the areola is brown before pregnancy. A peppering of nontender, nonsuppurative Montgomery tubercles is considered a normal finding (Fig. 10-5). The surface should be otherwise smooth. The peau d'orange skin associated with carcinoma is often seen first in the areola.

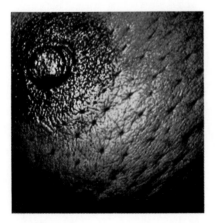

Fig. 10-4
Peau d'orange appearance from edema.
From Gallager, 1978.

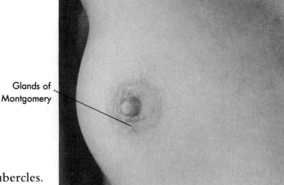

Glands of Montgomery

Fig. 10-5
Montgomery tubercles.
From Gallager, 1978.

The nipples should be bilaterally equal or nearly equal in size. Most nipples are everted, but one or both nipples may be inverted (Fig. 10-6). In these instances ask if there is a lifetime history of inversion. Recent unilateral inversion or retraction of a previously everted nipple suggests malignancy.

Simultaneous bilateral inspection is necessary to detect nipple retraction or deviation. Retraction is seen as a flattening, withdrawal, or inversion of the nipple and indicates inward pulling by inflammatory or malignant tissue (Fig. 10-7). The fibrotic tissue of carcinoma can also change the axis of the nipple, causing it to point in a direction different from that of the other nipple.

The nipples should be a homogenous color and match that of the areolae. Their surface may be either smooth or wrinkled, but should be free of crusting, cracking, or discharge.

Fig. 10-6
Simple nipple inversion.

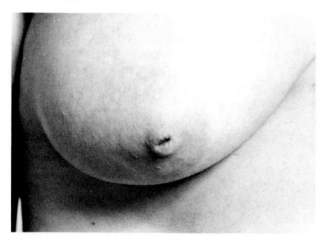

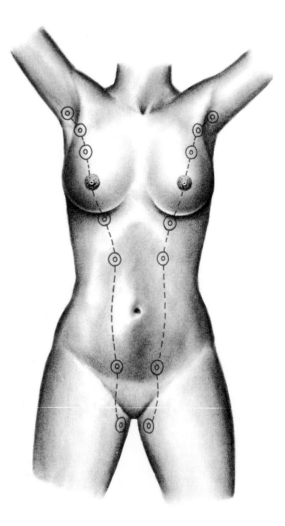

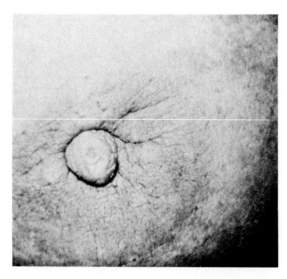

Fig. 10-7
Nipple retraction.
From Gallager, 1978.

Fig. 10-8
Supernumerary nipples and tissue may arise along the "milk line," an embryonic ridge.
From Thompson et al., 1986.

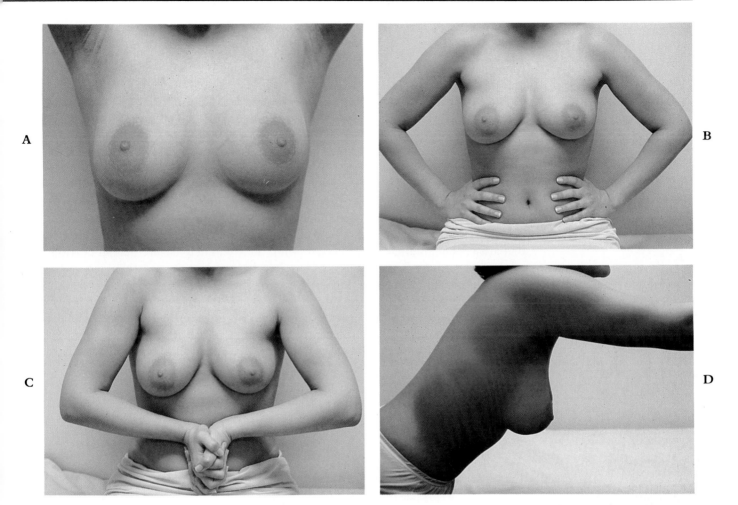

Fig. 10-9
Inspect the breasts in the following positions. **A,** Arms extended overhead. **B,** Hands pressed against hips. **C,** Pressing hands together (an alternate way to flex the pectoral muscles). **D,** Leaning forward from the waist.

Supernumerary nipples, which are sometimes present, appear as one or more extra nipples located along the embryonic mammary ridge (the "milk line") (Fig. 10-8). These nipples and areolae may be pink or brown, are usually small, and are commonly mistaken for moles. Infrequently, some glandular tissue may accompany these nipples.

Reinspect the woman's breasts with the patient in the following positions:

- Seated with arms over the head: This adds tension to the suspensory ligaments, accentuates dimpling, and may reveal variations in contour and symmetry (Fig. 10-9, *A*).
- Seated with hands pressed against hips (or alternatively have the patient push her palms together): This contracts the pectoral muscles, which can reveal deviations in contour and symmetry (Figs. 10-9, *B* and *C*).
- Seated and leaning forward from the waist: This also causes tension in the suspensory ligaments. The breasts should hang equally. This maneuver can be particularly helpful in assessing the contour and symmetry of large breasts, since the breasts fall away from the chest wall and hang freely. As the patient leans forward, support her by the hands (Fig. 10-9, *D*).

For all patient positions, the breasts should appear bilaterally equal, with an even contour and absence of dimpling, retraction, or deviation.

Palpation

Breast

After a thorough inspection, systematically palpate the breasts, axillae, and supraclavicular regions. Palpation of male breasts can be brief but should not be omitted.

Have the patient sit with arms hanging freely at the sides. Palpate all four quandrants of the breast, feeling for lumps or nodules. Use your finger pads because they are more sensitive than your finger tips.

Palpate systematically, pushing gently but firmly toward the chest with your fingers rotating in a clockwise or counterclockwise pattern. Fig. 10-10 illustrates two methods that are commonly used for palpation. Either method is acceptable, as long as every part of the breast is palpated. Early lesions can be very tiny and may be detected only through meticulous technique. The exact sequence you select for palpation is not critical, but it is essential for you to develop a systematic approach that always begins and ends at a fixed point. This will help ensure that all portions of the breast are examined. Do a complete light palpation and then repeat the examination with deeper, heavier palpation.

Press firmly enough to get a good sense of the underlying tissue, but not so firmly that the tissue is compressed against the rib cage, since this can give a false impression of a mass. In women a firm transverse ridge of compressed tissue (the inframammary ridge) may be felt along the lower edge of the breast. It is easy to mistake this for a breast mass.

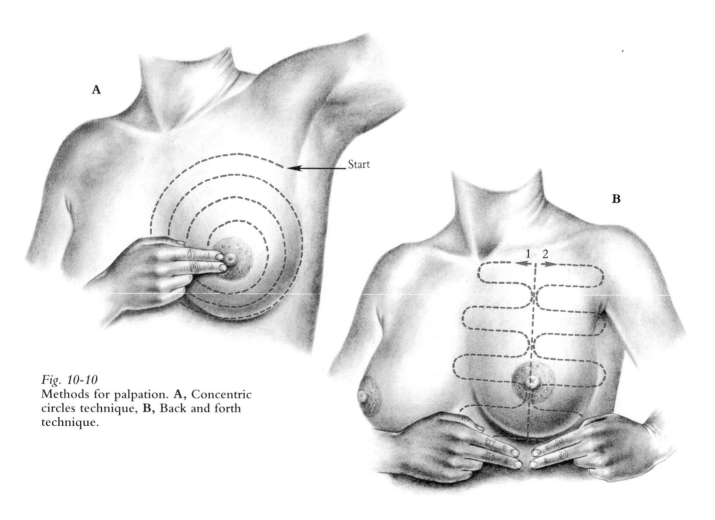

Fig. 10-10
Methods for palpation. **A,** Concentric circles technique, **B,** Back and forth technique.

Fig. 10-11
Palpating large breasts.

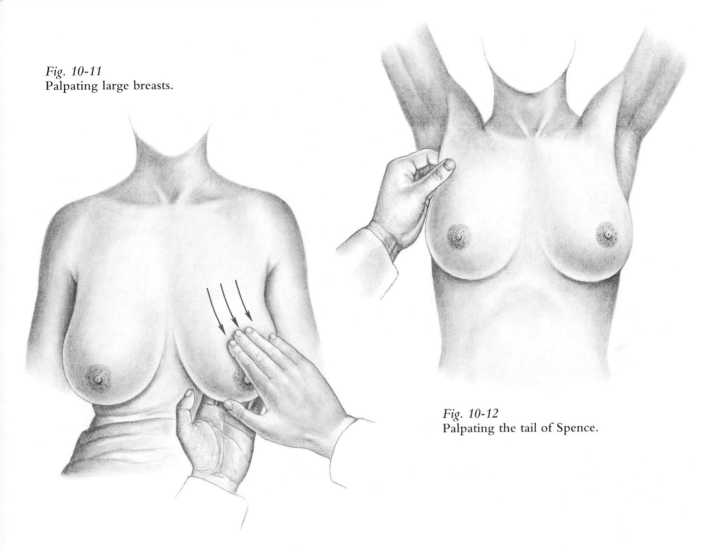

Fig. 10-12
Palpating the tail of Spence.

Try not to lift your fingers off the breast as you move from one point to another. For large breasts it may be helpful to immobilize the inferior surface of the breast with one hand while examining the superior surface with the other hand, (Fig. 10-11).

In most men expect to feel a thin layer of fatty tissue overlying muscle. Obese men may have a somewhat thicker fatty layer, giving the appearance of breast enlargement. A firm disk of glandular tissue can be felt in some men.

The breast tissue of adult women will feel dense, firm, and elastic. Expected variations include the lobular feel of glandular tissue (this feels like tiny granular bumps widely dispersed throughout the breast tissue) and the fine, granular feel of breast tissue in older women. A cyclical pattern of breast enlargement, increased nodularity, and tenderness is a common response to hormonal changes during the menstrual cycle. Be aware of where the woman is in her cycle, because these changes are most likely to occur premenstrually and during menses. They are least noticeable during the week following menstrual flow.

Palpate the tail of Spence in each breast (Fig. 10-12). With the patient still in a seated position, have her raise her arms over head and palpate the tail as it enters the axilla, gently compressing the tissue between your thumb and fingers.

Fig. 10-13
Supine position for palpation.

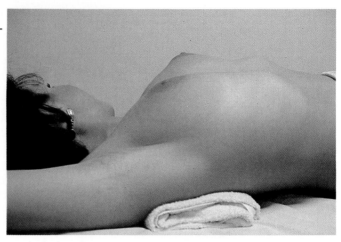

Fig. 10-14
A, Palpating for consistency of a breast lesion.
B, Palpating for delineation of borders of breast mass.
C, Palpating for mobility of breast mass.

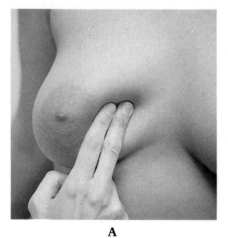

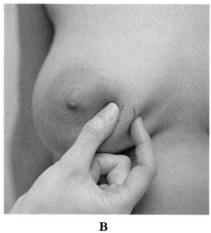

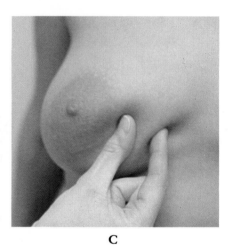

A

B

C

Fig. 10-15
Clinical signs of cancer: nipple retraction and dimpling of skin.

Breast cancer

Skin dimpling

Flattening of nipple

DESCRIPTION OF BREAST MASSES

Location: which quadrant, distance from nipple, show in an illustration
Size in centimeters: length, width, thickness
Shape: round, discoid, lobular, stellate, regular, irregular
Consistency: firmness, softness, hardness
Tenderness: to what degree
Mobility: moveable, in what directions, fixed to overlying skin or subadjacent fascia
Delimitation of borders: discrete, poorly defined
Retraction signs: presence or absence of dimpling, altered contour

Continue palpation with the patient in the supine position. Have her raise one arm behind her head and place a small pillow or folded towel under that shoulder to spread the breast tissue more evenly over the chest wall (Fig. 10-13). Palpate that breast, compressing the breast tissue between your fingers and the chest wall, using a rotary motion with your fingers. Repeat palpation with the woman's arm at her side. Breast tissue shifts with the change in arm position and allows palpation of a different portion of the breast overlying the ribs. Reverse these maneuvers for the other breast.

If a breast mass is felt, characterize it by its location, size, shape, consistency, tenderness, mobility, delimitation of borders, and retraction (Figs. 10-14 and 10-15). Transillumination can be used to confirm the presence of fluid in certain masses. These characteristics are not diagnostic by themselves, but in conjunction with a thorough history they provide a great deal of information for determining what course of action will be taken.

Nipple

The nipple should be palpated on both male and female patients. Compress the nipple between your thumb and index finger and inspect for discharge (Fig. 10-16, A). Do this gently because pinching can cause tissue trauma. Palpation may cause erection of the nipple and puckering of the areola. If discharge appears, note its color and try to determine the origin by massaging radially around the areola while watching for the discharge through the ductal opening on the nipple surface (Fig. 10-16, B). Prepare a smear of the discharge for cytologic examination. Spread a small amount on the glass slide and spray it with the cytologic fixative (Fig. 10-17).

Lymph Nodes

Palpate for lymph nodes in both male and female patients. To palpate the axillae, have the patient seated with arms flexed at the elbow. If you begin on the right, support the right lower arm with your right hand while examining the left axilla with your left hand, as shown in Fig. 10-18. With the palmar surface of your fingers, reach deeply into the axillary hollow, pushing firmly but not too aggressively upward. Then bring your fingers downward so that you gently roll the soft tissues against the chest wall and muscles of the axilla. Be sure to explore all sections of the axilla—the apex, the central or medial aspect along the ribcage, the lateral

Fig. 10-16
Palpation of the nipple (**A**)
and areolar area (**B**).

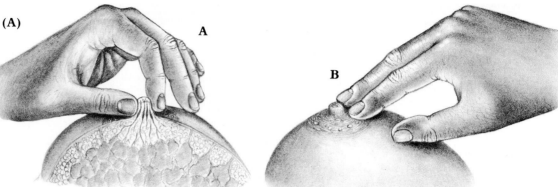

Fig. 10-17
Types of nipple discharge.
A, Milky discharge. **B,** Multi-
colored sticky discharge.
C, Purulent discharge.
D, Watery discharge.
E, Serous discharge.
F, Serosanguineous discharge.
From Gallager, 1978.

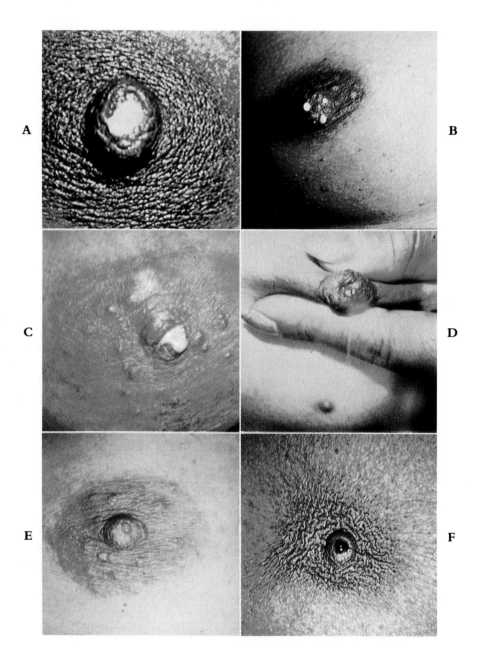

Fig. 10-18
Palpation of the axilla for lymph nodes. Note the technique for supporting the patient's arm.

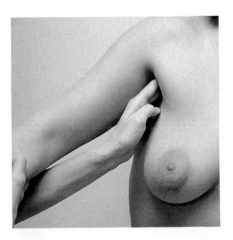

aspect along the upper surface of the arm, the anterior wall along the pectoral muscles, and the posterior wall along the border of the scapula. Then do a mirror image of this maneuver for the left axilla.

Nodes are not usually palpable in the adult. Palpable nodes may be the result of an inflammatory or malignant process. Nodes that are detected should be described according to location, size, shape, consistency, tenderness, fixation, and delimitation of borders. (See Chapter 15, Lymphatic System.)

The supraclavicular area should also be palpated for the presence of enlarged nodes. Hook your fingers over the clavicle and rotate them over the entire supraclavicular area. Have the patient turn his or her head toward the side being palpated and raise the same shoulder, allowing your fingers to reach more deeply into the fossa. You can also have the patient bend the head forward to relax the sternocleidomastoid muscle. These nodes are considered to be sentinal nodes (Virchow's nodes), so any enlargement is highly significant. Virchow's nodes are the first sign of invasion of the lymphatics by abdominal or thoracic carcinoma.

INFANTS

The breasts of many well infants, male and female, are enlarged for a relatively brief time during the newborn period. The enlargement may be noted at birth and is the result of passively transferred maternal estrogen. If you squeeze the breast bud gently, a small amount of clear or milky white fluid, commonly called "witch's milk," is sometimes expressed. The enlargement is rarely more than 1 to 1.5 cm in diameter and can be easily palpated behind the nipple. Usually disappearing within 2 weeks, it rarely lasts beyond 3 months of age.

ADOLESCENTS

The right and left breasts of the adolescent female may not develop at the same rate. Reassure the girl that this asymmetry is common and that her breasts are developing normally. Chapter 3, Growth and Measurement, describes the stages of breast development. Breast tissue of the adolescent female feels homogenous, dense, firm, and elastic.

Many males at puberty have transient unilateral or bilateral subareolar masses. These are firm, sometimes tender, and are often a source of great concern to the patient and his parents. Reassure them that these breast buds will most likely disappear, usually within a year. They seldom enlarge to a point of cosmetic difficulty.

Occasionally, however, pubescent males experience gynecomastia, an unusual and unexpected enlargement that is readily noticeable. Fortunately, it is usually

Fig. 10-19
Breast changes in pregnancy. Montgomery glands are prominent, and nipples and areolae are deeply pigmented. Accessory nipple beneath left breast is also pigmented.
From Willson et al., 1983.

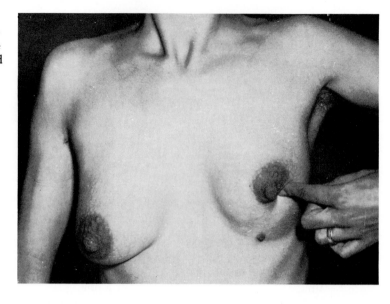

temporary, benign, and resolves spontaneously. If the enlargement is extreme it can be corrected surgically for psychologic or cosmetic reasons. Rarely, biopsy is required to rule out the presence of cancer.

PREGNANT WOMEN

Many changes in the breasts occur during pregnancy. Most become obvious during the first trimester. The woman may experience a sensation of fullness with tingling, tenderness, and a bilateral increase in size. It is important to ascertain that the woman is providing adequate support for her breasts with a properly fitting brassiere. As her breasts continue to enlarge, she may need to alter the size and style of the brassiere.

Generally, the nipples enlarge and are more erectile. As the pregnancy progresses the nipples sometimes become flattened or inverted, and instruction on nipple care is necessary if she plans to breast-feed. A crust caused by dried colostrum is often evident on the nipple. The colostrum, a clear viscous discharge that begins as early as the sixth week of gestation, becomes yellow and more viscous in later pregnancy. The areola begins to broaden and darken, and Montgomery tubercles may appear (Fig. 10-19).

Palpation reveals a generalized coarse nodularity, and the breasts feel lobular because of hypertrophy of the mammary alveoli. Dilated subcutaneous veins may create a network of blue tracing across the breasts.

During the second trimester vascular spiders may develop on the upper chest, arms, neck, and face as a result of elevated levels of circulating estrogen. The spiders are bluish in color and do not blanch with pressure. Striae may be evident on the breasts as a result of stretching as they increase in size.

LACTATING WOMEN

During the period of lactation it is important to assess adequate support of the breasts with a properly fitting brassiere. Palpate the breasts to determine their degree of softness. Full breasts, which are firm, dense, and slightly enlarged, may become engorged. Engorged breasts feel hard and warm and are enlarged, reddened, shiny, and painful.

If the woman is breast-feeding, examine the nipples for signs of irritation (redness and tenderness) and for blisters or petechiae, which are precursors of overt cracking. These are best seen with a magnifying glass. If the nipples are already cracked, they will be sore and may be bleeding.

After pregnancy and lactation, there is regression of most of these changes. The areolae and nipples tend to retain their darker color, and the breasts become less firm than their prepregnant state.

OLDER ADULTS

The breasts in postmenopausal women may appear flattened, elongated, and suspended more loosely from the chest wall as the result of glandular tissue atrophy and relaxation of the suspensory ligaments. The lobular feel of glandular tissue is replaced by a finer, granular feel upon palpation. The inframammary ridge thickens and can be felt more easily. The nipples become smaller and flatter.

Postmenopausal women should be encouraged to continue monthly breast self-examination. Since the breasts are no longer subject to hormonal changes of menstruation, these women should choose a convenient date and regularly examine their breasts on this date.

Common Abnormalities

Fibrocystic Disease

Benign cyst formation caused by ductal enlargement is associated with a long follicular or luteal phase of the menstrual cycle. The lesions are filled with fluid and are usually bilateral and multiple. Characteristically the cysts are tender and painful with an increase in these symptoms premenstrually. Fibrocystic disease occurs most commonly in women between the ages of 30 and 55. Table 10-2 details the differences between fibrocystic disease, fibroadenoma, and breast cancer.

Table 10-2
Differentiating Signs and Symptoms of Breast Masses

	Fibrocystic Disease	Fibroadenoma	Cancer
Age	20-49	15-55	30-80
Occurrence	Usually bilateral	Usually bilateral	Usually unilateral
Number	Multiple or single	Single; may be multiple	Single
Shape	Round	Round or discoid	Irregular or stellate
Consistency	Soft to firm; tense	Firm, rubbery	Hard, stone-like
Mobility	Mobile	Mobile	Fixed
Retraction Signs	Absent	Absent	Often present
Tenderness	Usually tender	Usually nontender	Usually nontender
Delimitation	Well delineated	Well delineated	Poorly delineated; irregular
Variation with Menses	Yes	Yes	No

Fibroadenoma

This benign neoplasm accounts for the majority of breast tumors in young women. Fibroadenomas are generally asymptomatic and do not change premenstrually. A sudden change in the size of an existing fibroadenoma may signal a malignant change. Biopsy is often performed to rule out carcinoma (see Table 10-3).

Malignant Breast Tumors

Peak incidence of malignancy is between ages 40 and 60, with two thirds of malignant breast tumors occuring in women under age 65. About 80% of patients with breast cancer have a painless lump in the breast as the initial symptom. Metastases occur through the lymph and vascular systems (see Table 10-3 and Fig. 10-20).

A 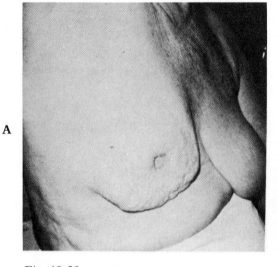 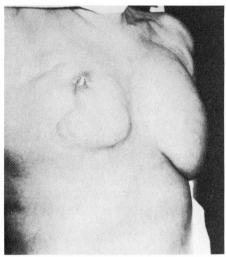 B

Fig. 10-20
A, Locally advanced carcinoma. Note nipple retraction, skin edema, and dimpling.
B, Locally advanced cancer. Note fixation and deformity of contour.
From Gallager, 1978.

Fat Necrosis

Fat necrosis is a response to local injury. It is felt as a firm irregular mass, often appearing as an area of discoloration.

Mastitis

Mastitis is inflammation and infection of the breast tissue characterized by sudden onset of swelling, tenderness, erythema, and heat. Most infections are staphylococcal. This is most common in lactating women, although it may occur at any age. Abscess formation can result and is probably related to duct obstruction. Trauma may cause noninfectious inflammatory masses. The usual symptoms are fever, chills, and malaise.

Intraductal Papillomas and Papillomatosis

These 2- to 3-cm tumors of the subareolar ducts may occur singly or in multiples. Papillomas are a common cause of serous or bloody nipple discharge. They need to be excised and examined to rule out malignancy.

Paget's Disease

Paget's disease of the breast is a surface manifestation of underlying ductal carcinoma. A red, scaling, crusty patch forms on the nipple, areola, and surrounding skin. The lesion appears eczematous but, unlike eczema, occurs unilaterally (Fig. 10-21).

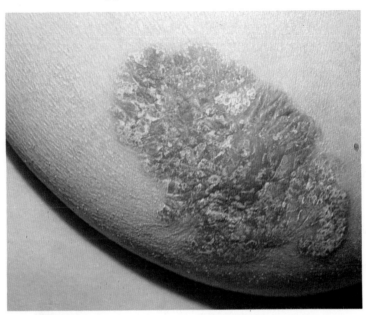

Fig. 10-21
Paget's disease.
From Habif, 1985.

Adult Gynecomastia

Gynecomastia is a smooth, firm, mobile, tender disk of breast tissue located behind the areola in males. It may be unilateral or bilateral. In adult men it can be caused by hormone imbalance, testicular or pituitary tumors, hormone-secreting tumors, liver failure, and antihypertensive medications, or those containing estrogens or steroids (Fig. 10-22).

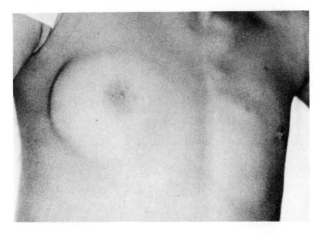

Fig. 10-22
Diffuse gynecomastia in adult male.
From Gallager, 1978.

Retention Cysts	Inflammation of the sebaceous glands in the areola result in retention cysts. They may become tender and suppurative.

Galactorrhea Lactation not associated with childbearing is most commonly caused by drugs, especially phenothiazines, tricyclic antidepressants, some antihypertensive agents, and estrogens. Intrinsic causes of galactorrhea include prolactin-secreting tumors, pituitary tumors, hypothyroidism, Cushing's syndrome, and hypoglycemia.

CHILDREN

Gynecomastia Enlargement of breast tissue in boys caused by normal puberty, hormonal imbalance, testicular or pituitary tumors, and medications containing estrogens or steroids (Fig. 10-23).

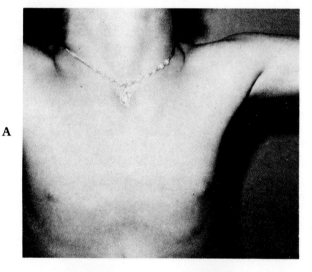

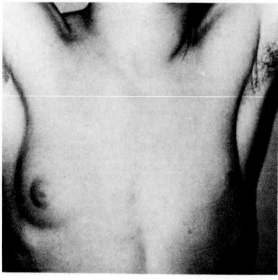

Fig. 10-23
A, Prepubertal gynecomastia, small and subareolar.
B, Adolescent gynecomastia (diffuse type).
From Gallager, 1978.

Premature Thelarche

Prepubertal breast enlargement of unknown etiology in girls can occur in the absence of other signs of sexual maturation. The degree of enlargement varies from very slight to fully developed breasts. It usually occurs bilaterally, with the breasts continuing to enlarge slowly throughout childhood until full development is reached during adolescence (Fig. 10-24).

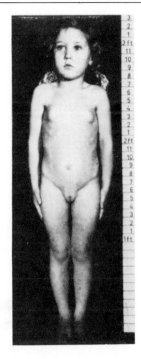

Fig. 10-24
Premature thelarche.
From Jolly, 1981.

OLDER ADULTS

Mammary Duct Ectasia

The subareolar ducts become blocked with desquamating secretory epithelium, necrotic debris, and chronic inflammatory cells. It occurs most frequently in menopausal women. Symptoms include pain, nipple retraction and discharge. Occasionally enlarged, easily palpable regional lymph nodes are found. There is no known association with malignancy.

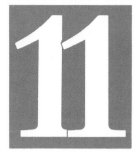

Abdomen

Anatomy and Physiology

The abdominal cavity contains several of the body's vital organs (Fig. 11-1). The peritoneum, a serous membrane, lines the cavity and forms a protective cover for many of the abdominal structures. Double folds of the peritoneum around the stomach comprise the greater and lesser omentum. The mesentery, a fan-shaped fold of the peritoneum, covers most of the small intestine and anchors it to the posterior abdominal wall.

Alimentary Tract

The alimentary tract is a tube approximately 27 ft long that runs from the mouth to the anus and includes the esophagus, stomach, small intestine, and large intestine. It functions to ingest and digest food; absorb nutrients, electrolytes, and water; and excrete waste products. Food and the products of digestion are moved along the length of the digestive tract by peristalsis, which is under autonomic nervous system control.

The esophagus is a collapsible tube about 10 in long, connecting the pharynx to the stomach. Passing just posterior to the trachea, the esophagus descends through the mediastinal cavity, travels through the diaphragm, and enters the stomach at the cardiac orifice.

The flask-shaped stomach lies transversely in the upper abdominal cavity, just below the diaphragm. It consists of three sections: the fundus, which lies above and to the left of the cardiac orifice; the middle two thirds, or body; and the pylorus, the most distal portion that narrows and terminates in the pyloric orifice. The stomach secretes hydrochloric acid and digestive enzymes that break down fats and proteins. Pepsin acts to digest proteins, while gastric lipase acts on emulsified fats. Very little absorption takes place in the stomach.

The small intestine, about 21 ft long, begins at the pyloric orifice. Coiled in the abdominal cavity, it joins the large intestine at the ileocecal valve. The first 12 in of the small intestine, the duodenum, forms a C-shaped curve around the head of the pancreas. The common bile duct and pancreatic duct open into the duodenum at the duodenal papilla, about 3 in below the pylorus of the stomach. The next 8 ft of intestine is the jejunum, which gradually becomes larger and thicker. The ileum makes up the remaining 12 ft of the small intestine. The ileocecal valve between the ileum and large intestine prevents backward flow of fecal material.

Digestion is completed in the small intestine through the action of pancreatic enzymes, bile, and several small intestine enzymes. Nutrients are absorbed through

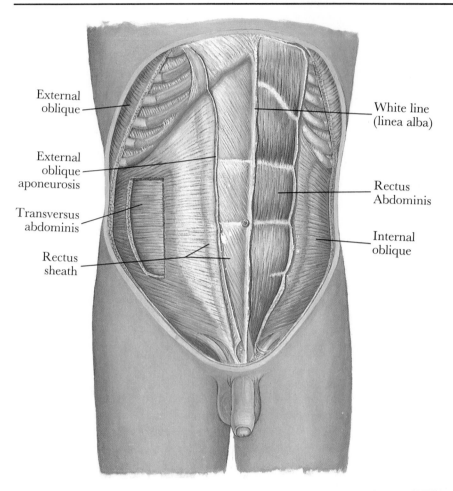

External
oblique

External
oblique
aponeurosis

Transversus
abdominis

Rectus
sheath

White line
(linea alba)

Rectus
Abdominis

Internal
oblique

Fig. 11-1
**Anatomic structures of the
abdominal cavity.**

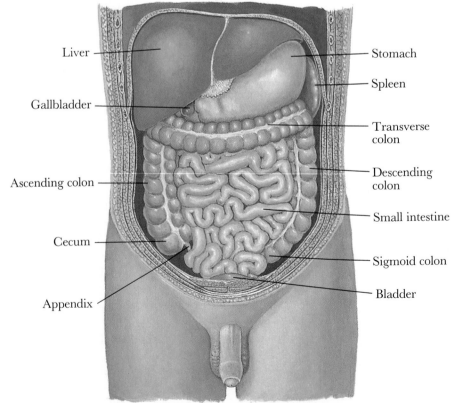

Liver

Gallbladder

Ascending colon

Cecum

Appendix

Stomach

Spleen

Transverse
colon

Descending
colon

Small intestine

Sigmoid colon

Bladder

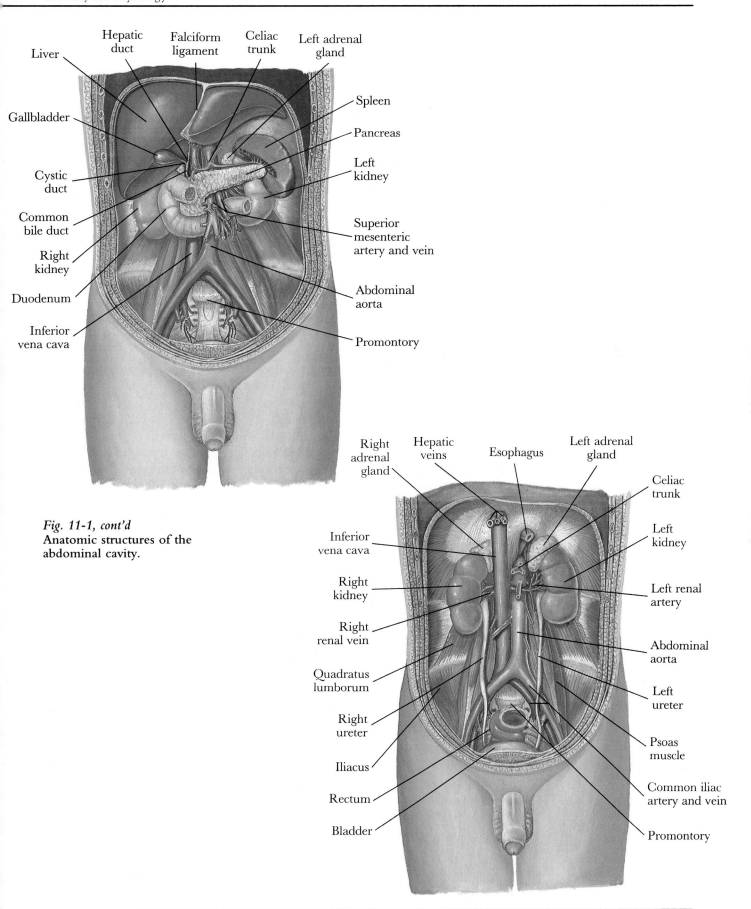

Fig. 11-1, cont'd
Anatomic structures of the abdominal cavity.

the walls of the small intestine, whose functional surface area is enormously increased by its circular folds and villi.

The large intestine begins at the cecum, a blind pouch about 2 to 3 in long. The ileal contents empty into the cecum through the ileocecal valve, and the veriform appendix extends from the base of the cecum. The ascending colon rises from the cecum along the right posterior abdominal wall to the undersurface of the liver where it turns toward the midline (the hepatic flexure), becoming the transverse colon. The transverse colon crosses the abdominal cavity toward the spleen, turning downward at the splenic flexure. The descending colon continues along the left abdominal wall to the rim of the pelvis, where it turns medially and inferiorly to form the S-shaped sigmoid colon. The rectum extends from the sigmoid colon to the muscles of the pelvic floor where it continues as the anal canal and terminates at the anus.

The large intestine is about 4½ to 5 ft long with a diameter of 2½ in. Water absorption takes place here. Mucous glands secrete large quantities of alkaline mucus that lubricate the intestinal contents and neutralize acids formed by intestinal bacteria. Live bacteria decompose undigested food residue, unabsorbed amino acids, cell debris, and dead bacteria through a process of putrefaction.

Liver

The liver lies in the right upper quadrant of the abdomen, just below the diaphragm. Its inferior surface almost embraces the gallbladder, stomach, duodenum, and heptic flexure of the colon. The heaviest organ in the body, the liver weighs about 3 lb in the adult. It is composed of 4 lobes containing lobules, the functional units. Each lobule is made up of liver cells radiating around a central vein. Branches of the portal vein, hepatic artery, and bile duct invest the periphery of the lobules. Bile secreted by the liver cells drains from the bile ducts into the hepatic duct, which joins the cystic duct from the gallbladder to form the common bile duct.

The hepatic artery transports blood to the liver directly from the aorta, and the portal vein carries blood from the digestive tract and spleen to the liver. Repeated branching of both vessels make the liver a highly vascularized organ. Three hepatic veins carry blood from the liver and empty into the inferior vena cava.

The liver plays an important role in the metabolism of carbohydrates, fats, and proteins. Glucose is converted and stored as glycogen until, in response to varying levels of insulin and regulator hormones, it is reconverted and released again as glucose. The liver also has the capacity to convert amino acids to glucose (gluconeogenesis). Fats, arriving at the liver in the form of fatty acids, are oxidized to two carbon components in preparation for entry into the tricarboxylic acid cycle. Cholesterol is used by the liver to form bile salts. Synthesis of fats from carbohydrates and proteins also occurs in the liver. Proteins are broken down to amino acids through hydrolysis, and their waste products are converted to urea for excretion.

Other functions of the liver include storage of several vitamins and iron, detoxification of potentially harmful substances, production of antibodies, conjugation and excretion of steroid hormones, and the production of prothrombin, fibrinogen, and other substances for blood coagulation. The liver is responsible for the production of the majority of proteins circulating in the plasma. It serves a vital role as an excretory organ through the synthesis of bile, the secretion of organic wastes into bile, and the conversion of fat-soluble wastes to water-soluble material for renal excretion.

Gallbladder

The gallbladder is a sac-like, pear-shaped organ about 4 in long lying recessed in the inferior surface of the liver. Its function is to concentrate and store bile from the liver. In response to cholecystokinin, a hormone produced in the duodenum, the gallbladder releases bile into the cystic duct, which, with the hepatic duct, forms the common bile duct. Contraction of the gallbladder propels bile along the common duct and into the duodenum at the duodenal papilla. Composed of cholesterol, bile salts, and pigments, bile serves to maintain the alkaline pH of the small intestine to permit emulsification of fats so that absorption can be accomplished.

Pancreas

The pancreas lies behind and beneath the stomach, with its head resting in the curve of the duodenum and its tip extending across the abdominal cavity to almost touch the spleen. In its function as an exocrine gland, the acinar cells of the pancreas produce digestive juices containing inactive enzymes for the breakdown of proteins, fats, and carbohydrates. Collecting ducts empty the juice into the pancreatic duct (duct of Wirsung), which runs the length of the organ. The pancreatic duct empties into the duodenum at the duodenal papilla, alongside the common bile duct. Once introduced into the duodenum, the digestive enzymes are activated. As an endocrine gland, islet cells scattered throughout the pancreas produce the hormones insulin and glucagon. These are secreted directly into the blood, to regulate the body's level of glucose. Insulin, the major anabolic hormone of the body, also serves several other vital functions.

Spleen

The spleen is in the left upper quadrant, lying above the left kidney and just below the diaphragm. White pulp (lymphoid tissue) comprises most of the organ and functions as part of the reticuloendothelial system to filter blood and to manufacture lymphocytes and monocytes. The red pulp of the spleen contains a capillary network and venous sinus system that allows for the storage and release of blood, permitting the spleen to accommodate up to several hundred milliliters at once.

Kidneys, Ureters, and Bladder

The two kidneys, the excretory organs responsible for the removal of water-soluble waste, are located in the retroperitoneal space of the upper abdomen. Each extends from about the vertebral level of T12 to L3. The right kidney is usually slightly lower than the left, presumably because of the large heavy liver just above it. Both kidneys are imbedded in fat and fascia, which anchor and protect these organs. Each contains more than one million nephrons, the structural and functional units of the kidneys. The nephrons are composed of a tuft of capillaries, the glomerulus, a proximal convoluted tubule, the loop of Henle, and a distal convoluted tubule. The distal tube empties into a collecting tubule.

Each kidney receives about one eighth of the cardiac output through its renal artery. The glomeruli filter blood at a rate of about 125 ml per minute in the adult male and about 110 ml per minute in the adult female. Most of the filtered material, including electrolytes, glucose, water, and small proteins, is actively resorbed in the proximal tubule. Some organic acids are also actively secreted in the distal tubule. Urinary volume is carefully controlled by antidiuretic hormone (ADH) to maintain a constant total body fluid volume. Urine passes into the renal pelvis via the collecting tubules and then into the ureter. Peristaltic waves move it on to a reservoir, the urinary bladder, which has a capacity of about 400 to 500 ml in the adult.

The kidney also serves as an endocrine gland responsible for the production of renin, which is important for the ultimate control of aldosterone secretion. It is the primary source of erythropoietin production in adults, thus influencing the body's red cell mass. In addition to synthesizing several prostaglandins, the kidney produces the biologically active form of vitamin D.

Musculature and Connective Tissues

The muscles that form and protect the abdominal cavity are composed of the recti abdomini muscles anteriorly and the internal and external oblique muscles laterally. The linea alba, a tendinous band, is located in the midline of the abdomen between the recti abdomini. It extends from the xiphoid process to the symphysis pubis and contains the umbilicus. The inguinal ligament (Poupart's ligament) extends from the anterior superior spine of the ilium to the pubis on each side.

Vasculature

The abdominal portion of the descending aorta travels from the diaphragm through the abdominal cavity, just to the left of midline. At about the level of the umbilicus the aorta branches into the two common iliac arteries. The splenic and renal arteries, which supply their respective organs, also branch off within the abdomen.

INFANTS

The pancreatic buds, liver, and gallbladder all begin to form during week 4 of gestation, by which time the intestine already exists as a single tube. The motility of the gastrointestinal tract develops in a cephalocaudal direction, permitting amniotic fluid to be swallowed by 16 weeks of gestation. Production of meconium, the end product of fetal metabolism, begins shortly thereafter. By 36 to 38 weeks of gestation the gastrointestinal tract is capable of adapting to extrauterine life. However, its elasticity, musculature, and control mechanisms continue to develop, reaching adult levels of function at 2 to 3 years of age.

During gestation the liver begins to form blood cells at about week 6, synthesize glycogen by week 9, and produce bile by week 12. The liver's role as a metabolic and glucogen storage organ accounts for its large size at birth. Its growth during infancy is not as rapid as skeletal growth, but it remains the heaviest organ in the body.

Pancreatic islet cells are developed by 12 weeks of gestation and begin producing insulin. The spleen is active in blood formation during fetal development and the first year of life. After that time, the spleen aids in the destruction of blood cells and the formation of hemoglobin.

Nephrogenesis begins during the second embryologic month. By 12 weeks the kidney is able to produce urine, and the bladder expands as a sac. Development of new nephrons ceases by 36 weeks of gestation. After birth the kidney increases in size incrementally because of the enlargement of the existing one million nephrons and adjoining tubules—a process that parallels body growth. The glomerular filtration rate is approximately 0.5 ml/min before 34 weeks of gestation and gradually increases in a linear fashion to 125 ml/min.

PREGNANT WOMEN

As the uterus enlarges, the muscles of the abdominal wall stretch and ultimately lose some tone. During the third trimester the rectus abdominis muscles may separate, allowing abdominal contents to protrude at the midline. The umbilicus flattens or protrudes. Striae may form as the skin is stretched. A line of pigmentation at the midline (linea nigra) often develops.

The colon is displaced laterally upward and posteriorly, and peristaltic activity decreases. As a result bowel sounds are diminished, and constipation, nausea, and vomiting are common. Blood flow to the pelvis increases as does venous pressure, contributing to hemorrhoid formation.

Following pregnancy, the muscles gradually regain tone, although separation of the rectus abdominis muscles may persist.

OLDER ADULTS

The process of aging brings about changes in the functional abilities of the gastro-intestinal tract. Motility of the intestine is the most severely affected; secretion and absorption are affected to a lesser degree. Altered motility may be caused in part by age-related changes in neurons of the central nervous system and by changes in collagen properties that increase the resistance of the intestinal wall to stretching. Reduced circulation to the intestine often follows other system changes associated with hypoxia and hypovolemia. Thus functional abilities of the intestine can decrease secondary to adverse changes occurring elsewhere in the older adult.

As a result of epithelial atrophy, the secretion of both digestive enzymes and protective mucus in the intestinal tract is decreased. Particular elements of the mucosal cells show a lesser degree of differentiation and are associated with reduction in secretory ability. These cells are also more susceptible to both physical and chemical agents, including ingested carcinogens. Bacterial flora of the intestine can undergo both qualitative and quantitative changes and become less biologically active. These changes may impair digestive ability and manifest food intolerances in the older adult.

Liver size decreases after age 50, which parallels the decrease in body weight. Hepatic blood flow decreases as a result of the decline in cardiac output associated with aging. The liver loses some ability to metabolize certain drugs.

The size of the pancreas is unaffected by aging, although the main pancreatic duct and its branches widen. The functional reserve of the pancreas may be reduced, although this can occur as a result of delayed gastric emptying rather than pancreatic changes.

Review of Related History

General Considerations

1. Nutrition: 24-hour recall intake, food preferences and dislikes, ethnic foods frequently eaten, religious food restrictions, food intolerances, lifestyle effects on food intake, weight gain or loss
2. Medications: laxatives, stool softeners, antiemetics, antidiarrheal agents, antacids, high doses of aspirin or acetaminophen, corticosteroids, antihypertensives, diuretics
3. Alcohol intake: frequency and usual amounts
4. Pregnancy: expected date of delivery, gestational weeks, or first day of last menstrual period
5. Recent stool characteristics: color, consistency, odor, frequency
6. Urinary characteristics: frequency, color, volume congruent with fluid intake, force of stream, ease of starting stream, ability to empty bladder
7. Recent stressful life events: physical and psychologic changes
8. Exposure to infectious diseases: hepatitis, flu; travel history
9. Trauma: through type of work, physical activity, accident

Present Problem

1. Abdominal pain
   a. Onset and duration: when it began; sudden or gradual; persistant, recurrent, intermittent
   b. Character: dull, sharp, burning, gnawing, stabbing, cramping, aching, colicky
   c. Location: of onset, change in location over time, radiating to another area, superficial or deep
   d. Associated symptoms: vomiting, diarrhea, constipation, passage of flatus, belching, jaundice, collapse, change in abdominal girth
   e. Relationship to: menstrual cycle, abnormal menses, urination, defecation, inspiration, change in body position, food or alcohol intake, aspirin or other drugs, stress, time of day
2. Indigestion
   a. Character: feeling of fullness, heartburn, discomfort, excessive belching, flatulence, loss of appetite, severe pain
   b. Location: localized or general, radiates to arms or shoulders
   c. Association with food intake: timing of food intake, amount, type
   d. Onset of symptoms: time of day or night, sudden or gradual
   e. Symptom relieved by antacids, rest, activity
3. Nausea: associated with vomiting; particular stimuli (odors, activities, time of day, food intake); date of last menstrual period
4. Vomiting
   a. Character: nature (color, fresh blood or coffee grounds, undigested food particles), quantity, duration, frequency, ability to keep any liquids or food in stomach
   b. Relationship to: previous meal, change in appetite, diarrhea or constipation, fever, weight loss, abdominal pain, medications, headache, nausea
5. Diarrhea
   a. Character: watery, copius, explosive; color; presence of blood, mucus, undigested food, oil or fat; odor; number per day, duration; change in pattern
   b. Associated symptoms: chills, fever, thirst, weight loss, abdominal pain or cramping
   c. Relationship to: timing and nature of food intake, stress
   d. Travel history
6. Constipation
   a. Character: presence of bright blood, black or tarry appearance of stool; diarrhea alternating with constipation; accompanied by abdominal pain or discomfort
   b. Pattern: last bowel movement, pain with passage of stool, change in pattern or size of stool
   c. Diet: recent change in diet, inclusion of high fiber foods
7. Jaundice: duration, abdominal pain, chills, fever, color of stools or urine, exposure to hepatitis, use of intravenous drugs, history of blood tranfusion
8. Dysuria
   a. Character: location (suprapubic, at end of urethra), pain or burning, frequency or volume changes
   b. Exposure to: tuberculosis, fungal or viral infection, parasitic infection, bacterial infection

9. Urinary frequency: change in usual pattern; changes in volume; associated with dysuria, incontinence, urgency; change in urinary stream; dribbling; nocturia
10. Urinary incontinence
    a. Character: amount and frequency, constant or intermittent, dribbling v frank incontinence
    b. Associated with: urgency, previous surgery, coughing, sneezing, walking up stairs, nocturia
11. Hematuria
    a. Character: color (bright red, rusty brown, cola-colored); present at beginning, end, or throughout voiding
    b. Associated symptoms: flank or costovertebral pain, passage of wormlike clots, pain on voiding
    c. Alternate possibilities: ingestion of foods containing red vegetable dyes (may cause red urinary pigment); ingestion of laxatives containing phenolphthalein
12. Chyluria (milky urine): exposure to parasitic infections through travel; exposure to tuberculosis

Past Medical History

1. Gastrointestinal disorder: peptic ulcer, polyps, ulcerative colitis, intestinal obstruction, pancreatitis
2. Hepatitis or cirrhosis of the liver
3. Abdominal or urinary tract surgery or injury
4. Urinary tract infection: number, treatment
5. Major illness: cancer, arthritis (steroids or aspirin use), kidney disease, cardiac disease

Family History

1. Familial Mediterranean fever (periodic peritonitis)
2. Gallbladder disease
3. Kidney disease: renal stone, polycystic disease, renal tubular acidosis, renal or bladder carcinoma
4. Malabsorption syndrome: cystic fibrosis, celiac disease
5. Hirschsprung's disease, aganglionic megacolon
6. Polyposis: Peutz-Jeghers syndrome, familial multiple polyposis
7. Colon cancer

INFANTS

1. Birth weight (less than 1500 gm at higher risk for necrotizing enterocolitis)
2. Passage of first meconium stool within 24 hours
3. Jaundice: in newborn period, exchange transfusions, phototherapy, breastfed infant, appearing later in first month of life
4. Vomiting: increasing in amount or frequency, forceful or projectile, failure to gain weight, insatiable appetite, blood in emesis (pyloric stenosis or gastroesophageal reflux)
5. Diarrhea, colic, failure to gain weight, weight loss, steatorrhea (malabsorption syndrome)
6. Apparent enlargement of abdomen, with or without pain, constipation, or diarrhea

1. Constipation: toilet training methods; diet; soiling; diarrhea; abdominal distention; pica; size, shape, consistency, and time of last stool; rectal bleeding; painful passage of stool
2. Abdominal pain: splinting of abdominal movement, resists movement, keeps knees flexed

1. Urinary symptoms: nocturia, change in stream, dribbling, frank incontinence
2. Change in bowel patterns, constipation, diarrhea
3. Dietary habits: inclusion of fiber in diet, change in ability to tolerate certain foods, change in appetite

Examination and Findings

- **Stethoscope**
- **Ruler or measuring tape**
- **Marking pen**

In order to perform the abdominal examination satisfactorily, you will need a good source of light, full exposure of the abdomen, warm hands with short fingernails, and a comfortable, relaxed patient. Have the patient empty his or her bladder before the examination begins. A full bladder interferes with accurate examination of nearby organs and makes the examination uncomfortable for the patient. Position the patient in a supine position with arms at sides. The patient's abdominal mus-

Fig. 11-2
Four quadrants of the abdomen.

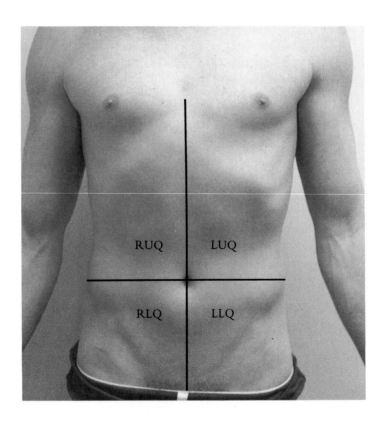

Fig. 11-3
Nine regions of the abdomen. *1*, Epigastric; *2*, umbilical; *3*, hypogastric (pubic); *4* and *5*, right and left hypochondriac; *6* and *7*, right and left lumbar; *8* and *9*, right and left inguinal.

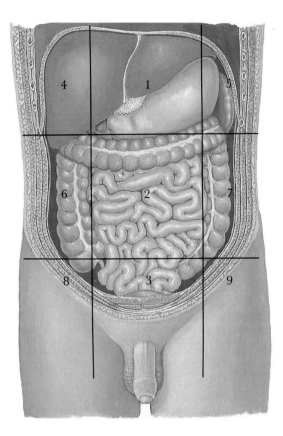

culature should be as relaxed as possible in order to allow access to the underlying structures. It may be helpful to place a small pillow under the patient's head and another small pillow under the slightly flexed knees. Ask the patient to breathe slowly through the mouth. Make your approach slow and gentle, avoiding sudden movements. Ask the patient to point to any tender areas and examine those last.

Landmarks

For the purposes of examination the abdomen can be divided into either four quadrants or nine regions. To divide the abdomen into quadrants, draw an imaginary line from the sternum to the pubis, through the umbilicus. Draw a second imaginary line perpendicular to the first, horizontally across the abdomen through the umbilicus (Fig. 11-2). The nine regions are created by two imaginary horizontal lines, one across the lowest edge of the costal margin and the other across the edge of the iliac crest, and by two vertical lines bilaterally from the midclavicular line to the middle of Poupart's ligament, approximating the lateral borders of the recti abdominis muscles (Fig. 11-3). Choose one of these mapping methods and use it consistently. Quadrants are the more common of the two methods. Table 11-1 lists the contents of the abdomen in each of the quadrants and regions. Become accustomed to mentally visualizing the underlying organs and structures in each of the zones as you proceed with the examination.

Certain other anatomic landmarks are useful in describing the location of pain, tenderness, and other findings. These landmarks are illustrated in Fig. 11-4.

Table 11-1
Landmarks for Abdominal Examination

Anatomical Correlates of the Four Quadrants of the Abdomen

Right upper quadrant	*Left upper quadrant*
Liver and gallbladder	Left lobe of liver
Pylorus	Spleen
Duodenum	Stomach
Head of pancreas	Body of pancreas
Right adrenal gland	Left adrenal gland
Portion of right kidney	Portion of left kidney
Hepatic flexure of colon	Splenic flexure of colon
Portions of ascending and transverse colon	Portions of transverse and descending colon

Right lower quadrant	*Left lower quadrant*
Lower pole of right kidney	Lower pole of left kidney
Cecum and appendix	Sigmoid colon
Portion of ascending colon	Portion of descending colon
Bladder (if distended)	Bladder (if distended)
Ovary and salpinx	Ovary and salpinx
Uterus (if enlarged)	Uterus (if enlarged)
Right spermatic cord	Left spermatic cord
Right ureter	Left ureter

Anatomical Correlates of the Nine Regions of the Abdomen

Right hypochondriac	*Epigastric*	*Left hypochondriac*
Right lobe of liver	Pyloric end of stomach	Stomach
Gallbladder	Duodenum	Spleen
Portion of duodenum	Pancreas	Tail of pancreas
Hepatic flexure of colon	Portion of liver	Splenic flexure of colon
Portion of right kidney		Upper pole of left kidney
Suprarenal gland		Suprarenal gland

Right lumbar	*Umbilical*	*Left lumbar*
Ascending colon	Omentum	Descending colon
Lower half of right kidney	Mesentery	Lower half of left kidney
Portion of duodenum and jejunum	Lower part of duodenum	Portions of jejunum and ileum
	Jejunum and ileum	

Right inguinal	*Hypogastric (pubic)*	*Left inguinal*
Cecum	Ileum	Sigmoid colon
Appendix	Bladder	Left ureter
Lower end of ileum	Uterus (in pregnancy)	Left spermatic cord
Right ureter		Left ovary
Right spermatic cord		
Right ovary		

From Malasanos et al., 1986.

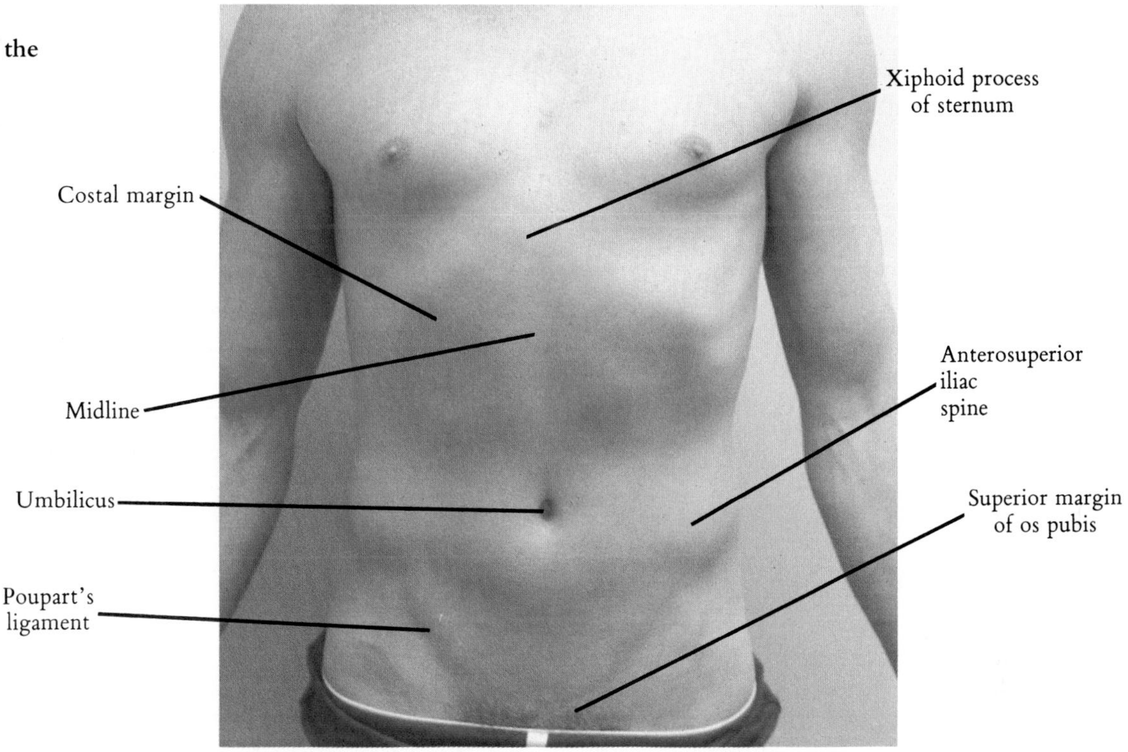

Fig. 11-4
Landmarks of the abdomen.

Costal margin

Xiphoid process
of sternum

Anterosuperior
iliac
spine

Midline

Umbilicus

Superior margin
of os pubis

Poupart's
ligament

Inspection

Begin by inspecting the abdomen from a seated position at the right side of the patient. This position allows a tangential view that enhances shadows and contouring. Observe the skin color and surface characteristics. The skin of the abdomen is subject to the same expected variations in color and surface characteristics as the rest of the body. The skin may be somewhat paler if it has not been exposed to the sun. Tanning lines are often visible on light colored skin. A fine venous network is often visible. Above the umbilicus venous return should be toward the head; below the umbilicus it should be toward the feet (Fig. 11-5, *A*). To determine the direction of venous return use the following procedure. Place the index finger of each hand side by side over a vein. Press laterally, separating the fingers and milking empty a section of vein. Release one finger and time the refill. Release the other finger and time the refill. The flow of venous blood is in the direction of the faster filling. Flow patterns are altered in some disease states (Fig. 11-5, *B* and *C*).

Unexpected findings include generalized color changes such as jaundice or cyanosis. A glistening taut appearance suggests ascites. Inspect for bruises and localized discoloration. Areas of redness may indicate inflammation. A bluish periumbilical discoloration (Cullen's sign) suggests intraabdominal bleeding. Striae often result from pregnancy or weight gain. Striae of recent origin are pink or blue in color but turn silvery white after time. Abdominal tumor or ascites that stretch the skin also produce striae. The striae of Cushing's disease remain purplish.

Inspect for any lesions, particularly nodules. Lesions are of particular importance since gastrointestinal diseases often produce secondary skin changes. A pearl-like enlarged umbilical node may signal intraabdominal lymphoma. Skin and gastroin-

Fig. 11-5
Abdominal venous
patterns. **A,** Normal.
B, Portal hypertension.
C, Inferior vena cava
obstruction.

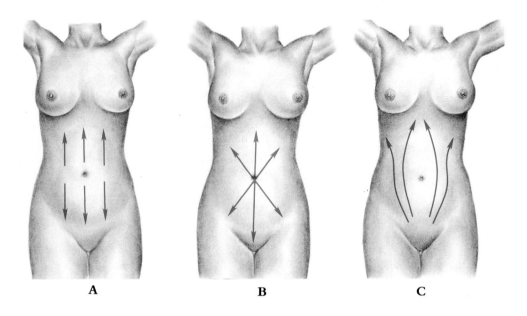

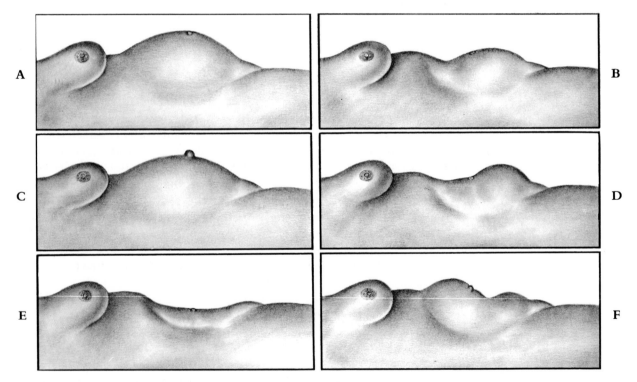

Fig. 11-6
Abdominal profiles. **A,** Fully rounded or distended, umbilicus inverted.
B, Distended lower half. **C,** Fully rounded or distended, umbilicus everted.
D, Distended lower third. **E,** Scaphoid. **F,** Distended upper half.

testinal lesions may arise from the same cause or occur without relationship to the other.

Note any scars and draw their location, configuration, and relative size on an illustration of the abdomen. If the cause of a scar was not explained during the history, now is a good time to pursue that information. The presence of scarring should alert you to the possibility of internal adhesions.

Inspect the abdomen for contour, symmetry, and surface motion, using tangential lighting to illuminate contour and visible peristalsis. Contour is the abdominal profile from the rib margin to the pubis, viewed on the horizontal plane. The expected contours can be described as flat, rounded, or scaphoid. (Fig. 11-6). A flat contour is common in well-muscled, athletic adults. The rounded or convex contour is characteristic of young children, but in adults it is the result of subcutaneous fat or poor muscle tone from inadequate exercise. The abdomen should be evenly rounded with the maximum height of convexity at the umbilicus. The scaphoid or concave contour is seen in thin adults.

Note the location and contour of the umbilicus. It should be centrally located without displacement upward, downward, or laterally. The umbilicus may be inverted or protrude slightly, but it should be free of inflammation, swelling, or bulges that may indicate a hernia.

Inspect for symmetry from a seated position at the patient's side, and then move to a standing position behind the patient's head. Contralateral areas of the abdomen should be symmetrical in appearance and contour. Look for any distention or bulges.

Generalized symmetrical distention may occur as a result of obesity, enlarged organs, and fluid or gas. Distention from the umbilicus to the symphysis can be caused by an ovarian tumor, pregnancy, uterine fibroids, or a distended bladder. Distention of the upper half, above the umbilicus, can mean carcinoma, pancreatic cyst, or gastric dilation. Asymmetrical distention or protrusion may indicate hernia, tumor, cysts, bowel obstruction, or enlargement of abdominal organs.

Ask the patient to take a deep breath and hold it. The contour should remain smooth and symmetrical. This manuever lowers the diaphragm and compresses the organs of the abdominal cavity, which may cause previously unseen bulges or masses to appear. Next ask the patient to raise his or her head from the table. This contracts the recti abdominis muscles, which produces muscle prominence in thin or athletic adults. Superficial abdominal wall masses may become visible. If an umbilical or incisional hernia is present, the increased abdominal pressure may cause it to protrude. Separation of the muscles may be apparent in patients with diastasis recti.

With the patient's head again resting on the table, inspect the abdomen for motion. Smooth, even movement should occur with respiration. Males exhibit primarily abdominal movement with respiration, whereas females show mostly costal movement. Limited abdominal motion associated with respiration in adult males may indicate peritonitis or disease. Surface motion from peristalsis is seen as a rippling movement across a section of the abdomen. It is usually not visible in either males or females and indicates a definite abnormality, most often an intestinal obstruction. Pulsation in the upper midline is often visible in thin adults. Marked pulsation may occur as the result of increased pulse pressure or abdominal aortic aneurysm.

Auscultation

Once inspection is completed, the next step is auscultation. This technique is used to assess bowel motility and to discover vascular sounds. Auscultation of the abdomen always precedes percussion and palpation, because percussion may alter the frequency and intensity of bowel sounds.

Place the diaphragm of a warmed stethoscope on the abdomen and hold it in place with only very light pressure. A cold stethoscope, like cold hands, may initiate contraction of the abdominal muscles. Listen for bowel sounds and note their frequency and character. They are usually heard as clicks and gurgles that occur irregularly and range from 5 to 35 per minute. Loud prolonged gurgles called borborygmi ("stomach growling") are sometimes heard. Increased bowel sounds may occur with gastroenteritis or early intestinal obstruction. High-pitched tinkling sounds suggest intestinal fluid and air under pressure, as in early obstruction. Decreased bowel sounds occur with peritonitis and paralytic ileus. The absence of bowel sounds is established only after 5 minutes of continuous listening. Auscultate all four quadrants to make sure that no sounds are missed and to localize specific sounds.

Listen with the diaphragm of the stethoscope in the epigastric region and each of the four quadrants for bruits in the aortic, renal, iliac, and femoral arteries (Fig. 11-7). Listen for friction rubs over the liver and spleen. Friction rubs are high-pitched and are heard in association with respiration. While friction rubs in the abdomen are rare, they indicate inflammation of the peritoneal surface of the organ from tumor, infection, or infarct.

Auscultate with the bell of the stethoscope in the epigastric region and around the umbilicus for a venous hum, which is soft, low-pitched, and continuous. A venous hum occurs with increased collateral circulation between portal and systemic venous systems.

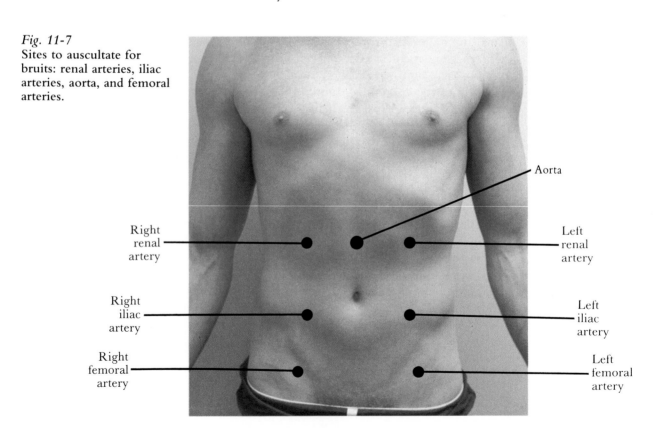

Fig. 11-7
Sites to auscultate for bruits: renal arteries, iliac arteries, aorta, and femoral arteries.

Percussion

Percussion is used to assess the size and density of the organs in the abdomen and to detect the presence of fluid (as with ascites), air (as with gastric distention), and fluid-filled or solid masses. Percussion is used either independently or concurrently with palpation while specific organs are evaluated, and it can validate palpatory findings. For simplicity, percussion and palpation will be discussed separately; however, either approach is acceptable.

First percuss all quadrants or regions of the abdomen for a sense of overall tympany and dullness (see Table 11-2). Tympany is the predominant sound because air is present in the stomach and intestines. Dullness is heard over organs and solid masses. A distended bladder produces dullness in the suprapubic area. Develop a systematic route for percussion, as shown in Fig. 11-8.

Table 11-2
Percussion Notes of the Abdomen

Note	Description	Location
Tympany	Musical note of higher pitch than resonance	Over air-filled viscera
Hyperresonance	Pitch lies between tympany and resonance	Base of left lung
Resonance	Sustained note of moderate pitch	Over lung tissue and sometimes over abdomen
Dullness	Short, high-pitched note with little resonance	Over solid organs adjacent to air-filled structures

Adapted from Percussion. In Gastrointestinal series: Physical examination of the abdomen, part 3, Richmond, Va., A.H. Robins Company.

Fig. 11-8
Systematic route for abdominal percussion.

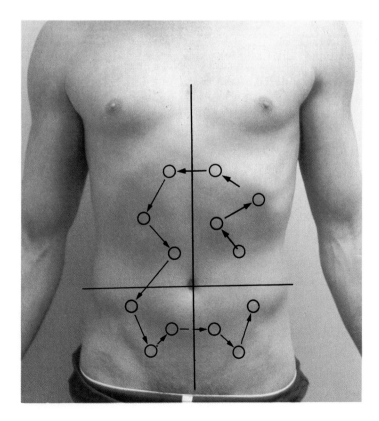

Fig. 11-9
Liver percussion route.

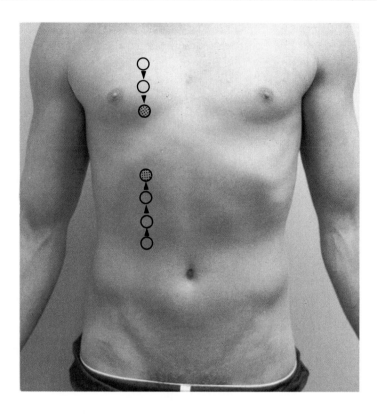

Now go back and percuss individually the liver, spleen, and stomach. Begin liver percussion at the right midclavicular line below the level of the umbilicus over an area of tympany. (Always begin with an area of tympany and proceed to an area of dullness, because that sound change is easier to detect than the change from dullness to tympany.) Percuss upward along the midclavicular line, as shown in Fig. 11-9, to determine the lower border of the liver. The area of liver dullness is usually heard at the costal margin or slightly below it. Mark the border with a marking pen. A lower liver border that is more than 2 to 3 cm (¾ to 1 in) below the costal margin may indicate organ enlargement or downward displacement of the diaphragm because of emphysema or other pulmonary disease.

To determine the upper border of the liver, begin percussion on the right midclavicular line at an area of lung resonance. Continue downward until the percussion tone changes to one of dullness, which marks the upper border of the liver. Mark the location with the pen. The upper border usually begins at the fifth to seventh intercostal space. An upper border below this may indicate downward displacement or liver atrophy. Dullness extending above the fifth intercostal space suggests upward displacement from abdominal fluid or masses.

Measure the distance between the marks to estimate the vertical span of the liver. The usual span is approximately 6 to 12 cm (2½ to 4½ in). A span greater than this may indicate liver enlargement, whereas a lesser span suggests atrophy. Age and sex influence liver size. Obviously, the liver will be larger in adults than in children. Liver span is usually greater in males and tall individuals than in females and short people. Interestingly, in the early years of life the liver tends to be somewhat larger in the female, but usually by about 4 years of age, the liver of the male will be larger. Of course, individuals at every age vary, and this will not hold true in all cases.

Although percussion provides the most accurate clinical measure of liver size, the measure remains only a gross estimate. Errors in estimating liver span can occur when the dullness of pleural effusion or lung consolidation obscures the upper liver border, leading to overestimation of size. Similarly, gas in the colon may produce tympany in the right upper quadrant and obscure the dullness of the lower liver border, leading to underestimation of liver size.

If liver enlargement is suspected, additional percussion maneuvers can provide further information. Percuss upward and then downward over the right midaxillary line. Liver dullness is usually detected in the fifth to seventh intercostal space. Dullness beyond those limits suggests a problem. You can also percuss along the midsternal line to estimate the midsternal liver span. Percuss upward from the abdomen and downward from the lungs, marking the upper and lower borders of dullness. The usual span at the midsternal line is 4 to 8 cm (1½ to 3 in). Spans exceeding 8 cm suggest liver enlargement.

It is best to report the size of the liver in two ways: by liver span as determined from percussing the upper and lower borders and by the extent of liver projection below the costal margin. When the size of a patient's liver is important in assessing the clinical condition, projection below the costal margin alone will not provide enough comparative information.

To assess the descent of the liver, ask the patient to take a deep breath and hold it while you percuss upward again from the abdomen at the right midclavicular line. The area of lower border dullness should move downward 2 to 3 cm. This maneuver will guide subsequent palpation of the organ.

The spleen is percussed just posterior to the midaxillary line on the left side. Percuss in several directions as shown in Fig. 11-10, beginning at areas of lung resonance. A small area of splenic dullness may be heard from the sixth to the tenth rib. A large area of dullness suggests spleen enlargement; however, a full stomach

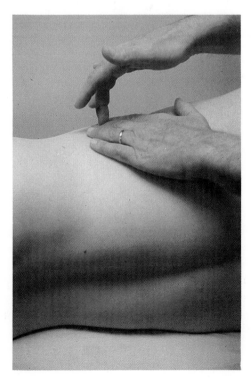

Fig. 11-10
Percussion of the spleen.

or feces-filled intestine may mimic the dullness of splenic enlargement. Percuss the lowest intercostal space in the left anterior axillary line before and after the patient takes a deep breath. The area should remain tympanic. With splenic enlargement, tympany changes to dullness as the spleen is brought forward and downward with inspiration. Remember that it is not possible to distinguish between the dullness of the posterior flank and that of the spleen. In addition, the dullness of a healthy spleen is often obscured by the tympany of colonic air.

Finally, percuss for the gastric air bubble in the area of the left lower anterior rib cage and left epigastric region. The tympany produced by the gastric bubble is lower in pitch than the tympany of the intestine.

Palpation

Palpation is used to assess the organs of the abdominal cavity and to detect muscle spasm, masses, fluid, and areas of tenderness. The abdominal organs are evaluated for size, shape, mobility, consistency, and tension. Stand at the patient's side (usually the right) with the patient in the supine position. Make certain that the patient is comfortable and that the abdomen is as relaxed as possible. Your hands should be warm to avoid producing muscle contraction and hinder further examination.

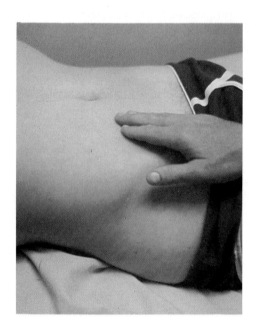

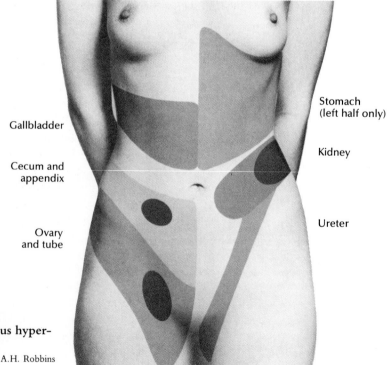

Fig. 11-11
Light palpation of the abdomen. With fingers extended and approximated, press in no more than 1 cm.

Gallbladder

Cecum and appendix

Ovary and tube

Stomach (left half only)

Kidney

Ureter

Fig. 11-12
Areas of cutaneous hypersensitivity.
From G.I. series, 1981, A.H. Robbins Co.

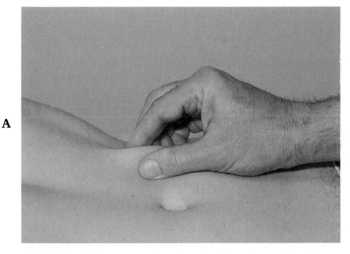

A

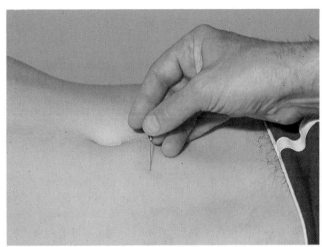

B

Fig. 11-13
Testing for cutaneous hypersensitivity. A, Lift a fold of skin away from underlying muscle or, B, stimulate the skin with a sharp point.

The ticklish patient can sometimes make it difficult for you to palpate the abdomen satisfactorily. However, there are ways to overcome this problem. Ask the patient to perform self-palpation, and place your hands over the patient's fingers, not quite touching the abdomen itself. After a bit, let your fingers drift slowly onto the abdomen while still resting primarily on the patient's fingers. You can learn a good deal, and ticklishness might not be so much of a problem. You might also use the diaphragm of the stethoscope (making sure that it is warm enough) as a palpating instrument. This serves as a beginning and, again, your fingers can drift over the edge of the diaphragm and palpate without eliciting an excessively ticklish response.

Begin with a light, systematic palpation of all four quadrants, initially avoiding any areas that have already been identified as problem spots. Lay the palm of your hand lightly on the abdomen, with the fingers extended and approximated (Fig. 11-11). With the palmar surface of your fingers, depress the abdominal wall no more than 1 cm, using a light and even pressing motion. Avoid short, quick jabs. The abdomen should feel smooth with a consistent softness. The patient's abdomen may tense if you press too deeply, if your hands are cold, if the patient is ticklish, or if inflammation is present. Guarding should alert you to move cautiously through the remainder of the examination.

Light palpation is particularly useful in identifying muscular resistance and areas of tenderness. A large mass or distended structure may be appreciated on light palpation as a sense of resistance. If resistance is present, try to determine whether it is voluntary or involuntary in the following way: place a pillow under the patient's knees and ask the patient to breathe slowly through the mouth as you feel for relaxation of the recti abdominis muscles upon expiration. If the tenseness remains, it is probably an involuntary response to localized or generalized rigidity. Rigidity is a boardlike hardness of the abdominal wall overlying areas of peritoneal irritation.

Specific zones of peritoneal irritation may be identified through cutaneous hypersensitivity (Fig. 11-12). To evaluate hypersensitivity, gently lift a fold of skin away from the underlying muscle or stimulate the skin with a pin or other object and have the patient describe the local sensation (Fig. 11-13). In the event of hypersensitivity, the patient will perceive pain or an exaggerated sensation in response to this maneuver.

Continue palpation of all four quadrants with the same hand position as for light palpation, exerting moderate pressure as an intermediate step to gradually approach deep palpation. Tenderness not elicited on gentle palpation may become evident with deeper pressure. An additional maneuver of moderate palpation is performed with the side of your hand (Fig. 11-14). This maneuver is useful in assessing organs that move with respiration, specifically the liver and spleen. Palpate during the entire respiratory cycle; as the patient inspires the organ is displaced downward, and you may be able to feel it as bumps gently against your hand.

Deep palpation is necessary to thoroughly delineate abdominal organs and to detect less obvious masses. Use the palmar surface of your extended fingers, pressing deeply and evenly into the abdominal wall (Fig. 11-15). Palpate all four quadrants, moving the fingers back and forth over the abdominal contents. (The abdominal wall may also slide back and forth as you do this.) Often you are able to feel the borders of the recti abdominis muscles, the aorta, and portions of the colon. Tenderness not elicited with light or moderate palpation may become evident. Deep pressure may also evoke tenderness in the healthy person over the cecum, sigmoid colon, aorta, and in the midline near the xiphoid process.

Identify any masses and note the characteristics: location, size, shape, consistency, tenderness, pulsation, mobility, and movement with respiration. To determine if a mass is superficial (located in the abdominal wall) or intraabdominal, have the patient lift his or her head from the examining table, thus contracting the abdominal

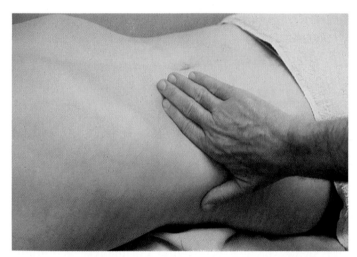

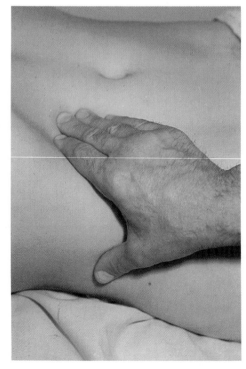

Fig. 11-14
Moderate palpation using the side of the hand.

Fig. 11-15
Deep palpation. Press deeply and evenly with the palmar surface of extended fingers.

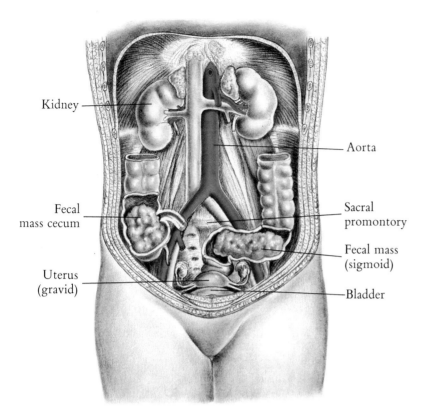

Fig. 11-16
**Abdominal structures
frequently felt as "masses."**

Kidney

Fecal
mass cecum

Uterus
(gravid)

Aorta

Sacral
promontory

Fecal mass
(sigmoid)

Bladder

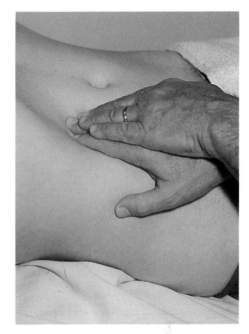

Fig. 11-17
Bimanual deep palpation.

muscles. Masses in the abdominal wall will continue to be palpable, while those located in the abdominal cavity will be more difficult to feel, since they are obscured by abdominal musculature. The presence of feces in the colon, often mistaken for an abdominal mass, can be felt as a soft, rounded, boggy mass in the cecum and in the ascending, descending, or sigmoid colons. Other structures that are sometimes mistaken for masses are the lateral borders of the recti abdominis muscles, the uterus, aorta, sacral promontory, and common iliac artery (Fig. 11-16). If you can mentally visualize the placement of the abdominal structures, it will be easier to distinguish between what you know ought to be there and an unexpected finding.

Palpate the umbilical ring and around the umbilicus. The area should be free of bulges, nodules, and granulation. The umbilical ring should be round and free of irregularities. Note whether it is incomplete or soft in the center, which suggests the potential of herniation. The umbilicus may be either slightly inverted or everted, but it should not protrude.

If deep palpation is difficult because of obesity or muscular resistance, you can use a bimanual technique with one hand atop the other as shown in Fig. 11-17. Exert pressure with the top hand while concentrating on sensation with the other hand. Some examiners prefer to use the bimanual technique for all patients.

Palpation of Specific Structures

LIVER. Place your left hand under the patient at the eleventh and twelfth ribs, pressing upward to elevate the liver toward the abdominal wall. Place your right hand on the abdomen, fingers pointing toward the head and extended so the tips rest on the right midclavicular line below the level of liver dullness, as shown in Fig. 11-18, *A*. Alternately, you can place your right hand parallel to the right costal margin, as shown in Fig. 11-18, *B*. In either case, press your right hand gently but deeply in and up. Have the patient breathe normally a few times and then take a deep breath. Try to feel the liver edge as the diaphragm pushes it down to meet your finger tips. Ordinarily, the liver is not palpable, although it may be felt in some thin persons even when no pathologic condition exists. If the liver edge is felt, it should be firm, smooth, even, and nontender. Feel for nodules, tenderness, and irregularity. If the liver is palpable, repeat the maneuver medially and laterally to the costal margin to assess the contour and surface of the liver.

An alternate technique is to hook your fingers over the right costal margin below the border of liver dullness, as shown in Fig. 11-19. Stand on the patient's right side facing his or her feet. Press in and up toward the costal margin with your fingers and ask the patient to take a deep breath. Try to feel the liver edge as it descends to meet your fingers.

If the abdomen is distended or the abdominal muscles tense, the usual techniques for determining the lower liver border may be unproductive. At such a point, the scratch test may be useful (Fig. 11-20). This technique uses auscultation to detect the differences in sound transmission over solid and hollow organs. Place the stethoscope over the liver and with the finger of your other hand scratch the abdominal surface lightly, moving toward the liver border. When you encounter the liver, the sound you hear in the stethoscope will be magnified.

To check for liver tenderness when the liver is not palpable, use indirect fist percussion. Place the palmar surface of one hand over the lower right rib cage, and then strike your hand with the ulnar surface of the fist of your other hand as shown in Fig. 11-21. The healthy liver is not tender to percussion.

A

B

Fig. 11-18
A, Palpating the liver. Fingers are extended with tips on right midclavicular line below level of liver tenderness and pointing toward the head. **B,** Alternate method for liver palpation with fingers parallel to the costal margin.

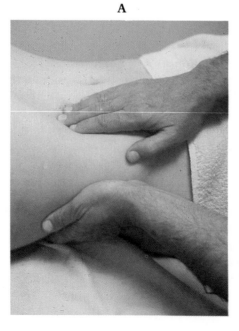
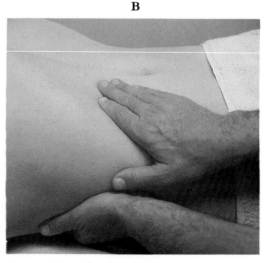

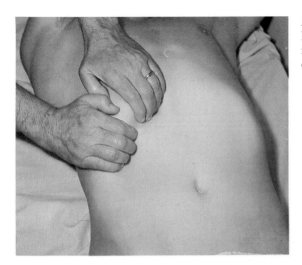

Fig. 11-19
Palpating the liver with
fingers hooked over the
costal margin.

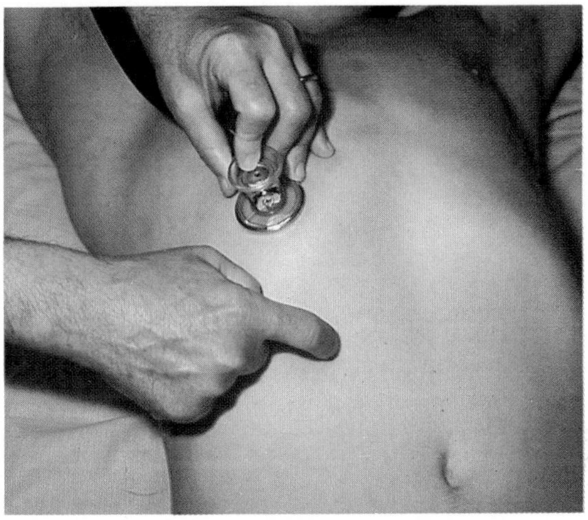

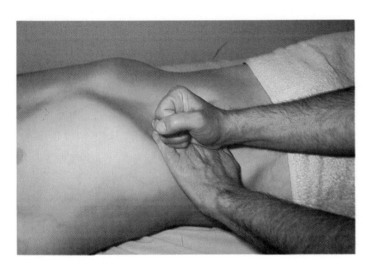

Fig. 11-20
Scratch technique for auscultating the liver.
With stethoscope over the liver, lightly
scratch the abdominal surface moving
toward the liver. The sound will be
magnified over the liver.

Fig. 11-21
Fist percussion of the
liver.

GALLBLADDER. Palpate below the liver margin at the lateral border of the rectus
muscle for the gallbladder. A healthy gallbladder will not be palpable. A palpable,
tender gallbladder indicates cholecystitis, while nontender enlargement suggests
common bile duct obstruction. If you suspect cholecystitis, have the patient take a
deep breath during deep palpation. As the inflamed gallbladder comes in contact
with the examining fingers, the patient will experience pain and abruptly halt inspiration (Murphy's sign).

SPLEEN. While still standing on the patient's right side, reach across with your left
hand and place it beneath the patient over the left costovertebral angle. Press
upward with that hand to lift the spleen anteriorly toward the abdominal wall.
Place the palmar surface of your right hand with fingers extended on the patient's
abdomen below the left costal margin (Fig. 11-22, *A*). Use findings from percussion as a guide. Press your fingertips inward toward the spleen as you ask the
patient to take a deep breath. Try to feel the edge of the spleen as it moves downward toward your fingers. The spleen is not usually palpable in an adult; if you can

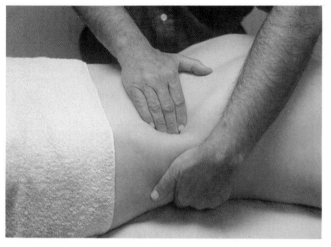
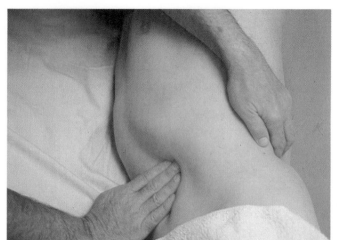

Fig. 11-22
A, Palpating the spleen. Press upward with the left hand at the patient's left costovertebral angle. Feel for the spleen with the right hand below the left costal margin. **B,** Palpating the spleen with the patient lying on the side. Press inward with the left hand and tips of the right fingers.

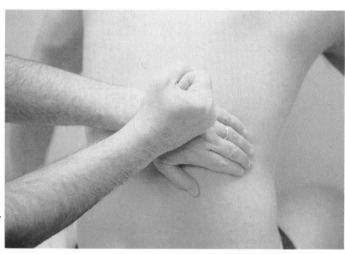

Fig. 11-23
Fist percussion of costovertebral angle for kidney tenderness.

feel it, it is probably enlarged. Be sure to palpate with your fingers below the costal margin so that you will not miss the lower edge of an enlarged spleen. Be gentle in palpation to avoid rupturing an enlarged spleen.

Repeat the palpation while the patient is lying on the right side with hips and knees flexed (Fig. 11-22, *B*). Still standing on the right side, press inward with your left hand to assist gravity in bringing the spleen forward and to the right. Press inward with the fingertips of your right hand and feel for the edge of the spleen. Again, you will not usually feel it, and if you can, it is probably enlarged.

KIDNEYS. To assess each kidney for tenderness, ask the patient to assume a sitting position. Place the palm of your hand over the right costovertebral angle and strike your hand with the ulnar surface of the fist of your other hand (Fig. 11-23). Repeat the maneuver over the left costovertebral angle. Direct percussion with the fist over each costovertebral angle may also be used. The patient should perceive the blow as a thud, but it should not cause tenderness or pain. For efficiency of time and motion, assessment for kidney tenderness is usually performed while examining the back rather than the abdomen.

Left kidney. Ask the patient to lie supine. Standing on the patient's right side, reach across with your left hand as you did in spleen palpation and place it over the left flank. Place your right hand at the patient's left costal margin. Have the patient take a deep breath, elevate the left flank with your left hand and palpate deeply (because of the retroperitoneal position of the kidney) with your right hand (Fig. 11-24). Try to feel the lower pole of the kidney with your fingertips as the patient inhales. The left kidney is ordinarily not palpable.

Another approach is to "capture" the kidney. Move to the patient's left side and position your hands as before, with the left hand over the patient's left flank and the right hand at the left costal margin. Ask the patient to take a deep breath. At the height of inspiration press the fingers of your two hands together to capture the kidney between the fingers. Ask the patient to breathe out and hold the exhalation while you slowly release your fingers. If you have captured the kidney you may feel it slip beneath your fingers as it moves back into place. Although the patient may feel the capture and release, the maneuver should not be painful. Again, a left kidney is rarely palpable.

Right kidney. Stand on the patient's right side, placing your left hand under the patient's right flank and your right hand at the right costal margin. Perform the same maneuvers as you did for the left kidney (Fig. 11-25). Because of the anatomic

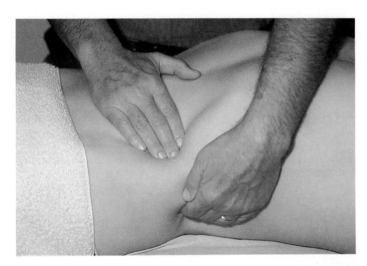

Fig. 11-24
Palpating the left kidney. Elevate the left flank with the left hand. Palpate deeply with the right hand.

Fig. 11-25
Capture technique for palpating the kidney (right kidney). As the patient takes a deep breath press the fingers of both hands together. As the patient exhales slowly release the fingers and feel for the kidney to slip between the examining fingers.

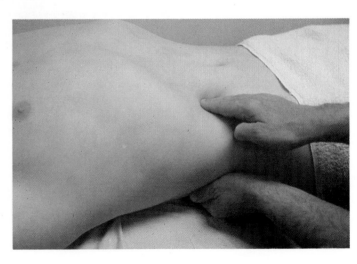

AN ENLARGED SPLEEN OR AN ENLARGED LEFT KIDNEY?

When an organ is palpable below the left costal margin, it may be difficult to differentiate an enlarged spleen from an enlarged left kidney. Percussion should help distinguish between the organs. The percussion note over an enlarged spleen is dull since the spleen displaces bowel. The usual area of splenic dullness will be increased downward and toward the midline. The percussion note over an enlarged kidney is resonant because the kidney is deeply situated behind the bowel. In addition, the edge of the spleen is sharper than that of the kidney. A palpable notch along the medial border suggests an enlarged spleen rather than an enlarged kidney.

position of the right kidney, it is more frequently palpable than the left kidney. If it is palpable, it should be smooth, firm, and nontender. It may be difficult to distinguish the kidney from the liver edge. The liver edge tends to be sharp while the kidney is more rounded. The liver also extends more medially and laterally and cannot be captured.

AORTA. With the patient in the supine position, palpate deeply slightly to the left of the midline and feel for the aortic pulsation. If the pulsation is prominent, try to determine the direction of pulsation. A prominent lateral pulsation suggests an aortic aneurysm. While the aortic pulse may be felt, particularly in thin adults, the pulse should be in an anterior direction.

If you are unable to feel the pulse on deep palpation, an alternate technique may help (Fig. 11-26). Place the palmar surface of your hands with fingers extended on the midline. Press the fingers deeply inward on each side of the aorta and feel for the pulsation. In thin individuals you can use one hand, placing the thumb on one side of the aorta and the fingers on the other side.

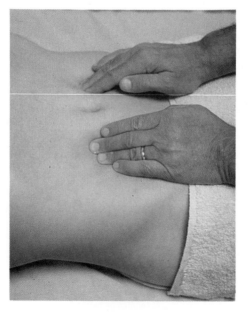

Fig. 11-26
Palpating the aorta. Press fingers deeply inward on each side of the aorta and feel for the pulsation.

ABDOMINAL REFLEXES. The technique for eliciting abdominal reflexes is described in Chapter 17 (Neurologic System and Mental Status). With each stroke expect to see contraction of the recti abdominis muscles and pulling of the umbilicus toward the stroked side. A diminished reflex may be present in patients who are obese or whose abdominal muscles have been stretched during pregnancy. Absence of the reflex may indicate a pyramidal tract lesion.

Additional Procedures

Ascites Assessment

Ascites may be suspected in patients who have protuberant abdomens or who have flanks that bulge in the supine position. Percuss for areas of dullness and resonance with the patient supine. Since ascites fluid settles with gravity, expect to hear dullness in the dependent parts of the abdomen and tympany in the upper parts where the relatively lighter bowel has risen. Mark the borders between tympany and dullness.

Then test for shifting dullness to help ascertain the presence of fluid. Have the patient lie on one side and again percuss for tympany and dullness and mark the borders. In the patient without ascites, the borders will remain relatively constant. In ascites, the border of dullness shifts to the dependent side (approaches the midline) as the fluid resettles through gravity (Fig. 11-27).

Another maneuver is to test for a fluid wave. This procedure requires three hands, so you will need assistance from the patient or another examiner (Fig. 11-28). With the patient supine, ask him or her or another person to press the edge of the hand and forearm firmly along the vertical midline of the abdomen. This positioning helps stop the transmission of a wave through adipose tissue. Place your hands on each side of the abdomen and strike one side sharply with your fingertips. Feel for the impulse of a fluid wave with the fingertips of your other hand. An easily detected fluid wave suggests ascites, but be cautioned that the findings of this maneuver are not conclusive. A fluid wave can sometimes be felt in people without ascites and, conversely, may not occur in people with early ascites.

Another maneuver allows you to test for fluid pooling (puddle sign). Ask the

Fig. 11-27
Testing for shifting dullness. Dullness shifts to the dependent side.

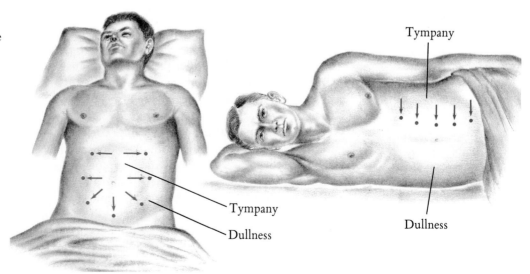

Tympany

Tympany

Dullness

Dullness

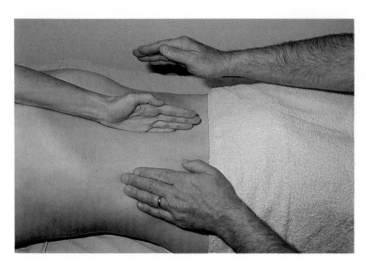

Fig. 11-28
Testing for fluid wave. Strike one side of the abdomen sharply with the fingertips. Feel for the impulse of a fluid wave with the other hand.

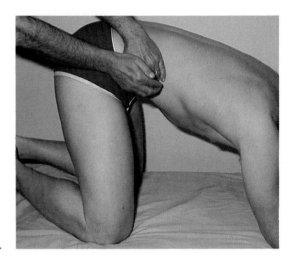

Fig. 11-29
Testing for pooling of abdominal fluid. Percuss the umbilical area for dullness.

patient to assume the knee-chest position and maintain that position for several minutes to allow any fluid to pool by gravity. Percuss the umbilical area for dullness to determine the presence of fluid (Fig. 11-29). The area will remain tympanic if no fluid is present.

None of these maneuvers is specific or reliable, and generally all have been replaced by sonographic examination of the abdomen. Their importance is now largely historic.

Pain Assessment

Abdominal pain is a common complaint, frequently difficult to evaluate. How bad is the pain? Is there an underlying physical cause? Pain that is severe enough to make the patient unwilling to move, accompanied by nausea and vomiting, and marked by areas of localized tenderness generally has an underlying physical cause. While examining the abdomen, keep your eyes on the patient's face. The facial response is as important in your evaluation as the patient's verbal response to questions about the quality and degree of pain. Ask the patient to cough or take a deep breath. Assess the patient's willingness to jump or to walk. Is the pain exacerbated? A time honored test is to ask the patient, "Do you want a hot dog?" It is unlikely that hunger will persist in the face of an acute intraabdominal infection.

Common causes of abdominal pain are described in Table 11-3. Careful assessment of the quality (Table 11-4) and location of pain (Table 11-5) can usually narrow the possible causes, allowing you to select additional diagnostic studies with greater efficiency.

Table 11-3
*Common Conditions Producing Abdominal Pain**

Condition	Usual Pain Characteristics	Possible Associated Findings
Appendicitis	Initially periumbilical or epigastric; colicky; later becomes localized to RLQ, often at McBurney's point	Guarding, tenderness; + iliopsoas and + obturator signs, RLQ skin hyperthesia; anorexia, nausea, or vomiting after onset of pain; low grade fever
Cholecystitis	Severe, unrelenting RUQ or epigastric; may be referred to right subscapular area	RUQ tenderness and rigidity, + Murphy's sign, palpable gallbladder, anorexia, vomiting, fever, possible jaundice
Pancreatitis	Dramatic, sudden, excruciating LUQ, epigastric, or umbilical pain; may be present in one or both flanks; may be referred to left shoulder	Epigastric tenderness, vomiting, fever, shock
Perforated gastric or duodenal ulcer	Abrupt RUQ; may be referred to shoulders	Abdominal free air and distention with increased resonance over liver; tenderness in epigastrum or RUQ; rigid abdominal wall, rebound tenderness
Diverticulitis	Epigastric, radiating down left side of abdomen especially after eating; may be referred to back	Flatulence, borborygmi, diarrhea, dysuria, tenderness on palpation
Intestinal obstruction	Abrupt, severe, spasmotic; referred to epigastrium, umbilicus	Distention, minimal rebound tenderness, vomiting, localized tenderness, visible peristalsis; bowel sounds absent (with paralytic obstruction) or hyperactive high pitched (with mechanical obstruction)
Volvulus	Referred to hypogastrium and umbilicus	Distention, nausea, vomiting, guarding; sigmoid loop volvulus may be palpable
Leaking abdominal aneurysm	Steady throbbing midline over aneurysm; may radiate to back, flank	Nausea, vomiting, abdominal mass, bruit
Biliary stones, colic	Episodic, severe, RUQ or epigastrium lasting 15 min to several hours; may be referred to subscapular area, especially right	RUQ tenderness, soft abdominal wall, anorexia, vomiting, jaundice, subnormal temperature
Salpingitis	Lower quadrant, worse on left	Nausea, vomiting, fever, suprapubic tenderness, rigid abdomen, pain on pelvic examination
Ectopic pregnancy	Lower quadrant; referred to shoulder	Hypogastric tenderness, symptoms of pregnancy, spotting, irregular menses, soft abdominal wall, mass on bimanual pelvic exam; ruptured: shock, rigid abdominal wall, distention
Pelvic inflammatory disease	Lower quadrant, increases with activity	Tender adnexa and cervix, cervical discharge, dyspareunia
Ruptured ovarian cyst	Lower quadrant, steady, increases with cough or motion	Vomiting, low grade fever, anorexia, tenderness on pelvic examination

*+, Positive; *RLQ,* right lower quadrant; *RUQ,* right upper quadrant; *LUQ,* left upper quadrant.

Table 11-4
Quality and Onset of
Abdominal Pain

Characteristic	Possible Related Condition
Burning	Peptic ulcer
Cramping	Biliary colic, gastroenteritis
Colic	Appendicitis with impacted feces
Aching	Appendiceal irritation
Knife-like	Pancreatitis
Gradual onset	Infection
Sudden onset	Duodenal ulcer, acute pancreatitis, obstruction, perforation

Adapted from Malasanos et al., 1986.

Table 11-5
Some Causes of Perceived
Pain in Anatomic Regions

Right Upper Quadrant		*Left Upper Quadrant*
Duodenal ulcer		Ruptured spleen
Hepatitis		Gastric ulcer
Hepatomegaly		Aortic aneurysm
Pneumonia		Perforated colon
	Periumbilical	Pneumonia
	Intestinal obstruction	
Right Lower Quadrant	Acute pancreatitis	*Left Lower Quadrant*
Appendicitis	Early appendicitis	Sigmoid diverticulitis
Salpingitis	Mesenteric thrombosis	Salpingitis
Ovarian cyst	Aortic aneurysm	Ovarian cyst
Ruptured ectopic	Diverticulitis	Ruptured ectopic
pregnancy		pregnancy
Renal/ureteral stone		Renal/ureteral stone
Strangulated hernia		Strangulated hernia
Meckel's diverticulitis		Perforated colon
Regional ileitis		Regional ileitis
Perforated cecum		Ulcerative colitis

Adapted from Judge et al., 1982.

Rebound Tenderness

If the patient is experiencing abdominal pain, this maneuver can be used to determine peritoneal irritation. Place the patient in the supine position. Hold your hand at a 90 degree angle to the abdomen with the fingers extended, then press gently and deeply into a region remote from the area of discomfort. Rapidly withdraw your hand and fingers (Fig. 11-30). The return to position (rebound) of the structures that were compressed by your fingers causes a sharp stabbing pain at the site of peritoneal inflammation. Rebound tenderness over McBurney's point in the lower right quadrant suggests appendicitis. The maneuver for rebound tenderness should be performed at the end of the examination, because a positive response produces pain and muscle spasm that can interfere with any subsequent examination. This maneuver is considered crude and unnecessary by many examiners, since light percussion produces a mild localized response in the presence of peritoneal inflammation.

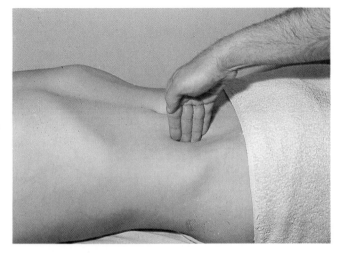

A

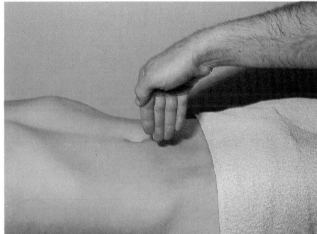

B

Fig. 11-30
Testing for rebound ten-
derness. **A,** Press deeply
and gently into the abdo-
men, then **B,** rapidly withdraw the hands and fingers.

Fig. 11-31
Iliopsoas muscle test. The
patient raises the leg from
the hip while the examiner
pushes downward against
it.

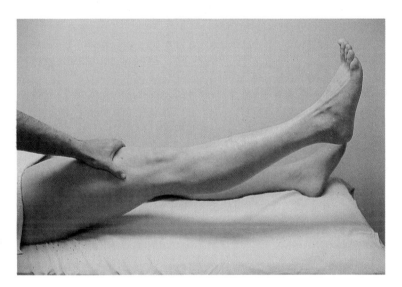

Iliopsoas Muscle Test

Perform this test when you suspect appendicitis, since an inflamed appendix may
cause irritation of the lateral iliopsoas muscle. Ask the patient to lie supine and then
place your hand over the lower thigh. Ask the patient to raise the leg, flexing at the
hip, while you push downward against the leg (Fig. 11-31). An alternate technique
is to position the patient on the left side and ask that the right leg be raised from the
hip while you press downward against it. A third technique is to hyperextend the
leg by drawing it backward while the patient is lying on the right side. In any of
these maneuvers, a patient with a positive iliopsoas sign will experience lower
quadrant pain.

Obturator Muscle Test

Perform this test when you suspect a ruptured appendix or a pelvic abscess, since
these conditions can cause irritation of the obturator muscle. The patient should be
supine for this test. Ask the patient to flex the right leg at the hip and knee to 90

degrees. Hold the leg just above the knee, grasp the ankle, and rotate the leg laterally and medially (Fig. 11-32). Pain in the hypogastric region is a positive sign indicating irritation of the obturator muscle.

Ballottement

Ballottement is a palpation technique used to assess a floating mass, such as the head of a fetus. To perform abdominal ballottement with one hand place your extended fingers, hand, and forearm at a 90-degree angle to the abdomen. Push in toward the mass with the fingertips (Fig. 11-33, *A*). If the mass is freely moveable it will float upward and touch the fingertips as fluid and other structures are displaced by the maneuver.

To perform bimanual ballottement, place one hand on the anterior abdominal wall and one hand against the flank. Push inward on the abdominal wall while palpating with the flank hand to determine the presence and size of the mass (Fig. 11-33, *B*).

Fig. 11-32
Obturator muscle test. With the right leg flexed at the hip and knee, rotate the leg laterally and medially.

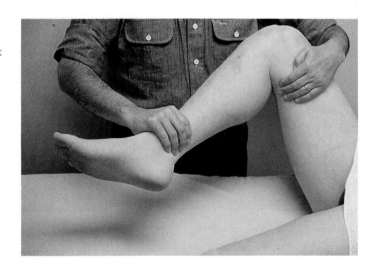

Fig. 11-33
Ballottement technique. **A,** Single-handed ballottement. Push inward at a 90-degree angle. If the object is freely movable it will float upward to touch the fingertips. **B,** Bimanual ballottement: *P,* pushing hand; *R,* receiving hand.

From G.I. series, 1981, A.H. Robbins Co.

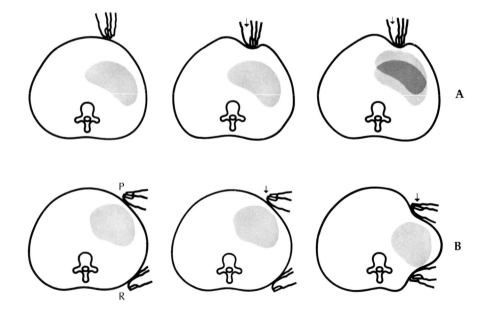

FINDINGS IN PERITONEAL IRRITATION

Rigid board-like abdomen
Tenderness and guarding
Severe localized pain
Absent bowel sounds
Positive obturator test
Positive iliopsoas test
Rebound tenderness

Adapted from Malasanos et al., 1985.

INFANTS AND CHILDREN

The infant's abdomen should be examined if possible during a time of relaxation and quiet. It is often best to do this at the start of the overall examination, especially before initiating any procedure that might cause distress (Fig. 11-34). Sucking a bottle or pacifier may help relax the infant. The parent's lap makes the best examining surface. Sit facing the parent, knees touching, and conduct the abdominal examination entirely on the parent's lap. This works well during the first several months, and often the first 2 to 3 years, of life. The infant will be most secure.

INSPECTION. Inspect the abdomen, noting its shape, contour, and movement with respiration. It should be rounded and dome-shaped because the abdominal musculature has not fully developed. Note any localized fullness. Abdominal and chest movements should be synchronous, with a slight bulge of the abdomen at the beginning of respiration. Note whether the abdomen protrudes above the level of the chest or is scaphoid. A distended or protruding abdomen can result from feces, a mass, or organ enlargement. A scaphoid abdomen suggests that the abdominal contents are displaced into the thorax.

Note any pulsations over the abdomen. Pulsations in the epigastric area are common in newborns and infants. Superficial veins are usually visible in the thin infant. However, distended veins across the abdomen are an abnormal finding

Fig. 11-34
Positioning to examine infant's abdomen.

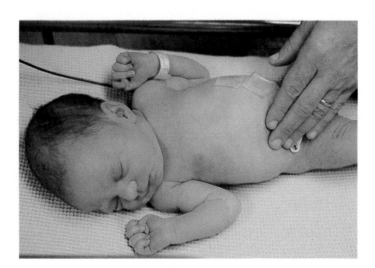

suggestive of vascular obstruction, abdominal distention, or abdominal obstruction. If any distended veins are present, identify the direction of blood flow. Spider nevi may indicate liver disease.

Inspect the umbilical cord of the newborn, counting the number of vessels present. Two arteries and one vein should be present. A single umbilical artery should alert you to the possibility of congenital anomalies. Any intestinal structure present in the umbilical cord or protruding into the umbilical area and visible through a thick transparent membrane suggests an omphalocele.

The umbilical stump area should be dry and odorless. Inspect it for discharge, redness, induration, and skin warmth. Once the stump has separated, serous or serosanguinous discharge may indicate a granuloma when no other signs of infection are present. Inspect all folds of skin in the umbilicus for a nodule of granulomatous tissue.

Note any protrusion through the umbilicus or recti abdominis muscles when the infant strains. The umbilicus is usually inverted. An umbilical hernia, the protrusion of omentum and intestine through the umbilical opening forming a visible and palpable bulge, is a common finding in infants (Fig. 11-35). Measure the diameter of the umbilical opening rather than the protruding contents to determine the size. The maximum size is generally reached by 1 month of age, and the hernia will generally close spontaneously by 1 to 2 years of age. Diastasis recti abdominis, a protrusion 1 to 4 cm wide in the midline that usually occurs between the xiphoid and the umbilicus, is a common finding in which the recti abdominis muscles do not approximate each other. Herniation through the recti abdominis muscles, however, is abnormal.

If the infant is vomiting frequently, use tangential lighting and observe the abdomen at eye level for peristaltic waves. Peristalsis is not usually visible. Peristaltic waves may sometimes be seen in thin, malnourished infants, but their presence usually suggests an intestinal obstruction, such as pyloric stenosis.

AUSCULTATION AND PERCUSSION. The procedures of auscultation and percussion of the abdomen do not differ from those used for adults. Peristalsis is detected when metallic tinkling is heard every 10 to 30 seconds, and bowel sounds should be present within 1 to 2 hours after birth. Since a scaphoid abdomen suggests a diaphragmatic hernia in the newborn, auscultate the chest for bowel sounds. No bruits or venous hums should be detected on abdominal auscultation.

Fig. 11-35
Umbilical hernia in infant.

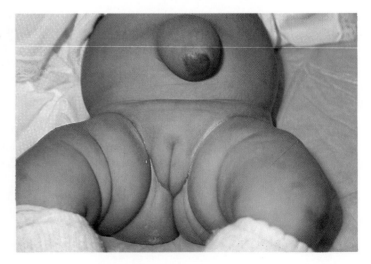

Table 11-6
Average Liver Spans for
Infants and Children

Age	Liver Span (cm)
6 months	2.4-2.8
12 months	2.8-3.1
24 months	3.5-3.6
3 years	4.0
4 years	4.3-4.4
5 years	4.5-4.8
6 years	4.8-5.1
8 years	5.1-5.6
10 years	5.5-6.1

The abdomen may produce more tympany on percussion than in adults, because infants swallow air when feeding or crying. As with adults, tympany in a distended abdomen is usually the result of gas, while dullness may indicate fluid or a solid mass. The upper edge of the liver should be detected within 1 cm of the fifth intercostal space at the right midclavicular line. Until 2 years of age females have a slightly larger liver span than males. The mean range of liver spans in infants and children is shown in Table 11-6.

PALPATION. Palpate the abdomen with the knees of the infant flexed to promote relaxation of the abdominal musculature. Begin with superficial palpation to detect the spleen, liver, and masses close to the surface. The spleen is usually palpable 1 to 2 cm below the left costal margin during the first few weeks after birth. A detectable spleen tip at the left costal margin is a common finding in well infants and young children. Any increase in spleen size may indicate blood dyscrasias or septicemia.

To assess the liver, superficially palpate at the right midclavicular line 3 to 4 cm below the costal margin. As the infant inspires, wait to feel a narrow mass tap your finger. Gradually move your fingers up the midclavicular line until the sensation is felt. The liver edge is usually palpable just below the right costal margin in the newborn. The liver edge may be palpable at 1 to 3 cm below the right costal margin in infants and toddlers. Hepatomegaly is present when the liver is more than 3 cm below the right costal margin, suggesting infection, cardiac failure, or liver disease.

Deep palpation is then performed in all quadrants. The location, size, shape, tenderness, and consistency of any masses should be noted. Transillumination should be used to distinguish cystic masses from solid masses. Fluid-filled masses will transilluminate, whereas solid masses will not. When pulsations are seen, palpate the aorta for any sign of enlargement. Fixed masses that are laterally mobile, pulsatile, or located along the vertebral column should be investigated further with special studies. If any suspicion of a neoplasm exists, limit palpation of the mass, because manipulation may cause injury or spread of malignancy.

A sausage-shaped mass in the left lower quadrant may indicate feces in the sigmoid colon associated with constipation. A midline suprapubic mass suggests Hirschsprung's disease in which feces fill the rectosigmoid colon. A sausage-shaped mass in the left or right upper quadrant may indicate intussusception. The almond-shaped mass of pyloric stenosis can often be detected with deep palpation in the right upper quadrant immediately after the infant vomits. It may be helpful to sit the infant in your lap, folding the upper body gently against your palpating hand, bringing the pyloric mass into opposition with your hand. Almost all other palpable masses in the abdomen of the newborn are renal in origin.

The bladder can usually be palpated and percussed in the infant and toddler in the suprapubic area. Determine the size of the bladder to detect any sign of distention. A distended bladder, felt as a firm, central dome-shaped structure in the lower abdomen, may indicate urethral obstruction or central nervous system defects.

Palpate the femoral arteries as described in Chapter 9 (Heart and Blood Vessels).

Tenderness or pain on palpation may be difficult to detect in the infant. However, pain and tenderness are assessed by behaviors such as change in the pitch of crying, facial grimacing, rejection of the opportunity to suck, and drawing the knees to the abdomen with palpation. When an infant will not stop crying, seize the quiet moment in the respiratory cycle to palpate in order to distinguish between a hard and soft abdomen. The abdomen should be soft during inspiration. If the abdomen remains hard with a noticeable rigidity or resistance to pressure during both respiratory phases, peritoneal irritation may be present. It is often necessary to delay examination of a distressed infant for a little while, waiting for a quieter moment, unless there is reason for urgency.

The abdomen of the young child protrudes slightly giving a potbellied appearance when standing, sitting, and supine (Fig. 11-36). After 5 years of age, the contour of the child's abdomen, when supine, may become convex and will not extend above an imaginary line drawn from the xiphoid process to the symphysis pubis. Respirations will continue to be abdominal until the child is 6 to 7 years old. Abdominal respiration beyond this age suggests thoracic problems. Restricted abdominal respiration in young children can be caused by peritoneal irritation or an acute abdomen. Diastasis recti abdominis should resolve by 6 years of age.

Fig. 11-36
Potbellied stance of a toddler.

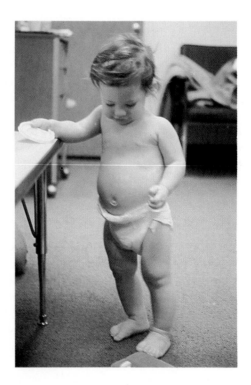

The upper edge of the liver should be detected by percussion at the sixth intercostal space. The lower edge of the liver may be palpated either at or 1 to 2 cm below the right costal margin.

Palpate the abdomen of a child who is ticklish with a firm rather than feathery touch. If that is unsuccessful, place the child's hand under the palm of your examining hand, leaving your fingers free to palpate. Localization of abdominal tenderness or pain may be difficult in the young child who cannot verbalize about the site or character of pain. Distract the child with a toy, or question the child about a favorite activity as you begin palpating in the abdominal region believed most distant from the area of pain. Observe for changes in facial expression and for constriction of the pupils during palpation to identify the location of greatest pain. Check for rebound tenderness and make the same observations of the child's facial expression and pupils.

The techniques of abdominal examination of the adolescent are the same as those used for adults. Do not overlook the possibility of pregnancy as a cause of a mass in the lower abdomen, even in young adolescent females.

PREGNANT WOMEN

Uterine changes that can be dectected on abdominal examination are discussed in Chapter 12 (Female Genitalia). Bowel sounds will be diminished as a result of decreased peristaltic activity. Striae and a midline band of pigmentation (linea nigra) may be present. Gastrointestinal complaints of nausea and vomiting are common in the first trimester. Constipation is a common occurrence and hemorrhoids often develop in later pregnancy.

Specific examination of the pregnant abdomen requires special maneuvers and measurement that are not addressed in this text.

OLDER ADULTS

The techniques of examination are the same as those used for younger adults. The abdominal wall of the older adult becomes thinner and less firm as a result of the loss of connective tissue and muscle mass that accompanies aging. Palpation may therefore be relatively easier and yield more accurate findings. Deposition of fat over the abdominal area is common, despite concurrent loss of fatty tissue over the extremities. The abdominal contour is often rounded as a result of loss of muscle tone.

The only modifications in examination techniques require some common sense. Use judgment in determining whether a patient is able to assume a particular position, such as the kneeling position to test for fluid pooling in assessing ascites. Similarly, remember that rotation of joints, such as with the obturator muscle test, may cause discomfort in patients who have decreased muscle flexibility or joint tenderness.

Be aware that respiratory changes can produce corresponding findings in the abdominal examination. The liver of patients with hyperexpanded lungs may be displaced downward. In this case, both the upper and lower borders of the liver may be detected 1 to 2 cm below the usual markers, but the liver span should still be between 6 and 12 cm. On the other hand, with the decrease in liver size after 50, you may find that the midclavicular liver span is somewhat less.

With decreased intestinal motility associated with aging, intestinal disorders are common in older adults, so be particularly sensitive to patient complaints and related findings in this regard. Constipation is a frequent complaint, and you are more likely to feel stool in the sigmoid colon. Accompanying complaints of gas and a sensation of bloatedness may be reflected with increased tympany on percussion.

Obstruction may be a problem with older adults, occurring as a result of hypokalemia, myocardial infarction, and infections such as pneumonia, septicemia, peritonitis, and pancreatitis. Vomiting, distention, and constipation can signal obstruction. The incidence of gastrointestinal cancer increases with age, with various symptoms that depend on the site of the tumor. Symptoms vary from dysphagia to nausea, vomiting, anorexia, and hematemesis to changes in stool frequency, size, consistency, or color. Most colon cancers are diagnosed by rectal examination, described in Chapter 14 (Anus, Rectum, and Prostate).

Pain perception may be altered as part of the aging process, and older patients may exhibit atypical pain symptoms, including less severe or totally absent pain with disease states that characteristically produce pain in younger adults. Therefore evaluation of pain in the older adult must take into account concurrent symptoms and accompanying findings.

Common Abnormalities

Musculature

Diastasis Recti Abdominis	Separation of the recti abdominis muscles is often caused by pregnancy or obesity. Raising the head and shoulders	from a supine position creates a visible midline bulge. The condition is of no clinical significance.
Incisional Hernia	This type of hernia is caused by a defect in the abdominal musculature that develops following surgical incision.	
Hernia of the Linea Alba	This type of hernia is felt as a small, tender, midline nodule, usually in the epigastrium.	
Strangulated Hernia	This is a nonreducible hernia in which the blood supply to the protruded tissue is obstructed. The condition requires immediate surgical intervention.	

Hepatobiliary System

Acute Hepatitis	Acute hepatitis is inflammation of the liver cells, often viral- or drug-induced, although it may result from a variety of causes. Symptoms include an enlarged	liver with a smooth, regular, tender border on palpation, abdominal discomfort, fatigue, nausea, malaise, and jaundice.
Chronic Hepatitis	Chronic inflammation of the liver may be self-limiting or progressive. Symptoms include fatigue, hepatomegaly,	abdominal discomfort, nausea, spider angiomas, and palmar erythema.

Cirrhosis	Cirrhosis is characterized by destruction of the liver parenchyma. The liver is usually enlarged with a firm nontender border on palpation. Associated symptoms include ascites, jaundice, prominent abdominal vasculature, cutaneous	spider angiomas, dark urine, light stools, and spleen enlargement. The patient often complains of fatigue, and in late stages muscle wasting may be evident.
Liver Carcinoma	Invasion of the liver by malignant cells produces liver enlargement and a hard, irregular border on palpation. Nodules may be present and palpable, and the	liver may be either tender or nontender. Associated symptoms can include ascites, jaundice, anorexia, fatigue, dark urine, and light-colored stools.
Cholelithiasis	Stone formation in the gallbladder is reponsible for most of the gallbladder diseases. Many patients are asymptomatic; however, symptoms of indiges-	tion, colic, and mild transient jaundice are not unusual. The condition commonly produces episodes of acute cholecystitis and pancreatitis.
Gallbladder Cancer	Invasion of the gallbladder by malignant cells produces abdominal pain, jaundice, and weight loss. A mass may be palpable in the upper abdomen.	

Pancreas

Chronic Pancreatitis	Chronic inflammation of the pancreas produces constant unremitting abdominal pain, epigastric tenderness, weight loss, and glucose intolerance.	
Pancreas Cancer	Invasion of the pancreas by malignant cells results in abdominal pain that radiates from the epigastrium to the upper quadrants or back, weight loss, anorexia, and jaundice.	

Kidneys

Glomerulonephritis	Inflammation of the capillary loops of the renal glomeruli usually produces nonspecific symptoms. The patient	complains of nausea, malaise, and arthralgias. Pulmonary infiltrates may be present.
Hydronephrosis	Hydronephrosis is the dilation of the renal pelvis from back pressure of urine that cannot flow past an obstruction in	the ureter. The patient experiences hematuria, pyuria, and fever, if secondary infection is present.
Pyelonephritis	Infection of the kidney and renal pelvis is characterized by flank pain, bacteriuria, pyuria, dysuria, nocturia, and fre-	quency. Costovertebral angle tenderness may be evident.

Renal Abscess	Renal abscess is a localized infection within the cortex of the kidney. The patient may complain of chills, fever,	and aching flanks. Fist percussion produces costovertebral angle tenderness.
Renal Calculi	Stone formation, usually in the renal pelvis, is characterized by hematuria, crystalluria, flank pain radiating to the	groin or genitals, and fever. The patient may pass one or more stones.
Acute Renal Failure	This is the sudden severe impairment of renal function causing an acute uremia episode. The impairment may be prerenal, renal, or postrenal. Urine output	may be normal, decreased, or absent. The patient may show signs of either fluid overload or deficit.
Chronic Renal Failure	Chronic renal failure is a slow, insidious, and irreversible impairment of renal function. Uremia usually develops	gradually. The patient may experience oliguria or anuria and have signs of fluid overload.
Renal Artery Emboli	Numerous small or a few major emboli produce occlusion of the renal artery, causing either acute or chronic renal failure. The condition may manifest itself	as a silent event or full blown syndrome of flank pain and tenderness, hematuria, hypertension, fever, and decreased renal function.
Urinary Incontinence	An involuntary release of urine may be temporary or chronic. Temporary incontinence may be the result of physio-	logic, psychologic, or mechanical factors. Chronic incontinence results from neurogenic factors.

INFANTS

Intussusception	The prolapse of one segment of the intestine into another causes intestinal obstruction. Intussusception commonly occurs in infants between 3 and 12 months of age. Symptoms include acute intermittent abdominal pain, abdominal distention, vomiting, and passage of one normal brown stool. Subsequent stools are mixed with blood and mucus with a red currant jelly appearance. A sausage-shaped mass may be palpated in	the right or left upper quadrant, while the lower quadrant feels empty. Intussusception in an infant can produce a dramatic onset. The apparently well child starts crying suddenly and excruciatingly, sometimes awakening from sleep. The child is inconsolable, sometimes doubling up with pain. The episode can cease abruptly, but the symptoms will most likely recur.
Umbilical Hernia	Some abdominal contents protrude through a congenital defect in the abdominal wall at the umbilical ring. The umbilicus often everts with increased abdominal pressure such as coughing or sneezing. Umbilical hernias can be very large and impressive. It is ordinarily easy to reduce them, pushing	the contents back into a more appropriate intraabdominal position. Usually, however, they pop right out again. The apparent size is not cause for alarm, and generally it pays to temporize. The greater number will resolve spontaneously with growth and development.

Pyloric Stenosis	Hypertrophy of the circular muscle of the pylorus leads to obstruction of the pyloric sphincter during the first month after birth. Symptoms include regurgitation progressing to projectile vomit-	ing, feeding eagerly (even after a vomiting episode), failure to gain weight, and signs of dehydration. A small rounded tumor is often palpable in the right upper quadrant after the infant vomits.
Meconium Ileus	A lower intestinal obstruction, caused by thickening and hardening of meconium in the lower intestine. It is identified by the failure to pass meconium in the	first 24 hours after birth and by abdominal distention. It is often the first manifestation of cystic fibrosis.
Biliary Atresia	Biliary atresia is a congenital obstruction or absence of a portion of the bile duct. Symptoms include jaundice that becomes apparent at 2 to 3 weeks of age,	hepatomegaly, abdominal distention, poor weight gain, and pruritis. Stools become lighter in color and urine darkens.
Meckel's Diverticulum	An outpouching of the ileum varies in size from a small appendiceal process to a segment of bowel several inches long, often in the proximity of the ileocecal valve. It is the most common congenital anomaly of the gastrointestinal tract.	The symptoms are those of intestinal obstruction or diverticulitis. In many cases the initial symptoms are bright or dark red rectal bleeding and little abdominal pain, although symptoms of acute appendicitis are not uncommon.
Gastroesophageal Reflux	Relaxation or incompetence of the lower esophagus persisting beyond the newborn period produces gastroesophageal reflux. Symptoms include vomit-	ing, which can be severe enough to cause weight loss and failure to thrive, respiratory problems from aspiration, and bleeding from esophagitis.
Necrotizing Enterocolitis	An inflammatory disease of the gastrointestinal mucosa, necrotizing enterocolitis is associated with prematurity and immaturity of the gastrointestinal tract.	Signs include abdominal distention, occult blood in stool, and respiratory distress. The condition is often fatal, complicated by perforation and septicemia.

CHILDREN

Neuroblastoma	The most common solid malignancy in early childhood, neuroblastoma frequently appears as a mass in the adrenal medulla of the young child, but a mass may occur anywhere along the craniospinal axis. A firm, fixed, nontender, irregular and nodular abdominal mass	that crosses the midline is often found. Symptoms include malaise, loss of appetite, weight loss, and protrusion of one or both eyes. Other symptoms arise from compression of the mass or metastases to adjacent organs.
Wilm's Tumor (Nephroblastoma)	Nephroblastoma, the most common intraabdominal tumor of childhood, usually appears at 2 to 3 years of age. It is a firm, nontender mass deep within the flank, only slightly moveable and	not usually crossing the midline. It is sometimes bilateral. Painless enlargement of the abdomen is the usual sign; however, a low-grade fever and hypertension may be present.

Hirschsprung's Disease (Congenital Aganglionic Megacolon)	The primary absence of parasympathetic ganglion cells in a segment of the colon interrupts the motility of the intestine. The absence of peristalsis causes feces to accumulate proximal to the defect, leading to an intestinal obstruction. Symptoms include failure	to thrive, constipation, abdominal distention, and episodes of vomiting and diarrhea. The newborn may fail to pass meconium in the first 24 to 48 hours after birth. Symptoms in older infants and young children are generally intestinal obstruction or severe constipation.

OLDER ADULTS

Diverticulitis	Inflammation of existing diverticula produces left lower quadrant pain, anorexia, nausea, vomiting, and altered bowel habits, usually constipation. The pain usually becomes localized at the site	of the inflammatory process. The abdomen may be distended and tympanic with decreased bowel sounds and localized tenderness.
Colon Cancer	Carcinoma of the colon usually occurs in the rectum, sigmoid, and lower descending colon, but it may also appear in the proximal colon. The earliest sign is usually occult blood in the stool. The patient often gives a history of changes in the frequency or character	of stool. There are few early physical findings unless a lesion is felt on rectal examination (see Chapter 14, Anus, Rectum, and Prostate). A tumor may be palpable in the right or left lower quadrant.

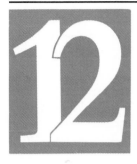
Female Genitalia

Anatomy and Physiology

External Genitalia

The vulva, or external genital organs, includes the mons pubis, labia majora, labia minora, clitoris, vestibular glands, vaginal vestibule, vaginal orifice, and urethral opening (Fig. 12-1). The symphysis pubis is covered by a pad of adipose tissue called the mons pubis or mons veneris, which in the postpubertal female is covered by coarse terminal hair. Extending downward and backward from the mons pubis are the labia majora, two folds of adipose tissue covered by skin. The labia majora vary in appearance, depending on the amount of adipose tissue present. The outer surfaces of the labia majora are also covered with hair in the postpubertal female.

Fig. 12-1
External female genitalia.
From Bobak and Jensen, 1984.

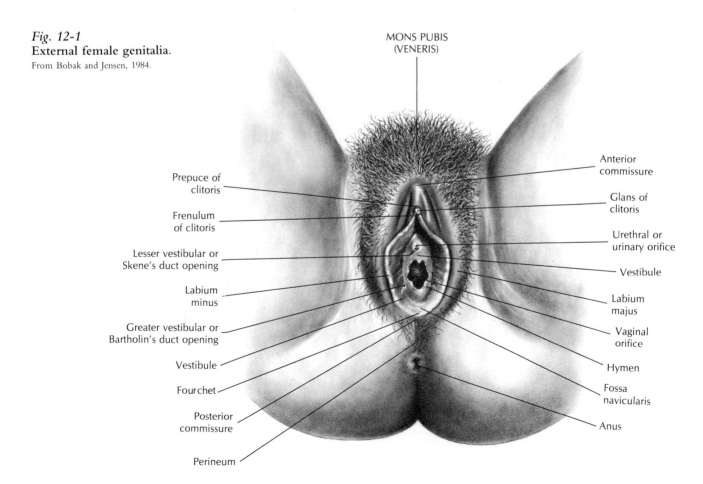

MONS PUBIS
(VENERIS)

Prepuce of clitoris

Frenulum of clitoris

Lesser vestibular or Skene's duct opening

Labium minus

Greater vestibular or Bartholin's duct opening

Vestibule

Fourchet

Posterior commissure

Perineum

Anterior commissure

Glans of clitoris

Urethral or urinary orifice

Vestibule

Labium majus

Vaginal orifice

Hymen

Fossa navicularis

Anus

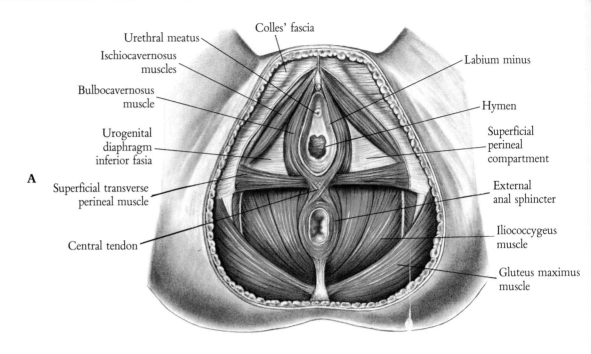

Fig. 12-2

A, Superficial musculature of the perineum. B, Deep musculature of the perineum.

From Thompson et al., 1986.

Lying inside and usually hidden by the labia majora are the labia minora, two hairless, flat, reddish folds. The labia minora meet at the anterior of the vulva where each labium divides into two lamellae, the lower pair fusing to form the frenulum of the clitoris and the upper pair forming the prepuce. Tucked in between the frenulum and the prepuce is the clitoris, a small bud of erectile tissue, the homologue of the penis and a primary center of sexual excitement. Posteriorly, the labia minora meet as two ridges that fuse to form the forchette.

The labia minora enclose the area designated as the vestibule, which contains six openings: the urethra, the vagina, two ducts of Bartholin's glands, and two ducts of Skene's glands. The lower two thirds of the urethra lies immediately above the anterior vaginal wall and terminates in the urethral meatus at the midline of the vestibule just above the vaginal opening and below the clitoris. Skene's ducts drain a group of urethral glands and open onto the vestibule on each side of the urethra. The ductal openings may be visible.

The vaginal opening occupies the posterior portion of the vestibule and varies in size and shape. Surrounding the vaginal opening is the hymen, a connective tissue membrane that may be circular, crescentic, or fimbriated. After the hymen tears and becomes permanently divided, the edges either disappear or cicatrize leaving hymenal tags. Bartholin's glands, located posteriorly on each side of the vaginal orifice, open onto the sides of the vestibule in the groove between the labia minora and the hymen. The ductal openings are not usually visible. During sexual excitement Bartholin's glands secrete mucus into the introitus for lubrication.

The pelvic floor consists of a group of muscles that form a supportive sling for the pelvic contents. The muscle fibers insert at various points on the bony pelvis and form functional sphincters for the vagina, rectum, and urethra (Fig. 12-2).

Internal Genitalia

The vagina is a musculomembranous tube that is transversely rugated during the reproductive phase of life. It inclines posteriorly at an angle of approximately 45 degrees with the vertical plane of the body (Fig. 12-3). The anterior wall of the vagina is separated from the bladder and urethra by connective tissue called the vesicovaginal septum. The posterior vaginal wall is separated from the rectum by the rectovaginal septum. Usually the anterior and posterior walls of the vagina lie in close proximity with only a small space between them. The upper end of the vagina is a blind vault into which the uterine cervix projects. The pocket formed around the cervix is divided into the anterior, posterior, and lateral fornices. These are of clinical importance since the internal pelvic organs can be palpated through their thin walls. The vagina carries menstrual flow from the uterus, serves as the terminal portion of the birth canal, and is the receptive organ for the penis during sexual intercourse.

The uterus sits in the pelvic cavity between the bladder and the rectum. It is an inverted pear-shaped muscular organ that is relatively mobile (Fig. 12-4). The uterus is covered by peritoneum and lined by the endometrium, which is shed during menstruation. The rectouterine cul-de-sac (pouch of Douglas) is a deep recess formed by the peritoneum as it covers the lower posterior wall of the uterus and upper portion of the vagina, separating it from the rectum. The uterus is flattened anteroposteriorly and usually inclines forward at a 45-degree angle, although it may be anteverted, anteflexed, retroverted, or retroflexed. In nulliparous women the size is approximately 5.5 to 8 cm long, 3.5 to 4 cm wide, and 2 to 2.5 cm thick. The uterus of a parous woman may be larger by 2 to 3 cm in any of the dimensions. The weight of a nonpregnant uterus is approximately 60 to 90 gm (Fig. 12-5).

Fig. 12-3
Midsagittal view of the female pelvic organs.

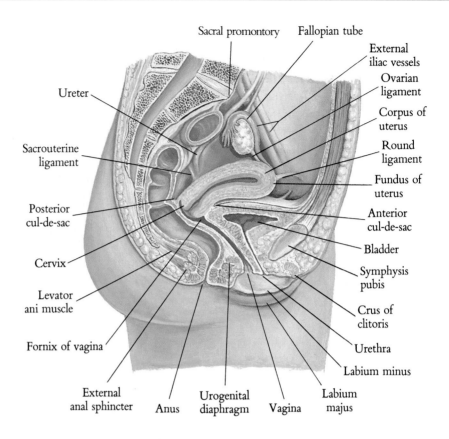

Fig. 12-4
Cross-sectional view of internal female genitalia and pelvic contents.

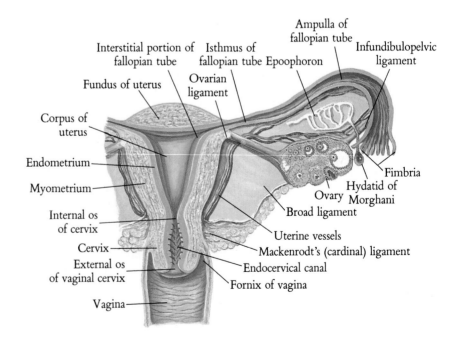

Fig. 12-5
Comparative sizes of pre-pubertal, adult nonparous, and multiparous uteri.
From Thompson et al., 1986.

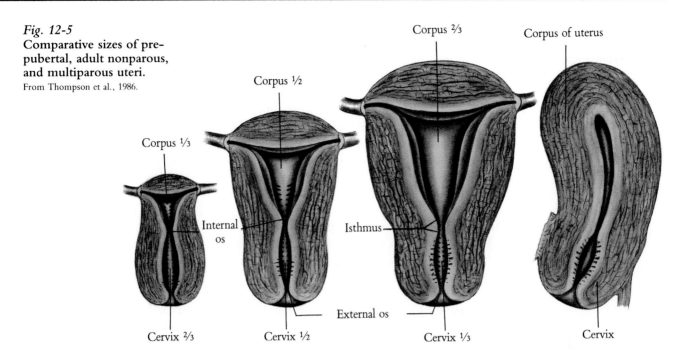

The uterus is divided anatomically into the corpus and cervix. The corpus consists of the fundus, which is the convex upper portion between the points of insertion of the fallopian tubes, the main portion or body, and the isthmus, which is the constricted lower portion adjacent to the cervix. The cervix extends from the isthmus into the vagina. The uterus opens into the vagina via the external cervical os.

The adnexae of the uterus are composed of the fallopian tubes and ovaries. The fallopian tubes insert into the upper portion of the uterus and extend laterally to the ovaries. Each tube ranges from 8 to 14 cm in length and is supported by a fold of the broad ligament called the mesosalpinx. The isthmus end of the fallopian tube opens into the uterine cavity. The fimbriated end opens into the pelvic cavity, with a projection that extends to the ovary and captures the ovum. Rhythmic contractions of the tubal musculature transport the ovum to the uterus.

The ovaries are a pair of oval organs resting in a slight depression on the lateral pelvic wall at the level of the anterosuperior iliac spine. The ovaries are approximately 3 cm long, 2 cm wide, and 1 cm thick in the adult woman during the reproductive years. Ovaries secrete estrogen and progesterone, which have several functions including controlling the menstrual cycle and supporting pregnancy.

The internal genitalia are supported by four pairs of ligaments: the cardinal, uterosacral, round, and broad ligaments.

INFANTS AND CHILDREN

The vagina of the female infant is a small narrow tube with fewer epithelial layers than that of the adult. The uterus is approximately 35 mm long with the cervix constituting about two thirds of the entire length of the organ. The ovaries are tiny and functionally immature. The labia minora are relatively avascular, thin, and pale. The labia majora are hairless and nonprominant. The hymen is a thin diaphragm just inside the introitus usually with a crescent-shaped opening in the midline. The clitoris is small.

During childhood the genitalia, except for the clitoris, grow incrementally at varying rates. Anatomic and functional development accelerates with the onset of puberty and the accompanying hormonal changes.

ADOLESCENTS

During puberty the external genitalia increase in size and begin to assume adult proportions. The clitoris becomes more erectile and the labia minora more vascular. The labia majora and mons pubis become more prominent and begin to develop hair, often occurring simultaneously with breast development. Chapter 3, Growth and Measurement, discusses growth changes and secondary sex characteristic developments that occur during puberty.

If the hymen is intact, the vaginal opening is about 1 cm in size. The vagina lengthens and the epithelial layers thicken. The vaginal secretions become acidic.

The uterus, ovaries, and fallopian tubes increase in size and weight. The uterine musculature and vascular supply increase. The endometrial lining thickens in preparation for the onset of menstruation (menarche), which usually occurs between the ages of 8 and 16 years. Just before menarche vaginal secretions increase. Functional maturation of the reproductive organs is reached during puberty.

PREGNANT WOMEN

The high levels of estrogen and progesterone that are necessary to support pregnancy are responsible for uterine enlargement during the first trimester. After the third month uterine enlargement is primarily the result of mechanical pressure of the growing fetus. As the uterus enlarges the muscular walls strengthen and become more elastic. As the uterus becomes larger and more ovoid, it rises out of the pelvis into the abdominal cavity. Uterine weight at term, excluding the fetus and placenta, will usually have increased more than tenfold, to a weight of about 1000 gm.

During pregnancy an increase in uterine blood flow and lymph causes pelvic congestion and edema. As a result, the uterus, cervix, and isthmus soften, and the cervix takes on a bluish color. The softness and compressibility of the isthmus results in exaggerated uterine anteflexion during the first 3 months of pregnancy, causing the fundus to press on the urinary bladder. The amount of vaginal secretions increase.

OLDER ADULTS

Concurrent with endocrine changes, ovarian function diminishes during a woman's 40s, and menstrual periods cease between 40 and 55 years of age (menopause). Just as menarche in the adolescent is one aspect of puberty, so menopause is only one aspect of this transitional phase of the life cycle. During this time, estrogen levels decrease causing the labia and clitoris to become smaller. The labia majora also become flatter as body fat is lost. Pubic hair turns gray and is usually more sparse.

The vaginal introitus gradually constricts. The vagina narrows, shortens, and loses its rugation, and the mucosa becomes thin, pale, and dry. The cervix becomes small and more pale. The uterus decreases in size, and the endometrium thins.

The ovaries also decrease in size to approximately 1 to 2 cm. Follicles gradually disappear, and the surface of the ovary convolutes. Ovulation usually ceases about 1 to 2 years before menopause.

The ligaments and connective tissue of the pelvis sometimes lose their elasticity and tone, thus weakening the supportive sling for the pelvic contents. The vaginal walls may lose some of their structural integrity.

Review of Related History

General Considerations

1. Menstrual history
   a. Age at menarche
   b. Date of last menstrual period: first day of last cycle
   c. Number of days in cycle and regularity of cycle
   d. Character of flow: amount (number of pads or tampons used in 24 hours), duration, presence of clots
   e. Dysmenorrhea: characteristics, duration, frequency (occur with each cycle?), relief measures
   f. Intermenstrual bleeding or spotting: amount, duration, frequency, timing in relation to phase of cycle
   g. Intermenstrual pain: severity, duration, timing
   h. Premenstrual symptoms: headaches, weight gain, edema, breast tenderness, irritability or mood changes, frequency (occur with every period?), interference with activities of daily living, relief measures
2. Obstetric history
   a. Gravity (number of pregnancies)
   b. Parity (number of births)
   c. Number of abortions: spontaneous or induced
   d. Complications of pregnancy, delivery, or abortion
   e. Number of living children
3. Douching history
   a. Frequency: length of time since last douche; number of years douching
   b. Method
   c. Solution used
   d. Reason for douching
4. Cleansing routines: use of sprays, powders, perfume, antiseptic soap, deodorants, or ointments
5. Contraceptive history
   a. Current method: length of time used, effectiveness, consistency of use, side effects, satisfaction with method
   b. Previous methods: duration of use for each, side effects, and reasons for discontinuing each
6. Sexual history
   a. Difficulties, concerns, problems
   b. Satisfaction with current practices and habits, with sexual relationship(s)
   c. Number of partners
   d. Sexual preference
7. Medications: prescription or over-the-counter
8. Date of last pelvic examination
9. Date of last Pap smear and results

Present Problem

1. Abnormal bleeding
    2. Character: shortened interval between periods (less than 19-21 days), lengthened interval between periods (more than 37 days), amenorrhea, prolonged menses (more than 7 days), bleeding between periods
    b. Change in flow: nature of change, number of pads or tampons used in 24 hours (tampons/pads soaked?), presence of clots
    c. Temporal sequence: onset, duration, precipitating factors, course since onset
    d. Associated symptoms: pain, cramping, abdominal distension, pelvic fullness, change in bowel habits, weight loss or gain
2. Pain
    a. Temporal sequence: date and time of onset, sudden *v* gradual onset, course since onset, duration, recurrence
    b. Character: specific location, type and intensity of pain
    c. Associated symptoms: vaginal discharge or bleeding, gastrointestinal symptoms, abdominal distention or tenderness, pelvic fullness
    d. Association with menstrual cycle: timing, location, duration, changes
    e. Relationship to body functions and activities: voiding, eating, defecation, flatus, exercise, walking up stairs, bending, stretching, sexual activity
    f. Aggravating or relief factors
    g. Previous medical care for this problem
    h. Effectiveness of treatment or medications (prescription or over-the-counter)
3. Vaginal discharge
    a. Character: amount, color, odor, consistency, changes in characteristics
    b. Occurrence: acute or chronic
    c. Medications: birth control pills, antibiotics
    d. Douching habits
    e. Clothing habits: use of cotton or ventilated underwear and pantyhose: tight pants or jeans
    f. Presence of discharge or symptoms in sexual partner
    g. Associated symptoms: itching; tender, inflamed, or bleeding external tissues; dyspareunia; dysuria or burning on urination; abdominal pain or cramping; pelvic fullness
4. Urinary symptoms: dysuria, burning or urination, frequency, urgency
    a. Character: acute or chronic; frequency of occurrence; last episode; onset; course since onset; feel like bladder is empty after voiding or not; pain at start, throughout, or at cessation of urination
    b. Description of urine: color, presence of blood or particles, clear or cloudy
    c. Associated symptoms: vaginal discharge or bleeding, abdominal pain or cramping, abdominal distention, pelvic fullness, flank pain

Past Medical History

1. Recent pregnancies, abortions, or gynecologic procedures
2. Past gynecologic procedures or surgery
3. Sexually transmitted diseases
4. Pelvic inflammatory disease
5. Vaginal infections
6. Diabetes
7. Cancer of reproductive organs

Family History

1. Diabetes
2. Cancer of reproductive organs
3. Mother received DES while pregnant with patient
4. Multiple pregnancies
5. Congenital anomalies

INFANTS AND CHILDREN

Usually no special questions are required unless there is a specific complaint from the parent or child.
1. Bleeding
   a. Character: onset, duration, precipitating factor if known, course since onset
   b. Age of menarche of mother
   c. Associated symptoms: pain, change in crying of infant, child fearful of parent or other adults
   d. Does the parent have any reason to suspect insertion of foreign objects by child?
   e. Does the parent have any reason to suspect sexual abuse?
2. Pain
   a. Character: type of pain, onset, course since onset, duration
   b. Specific location
   c. Associated symptoms: vaginal discharge or bleeding, urinary symtoms, gastrointestinal symptoms, child fearful of parent or other adults
   d. Contributory problems: use of bubble bath, irritating soaps or detergents; does parent have any reason to suspect insertion of foreign objects by child? does parent have any reason to suspect sexual abuse?
3. Vaginal discharge
   a. Relationship to diapers: use of powder or lotions, how frequently diapers are changed
   b. Associated symptoms: pain, bleeding
   c. Contributory problems: does parent have any reason to suspect insertion of foreign objects by child? does parent have any reason to suspect sexual abuse?

As the older child matures you should ask her the same questions that you ask any adult woman. You should not assume that youthful age precludes sexual activity or any of the related concerns. While taking the history it is necessary at some point to talk with the child alone while the parent is out of the room. Your questions should be posed gently, matter of factly, and nonjudgmentally.

OLDER ADULTS

1. Age at menopause or currently experiencing menopause
2. Menopausal symptoms: menstrual changes, mood changes, tension, back pain, hot flashes
3. Postmenopausal bleeding
4. Birth control measures during menopause
5. General feelings about menopause: self-image, effect on intimate relationships
6. Mother's experience with menopause
7. Symptoms related to physical changes: itching, urinary symptoms, dyspareunia
8. Changes in sexual desire or behavior: in self, in partner

Examination and Findings

- Speculum
- Gloves
- Water-soluble lubricant
- Lamp
- Sterile cotton swabs
- Glass slides
- Wooden or plastic spatula
- Cytologic fixative
- Culture plates

The pelvic examination is usually accompanied by some anxiety on the part of both the patient and the examiner. Some women may have had examinations in the past that were uncomfortable or embarrassing. There are several steps you can take to allay both your anxiety and the patient's. Explain in general terms what you are going to do. Ask the woman if she would like the opportunity to learn more about her own body during the examination. Maintain eye contact with the patient, both before and, as much as possible, during examination. This is a humanizing gesture that will not go unappreciated. Ask if this is her first pelvic examination. If she has not seen the equipment before, show it to her, and explain its use.

Assure the patient that you will explain to her what you are doing as the examination proceeds. Let her know that you will be as gentle as possible, and that if she feels any discomfort to let you know.

Make sure that the room is a comfortable temperature and that privacy is ensured. Lock the door if possible. A door or curtain that is left slightly ajar is unforgivable, and one that is opened suddenly and unexpectedly during the examination can undo all the rapport you may have established. Ask someone to be in the room with you to provide moral support for the patient and assistance for you, should you need it.

Have the patient empty her bladder before the examination. Bimanual examination is extremely uncomfortable for the woman if her bladder is full. A full bladder also makes it difficult to palpate the pelvic organs.

Assist the patient into the lithotomy position on the examining table. (If a table with stirrups is not available or if the woman is unable to assume the lithotomy position, examination can be performed, though less effectively, with the patient lying on her left side with her right thigh and knee drawn up to her chest.) Help the woman stabilize her feet in the stirrups and slide her buttocks down to the edge of the examining table. Place your hand at the edge of the table, and instruct her to move down until she touches your hand. If the patient is not positioned correctly, you will have difficulty with the speculum examination.

The patient can be draped in such a way that allows minimal exposure. A good method is to cover her knees and symphysis, depressing the drape between her knees. This allows you to see the woman's face (and she, yours) throughout the examination (Fig. 12-6).

Once the patient is positioned and draped, make sure that any equipment is nearby and in easy reach. Arrange the examining lamp so that the external genitalia are clearly visible. Wash your hands and put gloves on both hands.

Ask the woman to separate or spread her legs. Never try to spread her legs

Fig. 12-6
Draped patient in dorsal lithotomy position.

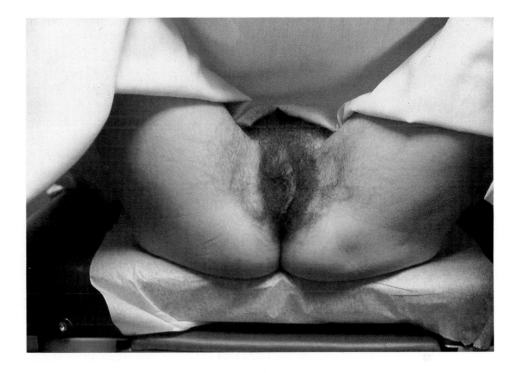

forcibly or even gently. The pelvic examination is an intrusive procedure, and you may need to wait a moment until the woman is ready. Tell her that you are going to begin, then start with a neutral touch on her lower thigh, moving your examining hand along the thigh without breaking contact to the external genitalia.

External Examination

Sit at the end of the examining table and inspect and palpate the external genitalia. Look at the hair distribution and notice the surface characteristics of the mons pubis and labia majora. The skin should be smooth and clean, the hair free of nits or lice. The labia majora may be gaping or closed and appear dry or moist. The labia majora are usually symmetric and may be either shriveled or full. The tissue should feel soft and homogeneous. Labial swelling, redness, or tenderness, particularly if unilateral, may be indicative of a Bartholin's gland abscess. Look for excoriation, rashes, or lesions, which suggest an infective or inflammatory process. If any of these signs are present, ask the woman if she has been scratching. Observe for discoloration, varicosities, obvious stretching, or signs of trauma or scarring.

Separate the labia majora with the fingers of one hand and inspect the labia minora. Use your other hand to palpate the labia minora between your thumb and second finger. Then separate the labia minora, and inspect and palpate the inside of the labia minora, the clitoris, urethral orifice, vaginal introitus, and perineum (Fig. 12-7).

The labia minora should appear symmetric, and the inner surface should be moist and dark pink. Note the fourchette. Hyperemia of the fourchette may indicate recent sexual activity. The tissue should feel soft and homogeneous, and no tenderness should be present. Look for inflammation, irritation, excoriation, or caking of discharge in the tissue folds, which suggests vaginal infection or poor hygiene. Discoloration or tenderness may be the result of traumatic bruising.

Ulcers or vesicles may be symptoms of a sexually transmitted disease. Feel for irregularities or nodules.

Inspect the clitoris for size and length. Generally the clitoris is about 2 cm or less in length and 0.5 cm in diameter. Enlargement may be a sign of a masculinizing condition. Observe also for atrophy, inflammation, or adhesions.

The urethral orifice appears as an irregular opening or slit. It may be close to or slightly within the vaginal introitus and is usually in the midline. Inspect for discharge, polyps, caruncles, and fistulas. Signs of irritation, inflammation, or dilation suggest repeated urinary tract infections or insertion of foreign objects. Ask questions regarding any findings at a later time—not during the pelvic examination when the woman feels most vulnerable.

The vaginal introitus can be a thin vertical slit or a large orifice with irregular edges from hymenal remnants (myrtiform caruncles). The tissue should be moist. Look for swelling, discoloration, discharge, lesions, fistulas, or fissures.

With the labia still separated, examine the Skene's glands and Bartholin's glands. Tell the woman you are going to insert one finger in her vagina and that she will feel you pressing forward with it. With your palm facing upward, insert the index finger of the examining hand into the vagina as far as the second joint of the finger. Exerting upward pressure, milk the Skene's glands by moving the finger outward. Do this on both sides of the urethra, and then directly on the urethra (Fig. 12-8). Look for discharge and note any tenderness. If a discharge occurs, note its color, consistency, and odor, and obtain a culture. Discharge from the Skene's glands or urethra usually indicates an infection, most frequently but not necessarily gonococcal.

Maintaining labial separation and with your finger still in the vaginal opening, tell the patient that she will feel you pressing around the entrance to the vagina. Palpate the lateral tissue between your index finger and thumb. Palpate the entire

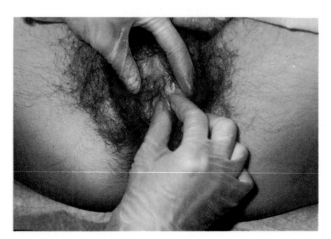

Fig. 12-7
Palpating the labia.

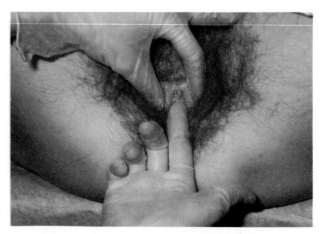

Fig. 12-8
Milking the urethra and paraurethral glands.

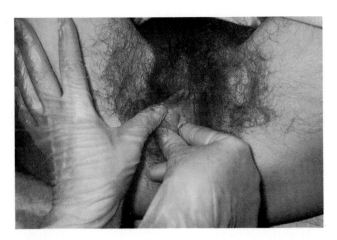

Fig. 12-9
Palpating around the vaginal introitus (Bartholin's glands).

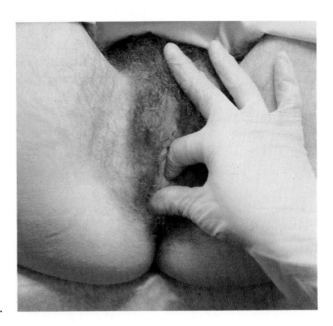

Fig. 12-10
Palpating the perineum.

area, paying particular attention to the posterolateral portion of the labia majora where the Bartholin's glands are located. Note any swelling, tenderness, masses, heat, or fluctuation. Observe for discharge from the opening of the Bartholin's gland duct. Palpate and observe bilaterally, since each gland is separate (Fig. 12-9). Note the color, consistency, and odor of any discharge, and obtain a specimen for culture. Swelling that is painful, hot to the touch, and fluctuant is indicative of an abscess of Bartholin's gland. The abscess is usually gonococcal or staphylococcal in origin and is pus filled. A nontender mass is indicative of a Bartholin's cyst, which is the result of chronic inflammation of the gland.

Ask the patient to squeeze the vaginal opening around your finger. Some nulliparous women can squeeze fairly tightly, some multiparous women less so. Then ask the patient to bear down as you watch for bulging and urinary incontinence. Bulging of the anterior wall and urinary incontinence indicate the presence of a cystocele. Bulging of the posterior wall indicates a rectocele. Uterine prolapse is marked by protrusion of the cervix or uterus on straining.

Inspect and palpate the perineum. The perineum surface should be smooth; episiotomy scarring may be evident in women who have borne children. The tissue will feel thick and smooth in the nulliparous women. It will be thinner and rigid in multiparous women. In either case, it should not be tender. Look for inflammation, fistulas, lesions, or growths (Fig. 12-10).

The anal surface is more darkly pigmented and the skin may appear coarse. It should be free of scarring, lesions, inflammation, fissures, lumps, skin tags, or excoriation. If you touch the anus or perianal skin, be sure to change your gloves so that you do not introduce bacteria into the vagina during the internal examination.

Internal Examination

Speculum

It is essential that you become familiar with how the speculum operates *before* you begin the examination, so that you do not inadvertently hurt the woman through mishandling of the instrument. Chapter 2, Examination Techniques and Equipment, details the proper use of the speculum. Become familiar with both the reuseable stainless steel and the disposable plastic specula, because the mechanism of action is somewhat different.

Lubricate the speculum (and the gloved fingers) with water only if you plan to obtain cytologic or any other studies, since gel lubricant interferes with specimen analysis. Otherwise, water-soluble lubricant may be used. Since studies may be indicated only after visualization of the vaginal walls and cervix, most clinicians routinely lubricate only with water. An added advantage of using water as a lubricant is that a cold speculum can be warmed by rinsing in warm (but not hot) water. A speculum can also be warmed by holding it in your hand or under the lamp for a few minutes.

Select the appropriate size speculum (see Chapter 2), and hold it in your hand with the index finger over the top of the proximal end of the anterior blade and the other fingers around the handle. This position controls the blades as the speculum is inserted into the vagina.

Tell the patient that she is going to feel you touching her again, and insert two fingers of your other hand just inside the vaginal introitus and apply pressure downward. Ask the woman to breathe slowly and to try to consciously relax her muscles. Wait until you feel the relaxation (Fig. 12-11, *A*). With fingers still in place, insert the closed speculum at an oblique angle over your fingers and directed at a 45-degree angle downward. The downward angle matches the anatomic angle of the vagina when the woman is in the lithotomy position and helps avoid trauma to the urethra and vaginal walls (Fig. 12-11, *B* and *C*).

Remove your fingers and rotate the speculum to a horizontal angle, inserting it the length of the vaginal canal. Avoid catching pubic hair or pinching labial skin. Maintaining downward pressure with the speculum, open it by pressing on the thumbpiece. Sweep the speculum slowly upward until the cervix comes into view. Adjust the light source. If the speculum was directed downward on insertion, you are assured of finding the cervix on the upward sweep, regardless of its position. This eliminates hunting for the cervix and avoids a lot of unnecessary up and down movement of the speculum, which is uncomfortable for the patient.

Once the cervix is visualized, manipulate the speculum a little further into the vagina so that the cervix is well exposed between the anterior and posterior blades. Tighten the thumbscrew on the thumbpiece to stabilize the distal spread of the blades. Adjust the proximal spread as needed (Fig. 12-11, *D*).

Inspect the cervix for color, position, size, surface characteristics, discharge, and size and shape of the os. The cervix should be pink, with the color evenly distributed. A bluish color indicates increased vascularity that may be a sign of pregnancy. Symmetric, circumscribed erythema around the os is a normal finding that indicates exposed columnar epithelium from the cervical canal. However, beginning practitioners should consider any reddened areas as an abnormal finding, especially if patchy or if the borders are irregular. A pale cervix is associated with anemia.

The position of the cervix correlates with the position of the uterus. A cervix that is pointing anteriorly indicates a retroverted uterus; one pointing posteriorly indicates an anteverted uterus. A cervix in the horizontal position indicates a uterus in midposition. The cervix should be located in the midline. Deviation to the right or

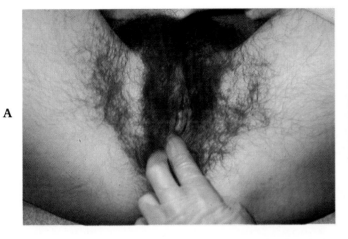

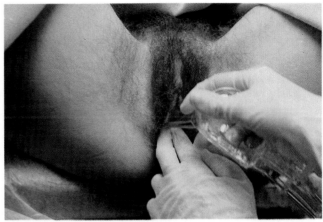

A   B

Fig. 12-11
A, Preparing for insertion of speculum: applying downward pressure in posterior vaginal opening with two fingers. **B,** Inserting closed speculum over fingers. **C,** Directing speculum downward at 45-degree angle. **D,** Speculum in place, locked, and stabilized. Note cervix in full view.

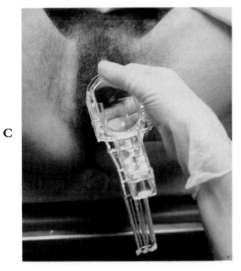

C

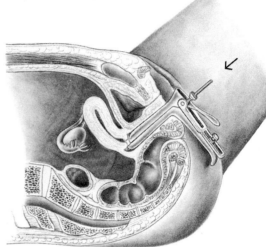

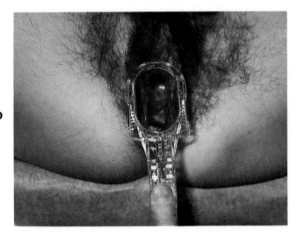

D

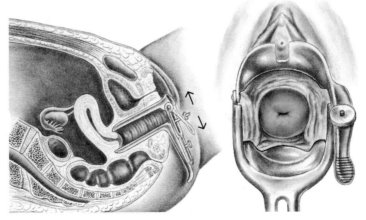

left may indicate a pelvic mass, uterine adhesions, or pregnancy. The cervix may protrude 1 to 3 cm into the vagina. Projection greater than 3 cm may indicate a pelvic or uterine mass. The cervix of a woman of childbearing age is usually 2 to 3 cm in diameter. An enlarged cervix is generally indicative of a cervical infection.

The surface of the cervix should be smooth. Some squamocolumnar epithelium of the cervical canal may be visible as a symmetric reddened circle around the os. Nabothian cysts may be observed as small, white or yellow, raised, round areas on

PROCEDURES FOR OBTAINING VAGINAL SMEARS AND CULTURES

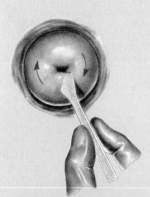

Scrape the cervix with the bifid end of the spatula for obtaining Papanicolaou smear.

Vaginal specimens are obtained after the cervix and surrounding tissue have been inspected and while the speculum is still in place in the vagina. Collect the Pap smear first, followed by gonococcal and other smears as indicated. It is important to label the specimen with the patient's name and a description of the specimen (e.g., cervical smear, vaginal smear, anal culture).

Papanicolaou smear. Insert the longer projection of the speculum into the cervical os. Rotate the spatula 360 degrees, keeping it flush against the cervical tissue. Withdraw the spatula and spread the specimen on a glass slide. A single light stroke with each side of the spatula is sufficient to thin the specimen out over the slide. Immediately spray with cytologic fixative and label the slide. Now introduce the rounded end of the spatula into the vagina and gently scrape over the posterior fornix to collect a vaginal pool specimen. Withdraw the spatula and prepare the glass slide as for the cervical specimen, labeling the slide as the vaginal pool specimen. Warn the patient that she may spot after this procedure.

Gonococcal culture specimen. Immediately after the Pap smear is obtained, introduce a sterile cotton swab into the vagina and insert it into the cervical os. Hold it in place for 10 to 30 seconds. Withdraw the swab and spread the specimen in a large **Z** pattern over the culture medium, rotating the swab at the same time. Label the tube or plate, and follow agency routine for transporting and warming the specimen. If indicated, a second specimen for culture from the anus can be obtained after the vaginal speculum has been removed. Insert a fresh sterile cotton swab about 2.5 cm into the rectum and rotate it full circle. Hold it in place for 10 to 30 seconds. Withdraw the swab and prepare the specimen as described for the vaginal culture.

Dry smear, wet prep, and KOH. Prepare the appropriate glass slides before you obtain the specimen. For *Haemophilus vaginalis* a dry glass slide is used; for *Trichomonas vaginalis* the secretions are mixed with a drop of saline on a glass slide; for *Candida albicans* the secretions are mixed with a drop of potassium hydroxide (KOH) solution on a glass slide. Introduce the plain wooden end of a sterile cotton swab into the vagina and roll it in the vaginal discharge. Withdraw the swab and smear the secretions on the dry slide or mix the sample in 2 drops of solution using a stirring, rolling motion. Cover the glass slides with coverslips and label the specimens. The slide is immediately examined under the microscope for characteristic cue cells of *H. vaginalis,* for trichomonads of *T. vaginalis,* or for mycelia and spores of *C. albicans.*

Fig. 12-12
A, Normal nulliparous
cervix. Note rounded os.
B, Normal parous cervix.
Note slit appearance of os.

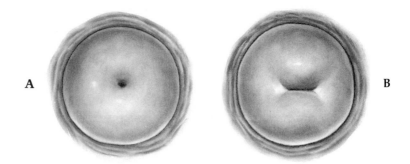

the cervix. These are retention cysts of the endocervical glands and are considered to be a normal finding. An infected nabothian cyst becomes swollen with fluid and distorts the shape of the cervix, giving it an irregular appearance. Look for friable tissue, red patchy areas, granular areas, and white patches that could indicate cervicitis, infection, or carcinoma.

Note any discharge. Determine whether the discharge comes from the cervix itself, or whether it is vaginal in origin and has only been deposited on the cervix. Normal discharge is odorless, may be creamy or clear, may be thick, thin, or stringy, and is often heavier at midcycle or immediately before menstruation. The discharge of a bacterial or fungal infection will more likely have an odor and will vary in color from white to yellow, green, or gray.

The os of the nulliparous woman is small, round, or oval. The os of a multiparous woman is usually a horizontal slit or may be irregular and stellate. Trauma from induced abortion or difficult removal of an intrauterine device may change the shape of the os to a slit (Fig. 12-12). Obtain specimens for Papanicolaou smear, culture, or other laboratory analysis.

Unlock the speculum and remove it slowly, rotating it during withdrawal so that you can inspect the vaginal walls. Note color, surface characteristics, and secretions. The color should be about the same pink as the cervix, or a little lighter. Reddened patches, lesions, or pallor indicates local or systemic pathology. The surface should be moist, smooth or rugated, and homogeneous. Look for cracks, lesions, bleeding, nodules, and swelling. Normal secretions that may be present are usually thin, clear or cloudy, and odorless. Secretions indicative of infection are often profuse; may be thick, curdy, or frothy; appear gray, green, or yellow; and may have a foul odor.

As the speculum is withdrawn, the blades will tend to close themselves. Avoid pinching the vaginal mucosa, and maintain downward pressure of the speculum to avoid trauma to the urethra. Hook your index finger over the anterior blade as it is removed. Note the odor of any vaginal discharge that has pooled in the posterior blade and obtain a specimen, if you have not already done so. Deposit the speculum in the proper container.

Bimanual Examination

Inform the woman that you are now going to examine her internally with your fingers. Remove the glove from one hand and lubricate the index and middle fingers of your examining hand. Insert the tips of the gloved index and middle fingers into the vaginal opening and press downward, again waiting for the muscles to relax. Gradually insert your fingers their full length into the vagina. Palpate the vaginal wall as you insert your fingers. It should be smooth, homogeneous, and nontender. Feel for cysts, nodules, masses, or growths.

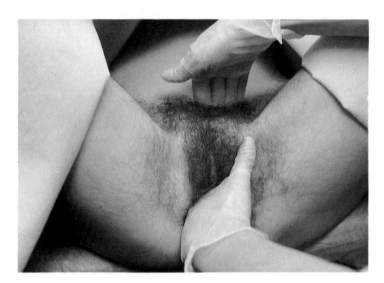

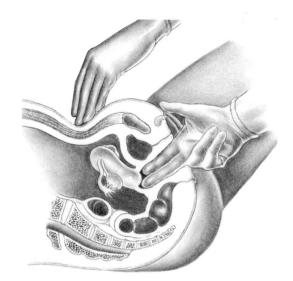

Fig. 12-13
Bimanual palpation of the uterus.

Be careful of where your thumb is during the bimanual examination. You can tuck it into the palm of your hand, but that will cut down on the distance you can insert your fingers. Just be aware of where it is and keep it from touching the clitoris, which is very uncomfortable for the woman (Fig. 12-13).

Locate the cervix with the palmar surface of your fingers, feel its end, and run your fingers around its circumference to feel the fornices. Feel the size, length, and shape, which should correspond with your observations from the speculum examination. The consistency of the cervix in a nonpregnant woman will be firm, like the tip of the nose, whereas during pregnancy the cervix is softer. Feel for nodules, hardness, and roughness. Note the position of the cervix as discussed in the speculum examination. The cervix should be in the midline and may be pointing anteriorly or posteriorly.

Grasp the cervix gently between your fingers and move it from side to side. Observe the patient for any expression of pain or discomfort with movement. The cervix should move 1 to 2 cm in each direction without discomfort. Painful cervical movement suggests a pelvic inflammatory process such as acute pelvic inflammatory disease or a ruptured tubal pregnancy. Insert the tip of one finger gently into the cervical os to evaluate its patency. The os should admit the fingertip 0.5 cm.

Palpate the uterus. Place the palmar surface of your other hand on the abdominal midline, midway between the umbilicus and the symphysis pubis. Place the intravaginal fingers in the anterior fornix. Slowly slide the abdominal hand toward the pubis pressing downward and forward with the flat surface of your fingers. At the same time, push inward and upward with the fingertips of the intravaginal hand while you push downward on the cervix with the backs of your fingers. Think of it as trying to bring your two hands together as you press down on the cervix. If the uterus is anteverted or anteflexed (the position of most uteri) you will feel the fundus between the fingers of your two hands at the level of the pubis (Fig. 12-14, *A* and *B*).

If you do not feel the uterus with the previous maneuver, place the intravaginal fingers together in the posterior fornix, with the abdominal hand immediately above the symphysis pubis. Press firmly downward with the abdominal hand while you press against the cervix inward with the other hand. A retroverted or retroflexed uterus should be felt with this maneuver (Fig. 12-14, *C* and *D*).

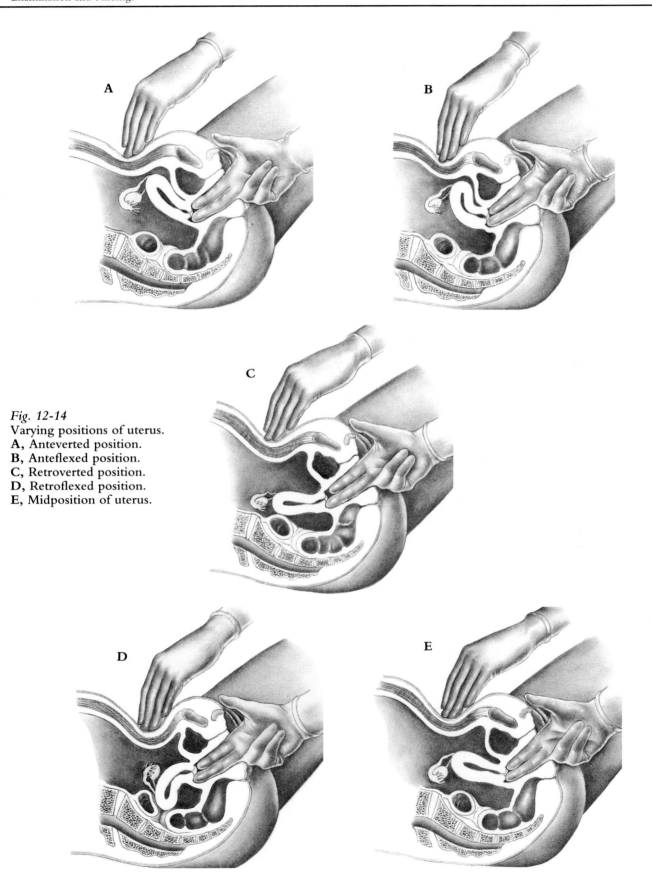

Fig. 12-14
Varying positions of uterus.
A, Anteverted position.
B, Anteflexed position.
C, Retroverted position.
D, Retroflexed position.
E, Midposition of uterus.

If you still cannot feel the uterus, move the intravaginal fingers to each side of the cervix. Keeping contact with the cervix, press inward and feel as far as you can. Then slide your fingers so that one is on top of the cervix and one is underneath. Continue pressing inward while moving your fingers to feel as much of the uterus as you can. When the uterus is in the midposition, you will not be able to feel the fundus with the abdominal hand (Fig. 12-14, E).

Confirm the location and position of the uterus by comparing your inspection findings with your palpation findings. The uterus should be located in the midline, regardless of its position. Deviation to the right or left is indicative of possible adhesions, pelvic masses, or pregnancy. Knowing the position of the uterus is essential before performing any intrauterine procedure, including insertion of an intrauterine contraceptive device.

Palpate the uterus for size, shape, and contour. It should be pear-shaped and 5.5 to 8 cm long, although it is larger in all dimensions in multiparous women. A uterus larger than expected in a woman of childbearing age is indicative of pregnancy or tumor. The contour should be rounded, and the walls should feel firm and smooth in the nonpregnant woman. The contour and smoothness will be interrupted by pregnancy or tumor.

Gently move the uterus between the intravaginal hand and abdominal hand to assess for mobility and tenderness. The uterus should be mobile in the anteroposterior plane. A fixed uterus indicates adhesions. Tenderness on movement suggests a pelvic inflammatory process or ruptured tubal pregnancy.

Palpate the adnexal areas and ovaries. Place the fingers of your abdominal hand on the right lower quadrant. With the intravaginal hand facing upward, place both fingers in the right lateral fornix. Press the intravaginal fingers deeply inward and upward toward the abdominal hand, while at the same time sweeping the flat surface of the fingers of the abdominal hand deeply inward and obliquely downward toward the symphysis pubis. Palpate the entire area by firmly pressing the abdominal hand and intravaginal fingers together. Repeat the maneuver on the left side (Fig. 12-15).

Fig. 12-15
Bimanual palpation of adnexa. Sweep abdominal fingers downward to capture ovary.

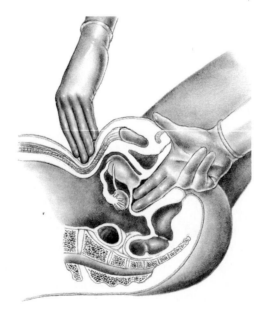

The ovaries, if palpable, should feel firm, smooth, ovoid, and approximately $3 \times 2 \times 1$ cm in size. The healthy ovary is slightly to moderately tender on palpation. Marked tenderness, enlargement, and nodularity are abnormal. Usually no other structures are palpable except for round ligaments. Fallopian tubes are usually not palpable, so a problem may exist if they are felt. You are also palpating for adnexal masses, and if any are found they should be characterized by size, shape, location, consistency, and tenderness.

The adnexae are frequently difficult to palpate because of their location and position, and the presence of excess adipose tissue in some women. If you are unable to feel anything in the adnexal areas with thorough palpation, you can assume that no abnormality is present, provided no clinical symptoms exist.

Rectovaginal Examination

The rectovaginal exploration is an important part of the total pelvic examination. It allows you to reach almost 2.5 cm (1 in) higher into the pelvis, which enables you to better evaluate the pelvic organs and structures. It is, however, an uncomfortable examination for the patient, and she may ask you to omit it. Nevertheless, it is important to perform, and you should explain to the woman why it is necessary.

As you complete the bimanual examination, withdraw your examining fingers. Some clinicians withdraw their fingers entirely, change gloves, and relubricate their fingers. Others leave their index finger in the vagina, withdraw their middle finger entirely, and relubricate it. Either method is acceptable, as long as there has been no clinical evidence of infection. If you suspect infection, change gloves to avoid introducing organisms into the rectum. Because of the risk of asymptomatic gonorrhea, it is more prudent in our view to change gloves as a matter of routine.

Tell the patient that the examination may be uncomfortable and that she may feel the urgency of a bowel movement. Assure her that she will not have one, and ask her to breathe slowly and consciously try to relax her sphincter, rectum, and buttocks, since tightening the muscles make the examination more uncomfortable for her.

Press your middle finger against the anus and ask the patient to bear down. As she does slip the tip of the finger into the rectum just past the sphincter. Palpate the area of the anorectal junction and just above it. Ask the woman to tighten and relax her anal sphincter. Observe sphincter tone. An extremely tight sphincter may be the result of anxiety about the examination, may be caused by scarring, or may indicate spasticity caused by fissures, lesions, or inflammation. A lax sphincter suggests neurologic deficit, while an absent sphincter may result from improper repair of third degree perineal laceration after childbirth or trauma.

Slide both your vaginal and rectal fingers in as far as they will go, then ask the woman to bear down. This will bring an additional centimeter within reach of your fingers. Rotate the rectal finger to explore the anterior rectal wall for masses, polyps, nodules, strictures, irregularities, and tenderness. The wall should feel smooth and uninterrupted. Palpate the rectovaginal septum along the anterior wall for thickness, tone, and nodules. You may feel the uterine body and occasionally the uterine fundus in a retroflexed uterus.

Press firmly and deeply downward with the abdominal hand just above the symphysis pubis while you position the vaginal finger in the posterior vaginal fornix, and press strongly upward against the posterior side of the cervix. Palpate as much of the posterior side of the uterus as possible, confirming your findings from

Fig. 12-16
Rectovaginal palpation.

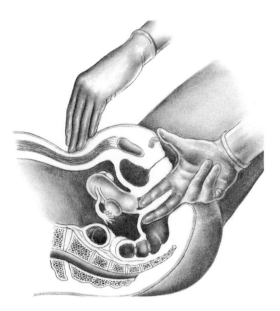

the vaginal examination regarding location, position, size, shape, contour, consistency, and tenderness of the uterus. This maneuver is particularly useful in evaluating a retroverted uterus (Fig. 12-16).

If you were unable to palpate the adnexal areas on bimanual examination or if the findings were questionable, repeat the adnexal examination using the same maneuvers described in the bimanual examination.

As you withdraw your fingers, rotate the rectal finger to evaluate the posterior rectal wall just as you did earlier for the anterior wall. Gently remove your examining fingers and observe for secretions and stool. Note the color and presence of any blood. Prepare a specimen for hemocult testing. Wipe off any secretions, discharge, and lubricating jelly from the woman's perineum, using a front-to-back stroke and a clean tissue for each stroke.

Assist the woman into a sitting position and give her the opportunity to regain her equilibrium and composure. Provide a sanitary pad if she is menstruating. Share with her the findings and ask her to voice her feelings about the examination. This conversation may be brief, but it should never be avoided.

INFANTS

The appearance of the external genitalia can help in the assessment of gestational age in the newborn. Examination is conducted with the infant's legs held in a frog position. The labia majora appear widely separated, and the clitoris is prominent up to 36 weeks of gestation, but by full term the labia majora completely cover the labia minora and clitoris.

The newborn's genitalia reflect the influence of maternal hormones. The labia majora and minora may be swollen, with the labia minora often more prominent. The hymen is often protruding, thick, and vascular, and it may simulate an extruding mass. These are all transient phenomena and will disappear in a few weeks (Fig. 12-17).

The clitoris may appear relatively large and usually has no significance. True hypertrophy is not common; however, an enlarged clitoris must always suggest adrenal hyperplasia when seen in the newborn.

Fig. 12-17
Female genitalia in infant.

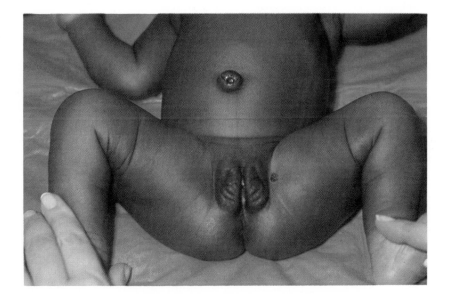

The central opening of the hymen is usually about 0.5 cm in diameter. It is important to determine the presence of an opening. However, make no effort to stretch the hymen. An imperforate hymen is rare but can cause difficulty later on, including hydrocolpos in the child, and hematocolpos in the adolescent.

Malformations in the external genitalia are often difficult to define. If the baby was a breech delivery, her genitalia may be swollen and bruised for many days after delivery. Any ambiguous appearance or unusual orifice in the vulvar vault or perineum must be expeditiously explored before the infant is inappropriately assigned a gender.

A mucoid whitish vaginal discharge is frequently seen during the newborn period and sometimes as late as 4 weeks after birth. The discharge is occasionally mixed with blood. This is the result of passive hormonal transfer from the mother and is an expected finding.

Thin but difficult to separate adhesions between the labia minora are often seen during the first few months or even years of life. Sometimes they completely cover the vulvar vestibule. There may be just the smallest of openings by which urine can escape. These may require separation, perhaps by the gentlest of teasing or the application of estrogen creams.

Vaginal discharges in infants and young children may occur as the result of irritation from the diaper or powder. These discharges are usually mucoid.

CHILDREN

The extent of the gynecologic examination depends on the child's age and complaints. For the well child the examination includes only inspection and palpation of the external genitalia. The internal vaginal examination is performed on a young child only when there is a specific problem. Speculum examination on a young child requires special equipment and an experienced and knowledgable gynecologist or pediatrician.

The young child usually cooperates with examination of the external genitalia if your approach is very matter of fact. The very young child can lie in the parent's lap, with the parent holding her legs in a frog position. The preschool child can be placed on the examining table, lying back against the head of the table, which should be raised about 30 degrees. The parent can help the child hold her legs up in a frog position.

A school-age child will not like the examination but is likely to cooperate if you take the time to reassure her that you will only look and touch the outside. You might have the child help by taking her hand and first having her touch herself. She should be positioned on the table on her back with her knees flexed and drawn up. The examination should be approached with the same degree of respect and caution as with the adult woman.

It is appropriate to have another person chaperone during examination of the genitalia. However, the older child should be consulted about this arrangement.

Inspect the perineum, all the structures of the vulvar vestibule, and the urethral and vaginal orifices by separating the labia with the thumb and forefinger of one hand.

Bartholin's and Skene's glands are usually not palable, and if they are, enlargement exists. This indicates infection, which is most often (but not always) gonococcal. Ask the girl to cough and observe the hymen. An imperforate hymen will bulge, whereas one with an opening will not.

A vaginal discharge often irritates the perineal tissues, causing redness and perhaps excoriation. Other sources of perineal irritation are bubble baths, soaps, detergents, and urinary tract infections. Carefully question the parent for a history of hematuria, dysuria, or other symptoms that would indicate urinary tract infection. A foul odor is more likely indicative of a foreign body (particularly in preschool children), especially if a secondary infection is present. Vaginal discharge may also result from trichomonal, gonococcal, or monilial infection.

Swelling of vulvar tissues, particularly if accompanied by bruising or foul smelling discharge should alert you to the possibility of sexual abuse, which unfortunately is common in our society. It must always be suspected if a young child has a sexually transmitted disease or if there is injury to the external genitalia. Injuries to the softer structure of the external genitalia are *not* caused by bicycle seats. A straddle injury from a bicycle seat is generally evident over the symphysis pubis where the structures are more fixed. The injuries resulting from sexual molestation are generally more posterior and may involve the perineum grossly. Such findings cannot be ignored, and careful questioning of the parent is mandatory.

Vaginal bleeding in children is often the result of injury, manipulation with foreign bodies, or sexual abuse. Occasionally there may be an ovarian tumor or carcinoma of the cervix. Remember, too, that some girls begin menstruation well before the expected time.

Occasionally, a rectal examination may be indicated to determine the presence or absence of the uterus or the presence of foreign bodies in the vagina. The rectal examination is performed with the patient lying on her back, feet held together, knees bent upon the abdomen. Place one hand on her knees to steady the child, slipping the examining finger into the rectum. Most examiners prefer the index finger, but this is not mandatory. Once your finger is introduced, you may release the legs and use your free hand to simultaneously palpate the abdomen. If the child is old enough to cooperate, have her pant like a puppy to relax the muscles. Foreign bodies will be palpable, as will the cervix. The ovaries are not usually felt. There may be bleeding and even a transient mild rectal prolapse after the examination, so be sure to warn the parent of this.

The adolescent requires the same examination and positioning as the adult. Ask if this is the young woman's first gynecologic examination. The first examination is perhaps the most important, because it will set the stage for how she views future examinations. Take all the time necessary to explain to her what you will be doing. Use models or illustrations to show her what will happen and what you will look for. An adolescent should be allowed the privacy, if she desires, of having the examination without her parent present. This can also provide an opportunity to talk with her in private.

Choose the appropriate size speculum. A pediatric speculum with blades that are 1 to 1.5 cm wide can be used and should cause minimal discomfort. If the adolescent is sexually active, a small adult speculum may be used.

As the girl goes through puberty you will see the maturational changes of sexual development (see Chapter 3, Growth and Measurement). Just before menarche there is a physiologic increase in vaginal secretions. The hymen may or may not be stretched across the vaginal opening. By menarche the opening should be at least 1 cm wide. As the adolescent matures, the findings are the same as those for the adult.

The gynecologic examination for the pregnant woman follows the same procedure as that for the nonpregnant adult woman. In early pregnancy you can feel a softening of the isthmus while the cervix is still firm (Hegar's sign). In the second month of pregnancy the cervix acquires its bluish color (Chadwick's sign) from increased vascularity. The cervix itself softens and will feel more like lips (Goodell's sign) rather than like the firmness of the nose tip. You will also notice increased vaginal secretions as a result of increased vascularity. None of these findings is perfectly sensitive or specific for detecting pregnancy and should not replace human chorionic gonadotropin (HCG) testing.

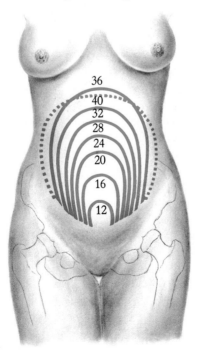

Fig. 12-18
Changes in fundal height with pregnancy.
Weeks 10-12: Uterus within pelvis; fetal heartbeat can be detected with Doppler.
Week 12: Uterus palpable just above symphysis pubis.
Week 16: Uterus palpable halfway between symphysis and umbilicus; ballottement of fetus possible by abdominal and vaginal examination.
Week 20: Uterine fundus at lower border of umbilicus; fetal heartbeat can be auscultated with fetoscope.
Weeks 24-26: Uterus changes from globular to ovoid shape; fetus palpable.
Week 28: Uterus approximately halfway between umbilicus and xiphoid; fetus easily palpable.
Week 34: Uterine fundus just below xiphoid.
Week 40: Fundal height drops as fetus begins to engage in pelvis.
Adapted from Malasanos et al., 1986.

The uterus may become more anteflexed during the first 3 months from softening of the isthmus. As a result the fundus may press on the urinary bladder, causing the woman to experience urinary frequency.

Early uterine enlargement may not be symmetric, and you may feel deviation of the uterus to one side and an irregularity in its contour at the site of implantation. This uterine irregularity occurs around week 8 to 10 (Piskacek's sign).

Changes in fundal height at the various weeks of gestation are shown in Fig. 12-18 along with some changes that are detectable on examination. Breast and skin changes that occur with pregnancy are discussed in Chapter 10. (Breasts and Axillae).

OLDER ADULTS

The examination procedure for the older adult is the same as that for the adult of childbearing age, with a few modifications for comfort. The older woman may require more time and assistance to assume the lithotomy position. She may need assistance from another individual to help hold her legs, since they may tire easily when the hip joints remain in abduction for an extended period. Patients with orthopnea will need to have their head and chest elevated during examination. You may need to use a smaller speculum depending upon the degree of introital constriction that occurs with aging.

Note that the labia appear flatter and smaller, corresponding with the degree of loss of subcutaneous fat elsewhere on the body. The skin is drier and shinier than that of a younger adult, and the pubic hair is gray and may be sparse. The clitoris is smaller than that of a younger adult.

The urinary meatus may appear as an irregular opening or slit. It may be located more posteriorly, very near, or within the vaginal introitus as a result of relaxed perineal musculature.

The vaginal introitus may be constricted and admit only one finger. In some multiparous older women the introitus may gape with the vaginal walls rolling toward the opening.

The vagina is narrower and shorter, and you will see and feel the absence of rugation. The cervix is smaller and paler than in younger women, and the surrounding fornices may be smaller or absent. The cervix may seem less mobile if it protrudes less far into the vaginal canal. The os may be smaller but should still be palpable.

The uterus diminishes in size and may not be palpable, and the ovaries are rarely palpable because of atrophy. Ovaries that are palpable should be considered suspicious for tumor, and additional workup, such as ultrasonography, to exclude cancer is required.

The rectovaginal septum will feel thin, smooth, and pliable. Anal sphincter tone may be somewhat diminished. Since the pelvic musculature relaxes, look particularly for stress incontinence and prolapse of the vaginal walls or uterus.

As with younger women, as you inspect and palpate you are evaluating for signs of inflammation (older women are particularly susceptible to atrophic vaginitis), infection, trauma, tenderness, growths, masses, nodules, enlargement, irregularity, and changes in consistency.

Common Abnormalities

Premenstrual Syndrome (PMS)	Premenstrual syndrome usually begins in a woman's late 20s and increases in incidence and severity as menopause approaches. It is characterized by edema, headache, weight gain, and behav-	ioral disturbances such as irritability, nervousness, dysphoria, and lack of coordination. Symptoms occur 5 to 7 days before menses and subside with onset of menses.

Infertility	The inability to conceive over a period of 1 year of unprotected intercourse has many causes, including both male and female conditions. Contributing factors in the woman include abnormalities of the vagina, cervix, uterus, fallopian tubes, and ovaries. Male infertility can be caused by insufficient, nonmotile, or	immature sperm; ductal obstruction of sperm; and transport-related factors. Factors influencing both women and men include stress, nutrition, chemical substances, chromosomal abnormalities, certain disease processes; sexual and relationship problems, and immunologic response.

Endometriosis

The presence and growth of endometrial tissue outside the uterus causes pelvic pain, dysmenorrhea, and heavy or prolonged menstrual flow. On bimanual examination tender nodules may be palpable along the uterosacral ligaments. Diagnosis is confirmed by laparoscopy (Fig. 12-19).

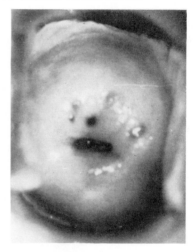

**Fig. 12-19
Superficial endometriosis of ectocervix, resembling hemorrhagic nabothian cysts.**
From Gardner and Kaufman, 1969.

Lesions from Sexually Transmitted Diseases

Condyloma Acuminatum (Venereal Warts)

Warty lesions on the labia, within the vestibule, or in the perianal region are the result of papilloma virus infection.

Venereal warts are sexually transmitted (Fig. 12-20).

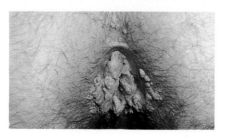

**Fig. 12-20
Condyloma acuminatum.**
Courtesy Antoinette Hood, M.D.

Condyloma Latum

Lesions of secondary syphilis appear about 6 to 12 weeks after infection. They are flat, round, or oval papules

covered by a gray exudate (Fig. 12-21).

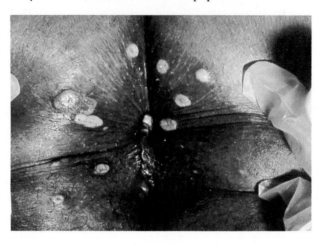

Fig. 12-21
Condyloma latum.
Courtesy Antoinette Hood, M.D.

Syphilitic Chancre (Primary Syphilis)

A syphilitic chancre is a firm, painless ulcer. Most chancres in women develop internally and often go undetected (Fig. 12-22).

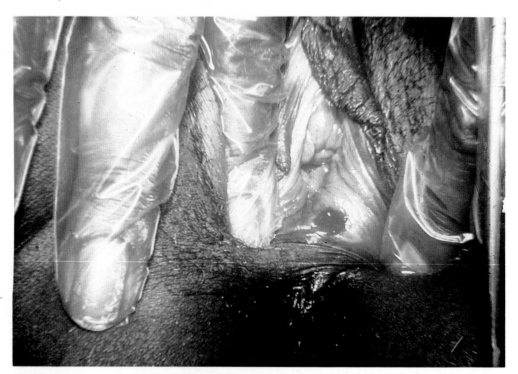

Fig. 12-22
Primary syphilitic chancre in vagina.
From Habif, 1985.

Herpes Lesions

Venereal herpes is a sexually transmitted disease that produces small red vesicles. The lesions may itch and are usually painful. Initial infection is often extensive, whereas recurrent infection is usually confined to a small localized patch on the vulva, perineum, vagina, or cervix (Fig. 12-23).

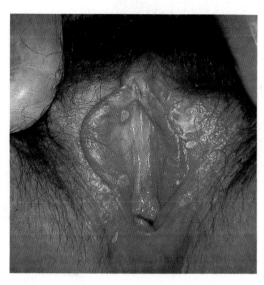

Fig. 12-23
Herpes lesions.
From Habif, 1985.

Vulva and Vagina

Inflammation of Bartholin's Gland

Inflamed Bartholin's glands are commonly but not always caused by gonococcal infection. It may be acute or chronic. Acute inflammation produces a hot, red, tender, fluctuant swelling that may drain pus. Chronic inflammation results in a nontender cyst on the labium (Fig. 12-24).

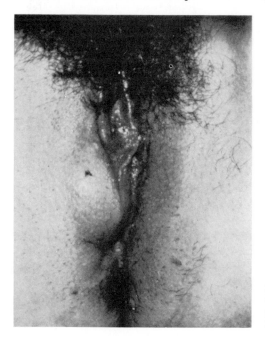

Fig. 12-24
Inflammation of Bartholin's glands.
From Gardner and Kaufman, 1969.

Cystocele

A cystocele is a hernial protrusion of the urinary bladder through the anterior wall of the vagina, sometimes even exiting the introitus. The bulging can be seen and felt as the woman bears down. More severe degrees of cystocele are accompanied by urinary stress incontinence (Fig. 12-25).

Fig. 12-25
Cystocele.

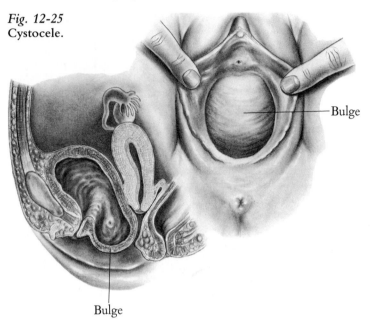

Bulge

Bulge

Rectocele

Hernial protrusion of part of the rectum through the posterior wall of the vagina is called rectocele or proctocele. Bulging can be observed and felt as the woman bears down. (Fig. 12-26).

Fig. 12-26
Rectocele.

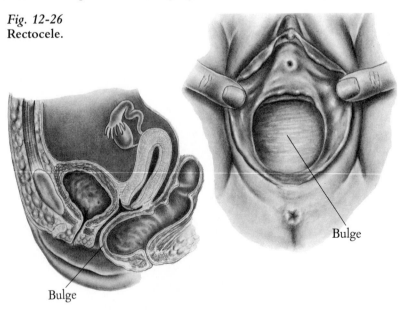

Bulge

Bulge

Carcinoma

Vaginal cancer in young women may be related to in utero DES exposure. Findings include vaginal discharge, lesions, and masses, and there may be a history of spotting, pain, and change in urinary habits. Cancer of the vulva appears as an ulcerated or raised red lesion on the vulva (Fig. 12-27).

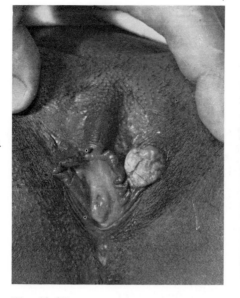
A

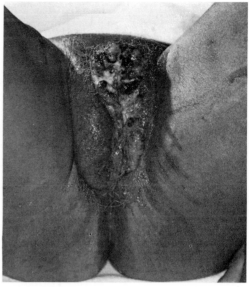
B

Fig. 12-27
A, Well-differentiated carcinoma of vulva. B, Advanced carcinoma of vulva, involving entire vagina, urethra, and rectum.
From Willson et al., 1983.

Urethral Caruncle

A bright red polypoid growth that protrudes from the urethral meatus, most urethral caruncles cause no symptoms (Fig. 12-28).

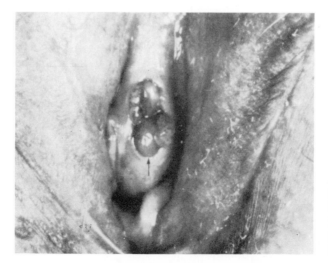

Fig. 12-28
Urethral caruncle, a red fleshy lesion at urethral meatus.
From Gardner and Kaufman, 1969.

Vaginal Infections

Vaginal infections often produce a vaginal discharge and may be accompanied by urinary and other symptoms. However, symptoms may be entirely absent.

Vaginal infections can be sexually transmitted, although candidal infections can result from antibiotics, oral contraceptives, and systemic disease.

Microorganism	Discharge	Erythema/ Itching	Associated Symptoms	Diagnosis
Neisseria gonorrhoeae	Yellow/green or may be absent; from cervical os	Cervix and vulva may be inflamed	Dysuria, frequency; discharge from Skene's glands on milking; symptoms of pelvic inflammatory disease (PID) may be present	Culture
Chlamydia trachomatis	Most infections are asymptomatic; may have muco-purulent discharge from cervical os; occurs with gono-coccal infection, urethritis, muco-purulent cervicitis, and PID			Tissue culture
Candida albicans	Scant to moderate; may be thin but usually thick, white, curdy, adherent	Mild to severe itching and erythema of labia, thighs, perineum; cervix may be red and edematous	Dysuria, frequency, dyspareunia	Potassium hydroxide (KOH)
Trichomonas vaginalis	Copius, frothy, yellow/green; strong, foul odor	Severe itching of vulva, with or without erythema; petechiae of cervix and vagina	Dysuria and dyspareunia with severe infection	Wet prep
Haemophilus vaginalis	Scant or moderate; homogeneous, grey, foul odor	Mild or absent		Wet prep

Cervix

Lacerations

Cervical lacerations are caused by trauma, most often childbirth. Lacerations can produce lateral transverse, bilateral transverse, or stellate scarring (Fig. 12-29).

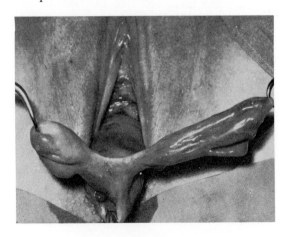

Fig. 12-29
Severely lacerated cervix with hypertrophy and prolapse.
From Willson et al., 1983.

Infected Nabothian Cysts	Enlarged fluid-filled retention cysts often distort the shape of the cervix. Infected nabothian cysts vary in size and may occur singly or in multiples.
Cervical Polyp	Cervical polyps are bright red, soft, and fragile. They usually arise from the endocervical canal.

Cervical Carcinoma

Cervical cancer produces a hard granular surface at or near the cervical os. The lesion can evolve to form an extensive irregular cauliflower growth that bleeds easily. Early lesions are indistinguishable from ectropion (Fig. 12-30).

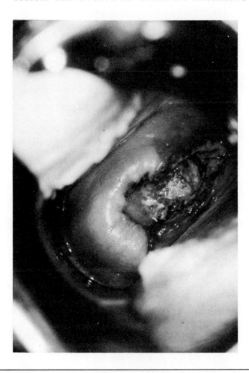

Fig. 12-30
Ulcerative squamous cell, carcinoma of the cervix.
From DiSaia and Creasman, 1984.

Ectropion

Columnar epithelium from the cervical canal appears as shiny red tissue around the os that may bleed easily. Ectropion is not an abnormality, but because it is indistinguishable from early cervical carcinoma, further diagnostic studies (Pap smear, biopsy) must be performed for differential diagnosis.

Uterus

Uterine Prolapse

The uterus prolapses as the result of weakening of the supporting structures of the pelvic floor, often occuring concurrently with a cystocele and rectocele. The uterus becomes progressively retroverted and descends into the vaginal canal. In first-degree prolapse the cervix remains within the vagina; in second-degree prolapse the cervix is at the introitus; in third-degree prolapse the cervix and vagina drop outside the introitus (Fig. 12-31).

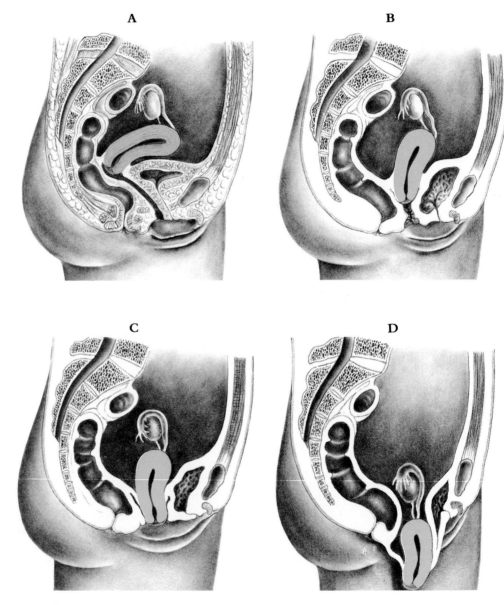

Fig. 12-31
Uterine prolapse. A, Normal uterus. **B,** First degree prolapse of the uterus.
C, Second degree prolapse of the uterus. **D,** Complete prolapse of the uterus.

Uterine Bleeding

Abnormality in menstrual bleeding and inappropriate uterine bleeding are common gynecologic problems. The following terms are used to describe unusual uterine bleeding:

amenorrhea Absent menses.

dysfunctional uterine bleeding (DUB) Abnormal uterine bleeding not associated with tumor, inflammation, pregnancy, trauma, or hormonal imbalance; a diagnosis given only after these causes are ruled out.

hypermenorrhea Excessive bleeding during a period of usual duration.

hypomenorrhea Decreased amount of menstrual flow.

menorrhagia Excessive bleeding during a period longer in duration than normal.

metrorrhagia Bleeding at irregular intervals, sometimes prolonged, but of normal amount.

oligomenorrhea Infrequent menstruation.

postmenopausal bleeding Bleeding occurring one year or more after menopause.

polymenorrhea Increased frequency of menstruation not consistently associated with ovulation.

spotting Small amounts of intermenstrual bloody vaginal discharge ranging from pink to dark brown.

The following are the types and common causes of uterine bleeding*

Type	Common Causes†
Midcycle spotting	Midcycle estradiol fluctuation associated with ovulation
Delayed menstruation with excessive bleeding	Anovulation or threatened abortion
Frequent bleeding	Chronic PID, endometriosis, DUB, anovulation
Profuse menstrual bleeding	Endometrial polyps, DUB, adenomyosis, submucous leiomyomas, IUD
Intermenstrual or irregular bleeding	Endometrial polyps, DUB, uterine or cervical cancer, oral contraceptives
Postmenopausal bleeding	Endometrial hyperplasia, estrogen therapy, endometrial cancer

*Adapted from Thompson et al., 1986.

†*DUB*, dysfunctional uterine bleeding; *IUD*, intrauterine device; *PID*, pelvic inflammatory disease.

Myomas (Leiomyomas, Fibroids)

Myomas are common, benign, uterine tumors that appear as firm, irregular nodules in the contour of the uterus. They may occur singly or in multiples and vary greatly in size. The uterus may become enlarged (Fig. 12-32).

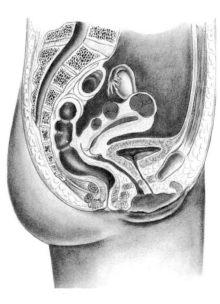

Fig. 12-32
Myomas of the uterus (fibroids).

Endometrial Carcinoma

Endometrial cancer occurs most often in postmenopausal women, particularly those receiving estrogen therapy. The symptom is postmenopausal bleeding.

Adnexae

Ovarian Cysts and Tumors

Ovarian growths can occur unilaterally or bilaterally. Cysts tend to be smooth and sometimes compressible, whereas tumors feel more solid and nodular; nei-ther is usually tender. A ruptured ovarian cyst will produce symptoms similar to those of ruptured tubal pregnancy (Fig. 12-33).

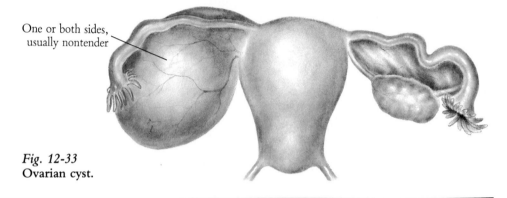

One or both sides, usually nontender

Fig. 12-33
Ovarian cyst.

Ovarian Carcinoma

Ovarian cancer is difficult to detect and often asymptomatic. An ovary that is enlarged should be considered suspi-cious for cancer, and further diagnostic tests are required.

Ruptured Tubal Pregnancy

A ruptured tubal pregnancy causes marked pelvic tenderness, with tenderness and rigidity of the lower abdomen. Motion of the cervix produces pain. A tender, unilateral adnexal mass may indicate the site of the pregnancy. Tachycardia and shock reflect the hemorrhage into the peritoneal cavity and cardiovascular collapse. This is a surgical emergency (Fig. 12-34).

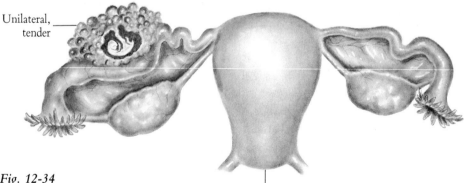

Unilateral, tender

Fig. 12-34
Ruptured tubal pregnancy.   Movement of cervix painful

Pelvic Inflammatory Disease (PID)

Often caused by gonococcal infection, pelvic inflammatory disease may be acute or chronic. Acute PID produces very tender, bilateral adnexal areas; the patient guards and usually cannot tolerate bimanual examination. The symptoms of chronic PID are bilateral, tender, irregular, and fairly fixed adnexal areas (Fig. 12-35).

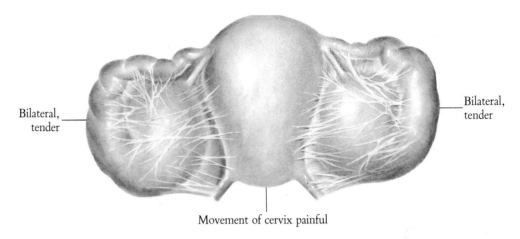

Bilateral, tender

Bilateral, tender

Movement of cervix painful

Fig. 12-35
Pelvic inflammatory disease.

Salpingitis

Inflammation or infection of the fallopian tube is often associated with PID. Salpingitis causes lower quadrant pain with tenderness on bimanual examination (Fig. 12-36).

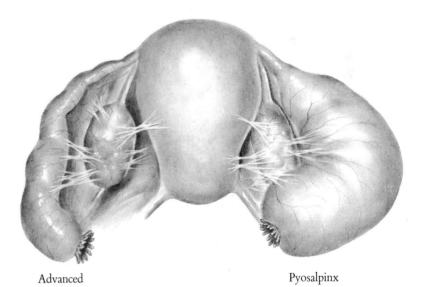

Advanced   Pyosalpinx

Fig. 12-36
Salpingitis.

Ambiguous Genitalia

Certain conditions of the labia and clitoris may indicate ambiguous genitalia. For example, partially fused labia suggests the presence of a scrotum; a urinary meatus that is not located behind the clitoris may indicate the presence of a penis (Fig. 12-37).

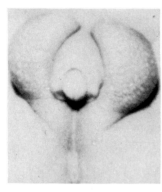

Fig. 12-37
Ambiguous external genitalia in 1-year-old girl.

From Gardner and Kaufman, 1969.

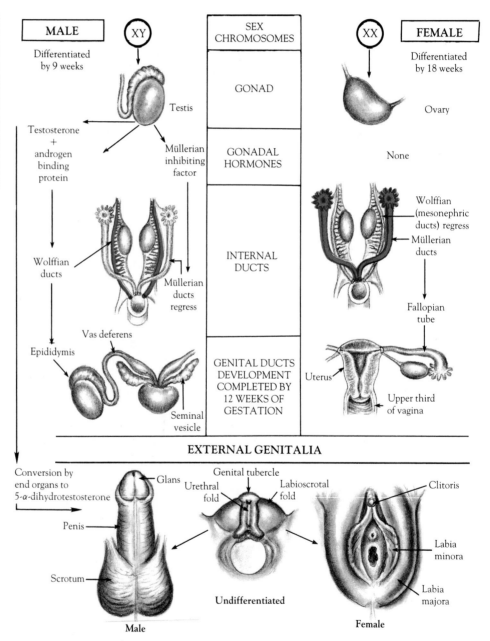

Fig. 12-38
Sexual differentiation in utero.

From Thompson et al., 1986.

Hydrocolpos

Vaginal secretions can collect behind an imperforate hymen. Hydrocolpos may be manifested by a small midline lower abdominal mass or a small cystic mass between the labia. The condition may resolve spontaneously or require surgical intervention.

Vulvovaginitis

Vaginal discharge that is accompanied by warm, erythematous, and swollen vulvar tissues is termed vulvovaginitis. Possible causes include trichomonal, monilial, or gonococcal infection; secondary infection from a foreign body; nonspecific infection from bubble baths, diaper irritation, urethritis, injury, and sexual abuse (Fig. 12-38).

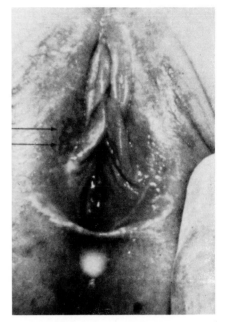
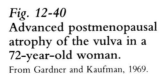

Fig. 12-39
Nonspecific vulvovaginitis in a 10-year-old girl.
From Gardner and Kaufman, 1969.

OLDER ADULTS

Atrophic Vaginitis

Atrophy of the vagina is caused by lack of estrogen. The vaginal mucosa is dry and pale, though it may become reddened and develop petechiae and superficial erosions. The accompanying vaginal discharge may be white, gray, yellow, green, or blood-tinged. It can be thick or watery, and although it varies in amount, the discharge is rarely profuse (Fig. 12-39).

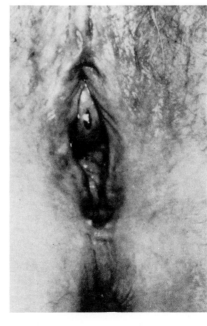

Fig. 12-40
Advanced postmenopausal atrophy of the vulva in a 72-year-old woman.
From Gardner and Kaufman, 1969.

CHAPTER

13

Male Genitalia

Anatomy and Physiology

The penis, testicles, epididymides, scrotum, prostate gland, and seminal vesicles comprise the male genitalia (Fig. 13-1).

The physiologic function of the penis is to serve as the final excretory organ for urine and, when erect, as the means of introducing sperm into the vagina. The penis consists of the two corpora cavernosa, which form the dorsum and sides, and the corpus spongiosum, which contains the urethra. The corpus spongiosum expands at its distal end to form the glans penis. The urethral orifice is a slit-like opening located approximately 2 mm ventral to the tip of the glans (Figs. 13-2 and 13-3). The skin of the penis is thin, redundant to permit erection, and free of subcutaneous fat. It is generally more darkly pigmented than body skin. Unless the patient has been circumcised, the prepuce (foreskin) covers the glans. In the uncircumcised male smegma is formed by the secretion of sebaceous material by the glans and the desquamation of epithelial cells from the prepuce. It appears as a cheesy white material on the glans and in the fornix of the foreskin.

The scrotum, like the penis, is generally more darkly pigmented than body skin. A septum divides the scrotum into two pendulous sacs, each containing a testis, epididymis, a spermatic cord, and a muscle layer that allows the scrotum to relax or contract (Fig. 13-4). Testicular temperature is controlled by altering the distance of the testis from the body through muscular action. Spermatogenesis requires maintenance of temperatures lower than 37° C.

The testicles are responsible for the production of both spermatozoa and testosterone. The adult testis is ovoid and measures approximately $4 \times 3 \times 2$ cm. The epididymis is a soft, comma-shaped structure located on the posterolateral and upper aspect of the testis in 90% of normal males. It provides for storage, maturation, and transit of sperm. The vas deferens begins at the tail of the epididymis, ascends the spermatic cord, travels through the inguinal canal, and unites with the seminal vesicle to form the ejaculatory duct.

The prostate gland, which resembles a large chestnut and is approximately the size of a testis, surrounds the urethra at the bladder neck. The physiologic function of the prostate and its secretions is not completely understood. It produces the major volume of ejaculatory fluid, which contains fibrinolysin. This enzyme liquifies the coagulated semen, a process that may be important for satisfactory sperm motility. The seminal vesicles extend from the prostate onto the posterior surface of the bladder.

Fig. 13-1
Male pelvic organs.

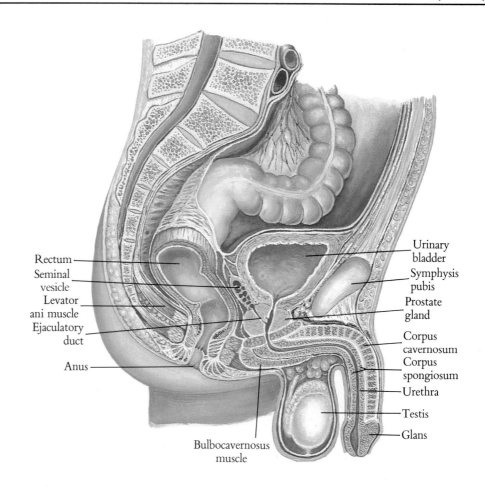

Rectum

Seminal
vesicle

Levator
ani muscle

Ejaculatory
duct

Anus

Bulbocavernosus
muscle

Urinary
bladder

Symphysis
pubis

Prostate
gland

Corpus
cavernosum

Corpus
spongiosum

Urethra

Testis

Glans

Fig. 13-2
Anatomy of the penis.

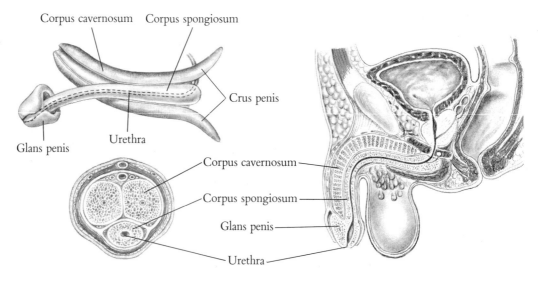

Corpus cavernosum   Corpus spongiosum

Crus penis

Glans penis

Urethra

Corpus cavernosum

Corpus spongiosum

Glans penis

Urethra

Fig. 13-3
Anatomy of urethra and penis.
From Bobak and Jensen, 1984.

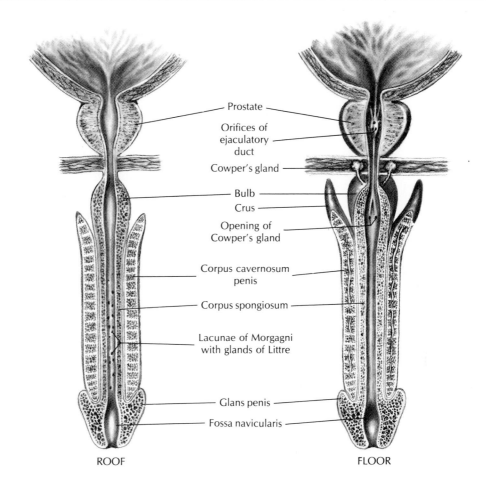

Prostate

Orifices of ejaculatory duct

Cowper's gland

Bulb

Crus

Opening of Cowper's gland

Corpus cavernosum penis

Corpus spongiosum

Lacunae of Morgagni with glands of Littre

Glans penis

Fossa navicularis

ROOF

FLOOR

Fig. 13-4
Scrotum and its contents.

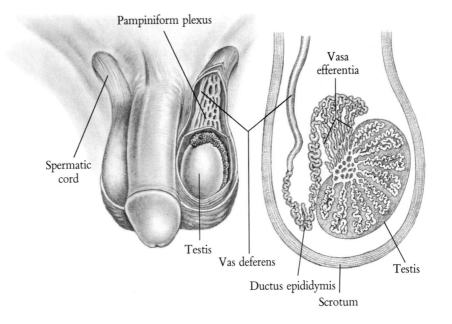

Pampiniform plexus

Vasa efferentia

Spermatic cord

Testis

Vas deferens

Ductus epididymis

Scrotum

Testis

Sexual Physiology

Erection of the penis occurs when the two corpora cavernosa become engorged with blood, generally 20 to 50 cc. Increased blood supply is produced by increased arterial dilation and decreased venous outflow; both processes are under the control of the autonomic nervous system.

Erection is a neurovascular reflex that can be induced by psychogenic and local reflex mechanisms. Local reflex mechanisms involve spinal reflex arcs that are initiated by tactile stimuli. Psychogenic erection can be initiated by any type of sensory input—auditory, visual, tactile, or imaginative stimuli. Cortical input can also serve to suppress sexual arousal.

Orgasm is a complex, pleasurable sensation accompanying ejaculation, the emission of secretions from the vas deferens, epididymides, prostate, and seminal vesicles. Orgasm is followed by constriction of the vessels supplying blood to the corpora cavernosa and gradual detumescence.

INFANTS AND CHILDREN

The external genitalia are identical for male and female at 8 weeks gestational age, but by 12 weeks gestation sexual differentiation has occurred. Any fetal insult during 8 or 9 weeks gestation may lead to major anomalies of the external genitalia. Minor morphologic abnormalities arise from injury after that period of development.

During the third trimester, the testes descend from the retroperitoneal space through the inguinal canal to the scrotum. At full term one or both testes may still lie within the inguinal canal, with the final descent into the scrotum occurring in the early postnatal period. Descent of the testicles may be arrested at any point, however, or may follow an abnormal path.

Small separations between the glans and the inner preputial epithelium begin during the third trimester. Separation of the prepuce from the glans is usually incomplete at birth, however, and often remains so until the age of 3 to 6 years.

ADOLESCENTS

With the onset of puberty sparse, downy, straight hair appears at the base of the penis; the scrotal skin reddens, thins, and becomes increasingly pendulous. The testes and penis begin enlarging. As maturation continues, the pubic hair darkens and extends over the entire pubic area, and the prostate gland enlarges. By the completion of puberty the pubic hair is curly, dense, coarse, and forms a diamond-shaped pattern from the umbilicus to the anus. The growth and development of the testes and scrotum are complete. The penis is enlarged in length and breadth. See Chapter 3, Growth and Measurement, for details of pubertal development.

OLDER ADULTS

Pubic hair becomes finer and less abundant with aging, and pubic alopecia may occur.

No change in the length of time necessary for the production of a mature spermatozoa occurs with aging. The viability of the sperm, however, probably decreases since the rate of conception declines with age. The ejaculatory volume may actually increase with age, perhaps because of decreased frequency of intercourse. The scrotum becomes more pendulous with aging, and the patient may complain about it.

Frequency of sexual activity declines with aging, although the rate of decline correlates most strongly with the frequency of sexual activity in youth—i.e., the man who was highly active in youth is more likely to maintain a higher level of sexual activity during later years. Erection may develop more slowly, and ejaculation may be less intense.

Review of Related History

General Considerations

1. Employment: risk of trauma to suprapubic region or genitalia, exposure to radiation or toxins
2. Exercise: use of protective device with contact sports
3. Concerns about genitalia: size, shape, surface characteristics, texture
4. Testicular self-examination practices
5. Concerns about sexual practices: sexual partners (single or multiple), sexual lifestyle (heterosexual, homosexual, bisexual)
6. Medications: prescription or over-the-counter drugs that might interfere with sexual performance (diuretics, sedatives, antihypertensive agents, tranquilizers, estrogen)
7. Reproductive function: number of children, form of contraception used

Present Problem

1. Difficulty achieving or maintaining erection
   a. Pain with erection, prolonged painful erection
   b. Constant or intermittent, with some or all sexual partners
   c. Associated with alcohol ingestion or medication
   d. Persistent erections unrelated to sexual stimulation
   e. Curvature of penis in any direction with erection
2. Difficulty with ejaculation
   a. Painful or premature, efforts to treat the problem
   b. Ejaculate color, consistency, odor, and amount
3. Discharge or lesion on the penis
   a. Character: lumps, sores, rash
   b. Discharge: color, consistency, odor, tendency to stain underwear
   c. Symptoms: itching, burning, stinging
   d. Exposure to sexually transmitted disease: multiple partners, infection in partners, failure to use condom
4. Infertility
   a. Lifestyle factors that may increase temperature of scrotum: tight clothing, briefs, hot baths, employment in high temperature environment (steel mill) or requiring prolonged sitting (truck driver)
   b. Length of time attempting pregnancy, sexual activity pattern, knowledge of fertile period of woman's reproductive cycle
   c. History of undescended testes
   d. Diagnostic evaluation to date: semen analysis, physical examination, sperm antibody titers
5. Enlargement in inguinal area
   a. Intermittent or constant, association with straining or lifting, duration, presence of pain

     b. Change in size or character of mass; ability to reduce the mass; if unable to reduce it, how long ago could it be reduced

     c. Pain in the groin: character (tearing, sudden searing, or cutting pain), associated activity (lifting heavy object, coughing, or straining at stool)

     d. Use of truss or other treatment

6. Testicular pain or mass

     a. Change in testicular size

     b. Events surrounding onset: noted casually while bathing, following trauma, during a sporting event

     c. Irregular lumps, soreness, or heaviness of testes

Past Medical History

1. Surgery of genitourinary tract: undescended testes, hypospadias, epispadias, hydrocele, varicocele, hernia, prostate, sterilization
2. Sexually transmitted diseases: single or multiple infections, specific organism (gonorrhea, syphilis, herpes, warts, chlamydia), treatment, effectiveness, residual problems
3. Chronic illness: testicular or prostatic cancer, neurologic or vascular impairment, diabetes mellitus, arthritis, cardiac or respiratory disease

Family History

1. Infertility in siblings
2. Hernias

INFANTS AND CHILDREN

1. Maternal use of sex hormones or birth control pills during pregnancy
2. Circumcised boy: complications from procedure
3. Uncircumcised boy: hygiene measures, ability to pull back and replace foreskin, interference with urinary stream
4. Scrotal swelling with crying or bowel movement
5. Congenital anomalies: hypospadias, epispadias, undescended testes, ambiguous genitalia
6. Concerns with masturbation, sexual exploration
7. Swelling, discoloration, or sores on the penis or scrotum, pain in the genitalia

ADOLESCENTS

1. Knowledge of reproductive function, source of information about sexual activity and function
2. Presence of nocturnal emissions, pubic hair, enlargement of genitalia, age at time of each occurrence
3. Sexual activity, contraception used

OLDER ADULTS

1. Change in frequency of sexual activity or desire: related to loss of spouse; no sexual partner; sexually restrictive environment; depression; physical illness resulting in fatigue, weakness, or pain
2. Change in sexual response: longer time required to achieve full erection, less forceful ejaculation, more rapid detumescence, longer interval between erections, prostatic surgery

Examination and Findings

EQUIPMENT	■ Gloves, if a sexually transmitted disease is suspected ■ Penlight for transillumination of any mass

Examination of the genitalia involves inspection, palpation, and transillumination of any mass found. The patient may be anxious about examination of his genitalia, so it is important to examine the genitalia carefully and completely but also briskly. The patient may be lying or standing for this part of the examination (Fig. 13-5).

First inspect the genital hair distribution. Genital hair is more coarse than scalp hair. It should be abundant in the pubic region and may continue in a narrowing midline pattern to the umbilicus (the male escutcheon pattern). Depending on how the patient is positioned, it may be possible to note that the distribution continues around the scrotum to the anal orifice. The penis itself is not covered with hair, and the scrotum generally has scant amounts.

Examine the penis. The dorsal vein should be apparent on inspection. If the patient is uncircumcised, retract the foreskin. It should retract easily, and a bit of white cheesy smegma may be seen over the glans. Occasionally the foreskin is tight and cannot be retracted. This condition is called phimosis (Fig. 13-6) and may occur normally during the first 6 years of age. It is usually congenital but may result from

Fig. 13-5
Normal appearance of male genitalia.

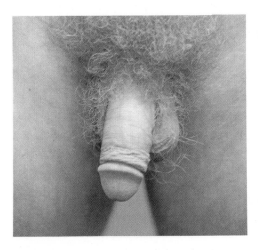
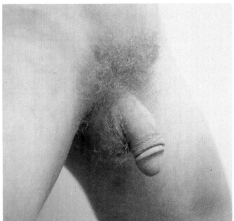

Fig. 13-6
Phimosis.
From 400 Self-assessment picture tests in clinical medicine, 1984.

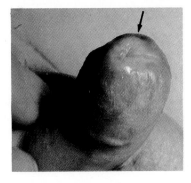

recurrent infections or balanoposthitis (inflammation of the glans penis and pre-puce). It may also be caused by previous unsuccessful efforts to retract the foreskin that have caused radial tearing of the preputial ring, resulting in adhesions of the foreskin to the glans. Balanitis, inflammation of the glans (Fig. 13-7), occurs only in uncircumcised individuals and is often associated with phimosis. It may be caused by either bacterial or fungal infections and is most commonly seen in men with poorly controlled diabetes mellitus and a candidal infection.

If the patient is circumcised, the glans is exposed and appears erythematous and dry. No smegma will be present.

Examine the external meatus of the urethra. The orifice should appear slit-like and be located on the ventral surface just millimeters from the tip of the glans. Press the glans between thumb and forefinger to open the urethral orifice (Fig. 13-8). The opening should be glistening and pink. Bright erythema or a discharge indicates inflammatory disease, whereas a pinpoint or round opening may result from meatal stenosis.

Palpate the shaft of the penis for tenderness and induration. Strip the urethra for any discharge by firmly compressing the base of the penis with your thumb and forefinger and moving them toward the glans. The presence of a discharge may well indicate a venereal infection. The texture of the flaccid penis should be soft and free of nodularity. Replace the foreskin after performing these maneuvers.

Rarely you may see a patient with a prolonged penile erection, called priapism (Fig. 13-9). It is often painful. While in the majority of cases the condition is idio-pathic, it can occur in patients with leukemia or hemoglobinopathies such as sickle cell disease.

Inspect the scrotum (Fig. 13-10). It should appear more deeply pigmented than the body skin, and the surface may be coarse. The scrotal skin is often reddened in red-haired individuals; however, reddened skin in other individuals may indicate an infectious process. The scrotum usually appears asymmetric, because the left testi-cle has a longer spermatic cord and is therefore often lower. The thickness of the scrotum definitely varies with temperature, age, and perhaps emotional state. Lumps in the scrotal skin are commonly caused by sebaceous cysts, also called epidermoid cysts. They appear as small lumps on the scrotum, but they may enlarge and discharge oily material (Fig. 13-11).

Occasionally you may observe unusual thickening of the scrotum caused by edema, often with pitting. This does not generally imply disease related to the genitalia but is more likely a consequence of general fluid retention associated with cardiac, renal, or hepatic disease.

Examine for evidence of a hernia. Fig. 13-16 shows the anatomy of the region and the three common types of hernias. With the patient standing, ask him to bear down as if having a bowel movement. While he is straining, inspect the area of the inguinal canal and the region of the fossa ovalis. After asking the patient to relax again, insert your examining finger into the lower part of the scrotum and carry it upward along the vas deferens into the inguinal canal (Fig. 13-12). Which finger you use depends on the size of the patient. In the young child the little finger is appropriate; in the adult the middle finger is generally used. You should be able to feel the oval external ring. Ask the patient to cough. If a hernia is present, you should feel the sudden appearance of a viscus against your finger. The hernia is described as indirect if it lies within the inguinal canal. It may also come through the external canal and even pass into the scrotum. This type of hernia occurs more frequently in young men and is the most common of the abdominal hernias. Since an indirect hernia on one side strongly suggests the possibility of bilateral hernia-tion, be sure to examine both sides thoroughly.

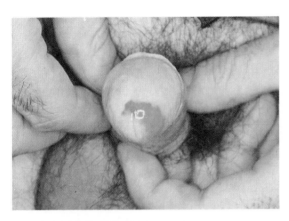

Fig. 13-7
Balanitis.
From Lloyd-Davies et al.: *Colour Atlas of Urology*, Year Book Medical Publishers.

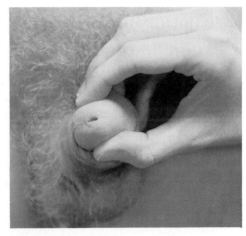

Fig. 13-8
Examination of urethral orifice.

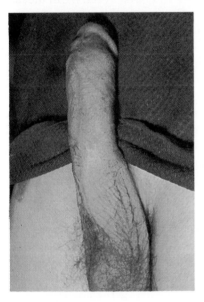

Fig. 13-9
Priapism.
From Lloyd-Davies et al.: *Colour Atlas of Urology*, Year Book Medical Publishers.

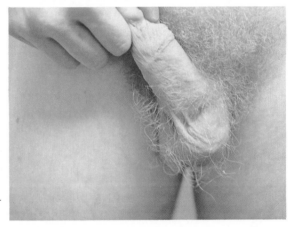

Fig. 13-10
Inspection of scrotum and ventral surface of penis.

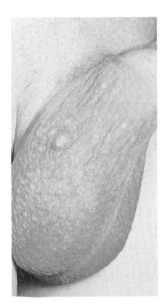

Fig. 13-11
Sebaceous cysts on scrotum.
From Lloyd-Davies et al.: *Colour Atlas of Urology*, Year Book Medical Publishers.

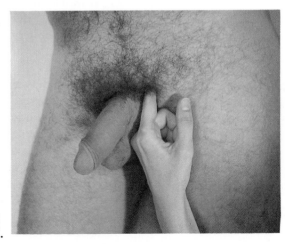

Fig. 13-12
Checking for inguinal hernia. Finger inserted through inguinal canal.

MINIMIZING THE PATIENT'S ANXIETY

The physical examination is laden with anxiety-provoking elements for most people, but no part of the body is likely to arouse as much psychic discomfort for the male patient as examination of his genitals. Adolescents and men are often fearful of having an erection during the examination. Boys and adolescents may worry about whether their genitals are normal, and misinformation on sexual matters (such as "the evils of masturbation") can add to their concerns. Your attitude and ability to communicate can reassure the apprehensive patient. Some important elements to remember:

- Know the language. It is inappropriate to talk down to anyone, but you and the patient must understand each other. You may not be entirely comfortable with some of the common words and phrases you may hear from the patients, but the common language may be appropriate in certain circumstances. You will not lose your dignity if you maintain your composure and you succeed in communicating effectively. Know the language and use it effectively, without apology, and in undemeaning fashion.
- Never make jokes. Light, casual talk or jokes about the genitalia or sexual function is always inappropriate, no matter how well you know the patient. Feelings about one's own sexuality run deep and are frequently well masked. Do not pull at the edges of a mask you may not suspect is there.
- Remember that your face is easily seen by the patient when you are examining the genitalia. An unexpected finding may cause a sudden change in your expression. You must guard against what you communicate by the unspoken.
- You need not be defensive if you are a woman examining a man, anymore than if you are a man examining a woman—an ordinary event historically. Here again, you communicate much by demeanor and hesitancy in speech. Do not be apologetic in any obvious or subtle way. Remember that you are a professional, doing the job of a professional.

The testes should be palpated using the thumb and first two fingers. The testes should be sensitive to gentle compression but not tender, and they should feel smooth, rubbery, and be free of nodules (Fig. 13-13). In some diseases such as syphilis and diabetic neuropathy, a testis may be totally insensitive to painful stimuli. Irregularities in texture or size may indicate an infection, cyst, or tumor.

The epididymis, located on the posterolateral surface of the testis, should be smooth, discrete, larger cephalad, and nontender. You may be able to feel the appendix epididymis as an irregularity on the cephalad surface.

Finally you need to palpate the vas deferens. It has accompanying arteries and veins, but they cannot be precisely identified by palpation. The vas itself feels smooth and discrete; it should not be beaded or lumpy in its course as you palpate from the testicle to the inguinal ring. The presence of such unexpected findings might indicate diabetes or old inflammatory changes, especially tuberculosis.

Examination of the prostate is detailed in Chapter 14 (Anus, Rectum, and Prostate).

INFANTS

Examine the newborn genitalia for congenital anomalies, incomplete development, and sexual ambiguity. Inspect the penis for size, placement of the urethral opening, and any anomalies. The non-erect length of the penis at birth is 2 to 3 cm. Transitory erection of the penis during infancy is common, and the penis should have a straight projection. A small penis (microphallus) may indicate other organ anomalies. The small penis must also be differentiated from the unusually large clitoris found in pseudohermaphrodism. A hooked, downward bowing of the penis suggests a chordee.

Inspect the glans penis of the neonate. The foreskin in the uncircumcised infant is commonly tight, but it should retract enough to permit a good urinary stream. Do not retract the foreskin more than necessary to see the urethra, especially if the neonate will not be circumcised. Do not force, because this can tear the prepuce from the glans, causing binding adhesions to form between the prepuce and the glans. Mobility of the foreskin increases with time, and it should be fully retractable by 3 or 4 years of age. The slit-like urethral meatus should be located near the tip. Inspect the glans of the circumcised infant for ulcerations, bleeding, and inflammation. The urinary stream should be strong with good caliber. Dribbling or a reduced force or caliber of the urinary stream may indicate stenosis of the urethral meatus.

Inspect the scrotum for size, shape, rugae, the presence of testicles, and any anomalies (Fig. 13-14). The scrotum of the premature infant may appear underdeveloped, without rugae, and without testes, while the full term neonate should have a loose, pendulous scrotum with rugae and a midline raphe. The proximal end of the scrotum should be the widest area. The scrotum in infants usually appears

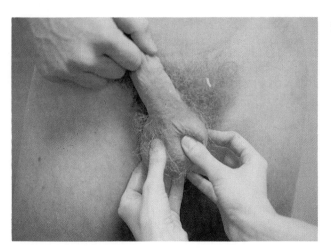

Fig. 13-13
Palpating contents of the scrotal sac.

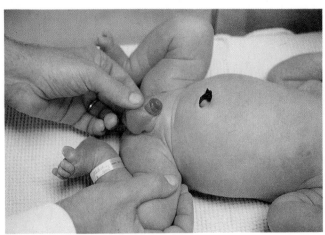

Fig. 13-14
Palpating scrotum of an infant.

CIRCUMCISION

There has been a lot of discussion recently about the value of circumcision. Although there is mounting opinion that circumcision is not a medically indicated procedure, attitudes on this vary and are highly personal. Circumcision is often performed on the basis of religious prescription.

large compared with the rest of the genitalia. Edema of the external genitalia is common, especially after a breech delivery. A deep cleft in the scrotum (bifid scrotum) is usually associated with other genitourinary anomalies or ambiguous genitalia.

When examining the scrotum, particularly in the young, make certain that your hands are warm and your touch is gentle. The cremasteric reflex—known as the yo-yo reflex—in which the scrotal contents retract is a response to cold hands and abrupt handling. Before you palpate the scrotum, place the thumb and index finger of one hand over the inguinal canals at the upper part of the scrotal sac. This maneuver helps prevent stimulating the cremasteric reflex. Palpate each side of the scrotum to detect the presence of the testes and other masses. The testicle of the newborn is approximately 1 cm in diameter.

If either of the testicles is not palpable, place a finger over the upper inguinal ring and gently push toward the scrotum. You may feel a soft mass in the inguinal canal. Try to push it toward the scrotum and palpate it with your thumb and index finger. If the testicle can be pushed into the scrotum, it is considered a descended testicle, even though it retracts to the inguinal canal. A testicle that is either palpable in the inguinal canal but cannot be pushed into the scrotum or is not palpable at all is an undescended testicle.

Palpate over the internal inguinal canal with the flat part of your fingers. Roll the spermatic cord beneath the fingers to feel the solid structure going through the ring. If the feeling of smoothness disappears as you palpate, the peritoneum is passing through the ring, indicating an invisible hernia. An apparent bulge in the inguinal area suggests a visible hernia. Palpation may elicit a sensation of crepitus.

When any mass other than the testicle or spermatic cord is palpated in the scrotum, determine if it is filled with fluid, gas, or solid material. It will most likely be a hernia or hydrocele. Attempt to reduce the size of the mass by pushing it back through the external inguinal canal. If a bright pen light transilluminates the mass and there is no change in size when reduction is attempted, it most likely contains fluid (hydrocele with a closed tunica vaginalis). A mass that does not transilluminate but does change in size when reduction is attempted is probably a hernia. A mass that neither changes in size nor transilluminates may represent an incarcerated hernia, which is a surgical emergency.

CHILDREN

The external genitalia of the toddler and preschooler are examined as described for infants. Preschoolers may have developed a sense of modesty, so you should gently and quickly complete the examination and reassure the child that he is developing normally.

Fig. 13-15
Position of child to push testicles into the scrotum.

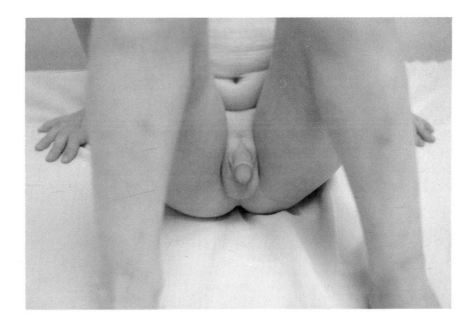

Inspect the penis for size, lesions, swelling, inflammation, and malformation. Retract the foreskin in the uncircumcised boy without forcing it, and inspect the glans for lesions, discharge, and the location and appearance of the urethral meatus. Some adherence of the prepuce to the glans may continue until 6 years of age. The penis may appear relatively small if obscured by fat in obese boys.

The scrotum is inspected for size, shape, color and the presence of testicles or other masses. Well formed rugae indicate that the testes have descended during infancy, even if the testes are not apparent in the scrotum. Palpate the scrotum to identify the testes and epididymides. The testes should be about 1 cm in size.

Some testes are very retractile and therefore hard to find. Warm hands, a warm room, and a gentle approach will help. If the patient is old enough to cooperate, ask him to sit in the tailor's position with legs crossed, or have the child sit on a chair with the heels of his feet on the chair seat and his hands on his knees. Either position places pressure on the abdominal wall that will help push the testicles into the scrotum. If an inguinal hernia exists, this maneuver is also useful in eliciting that finding (Fig. 13-15). A scrotum that remains small, flat, and undeveloped is a good indication of cryptorchidism (undescended testes).

A hard, enlarged, painless testicle may indicate a tumor. Acute swelling in the scrotum with discoloration can result from torsion of the spermatic cord or orchitis. Acute painful swelling without discoloration and a thickened or nodular epididymis suggests epididymitis. An enlarged penis without enlargement of the testes occurs with precocious puberty, adrenal hyperplasia, and central nervous system lesions.

ADOLESCENTS

The examination of older children and adolescents is performed as in the adult examination. Because of their great sensitivity to development and modesty, this portion of the physical examination is usually saved to the end. The adolescent boy needs to be reassured that his genital development is proceeding as expected. If the adolescent does have an erection, explain that this is a common response to touch and that you are not concerned by it.

Common Abnormalities

Hernia

A hernia is the protrusion of a peritoneal-lined sac through some defect in the abdominal wall. Fig. 13-16 shows the anatomy of the region and the three common types of pelvic hernias. Hernias occur because there is a potential space for protrusion of some abdominal organ, commonly the bowel but occasionally the omentum. These hernias arise along the course that the testicle traveled as it exited the abdomen and entered the scrotum during intrauterine life. Femoral hernias occur at the fossa ovalis, where the femoral artery exits the abdomen.

Fig. 13-16
Anatomy of region of common pelvic hernias.
A, Indirect inguinal hernia.

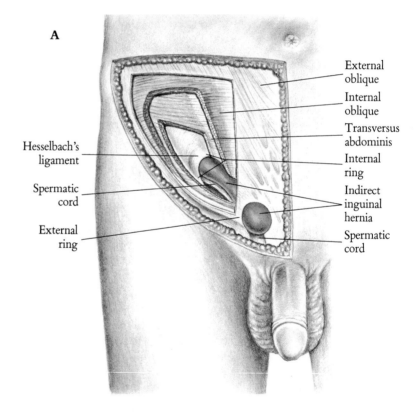

A

External oblique

Internal oblique

Transversus abdominis

Internal ring

Indirect inguinal hernia

Spermatic cord

Hesselbach's ligament

Spermatic cord

External ring

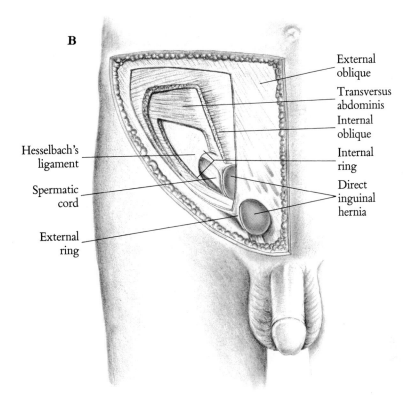

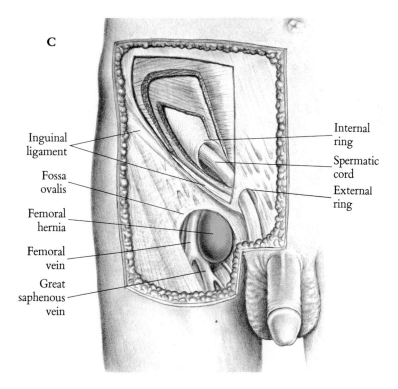

Fig. 13-16, cont'd
Anatomy of region of common pelvic hernias.
B, Direct inguinal hernia.
C, Femoral hernia.

Penis

Paraphimosis

Paraphimosis is the inability to replace the foreskin to its normal position after it has been retracted behind the glans. Impairment of local circulation can lead to edema or gangrene of the glans (Fig. 13-17).

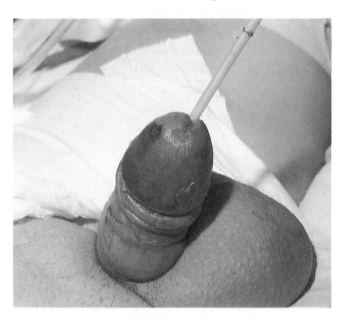

Fig. 13-17
Paraphimosis.
Courtesy Patrick C. Walsh, M.D.,
The Johns Hopkins University School
of Medicine, Baltimore.

Hypospadias

Hypospadias is a congenital defect in which the urethral meatus is located on the ventral surface of the glans, penile shaft, or the perineal area. If the orifice is ventral but within the substance of the glans, it is termed primary hypospadias. An orifice along the ventral shaft of the penis is termed secondary hypospadias, and one located at the base of the penis is termed tertiary hypospadias (Fig. 13-18). Rarely, the orifice may appear on the dorsal surface, a condition called epispadias.

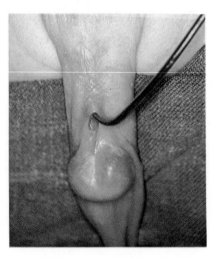

Fig. 13-18
Hypospadias.
From 400 Self-assessment picture tests
in clinical medicine, 1984.

Syphilitic Chancre

The lesion of primary syphilis generally occurs 2 weeks after exposure. It is most commonly located on the glans, is painless, and has indurated borders with a clear base. Scrapings from the ulcer show spirochetes when examined microscopically (Fig. 13-19).

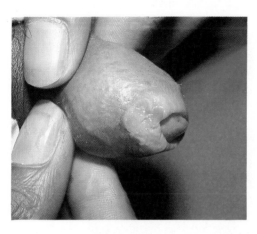

Fig. 13-19
Syphilitic chancre.
Courtesy Antoinette Hood, M.D.,
The Johns Hopkins University School
of Medicine, Baltimore.

Herpes

Venereal herpes is a viral infection that appears as superficial vesicles. The lesions may be located on the glans, penile shaft, or at the base of the penis. They are frequently quite painful, and at the time of primary infection are often associated with inguinal lymphadenopathy and systemic symptoms including fever (Fig. 13-20).

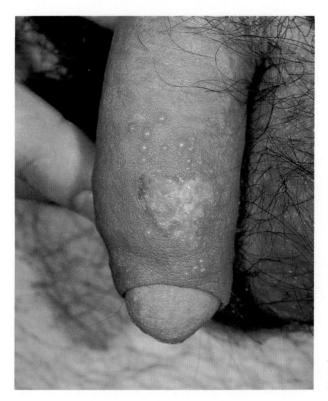

Fig. 13-20
Genital herpes.
From Habif, 1985.

Condyloma Acuminatum

A soft, reddish lesion that arises because of infection with a papovavirus is called condyloma acuminatum. The lesions are commonly present on the prepuce, glans penis, and penile shaft but they may be present within the urethra as well. The lesions may undergo malignant degeneration to squamous cell carcinoma (Fig. 13-21).

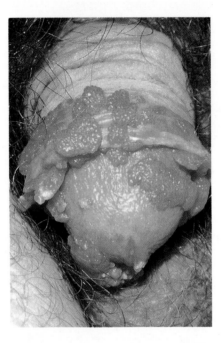

Fig. 13-21
Condylomata acuminata.
From Diagnostic Picture Tests in Clinical Medicine, 1984.

Lymphogranuloma Venereum

Lymphogranuloma verereum is a sexually transmitted disease caused by a chlamydial organism. Although the lesions appear on the genitalia, symptoms may be systemic. The initial lesion is a painless erosion at or near the coronal sulcus (Fig. 13-22). Subsequently local lymph nodes become involved; unless the infection is treated, draining sinus tracts may form. If lymphatic drainage is blocked, penile and scrotal lymphedema may ensue.

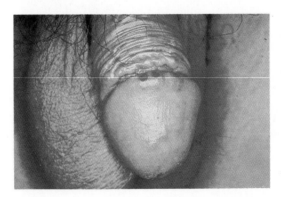

Fig. 13-22
Lymphogranuloma venereum.
Reprinted from Meheus, A., and Ursi, J.P.: *Sexually Transmitted Diseases*. Kalamazoo, Michigan, The Upjohn Company, 1982, with permission from the publisher.

Molluscum Contagiosum

Molluscum contagiosum is a sexually transmitted disease caused by a poxvirus. The lesions are smooth and dome shaped with discreet margins. They occur most commonly on the glans penis (Fig. 13-23).

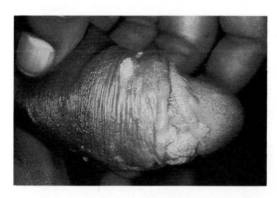

Fig. 13-23
Molluscum contagiosum (genital warts).
Reprinted from Meheus, A., and Ursi, J.P.: *Sexually Transmitted Diseases*. Kalamazoo, Michigan, 1982, with permission from the publisher.

Peyronie's Disease

A disorder of unknown etiology, Peyronie's disease is characterized by a fibrous band in the corpus cavernosum. It is generally unilateral and results in deviation of the penis during erection. Depending upon the extent of the fibrous band, the condition may make erection painful and intromission impossible. No treatment has been altogether successful. Vitamin E therapy has recently become popular, and corticosteroid injection has also been used. Occasionally surgery is required to remove the fibrous band (Fig. 13-24).

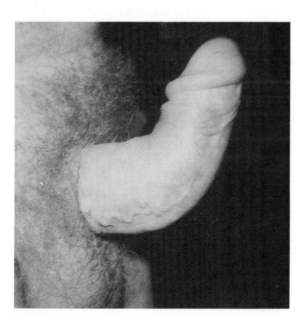

Fig. 13-24
Peyronie's disease.
Courtesy Patrick C. Walsh, M.D., The Johns Hopkins University School of Medicine, Baltimore.

Penile Carcinoma

Cancer of the penis is generally squamous and tends to occur in uncircumcised men who have poor hygiene practices. It often appears as a painless ulceration which, unlike a syphilitic chancre, fails to heal. The lesions are often extensive by the time help is sought, either because of fear or because the lesion is unnoticed under the foreskin (Fig. 13-25).

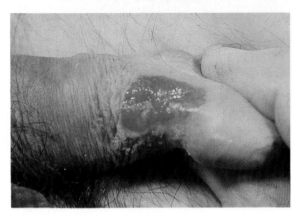

Fig. 13-25
Carcinoma of the penis.
Courtesy Patrick C. Walsh, M.D.,
The Johns Hopkins University School
of Medicine, Baltimore.

Scrotum

Hydrocele

The nontender, smooth, firm mass of the hydrocele results from fluid accumulation in the tunica vaginalis. Unless it has been present for a long time and is very large and taut, palpation of a hydrocele should reveal that it is confined to the scrotum and does not enter the inguinal canal. The mass will transilluminate. This condition is common in infancy. If the tunica vaginalis is not patent, the hydrocele will generally disappear spontaneously in the first 6 months of life (Fig. 13-26).

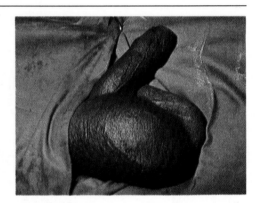

Fig. 13-26
Hydrocele.
From Lloyd-Davies et al.: *Colour Atlas of Urology*, Year Book Medical Publishers.

Spermatocele

A spermatocele is a cystic swelling occurring on the epididymis. It is not as large as a hydrocele, but it does transilluminate (Fig. 13-27).

Fig. 13-27
Spermatocele.
From Lloyd-Davies et al.: *Colour Atlas of Urology*, Year Book Medical Publishers.

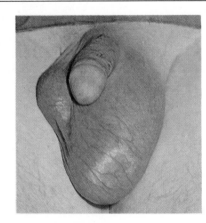

Varicocele

An abnormal tortuosity and dilation of veins of the pampiniform plexus within the spermatic cord is termed a varicocele. It is most common on the left side and may be associated with pain. It occurs in boys and young men and is associated with reduced fertility, proba-bly from increased venous pressure and elevated testicular temperature. The condition, often visible only when the patient is standing, is classically described as "bag of worms" (Fig. 13-28).

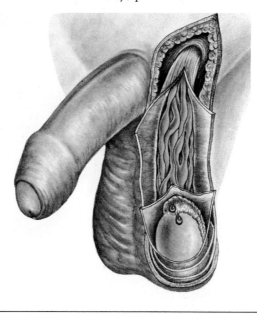

Fig. 13-28
Varicocele.

Epididymitis

Inflammation of the epididymis is often seen in association with a urinary tract infection. The epididymis is exquisitely tender, and the overlying scrotum may be markedly erythematous. Scrotal elevation may relieve the pain. A major consideration in the differential diagnosis is testicular tortion, a surgical emergency. Systemic symptoms such as fever and examination of the urine for white blood cells and bacteria may help to distinguish between these two conditions. Occasionally chronic epididymitis may occur as a consequence of tuberculosis. In the chronic form, the epididymis feels firm, lumpy, and may be slightly tender, and the vas deferens may be beaded (Fig. 13-29).

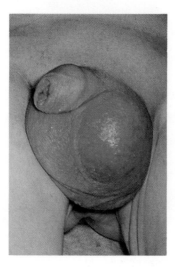

Fig. 13-29
Epididymitis.
From Lloyd-Davies et al.: *Colour Atlas of Urology,* Year Book Medical Publishers.

Orchitis

An acute inflammation of the testis, orchitis is uncommon except as a complication of mumps in the adolescent or adult. It is generally unilateral and results in testicular atrophy in 50% of the cases (Fig. 13-30).

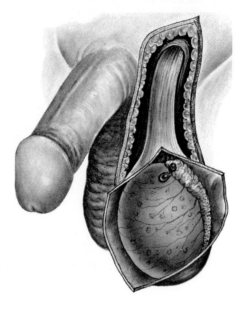

Fig. 13-30
Orchitis.

Testicular Tumor

A neoplasm arising from the testicle appears as an irregular, nontender mass fixed on the testis that does not transilluminate. It may be associated with inguinal lymphadenopathy. These tumors tend to occur in young men and is the most common tumor in males aged 15 to 30. Most testicular tumors are malignant (Fig. 13-31).

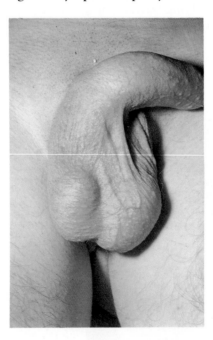

Fig. 13-31
Testicular tumor.
From 400 Self assessment picture tests in clinical medicine, 1984.

Klinefelter's Syndrome

Klinefelter's syndrome is a congenital anomaly associated with XXY chromosomal inheritance. It is associated with hypogonadism and lack of development of secondary sexual characteristics (Fig. 13-32).

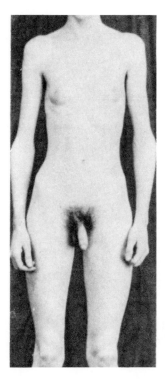

Fig. 13-32
Klinefelter's syndrome.
From Wilson and Walsh, 1979

INFANTS

Ambiguous Genitalia

A condition in which the examiner is uncertain whether the newborn has a very small penis with hypospadias or an enlarged clitoris. There may be partial fusion of the labioscrotal fold or a bifid scrotum. Testes cannot be palpated. The infant should have prompt chromosomal studies performed (Fig. 13-33; see also Fig. 12-38).

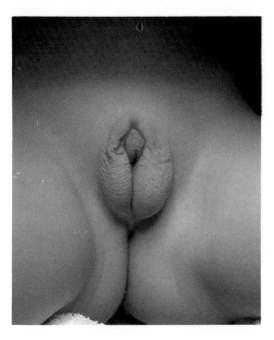

Fig. 13-33
Ambiguous genitalia in infant.
Courtesy Patrick C. Walsh, M.D.
The Johns Hopkins University School
of Medicine, Baltimore.

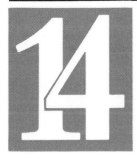

Anus, Rectum, and Prostate

Anatomy and Physiology

The rectum and anus form the terminal portions of the gastrointestinal tract (Fig. 14-1). The anal canal is approximately 2.5 to 4 cm in length and opens onto the perineum. The tissue visible at the external margin of the anus is moist hairless mucosa. Juncture with the perianal skin is characterized by increased pigmentation and, in the adult, the presence of hair.

The anal canal is normally kept securely closed by concentric rings of muscle, the internal and external sphincters. The internal ring of smooth muscle is under involuntary autonomic control. The urge to defecate occurs when the rectum fills with feces, which causes reflexive stimulation that relaxes the internal sphincter. Defecation is controlled by the striated external sphincter, which is under voluntary control. The lower half of the canal is supplied with somatic sensory nerves making it sensitive to painful stimuli, whereas the upper half is under autonomic control and is relatively insensitive. Therefore, conditions of the lower anus cause pain, while those of the upper anus may not.

Internally the anal canal is lined by columns of mucosal tissue (columns of Morgagni) that fuse to form the anorectal junction. The spaces between the columns are called crypts, into which anal glands empty. Inflammation of the crypts can result in fistula or fissure formation. Anastomosing veins cross the columns, forming a ring called the zona hemorrhoidalis. Internal hemorrhoids result from dilation of these veins. The lower segment of the anal canal contains a venous plexus that drains into the inferior rectal veins. Dilation of this plexus results in external hemorrhoids.

The rectum lies superior to the anus and is approximately 12 cm in length. Its proximal end is continuous with the sigmoid colon. The distal end, the anorectal junction, is visible on proctoscopic examination as a sawtooth-like edge, but it is not palpable. Above the anorectal junction, the rectum dilates and turns posteriorly into the hollow of the coccyx and sacrum, forming the rectal ampulla, which stores flatus and feces. The rectal wall contains three semilunar transverse folds (Houston's valves), the function of which is unclear. The lowest of these folds can be palpated by the examiner.

In males the prostate gland is located at the base of the bladder and surrounds the urethra. It is composed of muscular and glandular tissue and is approximately 4 × 3 × 2 cm. The posterior surface of the prostate gland is in close contact with the anterior rectal wall and is accessible by digital examination. It is convex and is divided by a shallow median sulcus into right and left lateral lobes. A third or median lobe, not palpable on examination, is composed of glandular tissue and lies between the ejaculatory duct and the urethra. It contains active secretory alveoli,

Fig. 14-1
Anatomy of the anus and rectum.

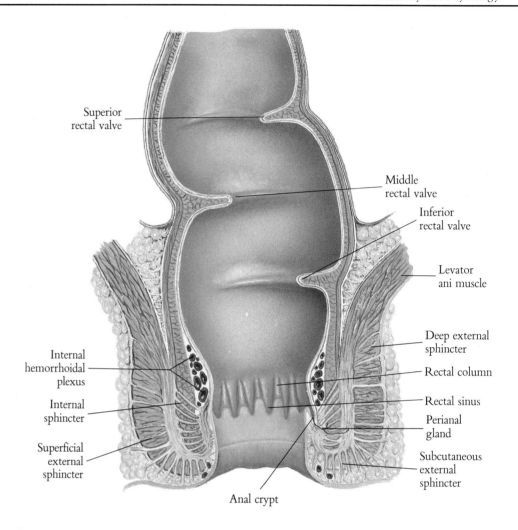

which contribute to ejaculatory fluid. The seminal vesicles extend outward from the prostate (Fig. 14-2).

In females the anterior rectal wall lies in contact with the vagina and is separated from it by the rectovaginal septum. See Chapter 12 (Female Genitalia) for a more detailed discussion.

INFANTS AND CHILDREN

At 7 weeks gestation a portion of the caudal hindgut is divided by an anorectal septum into a urogenital sinus and a rectum. The urogenital sinus is covered by a membrane that develops into the anal opening by 8 weeks gestation. Most anorectal malformations result from abnormalities in this partitioning process.

The first meconium stool is ordinarily passed within the first 24 to 48 hours of life and indicates anal patency. Thereafter, it is common for newborns to have a stool after each feeding (the gastrocolic reflex). Both the internal and external sphincters are under involuntary reflexive control, because myelination of the spinal cord is incomplete.

By the end of the first year the infant may have one or two bowel movements daily. Control of the external anal sphincter is gradually achieved between the ages of 18 and 24 months.

Fig. 14-2
**Anatomy of the prostate
gland and seminal vesicles.**

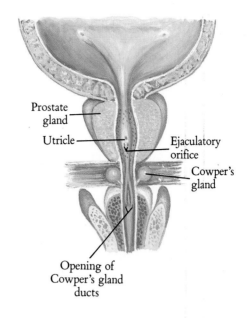

Prostate
gland

Utricle

Ejaculatory
orifice

Cowper's
gland

Opening of
Cowper's gland
ducts

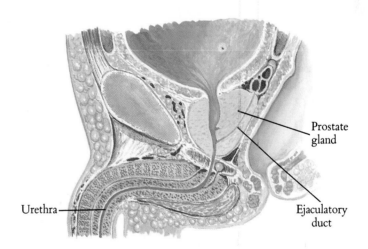

Prostate
gland

Urethra

Ejaculatory
duct

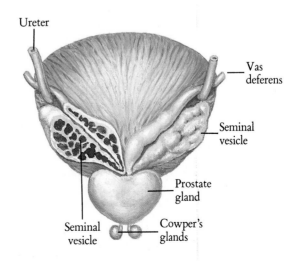

Ureter

Vas
deferens

Seminal
vesicle

Prostate
gland

Seminal
vesicle

Cowper's
glands

In males the prostate is undeveloped, small, inactive, and not palpable on rectal examination. The prostate remains undeveloped until puberty, at which time androgenic influences prompt its growth and maturation. The initially minimal glandular component develops active secretory alveoli, and the prostate becomes functional.

OLDER ADULTS Degeneration of afferent neurons in the rectal wall interferes with the process of relaxation of the internal sphincter in response to distention of the rectum. This can result in an elevated pressure threshold for the sensation of rectal distention in the older adult, with consequent retention of stool. Conversely, as the autonomically controlled internal sphincter loses tone, the external sphincter cannot by itself control the bowels, and the older adult may experience fecal incontinence.

In men the fibromuscular structures of the prostate gland atrophy, with loss of function of the secretory alveoli. However, the atrophy of aging is often obscured by benign hyperplasia of the glandular tissue. The muscular component of the prostate is progressively replaced by collagen.

Review of Related History

General Considerations

1. Bowel habits and characteristics: timing, frequency, number, consistency, shape, color, odor
2. Medications (prescription and over-the-counter): iron, laxatives, stool softeners, hemorrhoid preparations
3. Travel history: areas with high incidence of parasitic infestation
4. Diet: inclusion of fiber foods (cereals, breads, nuts, fruits, vegetables)

Present Problem

1. Changes in bowel function
   a. Character: number, frequency, consistency of stools; presence of mucus or blood; color (dark, bright red, black, light, or clay-colored); odor
   b. Onset and duration: sudden or gradual, relation to dietary change, relation to stressful events
   c. Accompanying symptoms: incontinence, flatus, pain, fever, nausea, vomiting, cramping, abdominal distention
2. Anal discomfort: itching, pain, stinging, burning
   a. Relation to body position and defecation
   b. Straining at stool
   c. Presence of mucus or blood
   d. Interference with activities of daily living or sleep
3. Rectal bleeding
   a. Color: bright or dark red, black
   b. Relation to defecation
   c. Amount: Spotting on toilet paper v active bleeding
   d. Accompanying changes in stool: color, frequency, consistency, shape, odor, presence of mucus
   e. Associated symptoms: incontinence, flatus, rectal pain, abdominal pain or cramping, abdominal distention, weight loss

*Past Medical
History*

1. Hemorrhoids
2. Spinal cord injury
3. Males: prostatic hypertrophy or carcinoma
4. Females: episotomy or fourth degree laceration during delivery

Family History

1. Rectal polyps
2. Colon cancer
3. Prostatic cancer

INFANTS AND CHILDREN

1. Newborns: age and characteristics of stool
2. Bowel movements accompanied by crying, straining, bleeding
3. Feeding habits: types of foods, milk (bottle or breast for infants), appetite
4. Age at which bowel control and toilet training were achieved
5. Associated symptoms: episodes of diarrhea or constipation; tenderness when cleaning after a stool; perianal irritations; weight loss; nausea, vomiting; incontinence in toilet trained child (association with convulsions)
6. Congenital anomaly: imperforate anus, myelomeningoccle, aganglionic megacolon

OLDER ADULTS

1. Changes in bowel habits or character: frequency, number, color, consistency, shape, odor
2. Associated symptoms: weight loss, rectal or abdominal pain, incontinence, flatus, episodes of constipation or diarrhea, abdominal distention, rectal bleeding
3. Dietary changes: intolerance for certain foods, inclusion of fiber foods, regularity of eating habits, appetite
4. Males: history of enlarged prostate, urinary symptoms (hesitancy, urgency, nocturia, force and caliber of urinary stream)

Examination and Findings

EQUIPMENT

- **Gloves**
- **Water-soluble lubricant**
- **Penlight**

Although the rectal examination is generally uncomfortable and often embarrassing for the patient, it provides such important information that it is a mandatory part of every thorough examination. Be calm, slowly paced, and gentle in your touch. Explain what will happen step by step and let the patient know what to expect. A hurried or rough examination can cause unnecessary pain and sphincter spasm, and you can easily lose the trust and cooperation of the patient.

The rectal examination can be performed in any of these positions: knee-chest, left lateral with hips and knees flexed, or standing with the hips flexed and the upper body supported by the examining table. In adult males, the latter two positions are satisfactory for most purposes and allow adequate visualization of the perianal and sacrococcygeal areas. In women the rectal examination is most often performed as part of the rectovaginal examination while the woman is in the lithotomy position (see Chapter 12, Female Genitalia).

Ask the patient to assume one of the examining positions, guiding gently with your hands when necessary. Use drapes but retain good visualization of the area. Glove one or both hands.

Inspect the sacrococcygeal (pilonidal) and perianal areas. The skin should be smooth and uninterrupted. Inspect for lumps, rashes, inflammation, excoriation, scars, pilonidal dimpling, and tufts of hair at the pilonidal area. Fungal infection and pinworm infestion can cause perianal irritation. Fungal infection is more common in adults with diabetes, and pinworms are more common in children. Palpate the area. The discovery of tenderness and inflammation should alert you to the possibility of a perianal abscess, anorectal fistula or fissure, pilonidal cyst, or pruritus ani.

Spread the patient's buttocks apart and inspect the anus. The use of a penlight or gooseneck lamp can assist in visualization. The skin around the anus will appear coarser and more darkly pigmented. Look for skin lesions, skin tags or warts, external hemorrhoids, fissures, and fistulas. Ask the patient to bear down. This will make fistulas, fissures, rectal prolapse, polyps, and internal hemorrhoids more readily apparent. Clock referents are used to describe the location of anal and rectal findings: 12:00 is in the ventral midline and 6:00 is in the dorsal midline.

Lubricate your index finger and press the pad of it against the anal opening (Fig. 14-3, A). Ask the patient to bear down to relax the external sphincter. As relaxation occurs, slip the tip of the finger into the anal canal (Fig. 14-3, B). Warn the patient that there may be a feeling of urgency for a bowel movement, assuring him or her that it will not happen. Ask the patient to tighten the external sphincter around your finger (Fig. 14-4), noting its tone; it should tighten evenly with no discomfort to the patient. A lax sphincter may indicate neurologic deficit. An extremely tight sphincter can result from scarring, spasticity caused by a fissure or other lesion, inflammation, or anxiety about the examination.

Fig. 14-3
A, Correct procedure for introducing finger into rectum. Press pad of finger against the anal opening. **B,** As external sphincter relaxes, slip the fingertip into the anal canal. Note that patient is in the hips-flexed position.

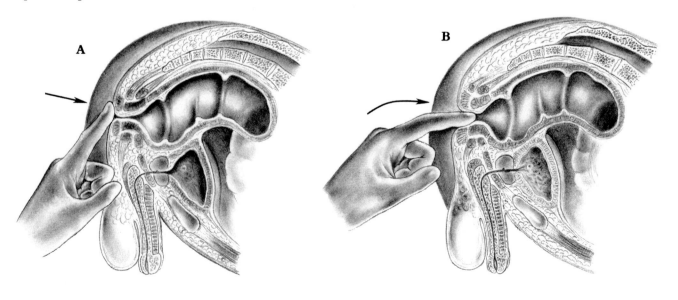

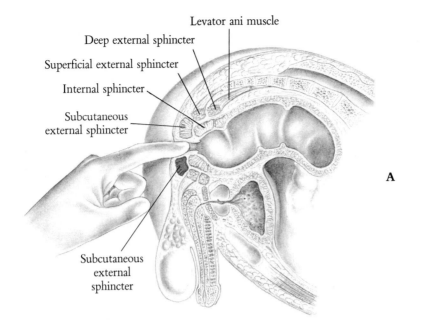

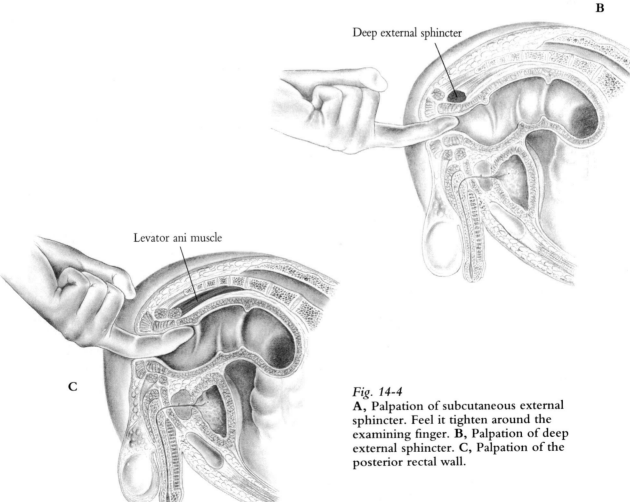

Fig. 14-4
A, Palpation of subcutaneous external sphincter. Feel it tighten around the examining finger. **B,** Palpation of deep external sphincter. **C,** Palpation of the posterior rectal wall.

Fig. 14-5
Palpation of the anterior
surface of the prostate
gland. Feel for the lateral
lobes and median sulcus.

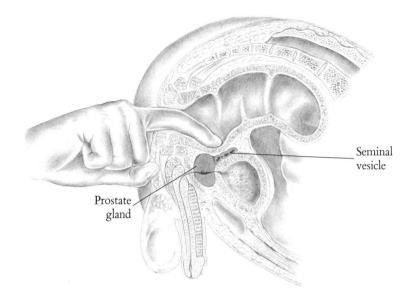

Seminal
vesicle

Prostate
gland

An anal fistula or fissure may produce such extreme tenderness that you are not able to complete the examination without local anesthesia. Rectal pain is almost always indicative of a local disease. Look for irritation, rock hard constipation, rectal fissures, or thrombosed hemorrhoids. Always inquire about previous episodes of pain. The patient with a really acute problem will often shift uncomfortably from side to side when sitting.

Rotate your finger to examine the muscular anal ring (Fig. 14-4, *B*). It should feel smooth and exert even pressure on the finger. Note any nodules or irregularities.

Insert your finger farther and palpate in sequence the lateral and posterior rectal walls, noting any nodules, masses, irregularities, polyps, or tenderness (Fig. 14-4, *C*). The walls should feel smooth, even, and uninterrupted. Internal hemorrhoids are not ordinarily felt unless they are thrombosed. The examining finger can palpate a distance of about 6 to 10 cm into the rectum.

Bidigital palpation with the thumb and index finger can sometimes reveal more information than palpating with the index finger alone. To perform bidigital palpation, lightly press your thumb against the perianal tissue and bring your index finger toward the thumb. This technique is particularly useful for detecting a perianal abscess.

Rotate the index finger to palpate the anterior rectal wall as above. In males you can palpate the posterior surface of the prostate gland (Fig. 14-5). Tell the patient that he may feel the urge to urinate but that he will not. Note the size, contour, consistency, and mobility of the prostate. The gland should feel like a pencil eraser—firm, smooth, and slightly moveable—and it should be nontender. A healthy prostate has a diameter of about 4 cm with less than 1 cm protrusion into the rectum. Greater protrusion denotes prostatic enlargement, which should be noted and the amount of protrusion recorded. Prostatic enlargement is classified by the amount of projection into the rectum; grade I is 1 to 2 cm of protrusion; grade II, 2 to 3 cm; grade III, 3 to 4 cm; and grade IV, more than 4 cm. The sulcus may be obliterated when the lobes are hypertrophied or neoplastic. A rubbery or boggy consistency is indicative of benign hypertrophy, while stony hard nodularity may indicate carcinoma, prostatic calculi, or chronic fibrosis. Fluctuant softness suggests prostatic abscess. Identify the lateral lobes and the median sulcus. The prostatic lobes should feel symmetric. The seminal vesicles are not palpable unless they are inflamed.

Palpation of the prostate can force secretions through the urethral orifice. Any secretions that appear at the meatus should be cultured and examined microscopically. Specimen preparation techniques are described in Chapter 12 (Female Genitalia).

In females the cervix may be palpable through the anterior rectal wall. A retroflexed or retroverted uterus is usually palpable through rectal examination (see Chapter 12). Do not mistake these structures or a tampon for a tumor.

After palpating the anterior wall in females and the prostate in males, ask the patient to bear down. This allows you to reach a few centimeters farther into the rectum. Because the anterior rectal wall is in contact with the peritoneum, you may be able to detect the tenderness of peritoneal inflammation and the nodularity of peritoneal metastases. The nodules, called shelf lesions, are papable just above the prostate in males and in the cul-de-sac of females.

Slowly withdraw your finger and examine it for any fecal material, which should be soft and brown. Note any blood or pus. Very light tan or gray stool could indicate obstructive jaundice, whereas tarry black stool should make you suspect upper intestinal tract bleeding. A more subtle blood loss can result in a virtually normal color of the stool, but even a small amount will yield a positive test for occult blood. Test any fecal material for blood using a chemical guaiac procedure. Proctoscopy is indicated if there is persistent anal or rectal bleeding, any interruption in the smooth contour of the rectal wall on palpation, persistent pain with negative findings on rectal examination, or unexplained persistent stool changes.

COMMON CAUSES OF RECTAL BLEEDING

There are numerous reasons that blood can appear in the feces, ranging from benign, self-limiting events to serious, life-threatening disease. Following are some common causes:

Swallowed blood	Regional enteritis
Hiatus hernia	Anal fissures
Meckel's diverticulum	Esophageal varices
Peptic ulcers, acute and chronic	Intussusception
Dysentery, acute and amoebic	Volvulus
Hookworm	Strangulated hernia
Aspirin-containing medications	Anaphylactoid purpura
Oral steroids	Familial telangiectasia
Iron poisoning	Bleeding disorders
Foreign body trauma	Thrombocytopenia
Polyps, single or multiple	Coagluation disorders
Neoplasms of any kind	Hemorrhoids
Colitis	

STOOL CHARACTERISTICS IN DISEASE

Changes in the shape, content, or consistency of the stool suggests that some disease process is at work. Knowing the stool characteristics can sometimes point to the type of disorder present. Intermittent, pencil-like stools suggest a spasmodic contraction in the rectal area. If persistent, permanent stenosis from scarring or from pressure of a malignancy is likely. Pipe-stem stools and ribbon stools indicate lower rectal stricture. A large amount of mucus in the fecal matter is characteristic of intestinal inflammation and mucous colitis. Small flecks of blood-stained mucus in liquid feces appear in amebiasis. Fatty stools are seen in pancreatic disease and malabsorption syndromes. Stools the color of aluminum, caused by a mixture of melena and fat, occur in tropical sprue, carcinoma of the hepatopancreatic ampulla, and children with diarrhea who are given sulfonamides.

INFANTS AND CHILDREN

Rectal examination is not automatically performed on infants and children unless there is a particular problem. An examination is required whenever there is any symptom that suggests an intraabdominal or pelvic problem, a mass or tenderness, bladder distention, bleeding, or rectal or bowel abnormalities. Deviation from the expected stool pattern (Table 14-1) in infants demands investigation.

It is imperative that you respect the child's modesty and apprehension. Careful explanation of each step in the process is necessary for the child who is old enough to understand.

Routinely inspect the anal region and perineum, examining the surrounding buttocks for redness, masses, and evidence of change in firmness. Inspect for swollen, tender perirectal protrusion, abscesses, and possibly rectal fistulae. There are a variety of problems that can be discovered by this inspection. Shrunken buttocks suggests a chronic debilitating disease. Asymmetric creases occur with congenital dislocation of the hips. Perirectal redness and irritation are suggestive of pinworms, *Candida,* or other irritants of the diaper area. Rectal prolapse results from constipation, diarrhea, or sometimes severe coughing or straining. Hemorrhoids are rare in children, and their presence suggests a serious underlying problem such as portal hypertension. Small flat flaps of skin around the rectum (condylomas) may be syphilitic in origin. Sinuses, tufts of hair, and dimpling in the pilonidal area may indicate lower spinal deformities.

Lightly touch the anal opening, which should produce anal contraction. Lack of contraction may indicate a lower spinal cord lesion.

Examine the patency of the anus and its position in all newborn infants. To determine patency, insert a lubricated catheter no more than 1 cm into the rectum. Patency is usually confirmed by passage of meconium. Occasionally a perianal fistula may be confused with a normal orifice. Be careful in making this judgment. Sometimes the anal orifice can seem appropriate, yet there may be atresia just inside or a few centimeters within the rectum. Rectal examination or inserting a catheter does not always provide definitive assessment, and radiologic studies may be necessary. If there is no evidence of stool in the newborn, suspect rectal atresia, Hirschsprung's disease (congenital megacolon), or cystic fibrosis.

Perform the rectal examination in infants and young children with the child lying on his or her back. You may hold the child's feet together and flex the knees and hips on the abdomen with one hand, using the gloved index finger of your other hand for the examination (Fig. 14-6). Some examiners are reluctant to use the index finger because of its size, choosing instead the fifth finger. However, even with the smallest of adult fingers, some bleeding and transient prolapse of the rectum often occur right after examination. Always warn the parents of this possibility.

Assess the tone of the rectal sphincter. It should feel snug but neither too tight nor too loose. A very tight sphincter can cause enough tension to produce a stenosis, which leads to stool retention and pain during a bowel movement. A lax sphincter is associated with lesions of the peripheral spinal nerves or spinal cord, *Shigella* infection, and previous fecal impactions.

Table 14-1
Sequence and Description of Stools in Infants

Infants	Type of Stool
Newborn	Meconium: greenish-black, viscous, contains occult blood; first stool is sterile; passed within 24 hours by 94% of newborns
3-6 days old	Transitional: thin, slimy, brown to green
Breast-fed	Mushy, loose, golden yellow; frequency varies from after each feeding to every few days; nonirritating to skin
Formula-fed	Light yellow, characteristic foul odor, irritating to skin

Adapted from Bobak and Jensen, 1984.

Fig. 14-6
Positioning the infant or child for rectal examination.

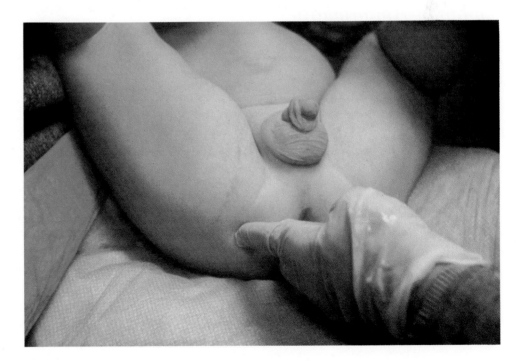

Feel for feces in the rectum. Chronic constipation in children with mental deficiency or emotional problems is often associated with a rectum distended with feces. A consistently empty rectum in the presence of constipation is a clue to the diagnosis of Hirschsprung's disease. A fecal mass in the rectum accompanying diarrhea suggests overflow diarrhea. Stool recovered on the examining finger should be tested for occult blood.

A rectal examination in the young female gives good access to information about the cervix and the uterus (see Chapter 12, Female Genitalia). The ovaries are not palpable on rectal examination.

In boys the prostate is usually not felt. A palpable prostate in preadolescent boys suggests precocious puberty or some virilizing disease.

The rectum can be further evaluated for suspected fissures, fistulae, or polyps by using a small proctoscope or even a wide-mouth speculum on the otoscope.

Rectal examination should be a usual part of the physical examination for adolescents. The same procedures and guidelines that are used for adults apply to adolescents. Be especially sensitive to a first examination, and spend additional time explaining what to expect. Illustrations and models can be very helpful.

OLDER ADULTS

The examination procedure and findings for the older adult are much the same as those for the younger adult. The older patient may be more limited in ability to assume a position other than the left lateral. Sphincter tone may be somewhat decreased. Older males are far more likely to have an enlarged prostate, which will be felt as smooth, rubbery, and symmetric. The median sulcus may or may not be obliterated. Older adults are more likely to have polyps and are at higher risk for carcinoma, making the rectal examination particularly important in this age group.

Common Abnormalities

Anus, Rectum, and Surrounding Skin

Pilonidal Cyst or Sinus

Most pilonidal cysts and sinuses are first diagnosed in young adults, although they are usually a congenital anomaly. Located in the midline, superficial to the coccyx and lower sacrum, the cyst or sinus is seen as a dimple with a sinus tract opening. The opening may contain a tuft of hair and be surrounded by erythema. A cyst may be palpable. The condition is usually asymptomatic, but it is sometimes complicated by an abscess, secondary infection, or fistula.

Perianal and Perirectal Abscesses

These abscesses appear as an area of swelling with variable degrees of erythema of the anus, both internally and externally. The abscess is painful and tender, and usually the patient has a fever (Fig. 14-7).

Fig. 14-7
Perianal/perirectal abscess.
Common sites of abscess
formation.

Supra-levator
ani muscle
abcess

Ischiorectal
abcess

Perirectal
abcess

Anorectal Fissure and Fistula

A tear in the anal mucosa *(fissure)* appears most often in the posterior midline, although it can also occur in the anterior midline. The fissure is usually caused by traumatic passage of large, hard stools. A sentinel skin tag may be seen at the lower edge of the fissure. There may be ulceration through which muscles of the internal sphincter are seen. The patient may have symptoms of pain, itching, or bleeding. The internal sphincter is spastic. Examination is painful and may require local anesthesia (Fig. 14-8).

An *anorectal fistula* is an inflammatory tract that runs from the anus or rectum and opens onto the surface of the perianal skin or other tissue. It is caused by drainage of a perianal or perirectal abscess. Serosanguinous or purulent drainage may appear with compression of the area. The external opening is usually seen as elevated red granular tissue.

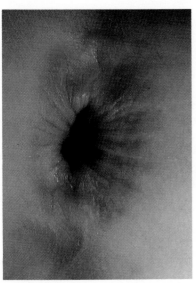

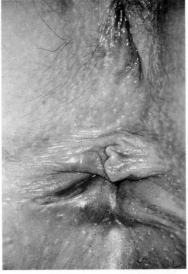

Fig. 14-8
A, Anal fissure in child.
B, Lateral anal fissure
in adult.

A from 400 Self-assessment picture tests, 1984. **B** courtesy Gershon Efron, M.D., Sinai Hospital of Baltimore.

A   **B**

Pruritus Ani

Chronic inflammation of perianal skin results in excoriation, thickening, and pigmentation. The patient complains of burning or itching that may interfere with sleep. It is commonly caused by fungal infection in adults and by parasites in children.

Hemorrhoids

External hemorrhoids are varicose veins that originate below the anorectal line and are covered by anal skin. They may cause itching and bleeding with defecation. Usually not visible at rest, they can protrude on standing and straining at stool. If not reduced, they can become edematous and thrombosed and may require surgical removal. Thrombosed hemorrhoids appear as blue, shiny masses at the anus. Hemorrhoidal skin tags, which can appear at the site of resolved hemorrhoids, are fibrotic or flaccid and painless (Fig. 14-9).

Internal hemorrhoids are varicose veins that originate above the anorectal junction and are covered by rectal mucosa. They produce soft swellings that are not palpable on rectal examination and are not visible unless they prolapse through the anus. They do not cause discomfort unless they are thrombosed, prolapsed, or infected. Bleeding may occur with or without defecation. Proctoscopy is usually required for diagnosis (Fig. 14-9).

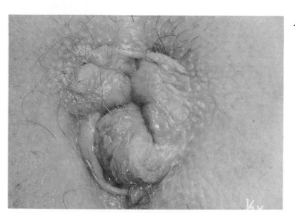

A

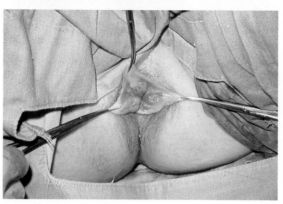

B

Fig. 14-9
**A, Prolapsed hemorrhoids.
B, Primary internal hemorrhoids.**
Courtesy Gershon Efron, M.D., Sinai Hospital of Baltimore.

Polyps

Occurring anywhere in the intestinal tract, polyps are a relatively common finding. They may be adenomas or inflammatory in origin and can occur singly or in profusion. Polyps are usually evidenced by rectal bleeding, and it is not uncommon to find a polyp protruding through the rectum. They are sometimes palpable on rectal examination as soft nodules and can be either pedunculated (on a stalk) or sessile (closely adhering to the mucosal wall). However, because of their soft consistency, polyps may be difficult to feel on palpation. Proctoscopy is usually required for diagnosis, and biopsy is performed to distinguish them from carcinoma (Fig. 14-10).

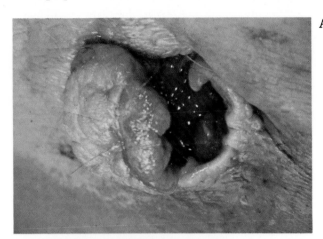

A

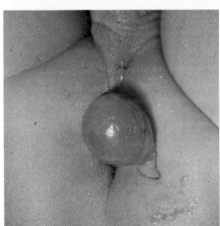

B

Fig. 14-10
A, Fibroepithelial polyp of the rectum. **B,** Infant with prolapsed rectal polyp.
Courtesy Gershon Efron, M.D., Sinai Hospital of Baltimore.

Rectal Carcinoma

Cancer of the rectum is usually felt as a sessile polypoid mass with nodular raised edges and areas of ulceration. The consistency is often stony, and the contour is irregular. Rectal carcinoma is often asymptomatic, so routine rectal examination is essential for adults.

Intraperitoneal Metastases

Malignant metastases may develop in the pelvis anterior to the rectum. These can be felt as a hard, nodular shelf at the tip of the examining finger.

Rectal Prolapse

The rectal mucosa, with or without the muscular wall, prolapses through the anal ring as the patient strains at stool. A prolapse of the mucosa is pink and looks like a doughnut or rosette. Complete prolapse involving the muscular wall is larger, red, and has circular folds. Rectal prolapse in children is associated with cystic fibrosis (Fig. 14-11).

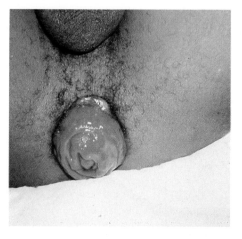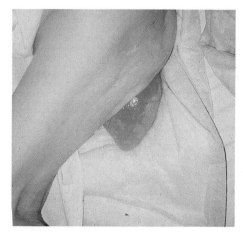

Fig. 14-11
Prolapse of the rectum.
Courtesy Gershon Efron, M.D., Sinai Hospital of Baltimore.

Prostate

Prostatitis

In *acute prostatitis* the prostate is enlarged, acutely tender, and often asymmetric. The patient may also have urethral discharge and fever. An abscess may develop, which is felt as a fluctuant mass in the prostate. The seminal vesicles are often involved and may be dilated and tender on palpation (Fig. 14-12).

Chronic prostatitis is usually asymptomatic. However, the prostate may feel boggy, enlarged, and tender or have palpable areas of fibrosis that simulate neoplasm.

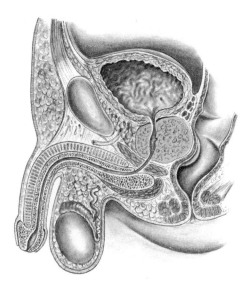

Fig. 14-12
Prostatitis.

CHILDREN

Imperforate Anus A variety of anorectal malformations can occur during fetal development. The rectum may end blindly, be stenosed, or have a fistulous connection to the perineum, urinary tract, or in females the vagina. The condition is usually diagnosed by rectal examination and confirmed by lack of passage of stool within the first 48 hours of life. Radiographic confirmation may be necessary (Figs. 14-13 to 14-15).

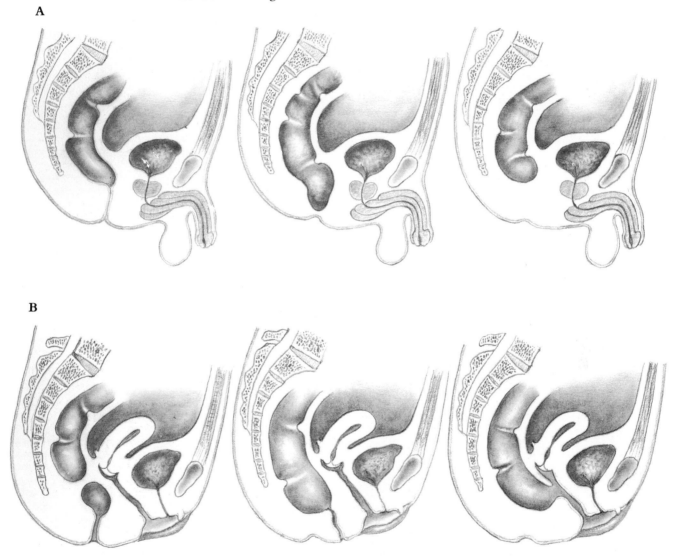

A

B

Fig. 14-13
Imperforate anus: various anorectal malformations. **A**, Left to right: congenital anal stenosis, anal membrane atresia, anal agenesis. **B**, Left to right: rectal atresia, retroperineal fistula, rectovaginal fistula.

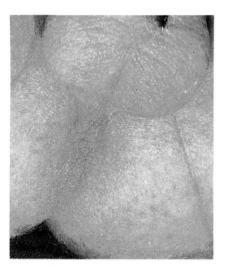

Fig. 14-14
Imperforate anus.
From Diagnostic picture tests in clinical medicine, 1984.

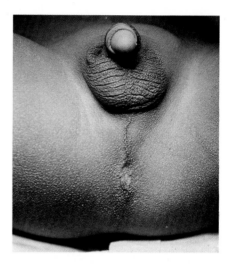

Fig. 14-15
Rectal atresia.
Courtesy Gershon Efron, M.D., Sinai Hospital of Baltimore.

Enterobiasis Infestation (Roundworm, Pinworm)

The adult nematode lives in the rectum or colon and emerges onto perianal skin to lay eggs while the child sleeps. The patient experiences intense itching of the perianal area, and perianal irritation often results from scratching. The parents often describe unexplained irritability in the infant or child, especially at night. The nematodes can be seen on microscopic examination. To obtain a specimen, press the sticky side of cellulose tape against the perianal folds and then press the tape on a glass side.

OLDER ADULTS

Benign Prostatic Hypertrophy (BPH)

A hypertrophic prostate is common in men over age 50. The gland begins to grow at age 45, continuing to enlarge with advancing age. Growth of the prostate parallels the increased incidence of BPH. Urinary symptoms include hesitancy, decreased force and caliber of stream, dribbling, incomplete emptying of the bladder, frequency, urgency, nocturia, and dysuria. On rectal examination the prostate feels smooth, rubbery, symmetric, and enlarged. The median sulcus may or may not be obliterated (Fig. 14-16).

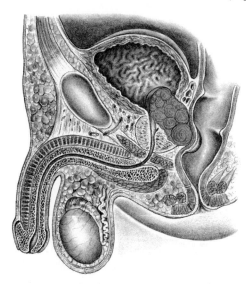

Fig. 14-16
Benign prostatic hypertrophy.

Prostatic Carcinoma

Rare before age 50, the incidence of prostatic cancer increases with age. Early carcinoma is asymptomatic. As the malignancy advances, symptoms of urinary obstruction occur. On rectal examination a hard, irregular nodule may be palpable. The prostate feels asymmetric, and the median sulcus is obliterated as the carcinoma enlarges. Prostatic calculi and chronic inflammation produce similar findings, and biopsy is required for differential diagnosis (Fig. 14-17).

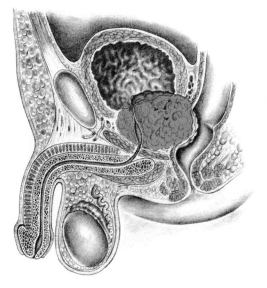

Fig. 14-17
Carcinoma of prostate.

C H A P T E R

Lymphatic System

Anatomy and Physiology

The lymphatic system is made up of lymph fluid, the collecting ducts, and various tissues including the lymph nodes, spleen, thymus, tonsils and adenoids, and Peyer's patches. Bits of lymph tissue are present in other parts of the body, including the mucosa of the stomach and appendix, bone marrow, and lungs (Fig. 15-1). The entire mass of the system is no more than 3% of the total body weight. The lymphatic system provides a network of defense against the invasion of microorganisms, allowing their capture and ultimate destruction.

Every tissue supplied by blood vessels has lymphatic vessels except the placenta and the brain. This wide-ranging presence is essential to the system's role in immunologic and metabolic processes. The activities of the lymphatic system, not yet completely understood, consist mainly of the following:
- Movement of lymph fluid in a closed circuit with the cardiovascular system
- Production of lymphocytes within the lymph nodes, tonsils, adenoids, spleen, and bone marrow
- Production of antibodies
- Phagocytosis, a specific function of cells that line the sinuses of lymph nodes
- Absorption of fat and fat-soluble substances from the intestinal tract
- Manufacture of blood when the primary sources are pathophysiologically compromised

In addition, the lymphatic system plays an unwanted role in providing at least one pathway for the spread of malignancy.

Lymph is a clear, sometimes opalescent and sometimes yellow-tinged fluid; it contains a variety of white blood cells (mostly lymphocytes) and occasional red blood cells. The lymphatic and cardiovascular systems are intimately related. The fluids and proteins that comprise lymphatic fluid originally move from the bloodstream into the interstitial spaces. They are then collected throughout the body by a profusion of microscopic tubules (Fig. 15-2). These tubules join together, forming larger ducts that collect lymph and carry it to the lymph nodes around the body.

The lymph nodes receive lymph from the collecting ducts in the various regions (Figs. 15-3 through 15-10), passing it on through efferent vessels. Ultimately the large ducts merge into the venous system at the subclavian veins.

The drainage point for the right upper body is a lymphatic trunk that empties into the right subclavian vein. The thoracic duct, the major vessel of the lymphatic system, drains lymph from the rest of the body into the left subclavian vein. It returns the various fluids and proteins to the cardiovascular system, forming a closed but porous circle. *Text continued on p. 498.*

Fig. 15-1
**Lymphatic system (lym-
phoreticular system).**

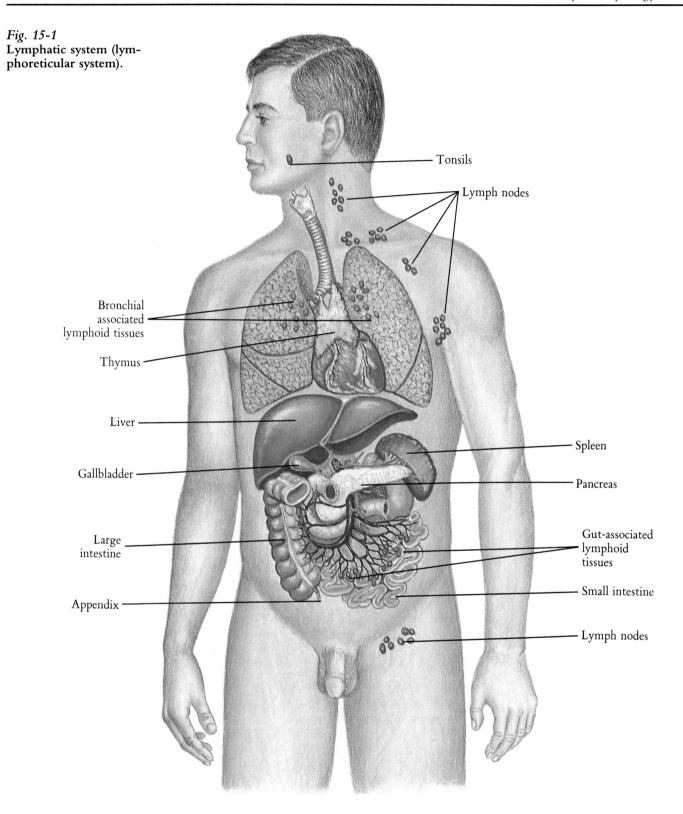

Tonsils

Lymph nodes

Bronchial
associated
lymphoid tissues

Thymus

Liver

Spleen

Gallbladder

Pancreas

Large
intestine

Gut-associated
lymphoid
tissues

Small intestine

Appendix

Lymph nodes

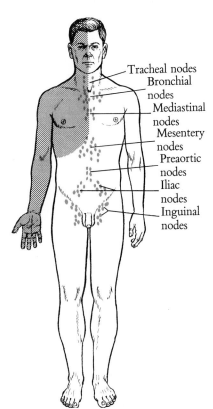

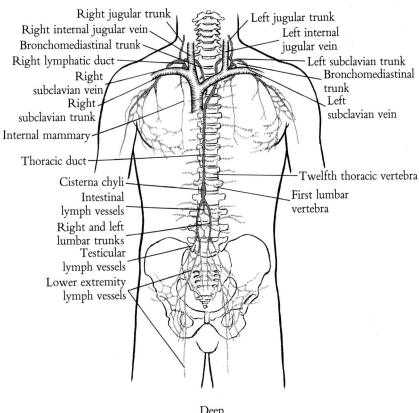

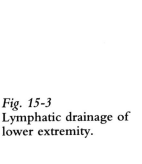

Fig. 15-2
Lymphatic drainage pathways. Shaded area of the body is drained via the right lymphatic duct, which is formed by the union of three vessels: right jugular trunk, right subclavian trunk, and right bronchomediastinal trunk. Lymph from the remainder of the body enters the venous system by way of the thoracic duct.

Adapted from Francis and Martin, 1975.

Fig. 15-3
Lymphatic drainage of lower extremity.

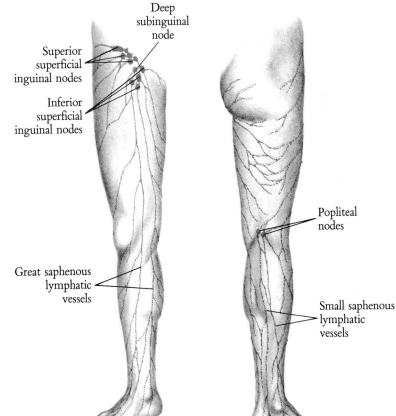

Fig. 15-4
System of deep and superficial collecting ducts, carrying lymph from upper extremity to subclavian lymphatic trunk. The only peripheral lymph center is the epitrochlear, which receives some of the collecting ducts from the pathway of the ulnar and radial nerves.

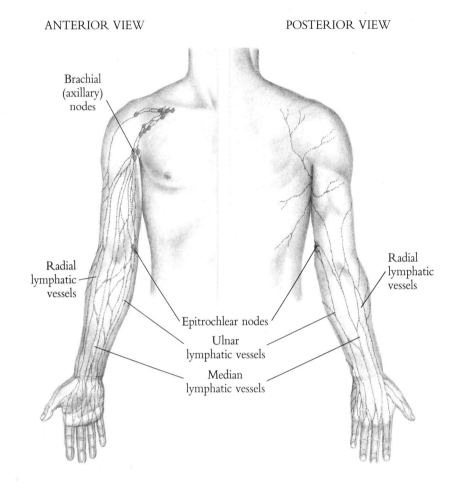

ANTERIOR VIEW   POSTERIOR VIEW

Brachial
(axillary)
nodes

Radial
lymphatic
vessels

Radial
lymphatic
vessels

Epitrochlear nodes

Ulnar
lymphatic vessels

Median
lymphatic vessels

Fig. 15-5
Six groups of lymph nodes may be distinguished in the axillary fossa.

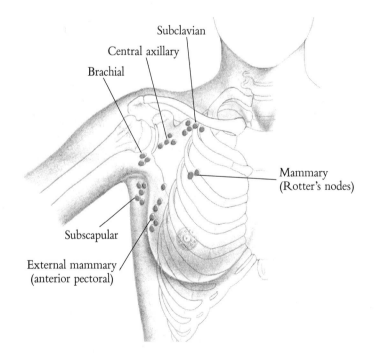

Subclavian

Central axillary

Brachial

Mammary
(Rotter's nodes)

Subscapular

External mammary
(anterior pectoral)

Fig. 15-6
Lymphatic drainage of breast.

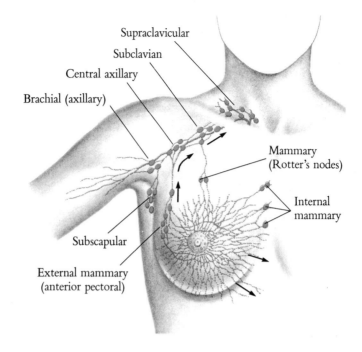

Fig. 15-7
Lymph nodes involved with the ear.

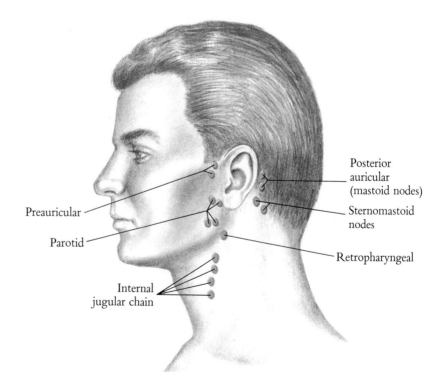

Fig. 15-8
Lymph nodes involved with the tongue.

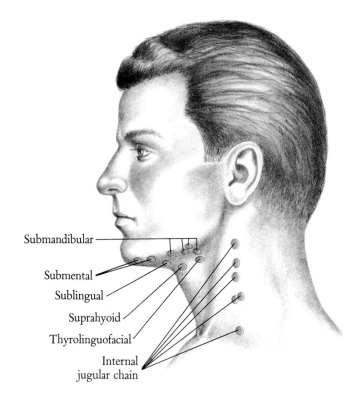

Submandibular

Submental

Sublingual

Suprahyoid

Thyrolinguofacial

Internal jugular chain

Fig. 15-9
Lymphatic drainage system of head and neck. If the group of nodes is often referred to by another name, the second name appears in parentheses.

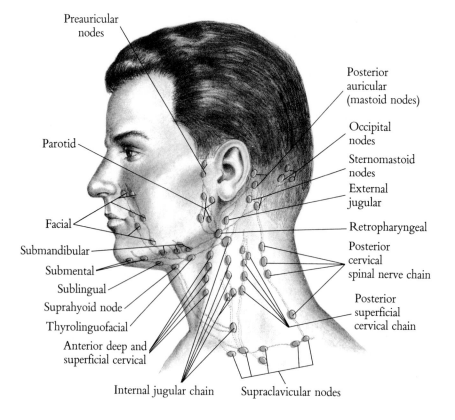

Preauricular nodes

Posterior auricular (mastoid nodes)

Occipital nodes

Sternomastoid nodes

External jugular

Retropharyngeal

Posterior cervical spinal nerve chain

Posterior superficial cervical chain

Parotid

Facial

Submandibular

Submental

Sublingual

Suprahyoid node

Thyrolinguofacial

Anterior deep and superficial cervical

Internal jugular chain

Supraclavicular nodes

Fig. 15-10
Lymph nodes of neck.
Note relationship to the
sternocleidomastoid
muscle.

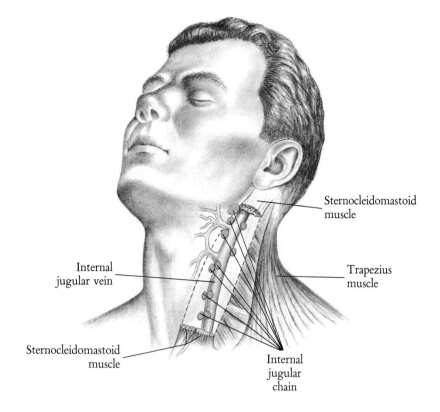

Sternocleidomastoid muscle

Internal jugular vein

Trapezius muscle

Sternocleidomastoid muscle

Internal jugular chain

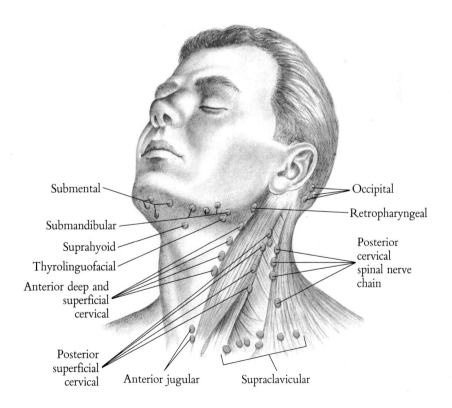

Submental

Submandibular

Suprahyoid

Thyrolinguofacial

Anterior deep and superficial cervical

Posterior superficial cervical

Anterior jugular

Supraclavicular

Occipital

Retropharyngeal

Posterior cervical spinal nerve chain

Because the lymphatic system has no pumping mechanisms of its own, it depends on the cardiovascular system for much of its impetus. The movement of lymph is sluggish compared with that of the blood. As lymph fluid volume increases, it flows faster in response to mounting capillary pressure, greater permeability of the capillary walls of the cardiovascular system, increased bodily or metabolic activity, and massage. Conversely, any mechanical obstruction will slow or stop the movement of lymph, dilating the system. The permeability of the lymphatic system is protective; if it is obstructed, lymph may diffuse into the vascular system, or collateral connecting channels may develop.

Lymph Nodes

The lymph nodes usually occur in groups. Superficial nodes are located in subcutaneous connective tissues, and deeper nodes lie beneath the fascia of muscles and within the various body cavities. They are numerous and tiny, but some of them may have diameters as large as 0.5 to 1 cm.

The superficial lymph nodes are the gateway to assessing the health of the entire lymphatic system. They are accessible to inspection and palpation, and they provide some of the earliest clues to the presence of infection or malignancy.

Lymphocytes

Lymphocytes are produced in the lymph nodes, tonsils, adenoids, spleen, and bone marrow. Lymphocytes arising from precursor cells in the nodes may stay in the node, never changing. Other lymphocytes differentiate into a variety of cells, remaining within lymphoid tissue or entering the lymph fluid and the blood.

Two types of lymphocytes enter the peripheral bloodstream: B lymphocytes have a 3- to 4-day life span and are relatively small in number; T lymphocytes have a lifespan of 100 to 200 days and are relatively numerous. An increased number of lymphocytes is a systemic response to most viral infections and some bacterial infections.

Thymus

The thymus is located in the superior mediastinum, extending upward into the lower neck. In early life the thymus is essential to the development of the protective immune function, but it serves little or no function in adults (Fig. 15-11).

Spleen

The spleen is situated in the left upper quadrant of the abdominal cavity between the stomach and the diaphragm. A highly vascular organ, it is essentially composed of two systems: the white pulp, made up of lymphatic nodules and diffuse lymphatic tissue, and the red pulp, made up of venous sinusoids. The spleen is a blood-forming organ early in life, a site for the storage of red corpuscles, and with its plethora of blood-filtering macrophages, part of the body's defense system. (See Chapter 11, Abdomen, for further discussion of the spleen.)

Tonsils and Adenoids

The palatine tonsils are commonly referred to as "the tonsils" without further description. Small and diamond shaped, they are set between the palatine arches on either side of the pharynx, just beyond the base of the tongue. Composed principally of lymphoid tissue, the tonsils are organized as follicles and crypts, covered by mucous membrane. The pharyngeal tonsils, or adenoids, are located at the nasopharyngeal border. When the adenoids are enlarged as a result of frequent bacterial or viral invasion, they can obstruct the nasopharyngeal passageway.

Fig. 15-11
Location of thymus gland
and its size relative to the
rest of the body during infancy (**A**) and adult life (**B**).

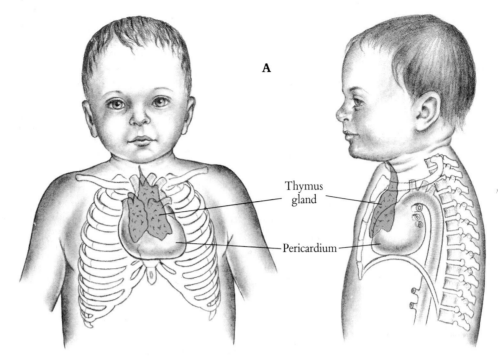

A

Thymus
gland

Pericardium

ANTERIOR VEIW

LATERAL VIEW

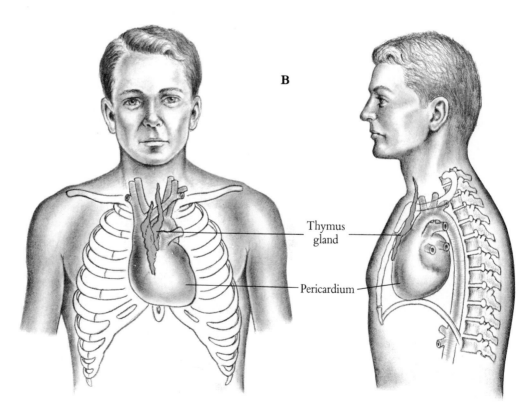

B

Thymus
gland

Pericardium

ANTERIOR VIEW

LATERAL VIEW

Peyer's Patches

Peyer's patches are small, elevated areas of lymph tissue on the mucosa of the small intestine. They actually consist of many lymphoid nodules grouped together, serving the intestinal tract.

INFANTS AND CHILDREN

The immune system and the lymphoid system begin developing at about 20 weeks gestation. The ability to produce antibodies is still immature at birth, which increases an infant's susceptibility to infection, particularly from bacteria, during the first few months of life. Lymphoid tissue is relatively plentiful in infants, increases during childhood especially between 6 to 9 years, and then regresses to adult levels by puberty (see Fig. 3-3, Chapter 3, Growth and Measurement).

The thymus is at its largest relative to the rest of the body shortly after birth, but reaches its greatest absolute weight at puberty. Then it begins to involute, replacing much of its tissue with fat and becoming a rudimentary organ in the adult.

The palatine tonsils, as all lymphoid tissue, are much larger during early childhood than after puberty. An enlargement of the tonsils in children is not indicative of problems.

The lymph nodes have the same distribution in children as in adults. Although not ordinarily palpable in the newborn, they react readily to any mild stimulus and may quickly become larger, particularly in the cervical and postauricular chains. It is possible that this relatively large mass of lymphoid tissue is needed to compensate for a rather immature ability to produce antibodies, thus adding to the demand for filtration and phagocytosis.

The lymphatic system gradually reaches adult competency during childhood (Fig. 15-12).

Fig. 15-12
Relative levels of presence and function of the immune factors.

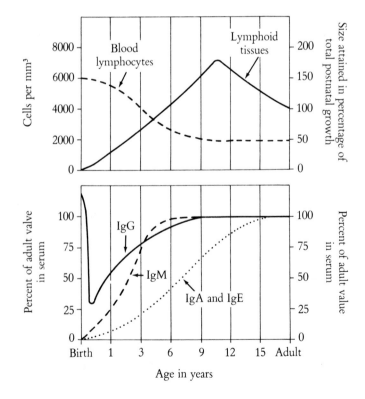

OLDER ADULTS The number of lymph nodes may diminish and decrease in size with advanced age, and some of the lymphoid elements are lost. The nodes of older patients are more likely to be fibrotic and fatty than those of the young, resulting in an impaired ability to resist infection.

Review of Related History

General Considerations

1. Environmental: exposure to radiation, toxic chemicals, infection, HTLV-III virus
2. Fatigue, weakness
3. Weight gain or loss
4. Travel to sites of infectious outbreaks
5. Medications: chemotherapy, antibiotics
6. Intravenous street drug use

Present Problem

1. Bleeding
   a. Site: nose, mouth, gums, rectal (blood in stools; black, tarry stools), skin (blood spots that do not blanch on pressure, easy bruising), in vomit
   b. Character: onset, frequency, duration, amount, color (bright red, brown, coffee-colored)
   c. Associated symptoms: pallor, dizziness, headache, shortness of breath
2. Enlarged nodes (bumps, kernels, swollen glands)
   a. Character: onset, location, duration, number, tenderness
   b. Associated symptoms: pain, fever, redness, warmth, red streaks, itching (some tumors cause pruritus)
   c. Predisposing factors: infection, surgery, trauma
3. Swelling of extremity
   a. Unilateral or bilateral, intermittent or constant, duration
   b. Predisposing factors: cardiac or renal disorder, surgery, infection, trauma, venous insufficiency
   c. Associated symptoms: warmth, redness or discoloration, ulceration
   d. Efforts at treatment and their effect: support stockings, elevation

Past Medical History

1. Chest x-rays
2. Tuberculosis and other skin testing
3. Blood transfusions, use of blood products
4. Chronic illness: cardiac, renal, malignancy, AIDS
5. Surgery: trauma to regional lymph nodes
6. Recurrent infections

Family History

1. Malignancy
2. Anemia
3. Recent infections
4. Tuberculosis
5. Agammaglobulinemia, severe combined immune deficiency
6. Hemophilia

INFANTS AND CHILDREN

1. Recurrent infections: tonsillitis, adenoiditis, bacterial infections, oral candidiasis, chronic diarrhea
2. Present or recent infections, trauma distal to nodes
3. Poor growth, failure to thrive
4. Loss of interest in play or eating
5. Immunization history

OLDER ADULTS

1. Present or recent infection or trauma distal to nodes
2. Delayed healing

Examination and Findings

EQUIPMENT

■ **Centimeter ruler**

The lymphatic system is examined by inspection and palpation, region by region, as you examine the other body systems. On occasion you may prefer to examine the entire lymphatic system at once, exploring all the areas in which the nodes are located, regardless of their widespread distribution. Individual chapters in this book discuss the lymphatic system in specific body areas.

Inspect each area of the body for apparent lymph nodes, edema, erythema, red streaks, and skin lesions. Using the pads of the second, third, and fourth fingers, gently palpate the superficial lymph nodes. Try to detect any inapparent enlargement, and note the consistency, mobility, tenderness, size, and warmth of the nodes. In areas where the skin is more mobile, move the skin over the area of the nodes. Press lightly at first, increasing pressure gradually. Heavier pressure alone can push nodes out of the way before you have had a chance to recognize their presence. Palpable lymph nodes are generally not found in healthy individuals.

Superficial nodes that are accessible to palpation but not large or firm enough to be felt are common. You may detect small, movable, discrete nodes less than a centimeter in diameter that move under your fingers. When the node seems fixed in its setting, there is a greater cause for concern.

When enlarged lymph nodes are encountered, explore the accessible adjacent areas and regions drained by those nodes for signs of possible infection or malignancy. Examine other regions for enlargement. Enlarged lymph nodes in any region should be characterized according to location, size, shape, consistency, tenderness, movability or fixation to surrounding tissues, and discreteness. Lymph nodes that are enlarged and juxtaposed so that they feel like a large mass rather than discrete nodes are described as matted.

Note if there is tenderness on touch or on rebound, the degree of discoloration or redness, and any unusual increase in vascularity, heat, or pulsations. (If bruits are audible with the stethoscope, it may be a blood vessel, not a lymph node.) Check to see if any large mass transilluminates when you are uncertain of its nature; as a rule, nodes do not and cysts do. Lymph nodes that are large, fixed or matted, inflamed, or tender indicate some problem. Tenderness is almost always indicative of inflammation; cancerous nodes are not usually tender. In bacterial infection, nodes may become warm or tender to the touch, matted, and much less discrete, particularly if the infection persists. It is possible to infer the site of an infection from the pattern of lymph node enlargement. For example, infections of the ear will usually drain to the preauricular, retropharyngeal, and deep cervical nodes (Fig. 15-7). A child with such an infection is apt to complain of an earache, although the pain originates in a node.

Lymph nodes to which a malignancy has spread are not usually tender. They vary greatly in size, from tiny to many centimeters in diameter. They are sometimes discrete and tend to be harder than expected. Involvement is often asymmetric; contralateral nodes in similar locations are not palpable.

In tuberculosis the lymph nodes are usually "cold" (actually, body temperature), soft, matted, and often not tender or painful.

Head and Neck

Palpate the entire neck lightly for nodes. The anterior border of the sternocleidomastoid muscle is the dividing line for the anterior and posterior triangles of the neck and serves as a useful landmark in describing location (see Fig. 5-4). Bending the patient's head slightly forward or to the side will ease taut tissues and allow better accessibility to palpation.

Feel for nodes in the head in the following six-step sequence: (1) the occipital nodes at the base of the skull, (2) the postauricular nodes located superficially over the mastoid process, (3) the preauricular nodes just in front of the ear (Fig. 15-13), (4) the tonsillar nodes at the angle of the mandible, (5) the submaxillary nodes halfway between the angle and the tip of the mandible, and (6) the submental nodes in the midline behind the tip of the mandible.

Then move down to the neck, palpating in this four-step sequence: (1) the superficial cervical nodes at the sternocleidomastoid, (2) the posterior cervical nodes along the anterior border of the trapezius (Fig. 15-14), and (3) the deep cervical

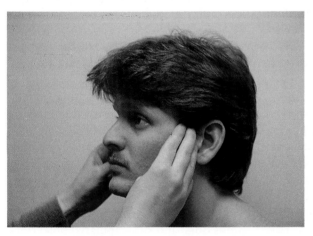

Fig. 15-13
Palpation of preauricular lymph nodes.

Fig. 15-14
Palpation of posterior cervical nodes. Dorsal surfaces (pads) of the fingertips are used to palpate along the anterior surface of the trapezius muscle and then moved slowly forward in a circular movement toward the posterior surface of the sternocleidomastoid muscle.

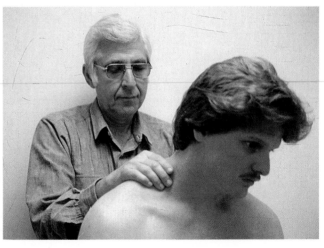

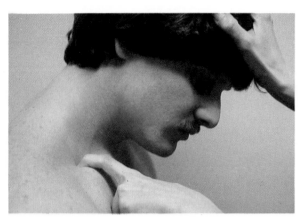

Fig. 15-15
Palpation of scalene triangle for supraclavicular lymph nodes. The patient is encouraged to relax the musculature of the upper extremities, so that the clavicles are dropped. The examiner's free hand is used to flex the patient's head forward to obtain relaxation of the soft tissues of the anterior neck. The left index finger is hooked over the clavicle lateral to the sternocleidomastoid muscle.

Fig. 15-16
Soft tissues of axilla are gently rolled against the chest wall and the muscles surrounding the axilla.

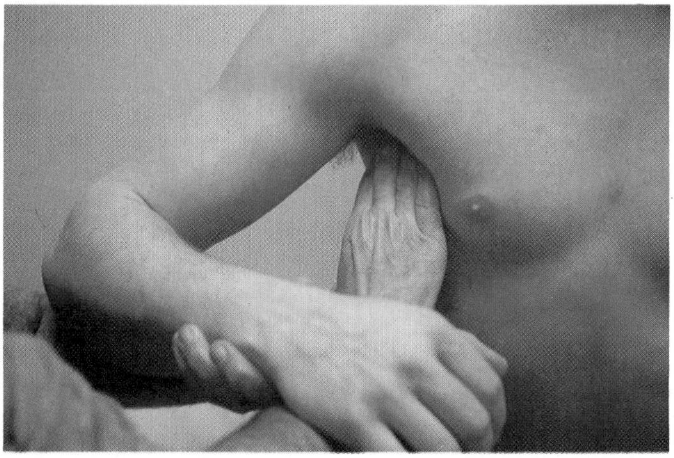

nodes deep to the sternocleidomastoid. The deep cervical nodes may be difficult to feel if you press too vigorously. Probe gently with your thumb and fingers around the muscle. (4) Finally, move to the supraclavicular areas, probing deeply in the angle formed by the clavicle and the sternocleidomastoid muscle, the area of Virchow's nodes (Fig. 15-15). Detection of these nodes should always be considered a cause for concern.

On occasion, postauricular nodes affected by ear infection, particularly external otitis, may be surrounded by some cellulitis. This may cause the ears to protrude.

Supraclavicular nodes are frequently the sites of metastatic disease, because they are located at the end of the thoracic duct and other associated lymphatic ducts. A Virchow's node in the left supraclavicular region may be the result of either abdominal or thoracic malignancy. Mediastinal collecting ducts from the lungs go to both sides of the neck, and supraclavicular nodes may be palpated on both sides.

Axillae

Think of the axillary examination by imagining a pentagonal structure: the pectoral muscles anteriorly, the back muscles (latissimus dorsi and subscapularis) posteriorly, the rib cage medially, the upper arm laterally, and the axilla at the apex. Let the soft tissues roll between your fingers and the chest walls and muscles as you palpate. A firm, deliberate yet gentle touch will feel less ticklish to the patient.

On palpation of the axillary lymph nodes, support the patient's forearm with your contralateral arm and bring the palm of your examining hand flat into the axilla, or alternatively let the patient's forearm rest on that of your examining hand (Fig. 15-16). Rotate your fingertips and palm, feeling the nodes; if they are palpable, attempt to glide your fingers beneath the nodes.

The examination of the breast, the axilla, and adjacent areas is described in Chapter 10 (Breast and Axillae).

Other Lymph Nodes

Use a systematic approach when palpating other sites of lymph node clusterings. Move the hand in a circular fashion, probing without pressing hard. Gently palpate and relieve tension by flexion of the extremity. To palpate the epitrochlear nodes, support the elbow in one hand as you explore with the other (Fig. 15-17). To palpate the inguinal and popliteal area, have the patient lie supine with the knee slightly flexed (Fig. 15-18).

Erythematous streaks arising from sites of infection or injury follow the course of the lymphatic vessels up the extremities, particularly the legs. In the early stage of inflammation, the streaks may be faint but discernible, if you are aware of the possibility. They suggest the presence of lymphangitis.

The lymphatic drainage of the testes is into the abdomen. Enlarged nodes there are not accessible to inspection and palpation. Nodes in the inguinal area enlarge if there are lesions of the penile and scrotal surfaces.

Similarly, the internal female genitalia drain into the pelvic and paraaortic nodes and are not accessible to inspection and palpation. However, the vulva and the lower one third of the vagina drain to the inguinal nodes.

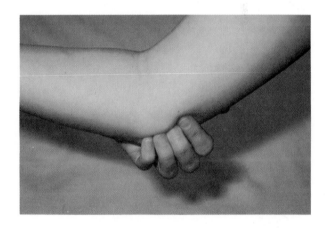

Fig. 15-17
Palpation for epitrochlear lymph nodes is performed in the depression above and posterior to the medial condyle of the humerus.

Fig. 15-18
A, Palpation of inferior superficial inguinal (femoral) lymph nodes. **B,** Palpation of superior superficial inguinal lymph nodes.

A

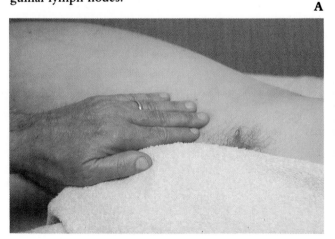

B

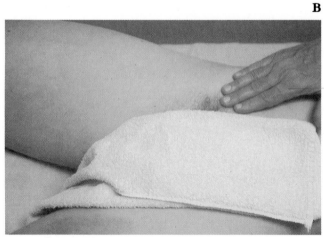

INFANTS AND CHILDREN

The technique of examination is similar for all ages. You will commonly find small, firm, discrete, and movable nodes that are neither warm nor tender located in the occipital, postauricular, cervical, and inguinal chains. The very thin child's inguinal nodes may even be readily visible. In children such nodes are not as worrisome as in the adult. The shape is usually globular or ovoid, sometimes flatter or more cylindrical.

The widespread occurrence of enlarged lymph nodes in children has been frequently documented and demonstrated to be unassociated with serious illness. It is not unusual to find enlarged postauricular and occipital glands in children younger than 2 years old. Past that age, such enlargement is relatively uncommon and may be significant. Conversely, cervical and submandibular nodal enlargement is relatively uncommon in children less than 1 year old and much more frequent in the older child. These age distributions should be considered in your decision to evaluate lymph node enlargement further (Herzog, 1983).

Nodes smaller than 0.5 cm are not generally cause for concern, and nodes with a diameter of 1 cm or less in the cervical and inguinal chains do not always indicate a problem. If nodes are suspiciously large, even mildly painful, or relatively immovable, investigate further.

The palatine tonsils may be enlarged in children, which is not in itself a problem. Excessive enlargement may, of course, obstruct the nasopharynx, increasing the risk of sleep apnea and, on rare occasions, pulmonary hypertension.

SOME CONDITIONS SIMULATING LYMPH NODE ENLARGEMENT

In the neck
   Cystic hygromas
   Thyroglossal duct cysts
   Branchial cleft cysts (sometimes accompanied by a tiny orifice in the
      neck on a line extending to the ear)
   Parotid swelling (e.g., from mumps or tumor)
Widespread
   Lymphangiomas
   Hemangiomas
      These lesions tend to feel spongy and may appear reddish-blue, depending on their size and the extent of the angiomatous involvement.

Common Abnormalities

Acute Lymphangitis	Acute lymphangitis is the inflammation of one or more lymphatic vessels. It is characterized by pain, a feeling of malaise and illness, and possibly fever. On inspection you may find a red streak following the course of the lymphatic collecting duct. It appears as a tracing of rather fine lines that progress up the extremity. The inflammation is sometimes palpable to gentle touch. Look distal to the inflammation for sites of infection, particularly interdigitally.
Lymphoma	Malignant neoplasms of the lymphatic system and the reticuloendothelial tissues are usually well-defined and solid. Histologically, their cells are often undifferentiated but resemble lymphocytes, histiocytes, or plasma cells. Lymphomas occur most often in lymph nodes, the spleen, and other sites in which lymphoreticular cells are found.
Hodgkin's Disease	Hodgkin's disease is a malignant lymphoma that occurs in the young of all races, generally in late adolescence and young adulthood, although it also occurs in people over 50. Males are twice as likely to develop Hodgkin's disease as females. Its clinical presentation is variable. Most commonly, there is a painless enlargement of the cervical lymph nodes that is generally asymmetric and inexorably progressive. Occasionally, pressure of the node on surrounding structures will produce symptoms that prompt the patient to seek medical care. The nodes are sometimes matted and generally feel very firm, almost rubbery. While asymmetry is the rule, nodes are occasionally enlarged in similar patterns on both sides of the body. The nodal size may fluctuate.
Acquired Immune Deficiency Syndrome (AIDS)	Acquired immune deficiency syndrome is characterized by the dysfunction of cell-mediated immunity. It is manifested clinically as the development of recurrent, often severe, opportunistic infections. The most common manifestations associated with full-blown AIDS are two life-threatening diseases: Kaposi's sarcoma and *Pneumocystis carinii* pneumonia. Initial symptoms include lymphadenopathy, fatigue, fever, and weight loss. AIDS is caused by the HTLV-III (HIV) virus.
AIDS-Related Complex (ARC)	A syndrome referred to as AIDS-related complex, pre-AIDS, or chronic lymphadenopathy syndrome has been described. It refers to the immunosuppression in a person from a high-risk group who has HTLV-III antibodies but has not yet developed the sequelae of recurrent infections and neoplastic disease. Signs and symptoms of ARC may include severe fatigue, malaise, weakness, persistent unexplained weight loss, persistent lymphadenopathy, fevers, arthralgias, and persistent diarrhea.

Lymphedema

Congenital lymphedema (Milroy's disease) is the hypoplasia and maldevelopment of the lymphatic system, resulting in swelling and often grotesque distortion of the extremities. The degree varies with the severity and distribution of the abnormality. Acquired lymphedema results from trauma to the ducts of regional lymph nodes (particularly axillary and inguinal) after surgery or metastasis. In each case obstruction and sometimes infection block the lymphatic ducts, producing lymphedema. Lymphedema does not pit, and the overlying skin will eventually thicken and feel tougher than usual.

Elephantiasis

Elephantiasis is a massive accumulation of lymphedema throughout the body that results from widespread inflammation and obstruction of the lymphatics by the filarial worms *Wuchereria bancrofti* or *Brugia malayi*. Adequate drainage is prevented, and the patient becomes more susceptible to infection, cellulitis, and fibrosis. The term is often loosely used to describe the result of any obstruction, congenital or acquired.

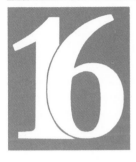

Musculoskeletal System

The musculoskeletal system provides the stability and mobility necessary for physical activity. Physical performance requires bones, muscles, and joints that function smoothly and effortlessly. Because the musculoskeletal system serves as the body's main line of defense against external forces, injuries are common, and all have the potential for producing permanent disability. Numerous disease processes affect the musculoskeletal system, including metabolic disorders, and can ultimately cause disability.

Disorders that affect the musculoskeletal system may also arise from the neurologic system. For example, delay in an expected muscle response can be caused by pain from a bone or muscle injury, or it may be the result of a cerebellar defect. A careful neurologic examination will help differentiate the cause.

Anatomy and Physiology

The musculoskeletal system is a bony structure with its joints held together by ligaments, attached to muscles by tendons, and cushioned by cartilage (Figs. 16-1 and 16-2). In addition to giving structure to the soft tissues of the body and allowing movement, the functions of the musculoskeletal system include protecting vital organs, providing storage space for minerals, producing blood cells (hematopoiesis), and resorbing and reforming itself.

Most joints are diarthrodial—freely moving articulations that are enclosed by a capsule of fibrous articular cartilage, ligaments, and cartilage covering the ends of the opposing bones. A synovial membrane lines the articular cavity and secretes the serous lubricating synovial fluid. Bursae develop in the spaces of connective tissue between tendons, ligaments, and bones to promote ease of motion at points where friction would otherwise occur. Table 16-1 describes the classification of joints.

The variability in size and strength of muscles among individuals is influenced by genetic constitution, nutrition, and exercise. At all ages, muscles increase in size with use and shrink with inactivity. Individual muscles must have intact neurologic innervation to function and to move joints through their full range of motion.

Table 16-1
Classification of Joints

Type of Joint	Example	Description
Synarthrosis		No movement is permitted
Suture	Cranial sutures	United by thin layer of fibrous tissue
Synchondrosis	Joint between the epiphysis and diaphysis of long bones	A temporary joint in which the cartilage is replaced by bone later in life
Amphiarthrosis		Slightly moveable joint
Symphysis	Pubic symphysis	Bones are connected by a fibrocartilage disk
Syndesmosis	Radius–ulna articulation	Bones are connected by ligaments
Diarthrosis (synovial)		Freely movable; enclosed by joint capsule, lined with synovial membrane
Ball and socket	Hip	Widest range of motion, movement in all planes
Hinge	Elbow	Motion limited to flexion and extension in a single plane
Pivot	Atlantoaxis	Motion limited to rotation
Condyloid	Wrist between radius and carpals	Motion in two planes at right angles to each other, but no radial rotation
Saddle	Thumb at carpal-metacarpal joint	Motion in two planes at right angles to each other, but no axial rotation
Glidding	Intervertebral	Motion limited to gliding

Continued.

Fig. 16-1
A, Bones of upper and lower extremities.

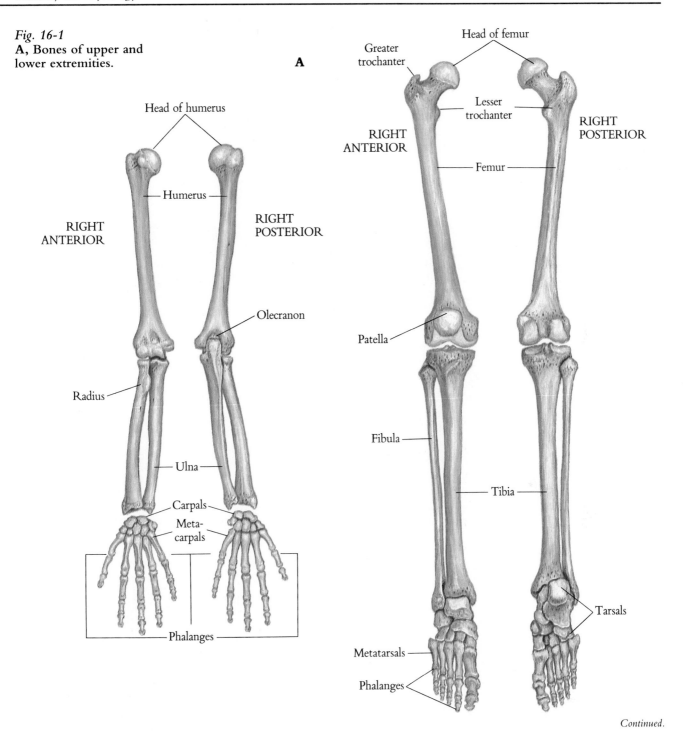

Fig. 16-1, cont'd
**B, Muscles of upper
extremities.**

ANTERIOR

B

POSTERIOR

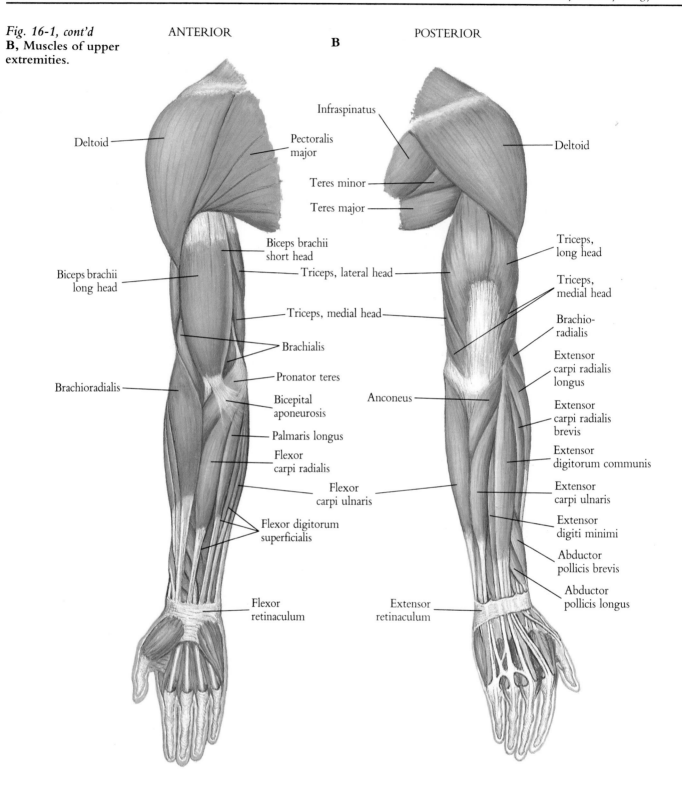

Deltoid

Biceps brachii
long head

Brachioradialis

Infraspinatus

Pectoralis
major

Teres minor

Teres major

Biceps brachii
short head

Triceps, lateral head

Triceps, medial head

Brachialis

Pronator teres

Bicepital
aponeurosis

Palmaris longus

Flexor
carpi radialis

Flexor
carpi ulnaris

Flexor digitorum
superficialis

Flexor
retinaculum

Anconeus

Extensor
retinaculum

Deltoid

Triceps,
long head

Triceps,
medial head

Brachio-
radialis

Extensor
carpi radialis
longus

Extensor
carpi radialis
brevis

Extensor
digitorum communis

Extensor
carpi ulnaris

Extensor
digiti minimi

Abductor
pollicis brevis

Abductor
pollicis longus

Fig. 16-1, cont'd
**C, Muscles of lower
extremities.**

ANTERIOR

POSTERIOR

C

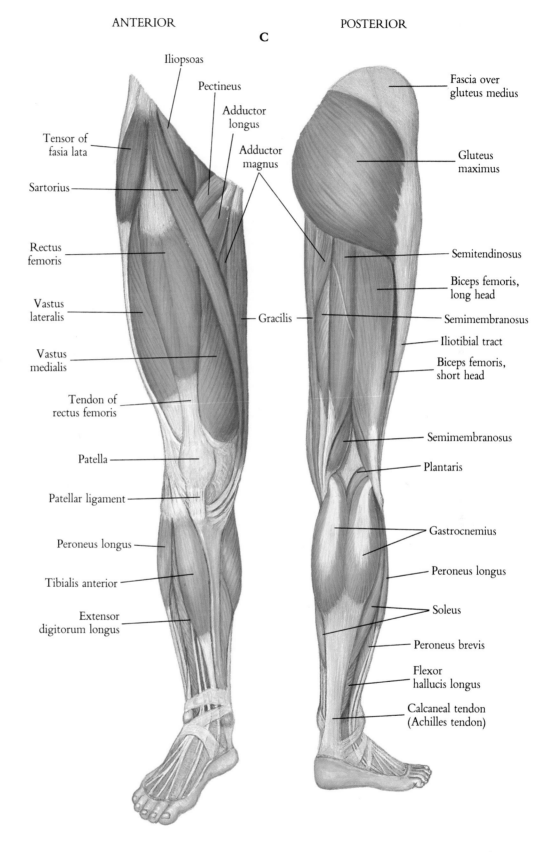

Iliopsoas

Pectineus

Adductor
longus

Adductor
magnus

Tensor of
fasia lata

Sartorius

Rectus
femoris

Vastus
lateralis

Gracilis

Vastus
medialis

Tendon of
rectus femoris

Patella

Patellar ligament

Peroneus longus

Tibialis anterior

Extensor
digitorum longus

Fascia over
gluteus medius

Gluteus
maximus

Semitendinosus

Biceps femoris,
long head

Semimembranosus

Iliotibial tract

Biceps femoris,
short head

Semimembranosus

Plantaris

Gastrocnemius

Peroneus longus

Soleus

Peroneus brevis

Flexor
hallucis longus

Calcaneal tendon
(Achilles tendon)

Fig. 16-2
A, Bones of trunk, anterior
view.

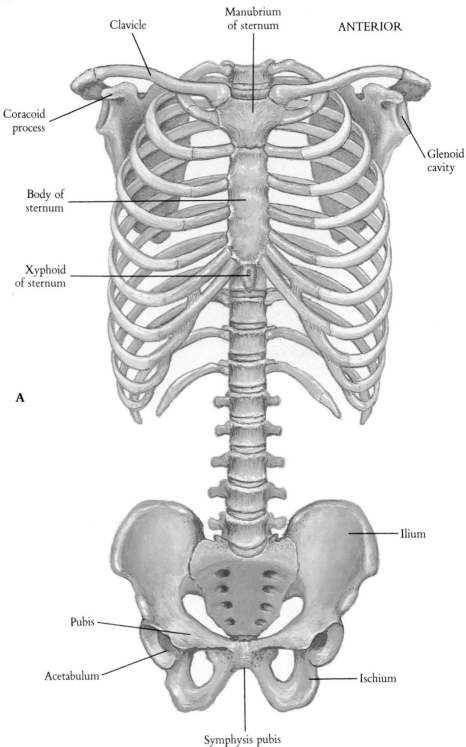

Clavicle

Manubrium
of sternum

ANTERIOR

Coracoid
process

Glenoid
cavity

Body of
sternum

Xyphoid
of sternum

A

Ilium

Pubis

Acetabulum

Ischium

Symphysis pubis

Fig. 16-2, cont'd
B, Bones of trunk, posterior
view.

POSTERIOR

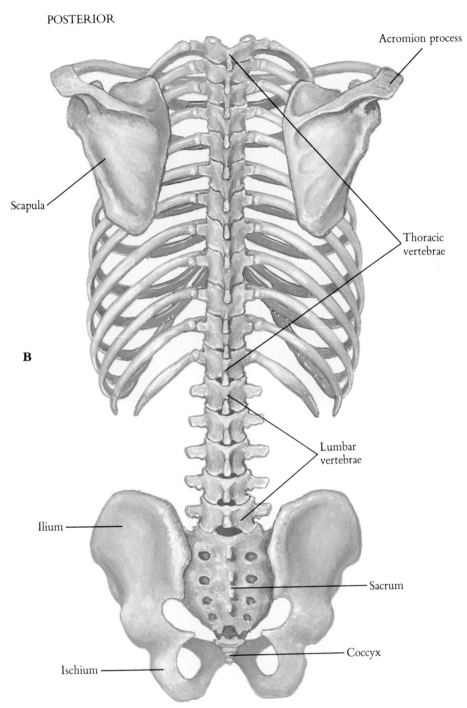

Acromion process

Scapula

Thoracic
vertebrae

B

Lumbar
vertebrae

Ilium

Sacrum

Coccyx

Ischium

Continued.

Fig. 16-2, cont'd
C, Superficial muscles of trunk, anterior view.

C

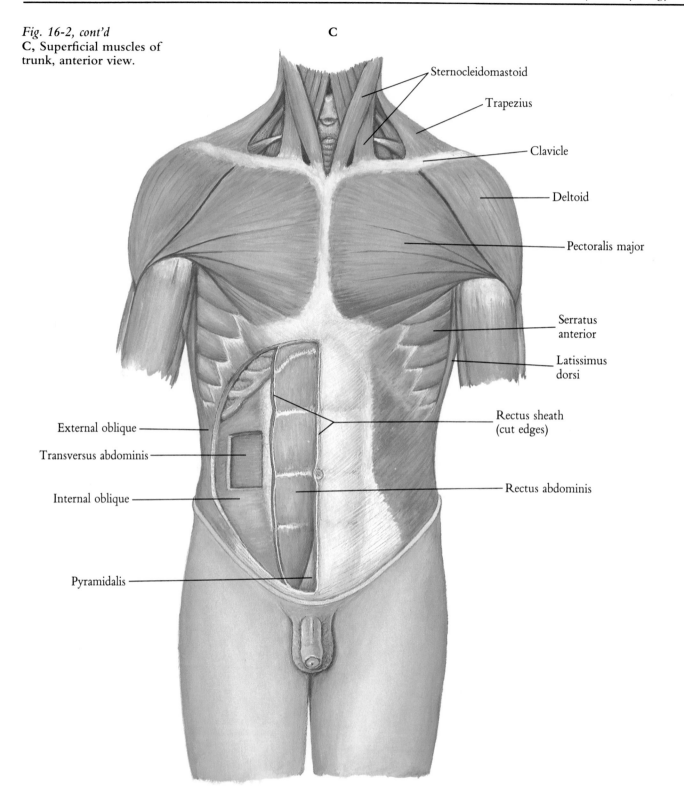

Sternocleidomastoid

Trapezius

Clavicle

Deltoid

Pectoralis major

Serratus anterior

Latissimus dorsi

Rectus sheath (cut edges)

Rectus abdominis

External oblique

Transversus abdominis

Internal oblique

Pyramidalis

Fig. 16-2, cont'd
D, Superficial muscles of trunk, posterior view.

D

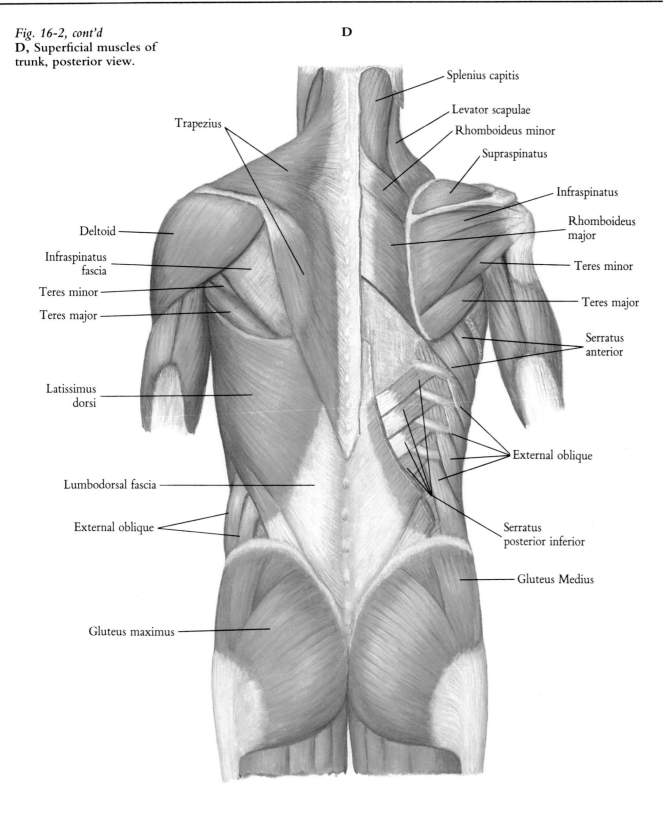

Splenius capitis

Levator scapulae

Rhomboideus minor

Supraspinatus

Infraspinatus

Rhomboideus major

Teres minor

Teres major

Serratus anterior

External oblique

Serratus posterior inferior

Gluteus Medius

Trapezius

Deltoid

Infraspinatus fascia

Teres minor

Teres major

Latissimus dorsi

Lumbodorsal fascia

External oblique

Gluteus maximus

Head and Spine

The temporomandibular joint forms the articulation between the mandible and the temporal bone in the cranium. Each is located in the depression just anterior to the tragus of the ear. The hinge action of the joint opens and closes the mouth, while the gliding action permits lateral movement, protrusion, and retraction of the mandible (Figs. 16-3 and 16-4). See Chapter 5 for a description of the fused bones of the cranium.

The spine is composed of cervical, thoracic, lumbar, and sacral vertebrae. Except for the sacral vertebrae, they are separated from each other by fibrocartilaginous disks. Each disk has a nucleus of fibrogelatinous material that cushions the vertebral bodies (Fig. 16-5). The vertebrae form a series of joints that glide slightly over the surface of each other, permitting movement on several axes. The cervical vertebrae are the most mobile. Flexion and extension occur between the skull and C1, while rotation occurs between C1 and C2. The sacral vertebrae are fused and with the coccyx form the posterior portion of the pelvis.

Fig. 16-3
Muscles of face and head, left lateral view.

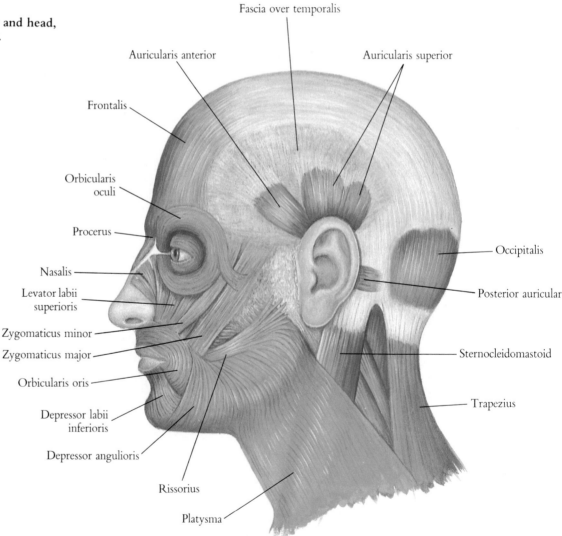

Fig. 16-4
**Structures of temporoman-
dibular joint.**

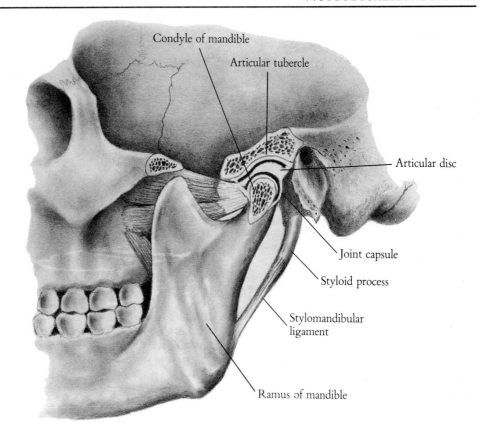

Fig. 16-5
**Structures of vertebral
joints.**
From Thompson et al., 1986.

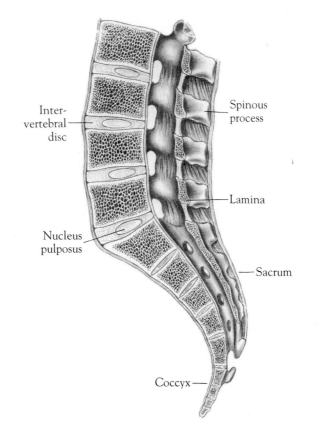

Upper Extremities

The glenohumoral joint (shoulder) forms the articulation of the humerus and the glenoid fossa of the scapula. The acromion and coracoid processes and the ligament between them form the capsule surrounding and protecting the joint. The shoulder is a ball and socket joint that permits movement of the humerus on many axes (Fig. 16-6).

Two additional joints adjacent to the glenohumeral joint compose the shoulder girdle. The acromioclavicular joint forms the articulation between the acromion process and the clavicle, and the sternoclavicular joint forms the articulation between the manubrium of the sternum and the clavicle.

The elbow forms the articulation of the humerus, radius, and ulna. Its three contiguous surfaces are enclosed in a single synovial cavity with the ligaments of the radius and ulna protecting the joint. A bursa lies between the olecranon and the skin (Fig. 16-7). The elbow is a hinge joint permitting movement of the humerus and ulna on one plane.

The radiocarpal joint (wrist) forms the articulation of the radius and the carpal bones. Articular disks separate the radius, ulna, and carpal bones, and the joint is further protected by ligaments and a fibrous capsule. The wrist is a condyloid joint, permitting movement in two planes. The hand has articulations between the carpals and metacarpals, metacarpals and proximal phalanges, and between the middle and distal phalanges. The metacarpophalangeal joints are condyloid (Fig. 16-8).

Fig. 16-6
Structures of glenohumoral and acromioclavicular joints.

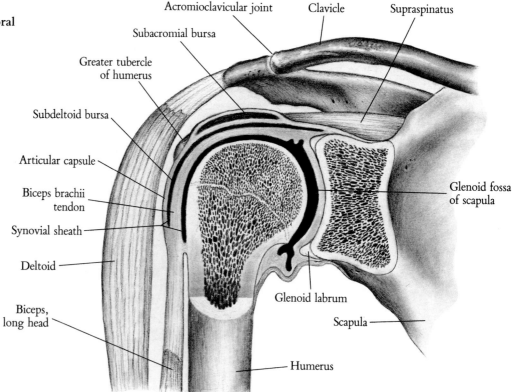

Fig. 16-7
Structures of left elbow joint, posterior view.

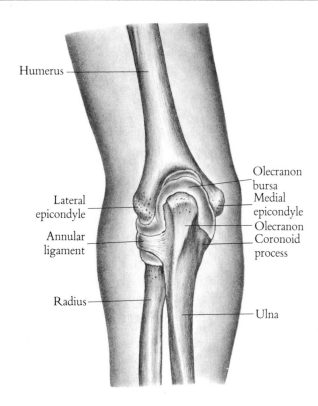

Fig. 16-8
Structures of wrist and hand joints.

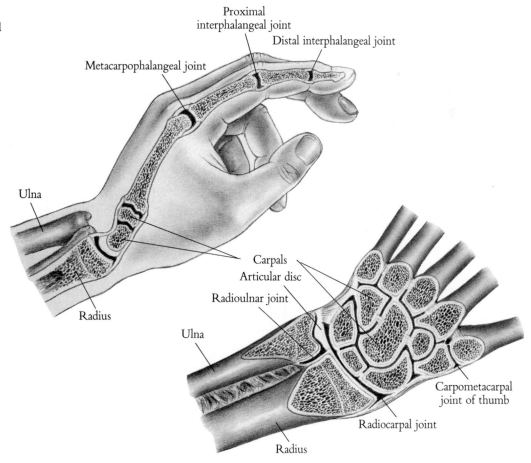

Lower Extremities

The joint of the hip forms the articulation between the acetabulum and the femur. The anterior iliac crest and acetabulum surround the fibrous capsule, protecting the joint, and three bursae reduce friction in the hip. The hip is a ball and socket joint, permitting movement of the femur on many axes (Fig. 16-9).

The knee forms the articulation of the femur, tibia, and patella. Fibrocartilaginous disks (medial and lateral menisci), which cushion the tibia and femur, are attached to the tibia and continuous with the articulated capsule. Collateral ligaments give medial and lateral stability to the knee. Two cruciate ligaments cross obliquely within the knee, adding anterior and posterior stability. Several bursae reduce friction. The suprapatellar bursa separates the patella, quadriceps tendon, and muscle from the femur. The knee is a hinge joint permitting movement between the femur and tibia on one plane (Fig. 16-10).

The tibiotalar joint (ankle) forms the articulation of the tibia, fibula, and talus. It is protected by ligaments on the medial and lateral surfaces. The tibiotalar joint is a hinge joint permitting flexion and extension in one plane. Additional joints in the ankle, the talocalcaneal joint (subtalar) and transverse tarsal joint, permit a pivot or rotation movement of the joint. Articulations of the foot between the tarsals and metatarsals, the metatarsal and proximal phalanges, and the middle and distal phalanges are condyloid (Fig. 16-11).

Fig. 16-9
Structures of hip.
From Thompson et al., 1986.

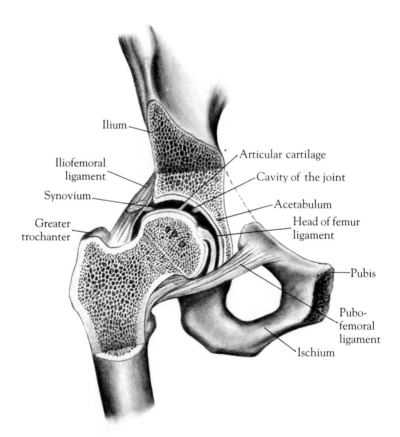

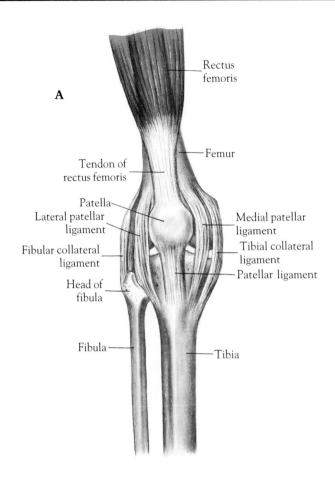

A

Rectus femoris

Femur

Tendon of rectus femoris

Patella

Lateral patellar ligament

Medial patellar ligament

Fibular collateral ligament

Tibial collateral ligament

Head of fibula

Patellar ligament

Fibula

Tibia

Fig. 16-10
Structures of knee, anterior view. A, Bones and ligaments of the joint. B, Muscles attaching at the knee.
A from Thompson et al., 1986.

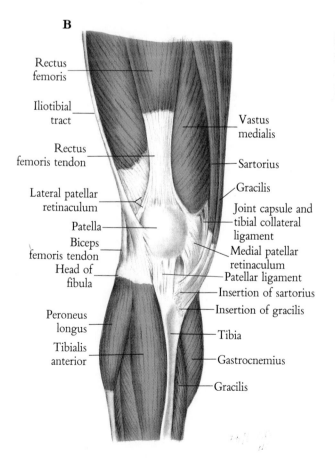

B

Rectus femoris

Iliotibial tract

Rectus femoris tendon

Lateral patellar retinaculum

Patella

Biceps femoris tendon

Head of fibula

Peroneus longus

Tibialis anterior

Vastus medialis

Sartorius

Gracilis

Joint capsule and tibial collateral ligament

Medial patellar retinaculum

Patellar ligament

Insertion of sartorius

Insertion of gracilis

Tibia

Gastrocnemius

Gracilis

Fig. 16-11
**Bones and joints of ankle
and foot.**

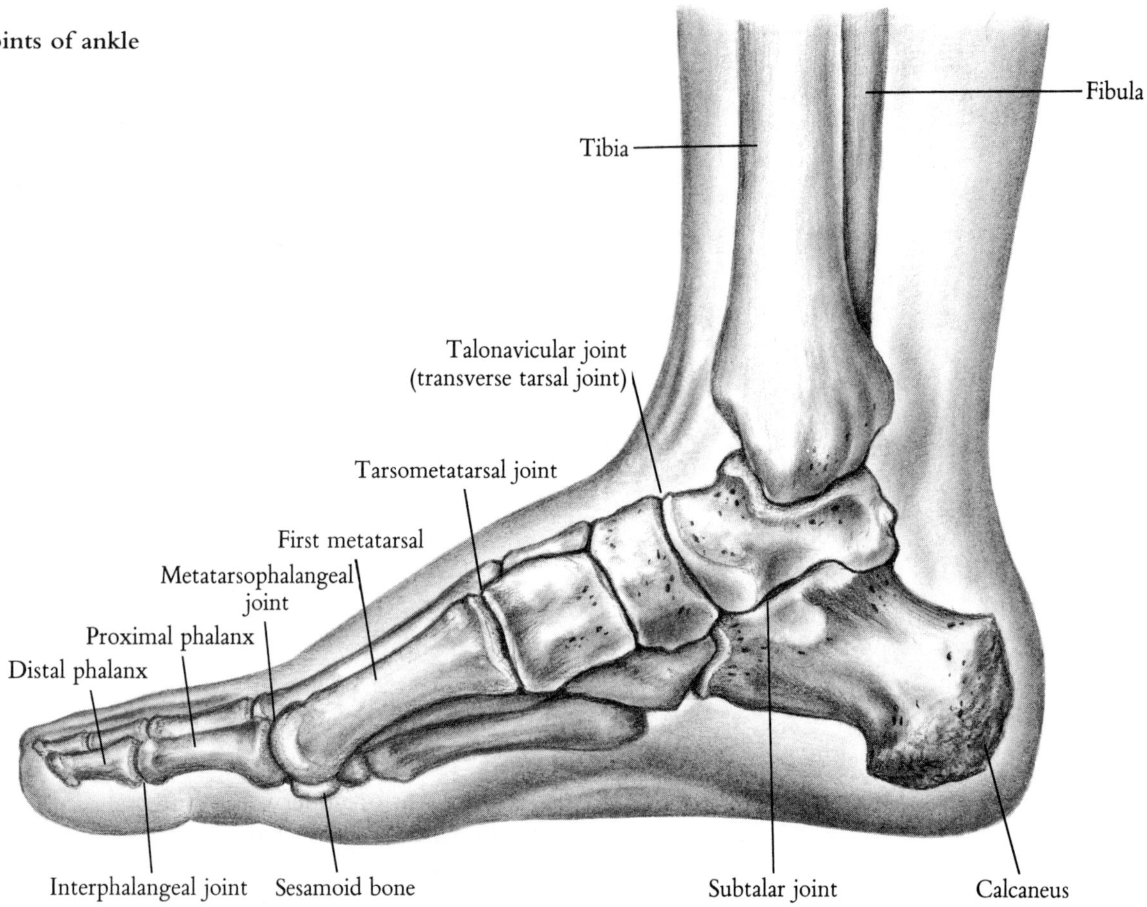

Fibula

Tibia

Talonavicular joint
(transverse tarsal joint)

Tarsometatarsal joint

First metatarsal

Metatarsophalangeal
joint

Proximal phalanx

Distal phalanx

Interphalangeal joint   Sesamoid bone   Subtalar joint   Calcaneus

During fetal development the skeletal system emerges from embryologic connective tissues to form cartilage that calcifies and eventually becomes true bone. Throughout infancy and childhood, long bones increase in diameter by the apposition of new bone tissue around the bone shaft. Increased length of long bones results from the proliferation of cartilage at the growth plates (epiphyses). In the smaller bones, such as the carpals, ossification centers form in calcified cartilage. There is a specific sequence and timing of bone growth and ossification during childhood. This is completed at about age 20 when the last epiphysis closes and becomes firmly fused to the bone shaft.

The number of muscle fibers an individual ultimately develops is established during fetal life. Muscle fibers lengthen during childhood as the skeletal system grows.

Increased levels of circulating hormones, estrogen and relaxin, contribute to the elasticity of ligaments and softening of the cartilages in the pelvis. This results in increased mobility of the sacroiliac, sacrococcygeal, and symphysis pubis joints. Protrusion of the abdomen as the uterus grows gives the pelvis a forward tilt, which places additional strain on the back and sacroiliac joints.

OLDER ADULTS With aging, the skeletal system undergoes an alteration in the equilibrium between bone deposition and bone resorption, and resorption dominates. The loss of bone density affects the entire skeleton, but the long bones and the vertebrae are particularly vulnerable. Weight-bearing bones may become predisposed to fractures. Bony prominences become more apparent with the loss of subcutaneous fat.

The muscle mass also undergoes alteration, as increased amounts of collagen collect in the tissues initially, followed by fibrosis of connective tissue. Tendons become less elastic. This results in a reduction of total muscle mass, tone, and strength. A progressive decrease in reaction time, speed of movements, agility, and endurance also occurs.

Any health problem that contributes to reduced physical activity promotes and hastens the musculoskeletal changes associated with aging. Routine exercise helps slow the progression of these changes.

Review of Related History

General Considerations

1. Employment: past and current, lifting and potential for accidental injury, safety precautions, chronic stress on joints
2. Exercise: extent, type, and frequency; stress on specific joints; overall conditioning
3. Activities of daily living: ability to perform personal care (eating, bathing, dressing, grooming, elimination), other activities (housework, walking, climbing stairs, caring for pet), communication
4. Weight: recent gain, overweight or underweight for body build
5. Height: maximum height achieved, any changes
6. Nutrition: amount of calcium, vitamin D, calories, and protein
7. Medications: antiinflammatory agents, aspirin, muscle relaxants

Present Problem

1. Joint complaints
   a. Character: stiffness or limitation of movement, change in size or contour, swelling or redness, pain or ache, unilateral or bilateral involvement, interference with daily activities
   b. Associated event: time of day, activity, specific movements, injury, strenuous activity, weather
   c. Temporal factors: change in frequency or character of episodes, better or worse as day progresses, nature of onset, slow *v* abrupt onset
   d. Efforts to treat: exercise, rest, weight reduction, physical therapy, heat, ice, splints, medications, joint injections
2. Muscular complaints
   a. Character: limitation of movement, weakness or fatigue, paralysis, tremor, tic, spasms, clumsiness, wasting, aching or pain
   b. Precipitating factors: injury, strenuous activity, sudden movement, stress
   c. Efforts to treat: heat, ice, splints, rest, medications
3. Skeletal complaints
   a. Character: difficulty with gait or limping; numbness, tingling, or pressure sensation; pain with movement, crepitus; abnormality or change in skeletal contour

b. Associated event: injury, recent fractures, strenuous activity, sudden movement, stress

c. Efforts to treat: rest, splints, medications

Past Medical History

1. Trauma: nerves, soft tissue, bones, joints; residual problems; bone infection
2. Surgery on joint
3. Chronic illness: cancer, arthritis, osteoporosis, renal or neurologic disorder
4. Skeletal deformities or congenital anomalies

Family History

1. Congenital abnormalities of hip or foot
2. Scoliosis or back problems
3. Arthritis: rheumatoid, osteoarthritis, ankylosing spondylitis, gout
4. Genetic disorders: osteogenesis imperfecta, dwarfing syndrome

INFANTS AND CHILDREN

1. Birth history
   a. Abnormal presentation, large for gestational age, birth injuries (may result in fractures or nerve damage)
   b. Low birth weight, premature, resuscitated, required special ventilator support (may result in anoxia leading to muscle tone disorders)
2. Fine and gross motor developmental milestones, appropriate for chronologic age
3. Quality of movement: spasticity, flaccidity, cog wheel rigidity
4. Leg pain
   a. Character: localized or generalized; in muscle or joint; limitation of movement; associated with movement, trauma, or growth spurt
   b. Onset: age, sudden or gradual, at night with rest, after activity

OLDER ADULTS

1. Weakness
   a. Onset: sudden or gradual, localized or generalized, occurred with activity or after sustained activity
   b. Associated symptoms: stiffness of joints, muscle spasms, muscle tension, any particular activity, dyspnea
2. Increases in minor injuries: stumbling, falls, limited agility; association with poor vision
3. Change in ease of movement: loss of ability to perform sudden movements, change in exercise endurance, pain, stiffness, localized to particular joints or generalized
4. Nocturnal muscle spasm: frequency, associated back pain, numbness or coldness of extremities
5. History of injuries or excessive use of a joint or group of joints, claudication, known joint abnormalities

Examination and Findings

EQUIPMENT	■ **Skin-marking pencil** ■ **Goniometer** ■ **Tape measure** ■ **Reflex hammer**

Begin your examination of the musculoskeletal system by observing the gait and posture when the patient enters the examining room. Note how the patient walks, sits, rises from sitting position, takes off his or her coat, and responds to other directions given during the examination.

As you give specific attention to bones, joints, and muscles, the body surface must be exposed and viewed with good lighting. Position the patient to provide the greatest stability to the joints. Examine each region of the body for limb and trunk stability, muscular strength and function, and joint function. Position the extremities uniformly as you examine and look for asymmetry.

Inspection

Inspect the anterior, posterior, and lateral aspects of the patient's posture (Fig. 16-12). Observe the patient's ability to stand erect, the symmetry of body parts, and the alignment of extremities. Note any lordosis, kyphosis, or scoliosis.

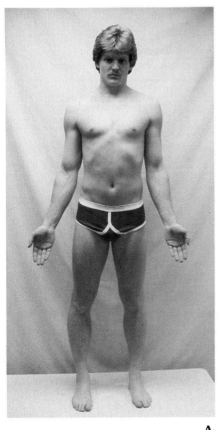
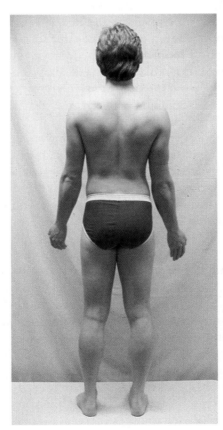
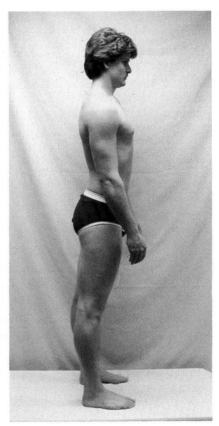

A **B** **C**

Fig. 16-12
Inspection of overall body posture. See the even contour of the shoulders, level scapulae and iliac crests, alignment of the head over the gluteal folds, and symmetry and alignment of extremities.
A, Anterior view. **B,** Posterior view. **C,** Lateral view.

Inspect the skin and subcutaneous tissues overlying the muscles, cartilage, bones, and joints for discoloration, swelling, and masses.

Observe the extremities for overall size, gross deformity, bony enlargement, alignment, contour, and symmetry of length and position. Expect to find bilateral symmetry in length, circumference, alignment, and the position and number of skin folds.

Inspect the muscles for gross hypertrophy or atrophy, fasciculations, and spasms. Muscle size should approximate symmetry bilaterally, without atrophy or hypertrophy. Bilateral symmetry should not be defined as absolute, since there is no perfect symmetry. For example, the dominant forearm is expected to be larger in athletes who play racquet sports and in manual laborers.

Palpation

Palpate all bones, joints, and surrounding muscles. Note any heat, tenderness, swelling, crepitus, and resistance to pressure. No discomfort should occur when you apply pressure to bones and joints. Muscle tone should be firm, not hard or doughy.

Range of Motion

Examine both the active and passive range of motion for each major joint and its related muscle groups. Adequate space for the patient to move each muscle group and joint through its full range is necessary and may be provided by pulling the examining table away from the wall. Instruct the patient in moving each joint through its range of motion as detailed under Specific Joints and Muscles. Pain, limitation of motion, spastic movement, joint instability, deformity, and contracture suggest a problem with the joint or related muscle group.

Direct the patient to relax and allow you to passively move the same joints through the ranges. Range of motion with active and passive maneuvers should be equal for each joint and between contralateral joints. Discrepancies between active and passive range of motion may indicate true muscle weakness or a joint disorder. No crepitation or tenderness with movement should be apparent.

When a joint appears to have an increase or limitation in its range of motion, a goniometer is used to precisely measure the angle. Begin with the joint in the fully extended or neutral position, and then flex the joint as far as possible. Measure the angles of greatest flexion and extension, comparing with the expected flexion and extension (Fig. 16-13).

Muscle Strength

Evaluating the strength of each muscle group, which is also considered part of the neurologic examination, is usually integrated with examination of the associated joint for range of motion. Ask the patient to first flex the muscle you direct and to then resist when you apply opposing force against that flexion (Fig. 16-14). Compare the muscle strength bilaterally. Expect muscle strength to be bilaterally symmetric with full resistance to opposition. Full muscle strength requires complete active range of motion.

Variations in muscle strength are graded from no voluntary contraction to full muscle strength, using one of the scales in Table 16-2. When muscle strength is grade 3 or less, disability is present. Activity cannot be accomplished in a gravity field, and external support is necessary to perform movements.

Table 16-2
Muscle Strength

Muscle Function Level	Scales		
	Grade	%Normal	Lovett Scale
No evidence of contractility	0	0	0 (zero)
Slight contractility	1	10	T (trace)
Full range of motion, gravity eliminated*	2	25	P (poor)
Full range of motion with gravity	3	50	F (fair)
Full range of motion against gravity, some resistance	4	75	G (good)
Full range of motion against gravity, full resistance	5	100	N (normal)

From Malasanos et al., 1986.
*Passive movement.

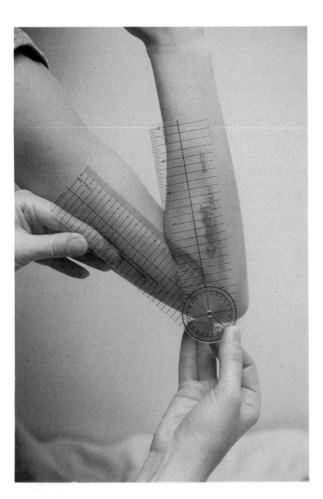

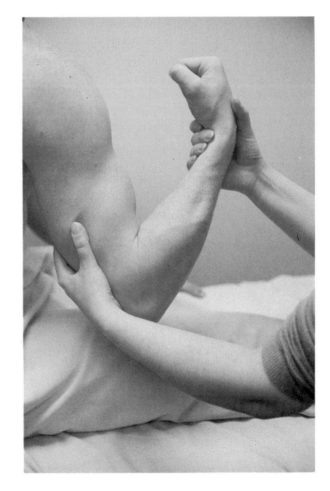

Fig. 16-13
Use of goniometer to measure joint range of motion.

Fig. 16-14
Evaluation of muscle strength: flexion of the elbow against opposing force.

Specific Joints and Muscles

Temporomandibular Joint

Locate the temporomandibular joints with your fingertips placed just anterior to the tragus of each ear. Allow your fingertips to slip into the joint space as the patient's mouth opens, and palpate the joint space (Fig. 16-15). An audible or palpable snapping or clicking in the temporomandibular joints is not unusual, but no pain, swelling, or crepitus should be present.

Range of motion is examined by asking the patient to perform the following movements:

- Open and close the mouth. Expect a space of 3 to 6 cm between the upper and lower teeth.
- Laterally move the lower jaw to each side. The mandible should move 1 to 2 cm in each direction (Fig. 16-16).
- Protrude and retract the chin. Expect both movements.

Strength of the temporalis muscles is evaluated by asking the patient to clench the teeth while you palpate the contracted muscles and apply opposing force. Cranial nerve V is simultaneously tested with this maneuver.

Cervical Spine

Inspect the patient's neck, both from an anterior and posterior position, observing for alignment of the head with the shoulders and symmetry of the skin folds and muscles. Expect the cervical spine to be straight with the head erect and in appropriate alignment. No asymmetric skin folds should be apparent.

Palpate the posterior neck, the cervical spine, and the paravertebral, trapezius, and sternocleidomastoid muscles. The muscles should have good tone and be symmetric in size with no palpable tenderness or muscle spasm.

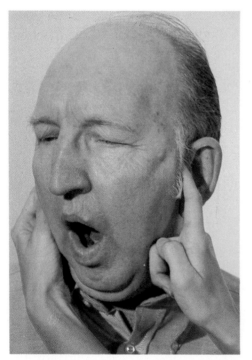

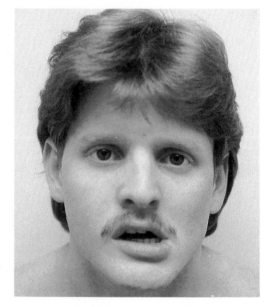

Fig. 16-15
Palpation of the temporo-mandibular joint.

Fig. 16-16
Lateral range of motion in the temporomandibular joint.

Fig. 16-17
Range of motion of the
cervical spine. **A,** Flexion
and hyperextension.
B, Lateral bending.
C, Rotation.

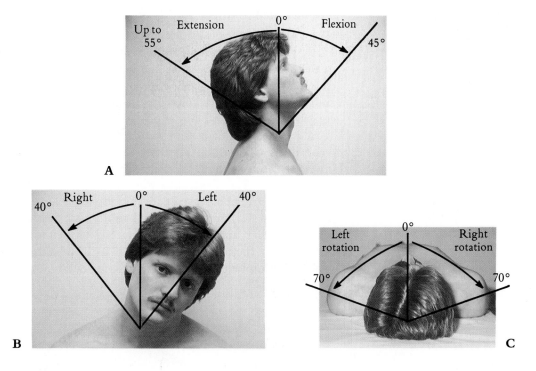

Fig. 16-18
Examining the strength
of the sternocleidomastoid
and trapezius muscles.
A, Flexion. **B,** Extension.
C, Rotation.

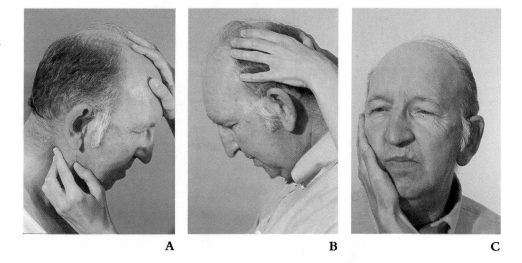

Evaluate range of motion in the cervical spine by asking the patient to perform the following movements (Fig. 16-17):
- Bend the head forward, chin to the chest. Expect flexion of 45 degrees.
- Bend the head backward, chin toward the ceiling. Expect hyperextension of 45 degrees.
- Bend the head to each side, ear to each shoulder. Expect lateral bending of 40 degrees.
- Turn the head to each side, chin to shoulder. Expect rotation of 70 degrees.

The strength of the sternocleidomastoid and trapezius muscles is evaluated with the patient maintaining each of the above positions while you apply opposing force. With rotation, cranial nerve XI is simultaneously tested (Fig. 16-18).

Thoracic and Lumbar Spine

Major landmarks of the back include each spinal process of the vertebrae (C7 and T1 are usually most prominent), the scapulae, the iliac crests, and the paravertebral muscles (Fig. 16-19). Expect the head to be positioned directly over the gluteal cleft, and the vertebrae to be straight as indicated by symmetric shoulder, scapular, and iliac crest heights. The curves of the cervical and lumbar spines should be concave, and the curve of the thoracic spine should be convex. The knees and feet should be in alignment with the trunk, pointing directly forward.

Lordosis is common in patients who are markedly obese. Kyphosis may be observed in aging adults. A sharp angular deformity, a gibbus, is associated with a collapsed vertebrae from osteoporosis (Fig. 16-20).

With the patient erect, palpate along the spinal processes and paravertebral muscles (Fig. 16-21). Percuss for spinal tenderness, first by tapping each spinal process with one finger, and then by rapping each side of the spine along the paravertebral muscles with the ulnar aspect of your fist. No muscle spasm or spinal tenderness with palpation or percussion should be elicited.

Fig. 16-19
Landmarks of the back.

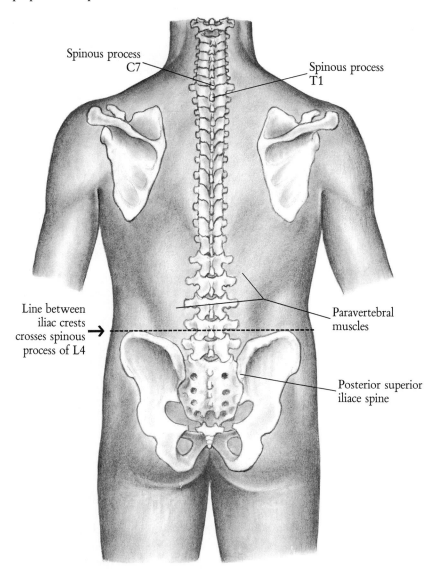

Spinous process C7

Spinous process T1

Line between iliac crests crosses spinous process of L4

Paravertebral muscles

Posterior superior iliace spine

Fig. 16-20
**Deviations in spinal
column curvatures.
A,** Expected spine
curvatures. **B,** Kyphosis.
C, Lordosis.
From Thompson et al., 1986.

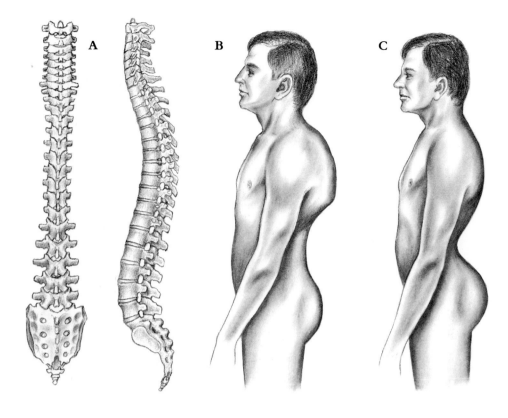

Fig. 16-21
Palpation of the spinal
processes of the vertebrae.

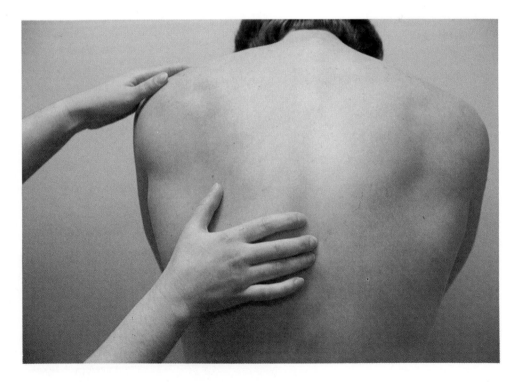

Fig. 16-22
Inspection of the spine for
lateral curvature and lum–
bar convexity.

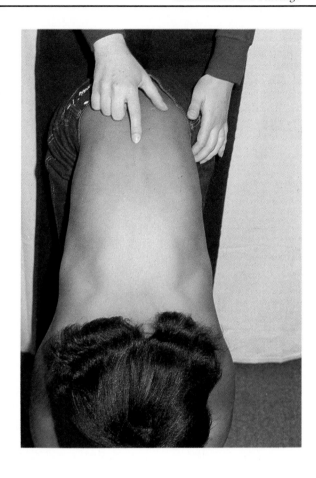

Fig. 16-23
Range of motion of the
thoracic and lumbar spine.
A, Flexion and hyperex–
tension. **B,** Lateral bend–
ing. **C,** Rotation of the
upper trunk.

A

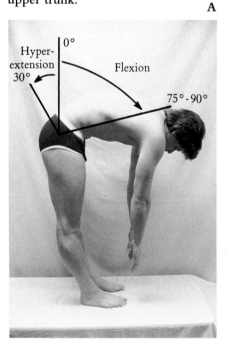

B

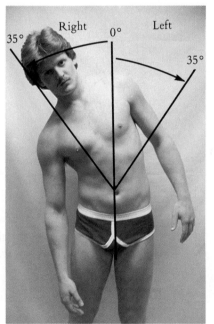

C

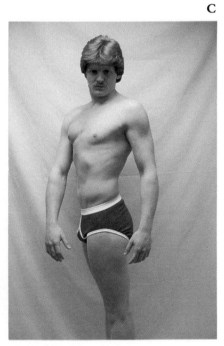

Ask the patient to bend forward and touch the toes while you observe from behind. Inspect the spine for unexpected curvature. (A mark with the skin pencil on each spinal process will enhance the inspection, especially if a curvature is suspected.) The patient's back should remain symmetrically flat as the concave curve of the lumbar spine becomes convex with forward flexion. A lateral curvature or rib hump should make you suspect scoliosis (Fig. 16-22).

Range of motion is evaluated by asking the patient to perform the following movements (Fig. 16-23):

- Bend forward at the waist and touch the toes. Expect flexion of 75 to 90 degrees.
- Bend back at the waist as far as possible. Expect hyperextension of 30 degrees.
- Bend to each side as far as possible. Expect lateral bending of 35 degrees bilaterally.
- Swing the upper trunk from the waist in a circular motion front to side to back to side, while you stabilize the pelvis. Expect rotation of the upper trunk 30 degrees forward and backward.

Shoulders

Inspect the contour of the shoulders, the shoulder girdle, the clavicles and scapulae, and the area muscles. There should be symmetry of size and contour of all shoulder structures. When the shoulder contour is asymmetric and one shoulder has hollows in the rounding contour, suspect a shoulder dislocation. Ask the patient to stand close to a wall and push against it with both hands. Observe for a winged scapula, an outward prominence of the scapula, indicating injury to the nerve of the anterior serratus muscle (Fig. 16-24).

Palpate the sternoclavicular joint, the acromioclavicular joint, clavicle, scapulae, coracoid process, greater trochanter of the humerus, the biceps groove, and the area muscles.

Examine the range of motion by asking the patient to perform the following movements (Fig. 16-25):

- Shrug the shoulders. Expect the shoulders to raise symmetrically.
- Raise both arms forward and straight up over the head. Expect forward flexion of 180 degrees.
- Extend and stretch both arms behind the back. Expect hyperextension of 50 degrees.
- Lift both arms laterally and straight up over the head. Expect shoulder abduction of 180 degrees.
- Swing each arm across the front of the body. Expect adduction of 50 degrees.
- Place both arms behind the hips, elbows out. Expect internal rotation of 90 degrees.
- Place both arms behind the head, elbows out. Expect external rotation of 90 degrees.

Have the patient maintain shrugged shoulders, forward flexion, and abduction while you apply opposing force to evaluate the strength of the shoulder girdle muscles. Cranial nerve XI is simultaneously evaluated with the shrugged shoulders maneuver.

Fig. 16-24
Contour changes of the
shoulder. **A,** With dislocation. **B,** Winging of the
scapula with abduction
of the arm.
B from DePalma, 1983.

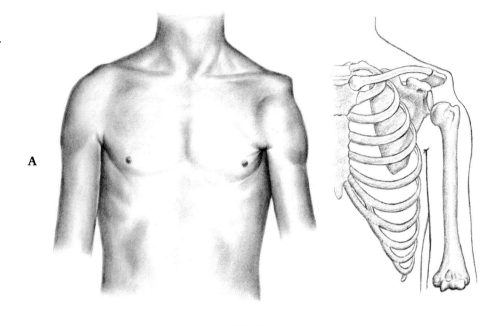

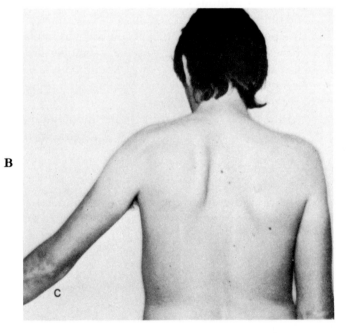

Fig. 16-25
Range of motion of the shoulder. **A,** Shrugged shoulders.
B, Forward flexion and hyperextension. **C,** Abduction and
adduction. **D,** Internal rotation. **E,** External rotation.

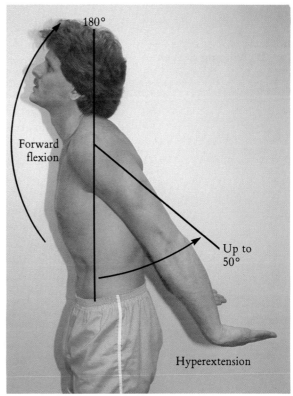

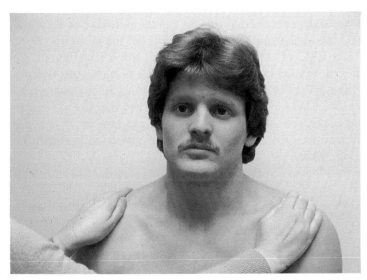

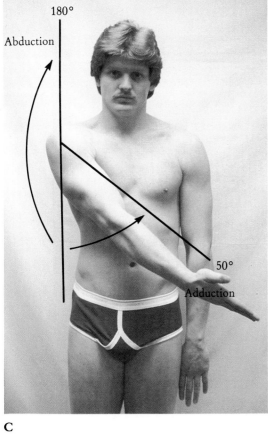

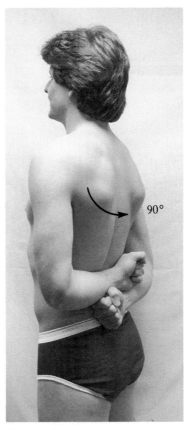

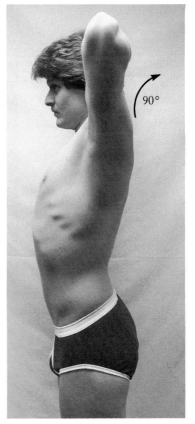

A

B

C

D

E

Elbows

Inspect the contour of the patient's elbows in both flexed and extended positions. Subcutaneous nodules along pressure points of the extensor surface of the ulna may indicate rheumatoid arthritis (Fig. 16-26).

Note any deviations in the carrying angle between the humerus and radius while the arm is passively extended, palm forward. The carrying angle is usually 5 to 15 degrees laterally. Variations in carrying angle are cubitus valgus, a lateral angle exceeding 15 degrees, and cubitus varus, a medial carrying angle (Fig. 16-27).

Flex the patient's elbow 70 degrees and palpate the extensor surface of the ulna, the olecranon process, and the medial and lateral epicondyles of the humerus. Then palpate the groove on each side of the olecranon process for thickening of the synovial membrane, tenderness, and swelling (Fig. 16-28). A boggy, soft, or fluctuant swelling, point tenderness at the lateral epicondyle or along the grooves of the olecranon process and epicondyles, and increased pain with pronation and supination of the elbow should make you suspect epicondylitis or tendinitis.

The elbow's range of motion is examined by asking the patient to perform the following movements (Fig. 16-29):
- Bend and straighten the elbow. Expect flexion of 160 degrees and full extension of 180 degrees.
- With the elbow flexed at a right angle, rotate the hand from palm side down to palm side up. Expect pronation of 90 degrees and supination of 90 degrees.

Have the patient maintain flexion and extension while you apply opposing force to evaluate the strength of the elbow muscles.

Fig. 16-26
Subcutaneous nodules on the extensor surface of the ulna.
Reprinted from the Revised Clinical Slide Collection of the Rheumatic Diseases. Copyright 1981. Used by permission of the American Rheumatism Association.

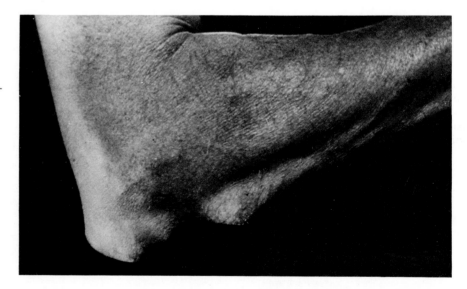

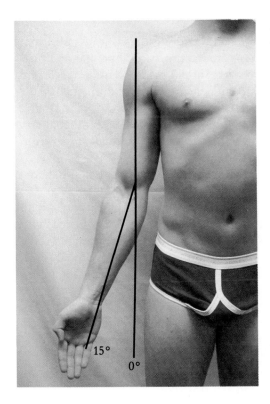

Fig. 16-27
Expected carrying angle of
the arm, at 5 to 15 degrees.

15°

0°

Fig. 16-28
Palpation of the olecranon
process grooves.

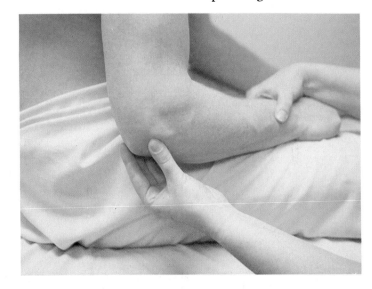

Fig. 16-29
Range of motion of the
elbow. **A,** Flexion and
extension. **B,** Pronation
and supination.

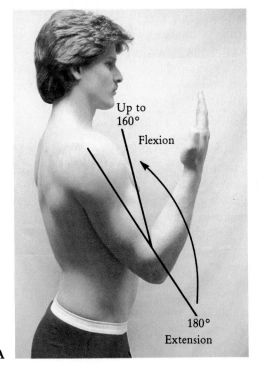

Up to
160°

Flexion

180°
Extension

A

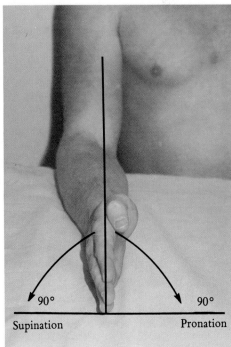

90°

Supination

90°

Pronation

B

Hands and Wrists

Inspect the dorsal and palmar aspects of the hands, noting the contour, position, shape, number, and completeness of digits. Note the presence of palmar and phalangeal creases. The palmar surface of each hand should have a central depression with a prominent, rounded mound (thenar eminence) on the thumb side of the hand and a less prominent hypothenar eminence on the little finger side of the hand. Expect the fingers to fully extend when in close approximation to each other and to be aligned with the forearm. The lateral finger surfaces should gradually taper from the proximal to the distal aspects (Fig. 16-30).

Deviation of the fingers to the ulnar side and swan neck or boutonnière deformities of the fingers usually indicate rheumatoid arthritis (Fig. 16-31).

Palpate each joint in the hand and wrist. Palpate the interphalangeal joints with your thumb and index finger. The metacarpophalangeal joints are palpated with both thumbs. Palpate the wrist and radiocarpal groove with your thumbs on the dorsal surface and your fingers on the palmar aspect of the wrist (Fig. 16-32). Joint surfaces should be smooth without nodules, swelling, bogginess, or tenderness.

Bony overgrowths in the distal interphalangeal joints, which are felt as hard, nontender nodules usually 2 to 3 mm in diameter but sometimes encompassing the entire joint, are associated with osteoarthritis. When located along the distal interphalangeal joints, they are called Heberden's nodes, and those along the proximal interphalangeal joints are called Bouchard's nodes. Painful swelling of the proximal interphalangeal joints, Haygarth's nodes, causes spindle-shaped fingers, which are associated with the acute stage of rheumatoid arthritis (Fig. 16-33). Cystic, round, nontender swellings along tendon sheaths or joint capsules that are more prominent with flexion may indicate ganglia.

With your index finger, strike the median nerve where it passes through the carpal tunnel, under the flexor retinaculum and volar carpal ligament (Fig. 16-34). A tingling sensation radiating from the wrist to the hand along the median nerve is a positive Tinel's sign, which is associated with carpal tunnel syndrome.

Examine the range of motion of the hand and wrist by asking the patient to perform these movements (Fig. 16-35):

- Bend the fingers forward at the metacarpophalangeal joint; then stretch the fingers up and back at the knuckle. Expect metacarpophalangeal flexion of 90 degrees and hyperextension as much as 20 degrees.
- Touch the thumb to each fingertip and to the base of the little finger; make a fist. All movements should be possible.
- Spread the fingers apart and then touch them together. Expect both movements.
- Bend the hand at the wrist up and down. Expect flexion of 90 degrees and hyperextension of 70 degrees.
- With the palm side down, turn each hand to the right and left. Expect radial motion of 20 degrees and ulnar motion of 55 degrees.

Have the patient maintain wrist flexion and hyperextension while you apply opposing force to evaluate strength of the wrist muscles. To evaluate hand strength, have the patient grip two of your fingers tightly. Finger extension, abduction, and adduction positions may also be used to evaluate hand strength.

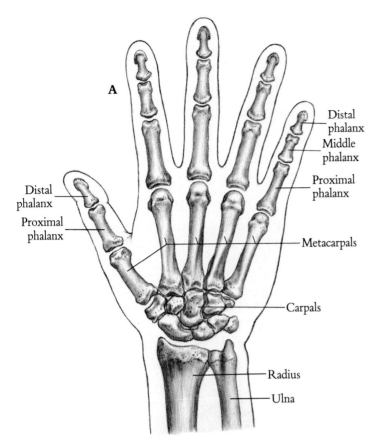

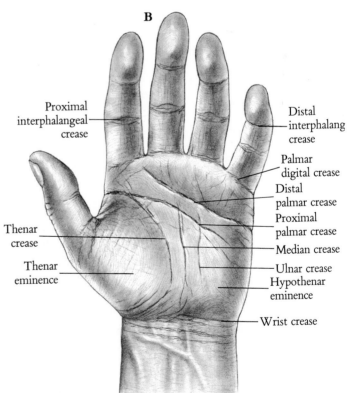

Fig. 16-30
A, Bony structure of the hand and wrist; note the alignment of the fingers with the radius. **B,** Features of the palmar aspect of the hand; note the creases, thenar eminence and hypothenar eminence, and gradual tapering of the fingers.

Fig. 16-31
Unexpected findings of the hand. **A,** Ulnar deviation of the fingers. **B,** Swan neck deformity of the fingers. **C,** Boutonnier deformity of the fingers.

A from Prior, 1981; **B** from Edmonson and Crenshaw, 1980; **C** from Milford, 1982.

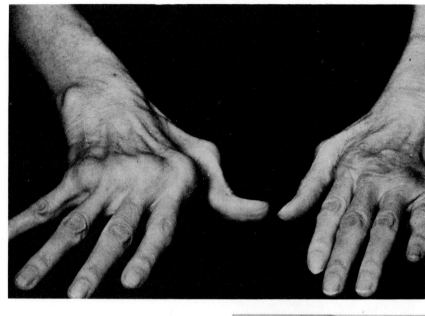

A

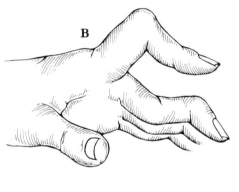

B

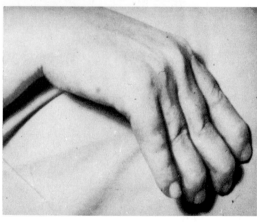

C

Fig. 16-32
Palpation of joints of the hand and wrist. **A,** Interphalangeal joints. **B,** Metacarpophalangeal joints. **C,** Radiocarpal groove and wrist.

A　　　　　　**B**　　　　　　**C**

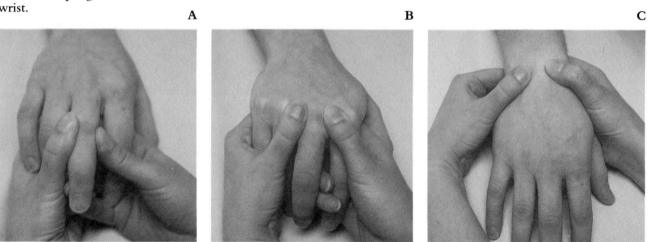

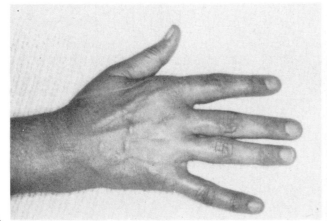

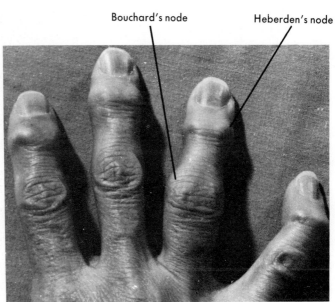

Bouchard's node   Heberden's node

A

B

Fig. 16-33
Unexpected findings of the fingers. **A,** Haygarth's nodes. Note swelling of the fourth proximal interphalangeal joint. **B,** Heberden's nodes at the distal interphalangeal joint and Bouchard's nodes at the proximal interphalangeal joint.

A from Kelley et al., 1973; **B** from Swanson, 1973.

Fig. 16-34
Elicitation of Tinel's sign.

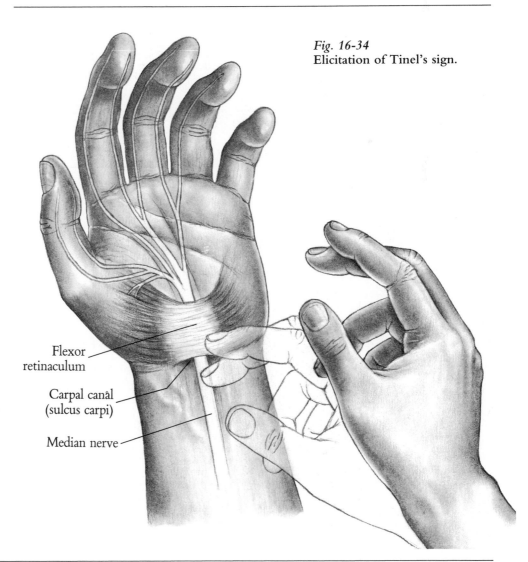

Flexor
retinaculum

Carpal canal
(sulcus carpi)

Median nerve

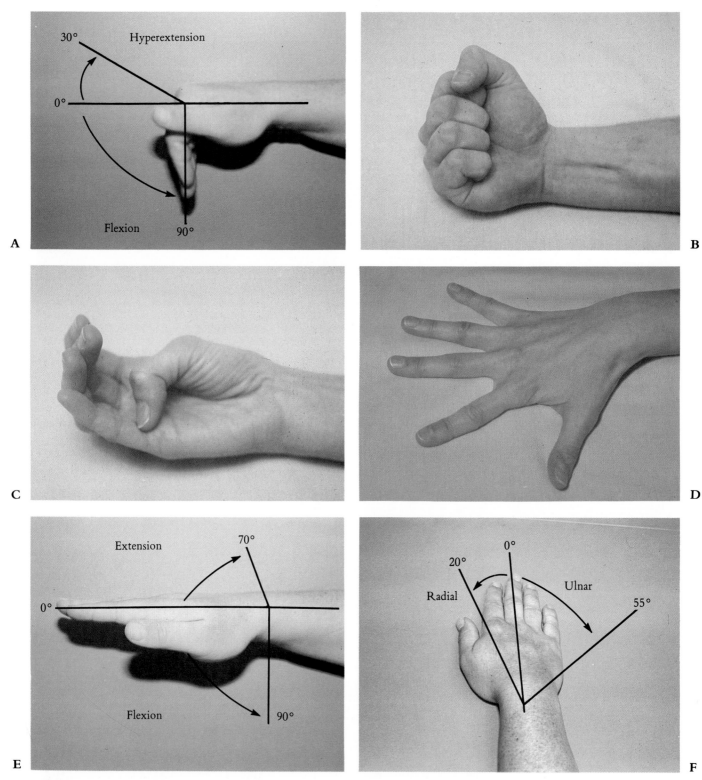

Fig. 16-35
Range of motion of the hand and wrist. **A,** Metacarpophalangeal flexion and hyperextension.
B, Finger flexion: fist formation. **C,** Finger flexion: thumb to each fingertip and to the base
of the little finger. **D,** Finger abduction. **E,** Wrist flexion and hyperextension. **F,** Wrist radial
and ulnar movement.

Hips

Inspect the hips anteriorly and posteriorly while the patient stands. Using the major landmarks of the iliac crest and the greater trochanter of the femur, note any asymmetry in the iliac crest height, the size of the buttocks, or the number and level of gluteal folds.

Palpate the hips and pelvis with the patient supine (Fig. 16-36). No instability, tenderness, or crepitus is expected.

Examine the hip's range of motion by asking the patient to perform the following movements (Fig. 16-37):

- While supine, raise the leg with the knee extended above the body. Expect up to 90 degrees of hip flexion.
- While either standing or prone, swing the straightened leg behind the body. Expect hip hyperextension of 30 degrees or less.
- While supine, raise one knee to the chest while keeping the other leg straight. Expect hip flexion of 120 degrees.
- While supine, swing the leg laterally and medially with knee straight. With the adduction movement, passively lift the opposite leg, to permit the examined leg full movement. Expect some degree of both abduction and adduction.
- While supine, flex the knee and rotate the leg inward toward the other leg. Expect internal rotation of 40 degrees.
- While supine, place the lateral aspect of the foot on the knee of the other leg; move the flexed knee toward the table. Expect 45 degrees of external rotation (Patrick's test).

Have the patient maintain flexion of the hip with knee in flexion and extension while you apply opposing force to evaluate strength of hip muscles. Muscle strength can also be evaluated during abduction and adduction, as well as by resistance to uncrossing the legs while seated.

Fig. 16-36
Palpating the pelvis for stability.

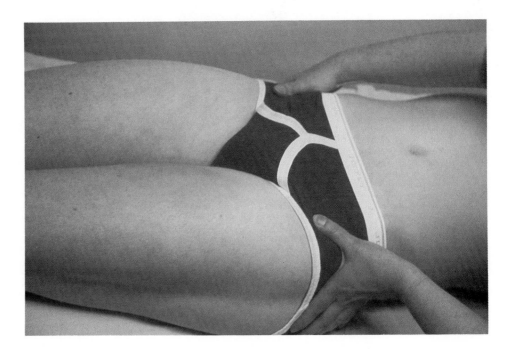

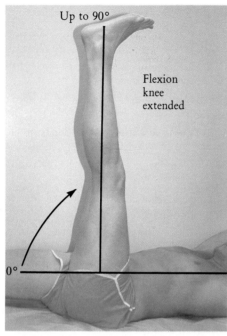

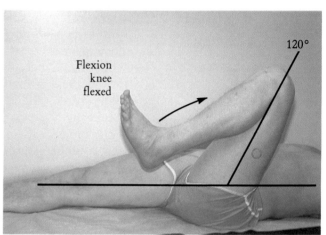

Fig. 16-37
Range of motion of the hip. **A,** Hip flexion, leg extended.
B, Hip flexion, knee flexed. **C,** Abduction.
D, Hip hyperextension, knee extended. **E,** Internal
rotation. **F,** External rotation.

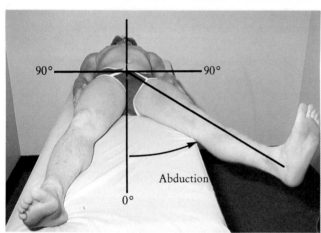

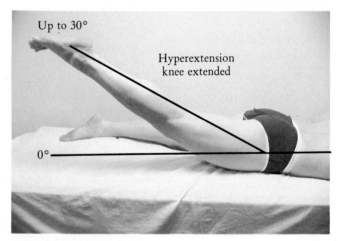

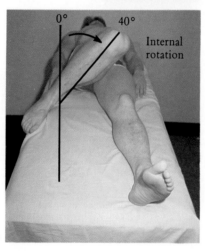

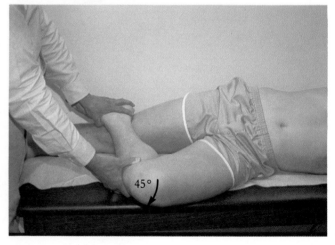

Knees

Inspect the knees and their popliteal spaces in both flexed and extended positions, noting the major landmarks: tibial tuberosity, medial and lateral tibial condyles, medial and lateral epicondyles of the femur, adductor tubercle of the femur, and the patella (see Fig. 16-10). Inspect the extended knee for its natural concavities on the anterior aspect, on each side, and above the patella.

Observe the lower leg alignment. The angle between the femur and tibia is expected to be less than 15 degrees. Variations in lower leg alignment are genu valgum (knock knees) and genu varum (bowlegs). Excessive hyperextension of the knee with weight bearing, genu recurvatum, may indicate weakness of the quadriceps muscles.

Palpate the popliteal space, noting any swelling or tenderness. Then palpate the tibiofemoral joint space, identifying the patella, the suprapatellar pouch, and the infrapatellar fat pad. The joint should feel smooth and firm, without tenderness, bogginess, nodules, or crepitus.

Examine the knee's range of motion by asking the patient to perform the following movements (Fig. 16-38):
- Bend each knee. Expect 130 degrees of flexion.
- Straighten the leg and stretch it. Expect full extension and up to 15 degrees of hyperextension.

The strength of the knee muscles is evaluated with the patient maintaining flexion and extension while you apply opposing force.

Fig. 16-38
Range of motion of the knee: flexion and extension.

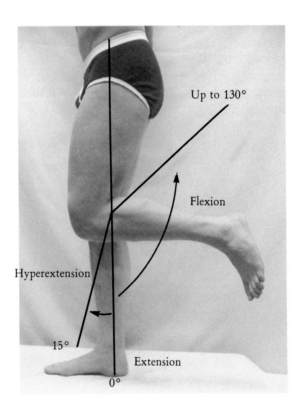

Up to 130°

Flexion

Hyperextension

15°

Extension

0°

Feet and Ankles

Inspect the feet and ankles while the patient is bearing weight (standing and walking) and sitting. Landmarks of the ankle include the medial malleolus, the lateral malleolus, and the Achilles tendon. Expect smooth and rounded malleolar prominences, prominent heels, and prominent metatarsophalangeal joints. Calluses and corns indicate chronic pressure or irritation.

Observe the contour of the feet and the position, size, and number of toes. The feet should be in alignment with the tibias. Pes varus (in-toeing) and pes valgus (out-toeing) are common alignment variations. Weight bearing should be on the midline of the foot, on an imaginary line from the heel midline to between the second and third toes. Deviations in forefoot alignment (metatarsus varus or metatarsus valgus), heel pronation, and pain or injury often cause a shift in weight-bearing position.

Expect the foot to have a longitudinal arch, although the foot may flatten with weight-bearing. Common variations include pes planus, a foot that remains flat even when not bearing weight, and pes cavus, a high instep (Fig. 16-39). Pes planus should not produce pain.

The toes should be straight forward, flat, and in alignment with each other. Several common deviations of the toes can occur (Fig. 16-40). Hyperextension of the metatarsophalangeal joint with flexion of the toe's proximal joint is called hammer toe. Claw toe is hyperextension of the metatarsophalangeal joint with flexion of the toe's proximal and distal joints. Hallux valgus is lateral deviation of the great toe that may cause overlapping with the second toe. A bursa often forms at the pressure point and, if it becomes inflamed, forms a painful bunion.

Heat, redness, swelling, and tenderness of the metatarsophalangeal joint of the great toe should make you suspect gouty arthritis. A draining tophus may occasionally be present.

Palpate the Achilles tendon and the anterior surface of the ankle. Using the thumb and fingers of both hands, compress the forefoot, palpating each metatarsophalangeal joint.

Fig. 16-39
Variations in the longitudinal arch of the foot.
A, Expected arch.
B, Pes planus (flatfoot).
C, Pes cavus (high instep).

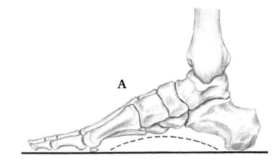
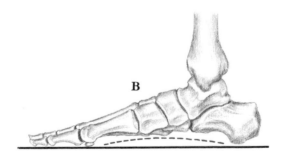
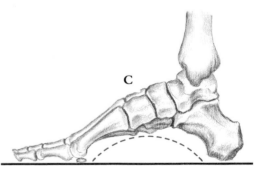

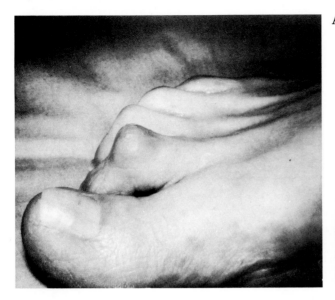

A

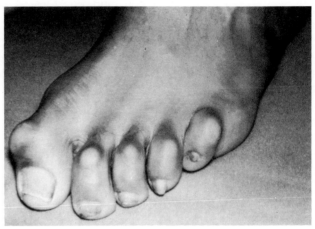

B

Fig. 16-40
Deviations of the toes.
A, Hammertoe. **B,** Claw
toe. **C,** Hallux valgus with
bunion.
A and **B** from Mann, 1986; **C** from
Thompson et al., 1986.

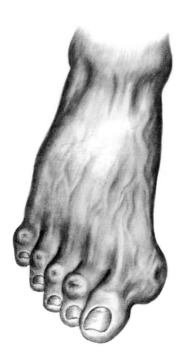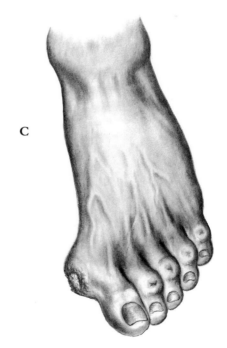

C

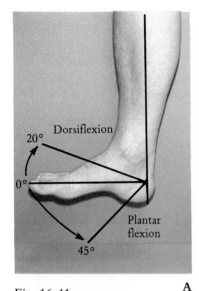 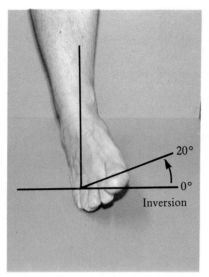 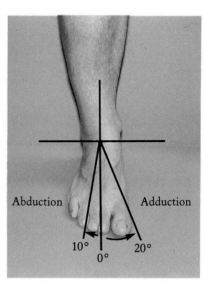

A   B   C

Fig. 16-41
Range of motion of the foot and ankle. **A,** Dorsiflexion and plantar flexion. **B,** Inversion and eversion. **C,** Abduction and adduction.

The range of motion of the foot and ankle is assessed by asking the patient to perform the following movements while sitting (Fig. 16-41):

- Point the foot toward the ceiling. Expect dorsiflexion of 20 degrees.
- Point the foot toward the floor. Expect plantar flexion of 45 degrees.
- Bending the foot at the ankle, turn the sole of the foot toward and then away from the other foot. Expect inversion of 30 degrees and eversion of 20 degrees.
- Rotating the ankle, turn the foot away from and then toward the other foot while the examiner stabilizes the leg. Expect abduction of 10 degrees and adduction of 20 degrees.
- Bend and straighten the toes. Expect flexion and extension, especially of the great toes.

Have the patient maintain dorsiflexion and plantar flexion while you apply opposing force to evaluate strength of the ankle muscles. Abduction and adduction of the ankle and flexion and extension of the great toe may also be used to evaluate muscle strength.

Additional Procedures

Various other procedures for further evaluation of specific joints of the musculoskeletal system are performed when problems are detected with routine procedures.

Limb Measurement

When a difference in length or circumference of matching extremities is suspected, measure and compare the size of both extremities. Leg length is measured from the anterior superior iliac spine to the medial malleolus of the ankle, crossing the knee on the medial side. Arm length is measured from the acromion process through the olecranon process to the distal ulnar prominence. The circumference of the extremities is measured in centimeters at the same distance on each limb from a major landmark (Fig. 16-42). Serious athletes who use the dominant arm almost exclusively in their activities (pitchers and tennis players) may have some discrepancy in circumference. For most people, no more than a 1 cm discrepancy in length and circumference between matching extremities should be found.

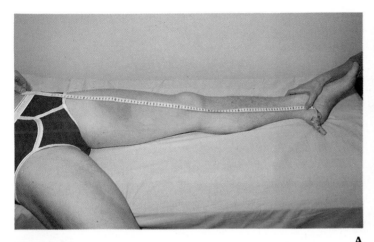

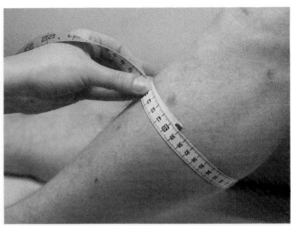

A

B

Fig. 16-42
Measuring limb length and circumference. A, Leg length. **B,** Leg circumference.

Knee Assessment

Ballottement is used to determine the presence of excess fluid or an effusion in the knee. With the knee extended, apply downward pressure on the suprapatellar pouch with the thumb and fingers of one hand, and then push the patella sharply backward against the femur with a finger of your other hand. Release the pressure suddenly against the patella, but keep your finger lightly touching the knee. A tap against your finger, as if a fluid wave were elicited, indicates an effusion (Fig. 16-43).

Examination for the bulge sign is also used to determine the presence of excess fluid in the knee. With the knee extended, milk the medial aspect of the knee upward two or three times, and then tap the lateral side of the patella. Observe for a bulge of returning fluid to the hollow area medial to the patella (Fig. 16-44).

McMurray's test is used to detect a torn meniscus. Have the supine patient flex one knee completely with the foot flat on the table near the buttocks. Maintain that flexion with your thumb and index finger stabilizing the knee on either side of the joint space. Hold the heel with your other hand and rotate the foot and lower leg to a lateral position. Extend the patient's knee to a 90-degree angle, noting any palpable or audible click or limited extension of the knee. Return the knee to full flexion, and repeat the procedure rotating the foot and lower leg to a medial position (Fig. 16-45). A palpable or audible click in the knee or lack of extension is a positive sign.

The drawer test is used to identify instability of the knee on the mediolateral or anteroposterior plane. Have the supine patient extend the knee. Stabilize the femur with one hand and hold the ankle with your other hand. Try to abduct and adduct the knee (Fig. 16-46, *A*). There should be no medial or lateral movement of the knee. Then have the patient flex the knee to 90 degrees, placing the foot flat on the table. Stabilize the foot with one hand and grasp the lower leg just below the knee with your other hand. Try to push the lower leg forward and backward (Fig. 16-46, *B*). Anterior or posterior movement of the knee is an unexpected finding.

When the patient complains of a knee locking, use Apley's test to detect a meniscal tear. Have the prone patient flex the knee to 90 degrees. Place your hand on the heel of the foot and press firmly, opposing the tibia to the femur. Then rotate the lower leg externally and internally (Fig. 16-47). Be cautious and do not cause the patient excess pain. Any clicks, locking, and pain in the knee is a positive Apley's sign.

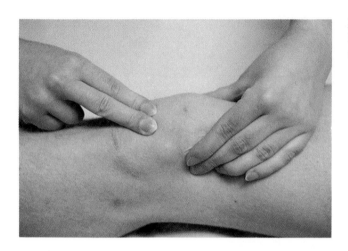

Fig. 16-43
Procedure for ballottement examination of the knee.

Fig. 16-44
Testing for the bulge sign in examination of the knee.

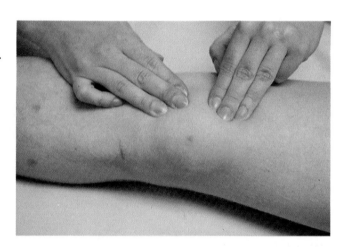

Fig. 16-45
Procedure for examination of the knee with McMurray's test.

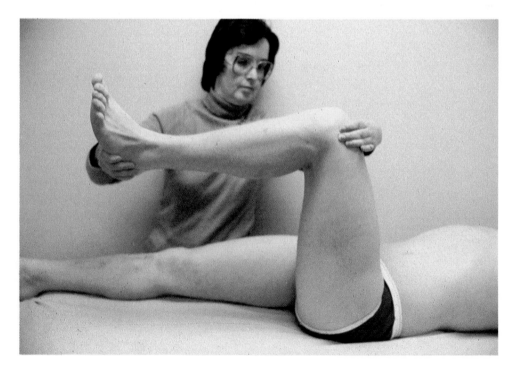

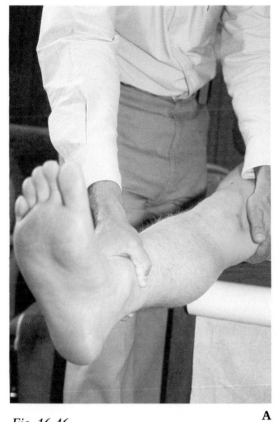

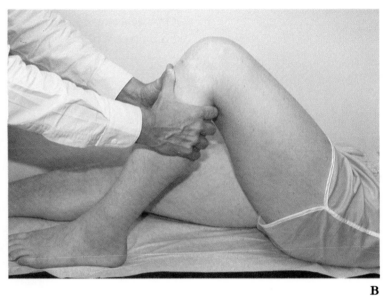

A

B

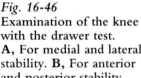

Fig. 16-46
Examination of the knee
with the drawer test.
A, For medial and lateral
stability. **B,** For anterior
and posterior stability.

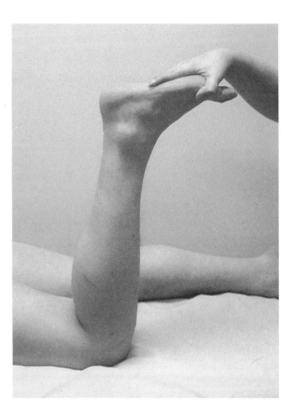

Fig. 16-47
Examination of the knee,
testing for Apley's sign.

Hip Assessment

The Thomas test is used to detect flexion contractures of the hip that may be masked by excessive lumbar lordosis. Have the supine patient fully extend one leg flat on the examining table and flex the other leg with the knee to the chest. Observe the patient's ability to keep the extended leg flat on the examining table (Fig. 16-48). Lifting the extended leg off the examining table indicates a hip flexion contracture in the extended leg.

Trendelenberg's test is a maneuver to detect hip dislocation. Ask the standing patient to balance first on one foot and then the other. Observing from behind, note any asymmetry of the iliac crests. When the iliac crest drops on the side opposite the weight-bearing leg, the weight-bearing hip is defective (Fig. 16-49).

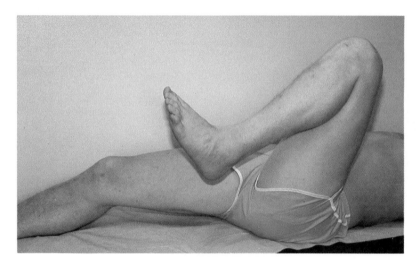

Fig. 16-48
Procedures for examination of the hip with Thomas test. Note the elevation of the extended leg off the examining table.

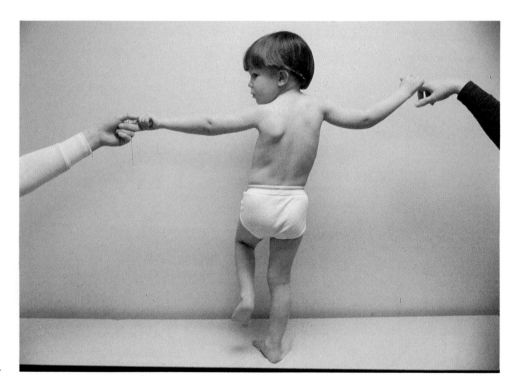

Fig. 16-49
Test for Trendelenberg's sign. Note any asymmetry in the level of the iliac crests with weight bearing.

Genetic and fetal insults can produce musculoskeletal anomalies. The fetus is exposed to various postural pressures that can be manifested in the infant as reduced extension of extremities and torsions of various bones.

Fully undress the infant and observe the posture and spontaneous generalized movements. (Use a warming table when examining newborns.) No localized or generalized muscular twitching is expected. Inspect the back for tufts of hair, dimples, discolorations, cysts, or masses near the spine. Transillumination of a mass near the spine should make you suspect a meningocele or myelomeningocele.

From about age 2 months, the infant should be able to lift the head and trunk from the prone position, giving you an indication of forearm strength. Assess the curvature of the spine and the strength of the paravertebral muscles with the infant in sitting position. Kyphosis of the thoracic and lumbar spine will be apparent in sitting position until the infant can sit without support (Fig. 16-50).

Inspect the extremities, noting symmetric flexion of arms and legs. The axillary, gluteal, femoral, and popliteal creases should be symmetric, and the limbs should be freely movable. No unusual proportions or asymmetry of limb length or circumference, constricted annular bands, or other deformities should be noted.

Place the newborn in a fetal position to observe how that may have contributed to any asymmetry of flexion, position, or shape of the extremities. Newborns have some resistance to full extension of the elbows, hips, and knees. Movements should be symmetric.

All babies are flat-footed, and many newborns have a slight varus curvature of the tibias (tibial torsion) or forefoot adduction (metatarsus adductus) from fetal positioning. The midline of the foot may bisect the third and fourth toes, rather than the second and third toes. The forefoot should be flexible, straightening with abduction. It is necessary to follow apparent problems carefully, but it is seldom necessary to intervene. As growth and development takes place, the expected body habitus is usually achieved.

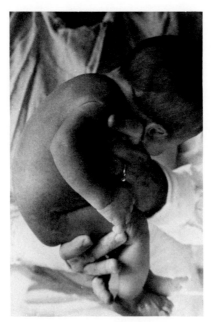

Fig. 16-50
Kyphosis, expected convex curvature of the newborn's spine.
From Bowers and Thompson, 1984.

The hands should open periodically with the fingers fully extended. When the hand is fisted, the thumb should be positioned inside the fingers. Open the fist and observe the dermatoglyphic features, noting the palmar and phalangeal creases on each hand. A simian crease is associated with Down's syndrome. Count the fingers and toes, noting polydactyly or syndactyly (Fig. 16-51).

Palpate the clavicles and long bones for fractures, dislocations, crepitus, masses, and tenderness. One of the most easily missed findings in the newborn is a fractured clavicle. It is embarrassing to have a parent ask what that lump is on the baby's collar bone. It is the callus that forms as the healing clavicle shapes and remolds itself. The tell-tale bony irregularity and crepitus may well have been detected during the neonatal examination.

Position the baby with the trunk flexed, and palpate each spinal process. Feel the shape of each, noting whether it is thin and well formed, as expected, or whether it is split, possibly indicating a bifid defect (Fig. 16-52).

Palpate the muscles to evaluate muscle tone, grasping the muscle to estimate its firmness. Observe for spasticity or flaccidity, and when detected, determine if it is localized or generalized. Use passive range of motion to examine joint mobility.

The Ortolani maneuver to detect hip dislocation or subluxation should be performed each time you examine the infant during the first year of life. Position yourself at the supine infant's feet, and flex the hips and knees to 90 degrees. Grasp a

Fig. 16-51
Anomalies of the newborn's hand. A, Simian crease. B, Syndactyly. C, Polydactyly.
Courtesy Mead Johnson, Evansville, Illinois.

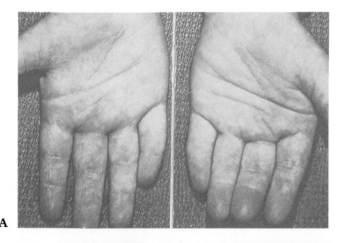

A

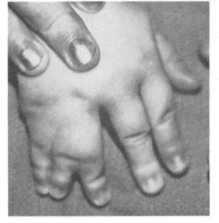

B

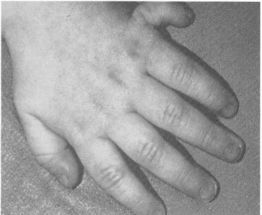

C

Fig. 16-52
Bifid defect of the vertebra, identified by palpation.

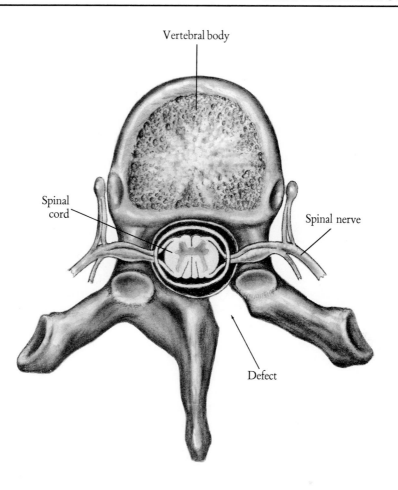

Vertebral body

Spinal cord

Spinal nerve

Defect

leg in each of your hands with your thumb on the inside of each thigh, the base of the thumb on each knee, and your fingers gripping the outer thigh with finger tips resting on the greater trochanter (Fig. 16-53). First, adduct the thighs to the maximum so that your thumbs touch. Next, slowly abduct the thighs while maintaining axial pressure. With the fingertips on the greater trochanter, exert a lever movement in the opposite direction so your fingertips press the head of the femur back toward the acetabulum center. If the head of the femur slips back into the acetabulum with a palpable clunk when pressure is exerted, suspect hip subluxation or dislocation. Asymmetric gluteal folds and abduction of the hips limited to less than 160 degrees may also indicate congenital hip dislocation (Fig. 16-54).

The test for Allis's sign is also used to detect hip dislocation or a shortened femur. With the infant supine on the examining table, flex both knees keeping the femurs aligned with each other. Position yourself at the child's feet, and observe the height of the knees (Fig. 16-55). When one knee appears lower than the other, Allis's sign is positive.

Muscle strength is evaluated by holding the infant upright with your hands under the axillae (Fig. 16-56). Adequate shoulder muscle strength is present if the infant maintains the upright position. If the infant begins to slip through your fingers, muscle weakness is present.

B

A

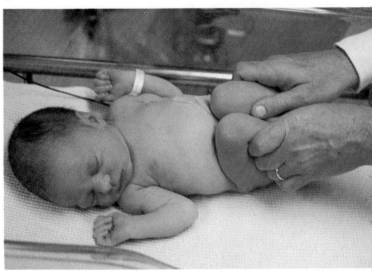
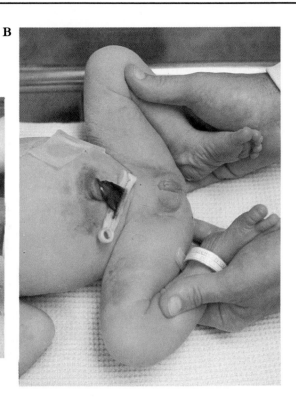

Fig. 16-53
Ortolani maneuver to detect congenital hip dislocation.
A, Phase I, adduction. **B,** Phase II, abduction.

Fig. 16-54
Signs of congenital hip
dislocation: limitation of
abduction and asymmetric
gluteal folds.

From Thompson et al., 1986.

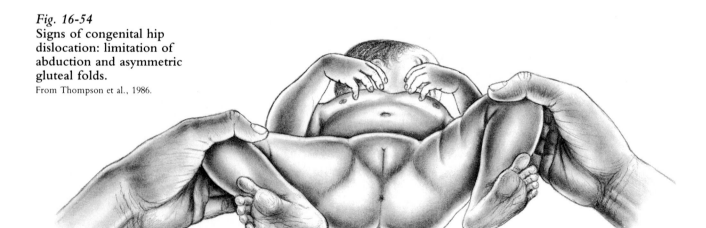

Fig. 16-55
Examination for Allis' sign.
From Thompson et al., 1986.

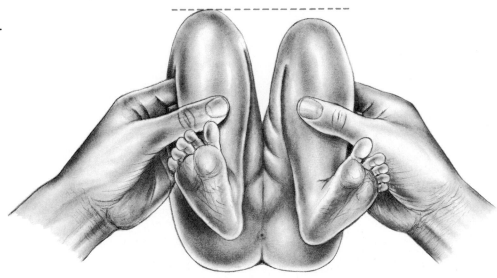

Fig. 16-56
Evaluation of shoulder muscle strength in the newborn.

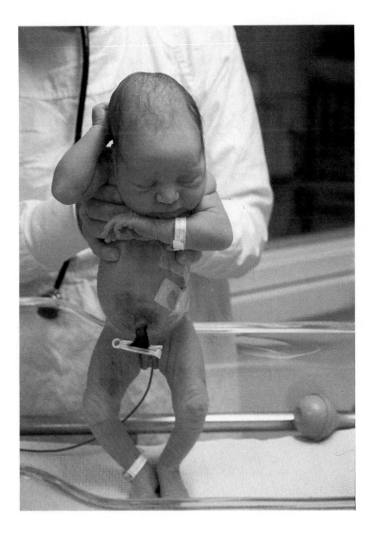

Fig. 16-57
Examination for tibial torsion.

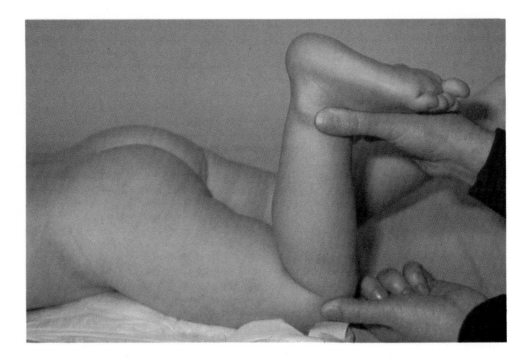

Tibial torsion is evaluated with the child prone on the examining table. Flex one knee 90 degrees and align the midline of the foot parallel to the femur. Using the thumb and index finger of one hand, grasp the medial and lateral condyles of the tibia. With the other hand, grasp the medial and lateral malleoli of the ankle, placing your thumb and index finger on the same sides of the leg. If your thumbs are not parallel to each other, tibial torsion is present (Fig. 16-57). Tibial torsion, a residual of fetal positioning, is expected to resolve after 6 months of weight bearing.

CHILDREN

Watching young children during play or while they are with the parent as the history is taken can provide a great deal of information about the child's musculoskeletal system. If the child has been able to pick up and play with toys, moving in unconstrained fashion without evidence of limitation, the laying on of hands is necessary but may not reveal any additional information. Suggest activities that will enhance your observations. The function of joints, range of motion, bone stability, and muscle strength can be adequately evaluated by observing the child climb, jump, hop, rise from a sitting position, and manipulate toys or other objects.

Position the young child to observe motor development and musculoskeletal function. Inspect the spine of the child while he or she is standing. Young children will have a lumbar curvature of the spine and a protuberant abdomen (Fig. 16-58). Observe the toddler's ability to sit, creep, and grasp and release objects during play. Knowledge of the expected sequence of motor development will facilitate your examination (Table 16-3).

As you inspect the bones, joints, and muscles, pay particular attention to the alignment of the legs and feet, because developmental stresses are placed on the musculoskeletal system. Remember to observe the wear of the child's shoes and ask about his or her favorite sitting posture. The reverse tailor position places stress on the joints of the hips, knees, and ankles. This could lead to future problems in lower limb alignment, such as femoral anteversion (Fig. 16-59).

Table 16-3
Expected Motor Development Sequence in Children, Birth to 9 Years of Age

Age	Fine Motor Development	Gross Motor Development
1 month		Turns head to side; keeps knees tucked under abdomen; gross head lag and rounded back when pulled to sitting position
2 months		Holds head in same plane as rest of body; can raise head and hold position
3 months	When supine, puts hands together; holds hands in front of face	Raises head to 45 degrees; may turn from prone to side position; slight head lag when pulled to sitting position
4 months	Grasps rattle; hands held together	Actively lifts head, looks around; rolls from prone to supine position; no head lag when pulled to sitting position; attempts to bear weight when held standing up
5 months	Can reach and pick up object; plays with toes	Able to push up from prone position with forearms and maintain position; rolls over prone to supine to prone; back straight when sitting
6 months	Drops object to reach for another offered; holds rattle or spoon	Sits, posture shaky, uses tripod position; raises abdomen off table when prone; when standing supports almost full weight
7 months	Transfers object between hands; holds object in each hand	Sits alone, uses hands for support; bounces in standing position; pulls feet to mouth
8 months	Begins thumb-finger grasping	Sits without support
9 months	Bangs objects together	Begins creeping, abdomen off floor; stands holding on when placed in position
10 months	Points with one finger; picks up small objects	Pulls self to standing position, unable to let self down; walks holding onto stable objects
11 months		Walks around room holding on to objects; stands securely, holding on with 1 hand
12 months	Feeds self with cup and spoon fairly well; offers toy and releases it	Sits from standing posture; twists and turns, maintaining posture; stands without support momentarily
15 months	Puts raisin into bottle; takes off shoes; pulls toys	Walks alone well; seats self in chair
18 months	Holds crayon, scribbles spontaneously	Walks up and down steps holding one hand, some running ability
2 years	Turns doorknob; takes off shoes and socks; builds 2-block tower	Walks up stairs alone, 2 feet on each step; walks backwards; kicks ball
30 months	Builds 4-block tower; feeds self more neatly; dumps raisin from bottle	Jumps from object; throws ball overhand; walking more stable
3 years	Unbuttons front buttons; copies vertical line within 30 degrees; copies circle; builds 8-block tower	Walks up stairs alternating feet; walks down steps 2 feet on each step; pedals tricycle; jumps in one place; performs broad jump
4 years	Copies cross; buttons large buttons	Walks down stairs alternating feet; balances on 1 foot for 5 seconds
5 years	Dresses self with minimal assistance; colors within lines; draws 3-part human	Hops on 1 foot; catches bounced ball 2 of 3 times; heel-toe walking
6 years	Copies square; draws 6-part human	Jumps, tumbles, skips, hops; walks straight line; skips rope with practice; rides bicycle; heel-toe walking backwards
7 years	Prints well, begins to write script	Skips and plays hopscotch; running and climbing more coordinated
8 years	Mature handwriting skill	Movements more graceful
9 years		Eye-hand coordination developed

Adapted from Bowers and Thompson, 1984.

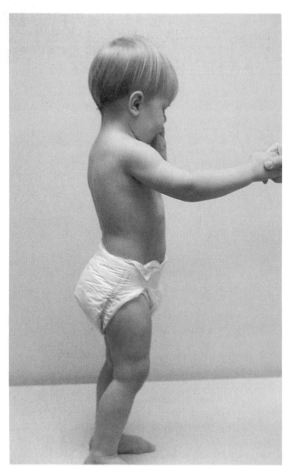

Fig. 16-58
Lumbar curvature of the
toddler's spine.

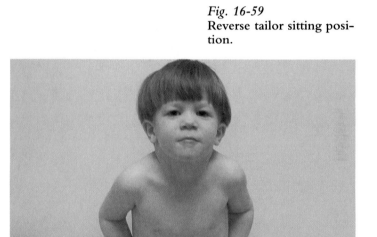

Fig. 16-59
Reverse tailor sitting position.

Inspect the longitudinal arch of the foot and the position of the feet with weight bearing. The longitudinal arch of the foot is obscured by a fat pad until about 3 years of age, and after that time, it should be apparent when it is not bearing weight. Metatarsus adductus should be resolved. The feet of the toddler will often pronate slightly inward until about 30 months of age. After that time weight bearing should shift to the midline of the feet.

Bowleg (genu varum) is evaluated with the child standing, facing you, knees at your eye level. Measure the distance between the knees when the medial malleoli of the ankles are together. Genu varum is present if a space of 2.5 cm (1 in) exists between the knees. The expected 10- to 15-degree angle at the tibiofemoral articulation increases with genu varum but remains bilaterally symmetric. On future examinations, note any increase in the angle or increased space between the knees. Genu varum is a common finding of toddlers until 18 months of age. Asymmetry of the tibiofemoral articulation angle or space between the knees should not exceed 1½ in.

Knock knee (genu valgum) is also evaluated with the child standing, facing you, knees at your eye level. Measure the distance between the medial malleoli of the ankles with the knees together. Genu valgum is present if a space of 2.5 cm (1 in) exists between the medial malleoli. As with genu varum, the tibiofemoral articulation angle will increase with genu valgum. On future examinations, note any increase in the angle or increased space between the ankles. Genu valgum is a common finding of children between 2 and 4 years of age (Fig. 16-60). Asymmetry of the tibiofemoral articulation angle or a space between the medial malleoli should not exceed 2 in.

Subluxation of the head of the radius is often called nursemaid's elbow. Tugging on a child's arm in removing clothing or lifting a child by grabbing the hand can lead to this dislocation. The injury is relatively easy to cause and fortunately easy to reduce, but it is better to prevent it. A toddler should not dangle in the air suspended by an adult's grasp on the hand.

Palpate the bones, muscles, and joints, paying particular attention to asymmetric body parts. Use passive range of motion to examine a joint and muscle group if some limitation of movement is noted while the child is playing.

Ask the child to stand, rising from a supine position. The child with good muscle strength will rise to a standing position without using the arms for leverage. Generalized muscle weakness is indicated by Gowers' sign in which the child rises from a sitting position by placing hands on the legs and pushing the trunk up (Fig. 16-61).

Fig. 16-60
Genu valgum (knock knee) in the young child.

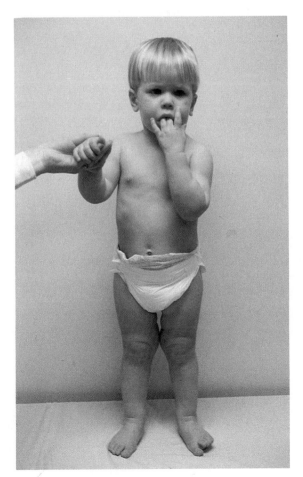

A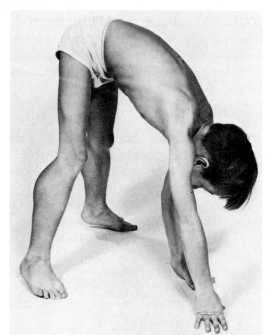

B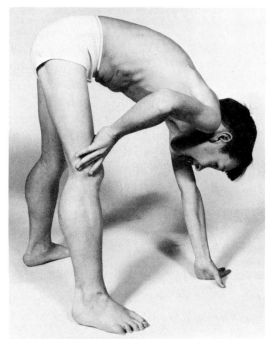

Fig. 16-61
Gower's sign of general-
ized muscle weakness.
A, Maneuvers to position
supported by both arms
and legs. **B,** Pushes off
floor to rest hand on knee.
C, Then pushes self upright.
From Swaiman and Wright, 1982.

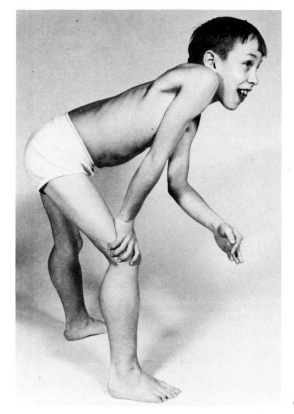

C

ADOLESCENTS

Examine older children and adolescents with the same procedures used for adults. Remember to use caution when examining sports-related injuries.

The spine should be smooth with balanced concave and convex curves. No lateral curvature or rib hump with forward flexion should be apparent. The shoulders and scapulae should be level with each other within ½ in, and a distance between the scapulae of 3 to 5 in is usual. Adolescents may have slight kyphosis and rounded shoulders with an interscapular space of 5 or 6 in.

PREGNANT WOMEN

Postural changes with pregnancy are common. The growing fetus shifts the woman's center of gravity forward, leading to increased lordosis and a compensatory forward cervical flexion. Stooped shoulders and large breasts exaggerate the spinal curvature. Increased mobility and instability of the sacroiliac joints and symphysis pubis contribute to the "waddling" gait of late pregnancy.

Carpal tunnel syndrome is experienced by some women during the last trimester.

OLDER ADULTS

The older adult should be able to participate in the physical examination as described for the adult, but the response to your requests may be more slow and deliberate. Fine and gross motor skills required to perform activities of daily living such as dressing, grooming, climbing steps, and writing will provide an evaluation of the patient's joint and muscle agility. Joint and muscle agility will vary among older adults (Fig. 16-62).

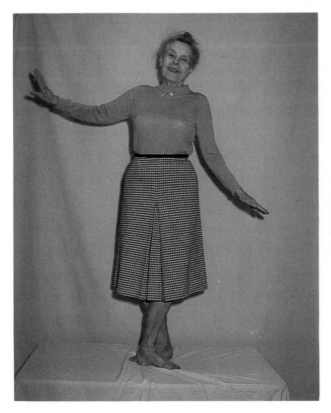

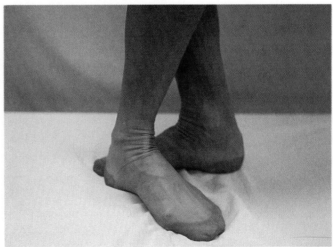

Fig. 16-62
Agility in the older adult. Note the flexibility and ability to balance in this 83-year-old woman.

The patient's posture may display increased dorsal kyphosis, accompanied by flexion of the hips and knees. The head may tilt backward to compensate for the increased thoracic curvature (see Fig. 16-20, *B*). The extremities may appear to be relatively long if the trunk has diminished in length. The base of support may be broader with the feet more widely spaced, and the patient may hold the arms away from the body to aid balancing.

The reduction in total muscle mass is often related to atrophy, either from disuse, as in patients with arthritis, or from loss of nervous innervation, as in patients with diabetic neuropathy.

Common Abnormalities

Ankylosing Spondylitis

A hereditary, chronic inflammatory disease, ankylosing spondylitis initially affects the lumbar spine and adjacent structures. Initial symptoms of stiffness, loss of lumbar lordosis, and decreased spinal mobility commonly progress to eventual fusion and deformity of the spine. The joints of the hip, shoulder, neck, ribs, and jaw may also be involved (Fig. 16-63).

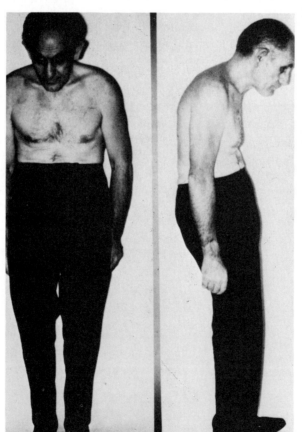

Fig. 16-63
Posture of patient affected by ankylosing spondylitis.
From Prior, 1981.

Carpal Tunnel Syndrome	Compression on the median nerve caused by thickening of its flexor tendon sheath often results from trauma. During pregnancy, edematous swelling of the hands is thought to contribute. The symptoms of numbness, burning,	and tingling often occur at night, but they can also be elicited by rotational movements of the wrist. Weakness of the hand and flattening of the thenar eminence of the palm may result.
Gout	Gout is an inflammatory arthritis caused by abnormalities in purine metabolism that results in prolonged hyperuricemia and uric acid deposition in joint spaces. Joint involvement is almost always monarticular. The classical joint affected is the proximal phalanx of the great	toe, although other joints of the foot, ankle, and knee are sometimes affected. Symptoms include exquisite pain, knobby swelling at the joint, and sometimes drainage of a tophus. Gout primarily affects men over age 40 (Fig. 16-64).

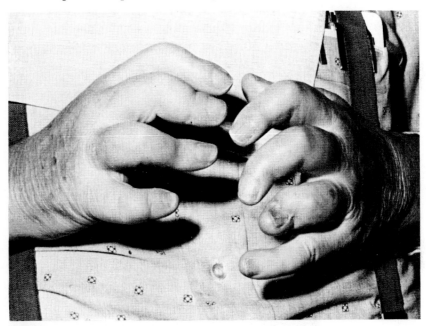

Fig. 16-64
Gout in the hands without apparent tophi.
From Halstead, 1982.

Paget's Disease (Osteitis Deformans)

An inflammatory focal disorder of the bone, Paget's disease appears in persons over 45 years of age. Excessive bone resorption and excessive bone formation produces a mosaic pattern of lamellar bone. Bowed tibias, misshaped pelvis or skull, shortened thorax, and frequent fractures occur. The bones of the skull are often affected, which can produce symptoms of vertigo, headache, and progressive deafness from involvement of the ossicles or neural elements. The cause is unknown, although a slow acting virus is suspected.

Osteoarthritis

Osteoarthritis results from gradual deterioration of the articular cartilages. It affects both weight-bearing and non-weight-bearing joints, but the knees, hips, and spine are most likely to become symptomatic. The incidence of the disease increases with age, and most older adults have some degree of osteoarthritis. Both acute and chronic trauma and inflammation are precipitating factors. Osteoarthritis is slightly more common in women. The affected joint is painful, enlarged, and limited in motion (Fig. 16-65).

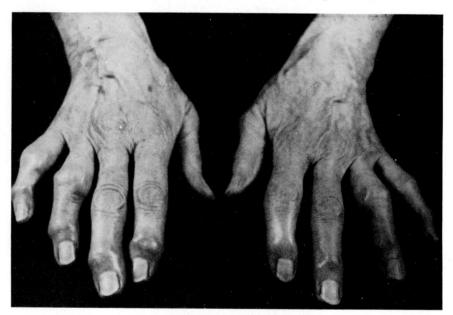

Fig. 16-65
Osteoarthritis signs in the hand.
Reprinted from the Revised Clinical Slide Collection on the Rheumatic Disease.
Copyright 1981. Used by permission of the American Rheumatism Association.

Rheumatoid Arthritis

A chronic, destructive disease in which inflammation of the synovium and increased synovial exudate lead to thickening of the synovium and swelling of the involved joints. Usually the disease is bilateral, symmetric, and polyarticular. Initially the joints of the hands, wrists, knees, and feet are involved. Fingers may deviate to the ulnar side, and swan neck or boutonnière deformities occur as the disease progresses. Rheumatoid nodules develop at pressure points. Joint pain, tenderness, stiffness, and swelling of symmetric joints are often accompanied by systemic changes such as major organ involvement, weight loss, malaise, and fatigue. (Fig. 16-66).

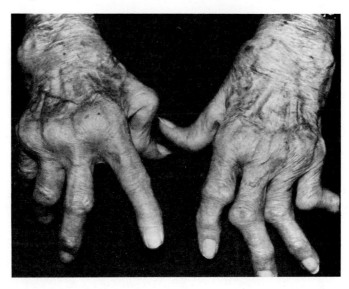

Fig. 16-66
Rheumatoid arthritis in the hand.
From Kiene and Johnson, 1983.

INFANTS AND CHILDREN

Meningomyelocele, Spina Bifida

Congenital neural tube defects, with incomplete closure of the vertebral column, permit the meninges and sometimes the spinal cord to protrude into a saclike structure (Fig. 16-67).

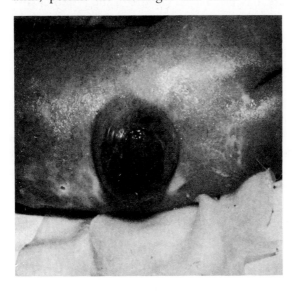

Fig. 16-67
Meningomyelocele of the lumbar spine.
From Whaley and Wong, 1983.

Clubfoot (Talipes Equinovarus)	Clubfoot is a fixed congenital defect of the ankle and foot. The most common combination of position deformities in-	clude inversion of the foot at the ankle and plantar flexion with the toes lower than the heel (Fig. 16-68).

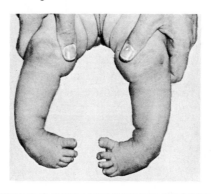

Fig. 16-68
Clubfoot deformity, talipes equinovarus.
From Brashear and Raney, 1978.

Metatarsus Adductus (Metatarsus Varus)	The most common congenital foot deformity, metatarsus adductus can be either fixed or flexible. This defect is caused by intrauterine positioning. Medial adduction of the toes and forefoot results from angulation at the tarso-	metatarsal joint. The lateral border of the foot is convex, and a crease is sometimes apparent on the medial border of the foot. The heel and ankle are uninvolved.
Congenital Hip Dislocation	Hip dislocation is a common congenital defect with varying degrees of involvement. Acetabular dysplasia arises from delay in ossification of the acetabulum, which is oblique and shallow, but the femoral head remains in the acetabulum. Subluxation is an incomplete dislocation in which the femoral head	remains in contact with the acetabulum, but the joint ligaments and capsule are stretched, which allows displacement of the femoral head. Dislocation indicates that the femoral head loses contact completely with the acetabular capsule and is displaced over the fibrocartilaginous rim.
Rickets	Bony, painless swelling at the epiphyses is often attributed to vitamin D deficiency. There may be delayed closure of the fontanels, enlargement of the costo-	chondral junction of the ribs (rachitic rosary), bowing of the arms and legs, and enlargement of the epiphysis at the ends of the long bones.
Juvenile Rheumatoid Arthritis	Juvenile rheumatoid arthritis is actually a group of inflammatory disorders that begin during childhood and adolescence. Onset may be systemic, polyarticular, or pauciarticular. Inflammation of the synovium and joint effusion lead to erosion, destruction, and fibrosis of	articular cartilages in the affected joints. Stiffness, swelling, and loss of motion develop in the affected joints. The severe types of disease produce extraarticular symptoms (iridocyclitis, fever, anemia, pericarditis) and can cause severe disability.
Sprengel's Deformity	Congenital elevation of the scapula causes the affected side of the neck to be fuller and shorter. Abduction of the shoulder is limited.	

Cleidocranial Dysostosis	Cleidocranial dysostosis is the congenital complete or partial absence of the clavicles. It is accompanied by defective	ossification of the cranium, with large fontanels and delayed closing of the sutures (Fig. 16-69).

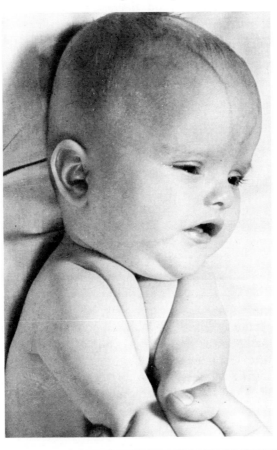

Fig. 16-69
Cleidocranial dysostosis, congenital absence of the clavicles.
From Swaiman and Wright, 1982.

Osgood-Schlatter Disease	A self-limiting disorder of the knee, Osgood-Schlatter disease occurs during adolescence. It is thought to result from repetitive stress on the patellar tendon.	Pain and a lump on the tibial tuberosity just below the knee are the usual symptoms. Pain with resistance to extension of the knee also occurs.
Muscular Dystrophy	Muscular dystrophy is a group of genetic disorders involving gradual degeneration of the muscle fibers. The disorders are characterized by progressive weakness and muscle atrophy or pseudohy-	pertrophy from fatty infiltrates. Some forms cause mild disability, and these patients can expect a normal life span. Other types produce severe disability, deformity, and death.
Radial Head Subluxation	A dislocation injury caused by jerking the arm upward while the elbow is flexed. This injury is common in children 1 to 4 years of age. The child com-	plains of pain in the elbow and wrist, refuses to move the arm, and holds it slightly flexed and pronated. Supination motion is resisted.

Femoral Anteversion

In femoral anteversion the femurs twist medially with the patella facing inward. Increased internal rotation of the hip of more than 70 degrees and decreased external hip rotation contribute to or result from the condition. In-toeing of the feet often occurs, and to compensate, the tibias may twist laterally to permit correct positioning of the feet. Femoral anteversion is often associated with reverse tailor sitting (Fig. 16-70).

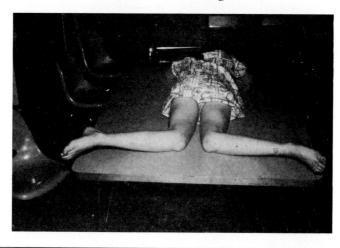

Fig. 16-70
Femoral anteversion.
From Mann, 1986.

Scoliosis

Lateral curvature of the spine may be either functional because of a leg length discrepancy or structural with a genetic component. Structural scoliosis progresses during childhood with growth. It produces uneven shoulder and hip levels and a rotational deformity leading to a rib hump and flank asymmetry on forward flexion. Physiologic alterations in the spine, chest, and pelvis result (Fig. 16-71).

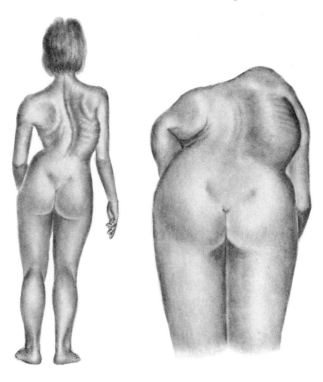

Fig. 16-71
Scoliosis, lateral curvature of the spine.

Legg-Calvé-Perthes Disease

Osteochondrosis of the femoral head appears in boys primarily between the ages of 3 and 10. A circulatory disorder or inflammatory process causes necrosis of the femoral capital epiphysis. This results in flattening of the upper surface of the femoral head. Revascularization and regeneration of the femoral head lead to varying degrees of hip deformity and dysfunction. The child usually complains of persistent pain that may be accompanied by joint dysfunction such as a limp or limited motion.

OLDER ADULTS

Osteoporosis

Osteoporosis is the decrease in bone mass that occurs when bone resorption is more rapid than bone deposition. The bones become fragile and susceptible to fractures. The disorder occurs most frequently in white and Asian postmenopausal women. The most common fracture sites are vertebrae, wrist, and hip.

Dupuytren's Contracture

Dupuytren's contracture affects the palmar fascia of one or more fingers and tends to be bilateral. Although the cause is unknown, there appears to be a hereditary component. A gradual increase in incidence occurs with age. It is also seen with increased frequency in patients with diabetes, alcoholic liver disease, and epilepsy (Fig. 16-72).

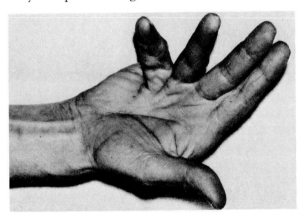

Fig. 16-72
Dupuytren's contracture.
From Edmonson and Crenshaw, 1980.

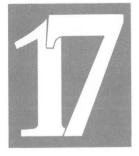

Neurologic System

The nervous system with its central and peripheral divisions maintains and controls all body functions by its voluntary and autonomic responses. Evaluation of motor, sensory, autonomic, cognitive, and behavioral elements makes neurologic assessment one of the most complex portions of the physical examination.

Anatomy and Physiology

The central nervous system (brain and spinal cord) is the main network of coordination and control for the body (Fig. 17-1). The peripheral nervous system, composed of motor and sensory nerves and ganglia outside the central nervous system, carries information to and from the central nervous system. The autonomic nervous system regulates the internal environment of the body, over which a person has no voluntary control. It has two divisions, each tending to balance the impulses of the other. The sympathetic division prods the body into action during times of physiologic and psychologic stress. The parasympathetic division functions in a complementary and a counterbalancing manner to conserve body resources and maintain day-to-day body functions such as digestion and elimination.

The intricate interrelationship of the nervous system permits the body to:

- Receive sensory stimuli from the environment
- Identify and integrate the adaptive processes needed to maintain current body functions
- Orchestrate body function changes required for adaptation and survival
- Integrate the rapid responsiveness of the central nervous system with the more gradual responsiveness of the endocrine system
- Control cognitive and voluntary behavioral processes
- Control subconscious and involuntary body functions

The brain and spinal cord are protected by the skull and vertebrae, the meninges, and cerebrospinal fluid. Three layers of meninges surround the brain and spinal cord, assisting in the production and drainage of cerebrospinal fluid (Fig. 17-2). Cerebrospinal fluid circulates between an interconnecting system of ventricles in the brain and around the brain and spinal cord, serving as a shock absorber.

Fig. 17-1
Base view of brain and cross-section of spinal cord.

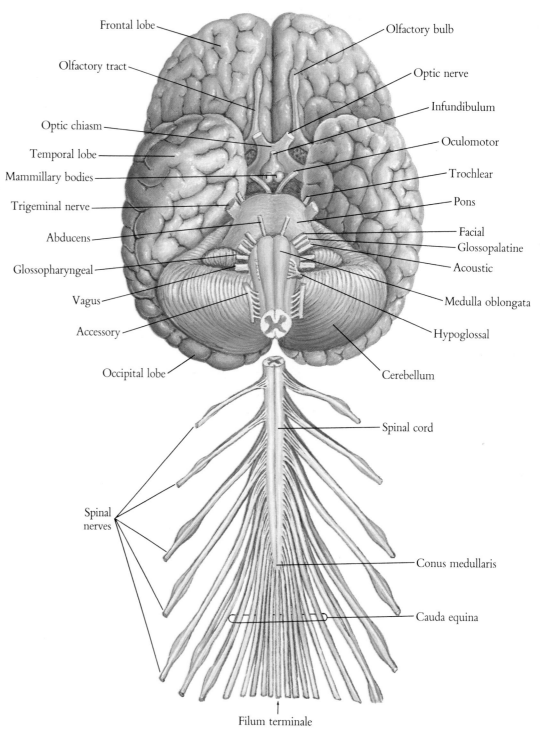

Frontal lobe

Olfactory bulb

Olfactory tract

Optic nerve

Infundibulum

Optic chiasm

Oculomotor

Temporal lobe

Trochlear

Mammillary bodies

Pons

Trigeminal nerve

Facial

Abducens

Glossopalatine

Acoustic

Glossopharyngeal

Medulla oblongata

Vagus

Hypoglossal

Accessory

Occipital lobe

Cerebellum

Spinal cord

Spinal nerves

Conus medullaris

Cauda equina

Filum terminale

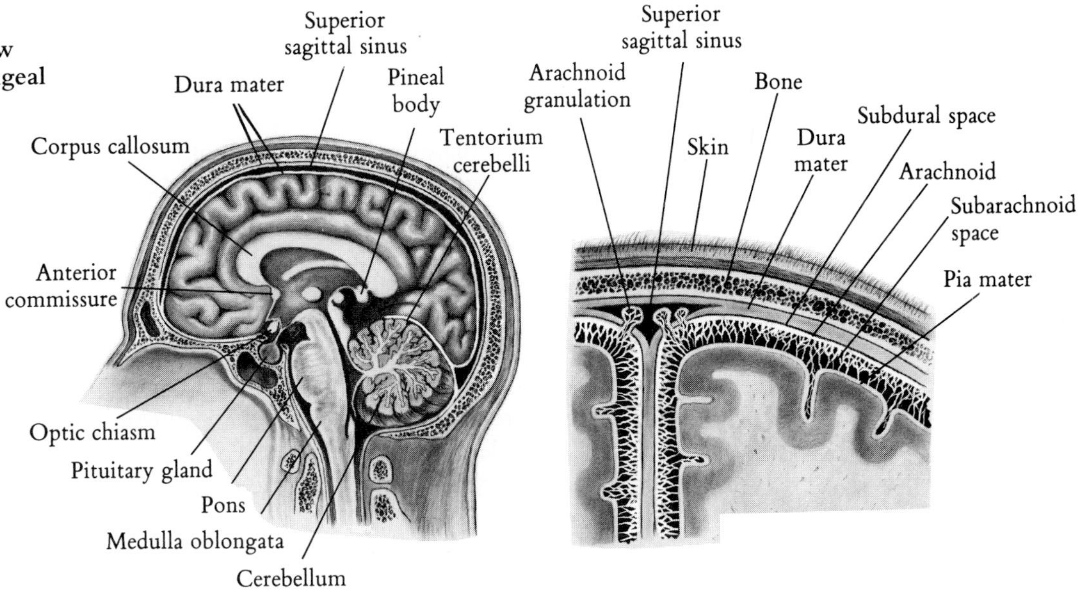

Fig. 17-2
Cross-sectional view of brain and meningeal layers.
From Rudy, 1984.

Corpus callosum · Dura mater · Superior sagittal sinus · Pineal body · Tentorium cerebelli · Anterior commissure · Optic chiasm · Pituitary gland · Pons · Medulla oblongata · Cerebellum · Superior sagittal sinus · Arachnoid granulation · Skin · Bone · Dura mater · Subdural space · Arachnoid · Subarachnoid space · Pia mater

Brain

The brain receives its blood supply from the two internal carotid arteries, two vertebral arteries, and the basilar artery (Fig. 17-3). Blood drains from the brain through venous sinuses that empty into the internal jugular veins. The three major units of the brain are the cerebrum, the cerebellum, and the brainstem.

Cerebrum

Two cerebral hemispheres, each divided into lobes, form the cerebrum. The gray outer layer, the cerebral cortex, houses the higher mental functions and is responsible for general movement, visceral functions, perception, behavior, and the integration of these functions. Commissural fibers interconnect the counterpart areas in each hemisphere, unifying its higher sensory and motor function (Fig. 17-4).

The *frontal lobe* contains the motor cortex associated with voluntary skeletal movement and speech formation (Broca's area). The association areas related to emotions, affect, drive, awareness of self, and the autonomic responses related to emotional states also originate here.

The *parietal lobe* is primarily responsible for processing sensory data as it is received. It assists with the interpretation of tactile sensations (temperature, pressure, pain, size, shape, texture, and two-point discrimination), as well as visual, gustatory, olfactory, and auditory sensations. Comprehension of written words, recognition of body parts, and awareness of body position (proprioception) are dependent on the parietal lobe.

The *occipital lobe* contains the primary vision center and provides interpretation of visual data.

The *temporal lobe* is responsible for the perception and interpretation of sounds and determination of their source. It contains Wernicke's speech area, permitting comprehension of spoken and written language. It is also involved in the integration of taste, smell, and balance, as well as behavior, emotion, and personality.

The *limbic system* mediates certain patterns of behavior that determine survival, such as mating, aggression, fear, and affection. Memory functions depend on the limbic system, particularly short-term memory and the ability to store and retrieve information. Interference with the physiology of the limbic system results in distorted perception and inappropriate behavior.

Cerebellum

The cerebellum aids the motor cortex of the cerebrum in the integration of voluntary movement. It processes sensory information from the eyes, ears, touch receptors, and musculoskeleton. Integrated with the vestibular system, the cerebellum utilizes the sensory data to control muscle tone, equilibrium, and posture.

Brainstem

The brainstem is the pathway between the cerebral cortex and the spinal cord, and it controls many involuntary functions. Its structures include the medulla oblongata, pons, midbrain, and diencephalon. The nuclei of the 12 cranial nerves arise from these structures (Fig. 17-5 and Table 17-1).

Fig. 17-3
Arterial blood supply to the brain.
From Rudy, 1984.

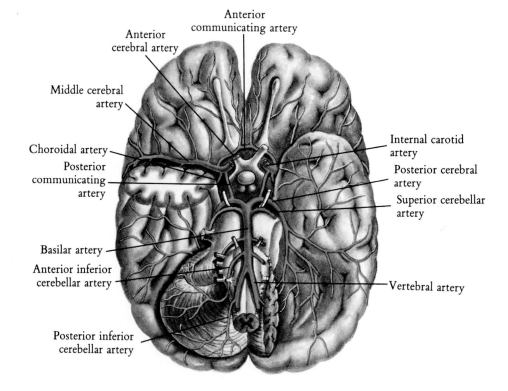

Fig. 17-4
A, Lobes and principle fissures of cerebral cortex, cerebellum, and brainstem.
B, Functional subdivisions of the cerebral cortex.

From Rudy, 1984.

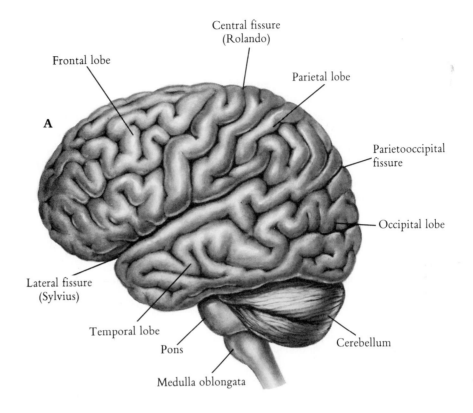

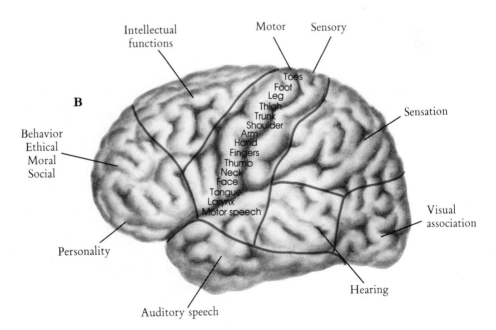

Table 17-1
Structures of the Brainstem and Their Functions, Including the Origin of Cranial Nerve (CN) Nuclei

Structure	*Function*
Medulla Oblongata CN IX–XII	Respiratory, circulatory, and vasomotor activities; houses respiratory center
	Reflexes of swallowing, coughing, vomiting, sneezing, and hiccupping
	Relay center for major ascending and descending spinal tracts that decussate at the pyramid
Pons CN V–VIII	Reflexes of pupillary action and eye movement
	Regulates respiration, houses a portion of the respiratory center
	Controls voluntary muscle action with corticospinal tract pathway
Midbrain CN III–IV	Reflex center for eye and head movement
	Auditory relay pathway
	Corticospinal tract pathway
Diencephalon CN I–II	Relays impulses between cerebrum, cerebellum, pons, and medulla (Fig. 17–5)
Thalamus	Conveys all sensory impulses (except olfaction) to and from cerebrum before their distribution to appropriate associative sensory areas
	Integrates impulses between motor cortex and cerebrum, influencing voluntary movements and motor response
	Controls state of consciousness, conscious perceptions of sensations, and abstract feelings
Epithalamus	Houses the pineal body
	Sexual development and behavior
Hypothalamus	Major processing center of internal stimuli for autonomic nervous system
	Maintains temperature control, water metabolism, body fluid osmolarity, feeding behavior, and neuroendocrine activity
Pituitary gland	Hormonal control of growth, lactation, vasoconstriction, and metabolism

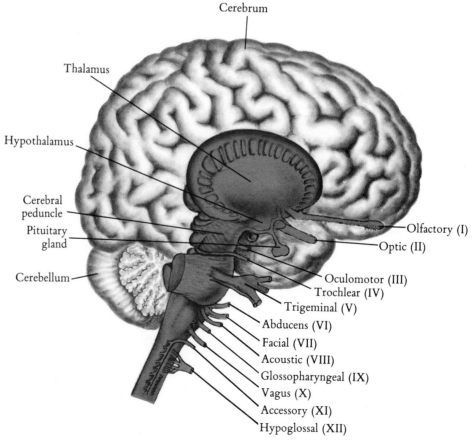

Fig. 17-5
Structures of the diencephalon and location of the cranial nerve roots.

From Rudy, 1984.

Cerebrum

Thalamus

Hypothalamus

Cerebral peduncle

Pituitary gland

Cerebellum

Olfactory (I)

Optic (II)

Oculomotor (III)

Trochlear (IV)

Trigeminal (V)

Abducens (VI)

Facial (VII)

Acoustic (VIII)

Glossopharyngeal (IX)

Vagus (X)

Accessory (XI)

Hypoglossal (XII)

Cranial Nerves

Cranial nerves are peripheral nerves that arise from the brain rather than the spinal cord. Each nerve has motor or sensory functions, and four cranial nerves have parasympathetic functions (Table 17-2).

Basal Ganglia

The basal ganglia function as the pathway and processing station between the cerebral motor cortex and the upper brainstem. They contribute input from visual, labyrinthine, and proprioceptive sources that allow gross intentional movement without conscious thought.

Table 17-2
The Cranial Nerves and Their Function

Cranial Nerves	Function
Olfactory (I)	Sensory: smell reception and interpretation
Optic (II)	Sensory: visual acuity and visual fields
Oculomotor (III)	Motor: pupillary constriction, change lens shape, raise eyelids, most extraocular movements
Trochlear (IV)	Motor: downward, inward eye movement
Trigeminal (V)	Motor: jaw opening and clenching, chewing and mastication Sensory: sensation to cornea, iris, lacrimal glands, conjunctiva, eyelids, forehead, nose, nasal and mouth mucosa, teeth, tongue, ear, facial skin
Abducens (VI)	Motor: lateral eye movement
Facial (VII)	Motor: movement of facial expression muscles except jaw, close eyes, labial speech sounds (b, m, w, and rounded vowels) Sensory: taste, anterior two thirds of tongue, sensation to pharynx Parasympathetic: secretion of saliva and tears
Acoustic (VIII)	Sensory: hearing and equilibrium
Glossopharyngeal (IX)	Motor: voluntary muscles for swallowing and phonation Sensory: sensation of nasopharynx, gag reflex, taste posterior one third of tongue Parasympathetic: secretion of salivary glands, carotid reflex
Vagus (X)	Motor: voluntary muscles of phonation (gutteral speech sounds) and swallowing Sensory: sensation behind ear and part of external ear canal Parasympathetic: secretion of digestive enzymes, peristalsis, carotid reflex, involuntary action of heart, lungs, and digestive tract
Spinal accessory (XI)	Motor: turn head, shrug shoulders, some actions for phonation and swallowing
Hypoglossal (XII)	Motor: tongue movement for speech sound articulation (l, t, n) and swallowing

Adapted from Rudy, 1984.

Spinal Cord

The spinal cord begins at the foramen magnum and is a continuation of the medulla oblongata, terminating at L1 to L2 of the vertebral column. Fibers, grouped into tracts, run through the spinal cord carrying sensory, motor, and autonomic impulses between higher centers in the brain and the body. The myelin-coated, white matter of the spinal cord contains the ascending and descending tracts (Fig. 17-6). The gray matter, which contains the nerve cell bodies, is arranged in a butterfly shape with anterior and posterior horns.

The descending spinal tracts originate in the brain and convey impulses to various muscle groups with inhibitory or facilitory actions. They also have a role in the control of muscle tone and posture. The pyramidal tract is the great motor pathway that carries impulses for voluntary movement, especially those requiring skill.

The ascending spinal tracts mediate various sensations. They facilitate the sensory signals necessary for complex discrimination tasks and are capable of transmitting precise information about the type of stimulus and its location. The posterior (dorsal) column spinal tract carries the fibers for the discriminatory sensations of touch, deep pressure, vibration, position of the joints, stereognosis, and two-point discrimination. The spinothalamic tracts carry the fibers for the sensations of light and crude touch, pressure, temperature, and pain.

Fig. 17-6
Pathway of spinal tracts from spinal cord to motor cortex. Note decussation of the pyramids at the level of the medulla.
From Rudy, 1984.

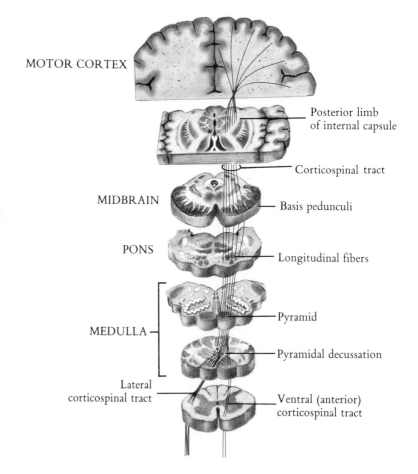

MOTOR CORTEX

Posterior limb of internal capsule

Corticospinal tract

MIDBRAIN

Basis pedunculi

PONS

Longitudinal fibers

Pyramid

MEDULLA

Pyramidal decussation

Lateral corticospinal tract

Ventral (anterior) corticospinal tract

Upper motor neurons, all originating and terminating within the central nervous system, make up the descending pathways from the brain to the spinal cord. The lower motor neurons originate in the anterior horn of the spinal cord and terminate in the muscle fibers.

Spinal Nerves

Thirty-one pairs of spinal nerves arise from the spinal cord and exit at each intervertebral foramen (Fig. 17-7). The sensory and motor fibers of each spinal nerve supply and receive information in a specific body distribution called a dermatome (Fig. 17-8). The anterior branches of several spinal nerves combine to form nerve plexi, so that a spinal nerve may lose its individuality to some extent. The spinal nerve may also complement the effort of an anatomically related nerve or even help compensate for some loss of function. A multitude of peripheral nerves originate from these nerve plexi (Fig. 17-9).

Text continued on p. 588.

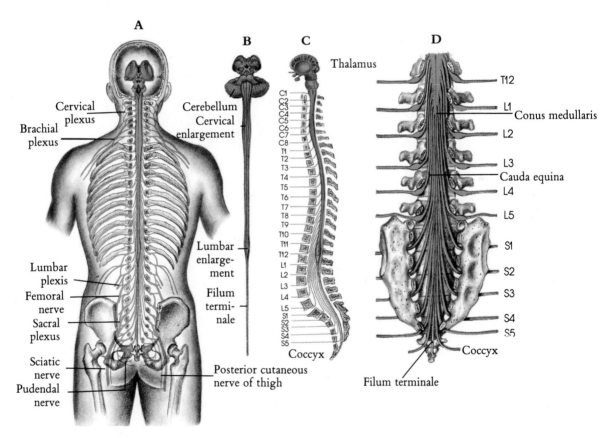

Fig. 17-7
Location of exiting spinal nerves in relation to the vertebrae. **A,** Posterior view. **B,** Anterior view of brainstem and spinal cord. **C,** Lateral view showing relationship of spinal cord to vertebrae and, **D,** enlargement of caudal area with group of nerve fibers composing the cauda equina.
From Rudy, 1984.

ANTERIOR VIEW

Fig. 17-8
Dermatomes of the body, the area of body surface innervated by particular spinal nerves; C1 usually has no cutaneous distribution. **A,** Anterior view.

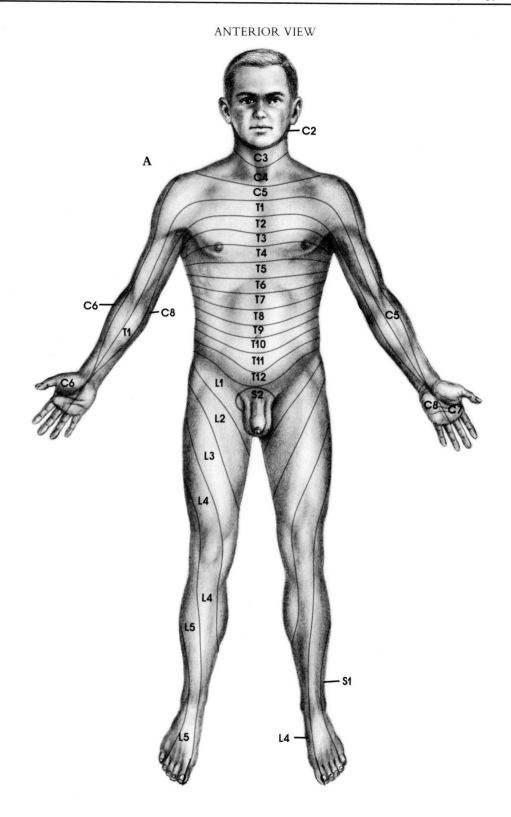

POSTERIOR VIEW

Fig. 17-8, cont'd
B, Posterior view. It appears that there is a distinct separation of surface area controlled by each dermatome, but there is almost always overlap between spinal nerves.

From Rudy, 1984.

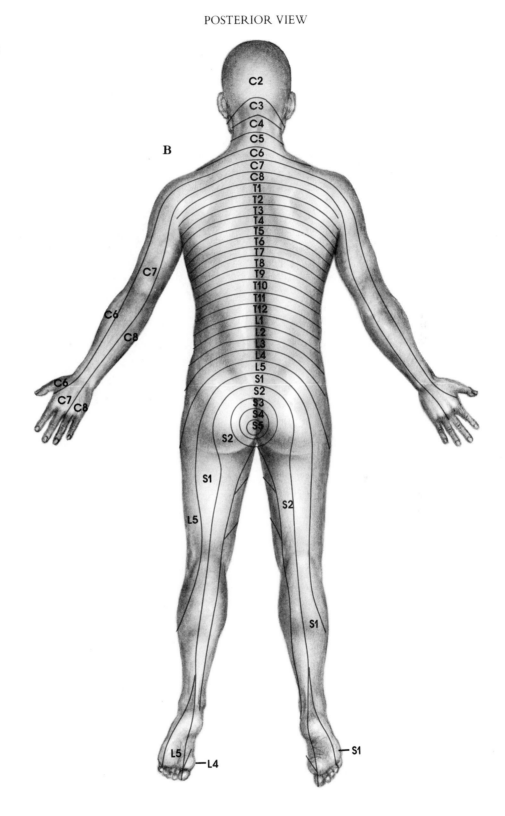

Fig. 17-9
Area of sensory innervation by certain peripheral nerves. A, Anterior view. B, Posterior view.
From Rudy, 1984.

ANTERIOR VIEW

A

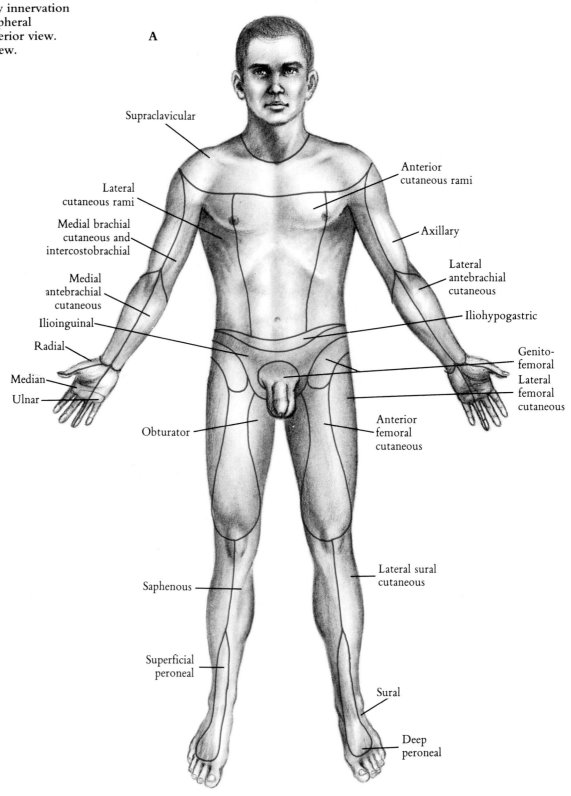

Supraclavicular

Anterior cutaneous rami

Lateral cutaneous rami

Medial brachial cutaneous and intercostobrachial

Axillary

Lateral antebrachial cutaneous

Medial antebrachial cutaneous

Ilioinguinal

Iliohypogastric

Radial

Median

Genito-femoral

Ulnar

Lateral femoral cutaneous

Obturator

Anterior femoral cutaneous

Saphenous

Lateral sural cutaneous

Superficial peroneal

Sural

Deep peroneal

POSTERIOR VIEW

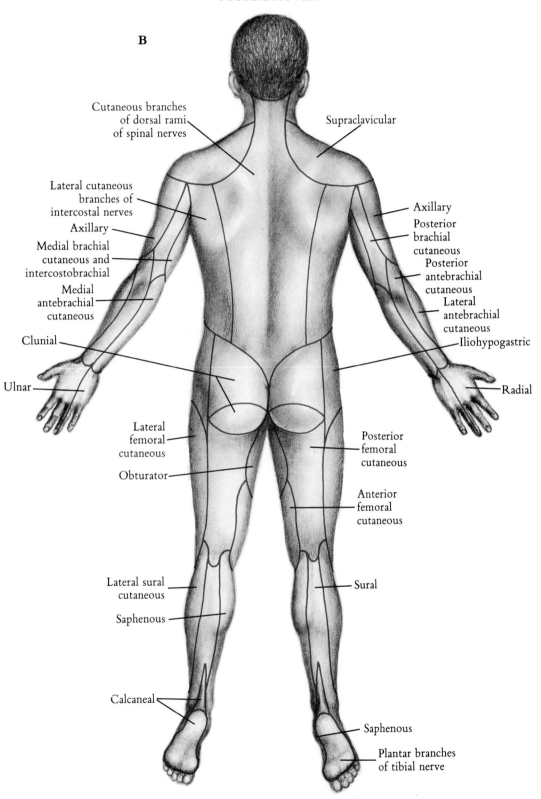

B

Cutaneous branches
of dorsal rami
of spinal nerves

Supraclavicular

Lateral cutaneous
branches of
intercostal nerves

Axillary

Medial brachial
cutaneous and
intercostobrachial

Medial
antebrachial
cutaneous

Clunial

Ulnar

Axillary
Posterior
brachial
cutaneous
Posterior
antebrachial
cutaneous
Lateral
antebrachial
cutaneous
Iliohypogastric

Radial

Lateral
femoral
cutaneous

Obturator

Posterior
femoral
cutaneous

Anterior
femoral
cutaneous

Lateral sural
cutaneous

Saphenous

Sural

Calcaneal

Saphenous

Plantar branches
of tibial nerve

Fig. 17-10
Cross-section of the spinal cord showing a simple reflex arc.
From Rudy, 1984.

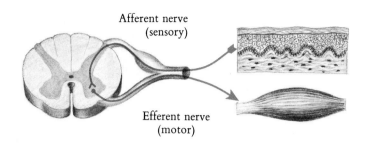

Afferent nerve
(sensory)

Efferent nerve
(motor)

Within the spinal cord, each spinal nerve separates into ventral and dorsal roots. The motor fibers of the ventral root carry impulses from the spinal cord to the muscles and glands of the body. The sensory fibers of the dorsal root carry impulses from sensory receptors of the body to the spinal cord. From here the impulses travel to the brain for interpretation by the cerebral sensory cortex. The impulse may alternatively initiate a reflex action when it synapses immediately with the motor fiber after a stimulus such as a tap on a stretched muscle tendon. In this case, the impulse is transmitted outward by the motor neuron in the anterior horn of the spinal cord via the spinal nerve and peripheral nerve of the skeletal muscle, stimulating a brisk contraction (Fig. 17-10). Such a reflex is dependent upon intact afferent nerve fibers, functional synapses in the spinal cord, intact motor nerve fibers, functional neuromuscular junctions, and competent muscle fibers.

INFANTS AND CHILDREN

The major portion of brain growth occurs in the first year of life, along with myelinization of the brain and nervous system. Any intruding event (infection, biochemical imbalance, or trauma) that upsets brain development and growth during this period can have profound effects on eventual brain function.

The following primitive reflexes are present in the newborn: yawn, sneeze, hiccup, blink at bright light and loud sound, pupillary constriction with light, and withdrawal from painful stimuli. As the brain develops, some primitive reflexes are inhibited when more advanced cortical functions and voluntary control take over.

Motor maturation proceeds in a cephalocaudal direction. Motor control of the head and neck develops first, followed by the trunk and extremities. Motor development is a succession of integrated milestones, each leading to more complex and independent function. There is an orderly sequence to development, but considerable variation in timing exists in children. Many capabilities may be developing simultaneously in any one child.

OLDER ADULTS

The changes that occur with aging are more physiologic than anatomic. The number of brain cells is thought to decrease by 1% a year beginning at 50 years of age. However, the vast number of reserve cells inhibits the appearance of clinical signs. The velocity of nerve impulse conduction declines 10% between 30 and 90 years of age, so responses to various stimuli take longer. Sensory perceptions of touch and pain stimuli may also be diminished.

No decline in general intelligence is evident unless a systemic or neurologic disorder develops. Problem solving skills may decline, probably from disuse, but vocabulary skills and inventories of available information do not significantly change. Remote memory may be more efficient than recent memory, but that may be a function of the individual's overall health.

Review of Related History

**General
Considerations**

1. Environmental or occupational hazards: exposure to lead, arsenic, insecticides, organic solvents, other chemicals; operates dangerous equipment; works at heights or in water
2. Emotional status: feelings about self, ability to cope with current stressors in life, level of stress, goals, frustrations, attitudes, relationship with family members
3. Intellectual level: educational history, any cognitive changes, communication pattern (understands questions, speech is coherent and appropriate), change in memory or thought processes, access to information
4. Use of alcohol or mood-altering drugs
5. Hand, eye, and foot dominance; family patterns of dexterity and dominance
6. Chronic illness: neurologic, cardiovascular, or respiratory disorder; epilepsy
7. Acute infection or trauma
8. Medications: anticonvulsants, antidepressants, tranquilizers, antivertigos, antitremor drugs

Present Problem

Seizures or Convulsions

1. Sequence of events (get independent observer's report): aura, fall to ground, shrill cry, motor activity (where spasm began and moved through the body, unilateral or bilateral), transition phase (change in character of motor activity), change in color of face or lips, pupil changes or eye deviations, loss of consciousness, incontinence, postictal phase, total length of seizure activity and postictal phase
2. Character of symptoms
   a. Aura: irritability, tension, confusion, blurred vision, mood changes, focal motor seizure activity, gastrointestinal distress
   b. Level of consciousness: loss, impairment, absence; duration
   c. Automatisms: eyelid fluttering, chewing, lip smacking, swallowing
   d. Muscle tone: flaccid, stiff, tense, twitching
   e. Postictal behavior: weakness, paralysis, confusion, drowsiness, headaches, muscle aching, time sleeping after seizure; lateralizing quality of these signs
3. Relationship to time of day, meals, fatigue, emotional stress, excitement, menses, discontinuing medication; activity before attack, frequency of occurrence

Pain

1. Quality and intensity: deep or superficial; aching, boring, throbbing, sharp or stabbing, burning, pressing, stinging, cramping, gnawing, prickling, shooting; radiating from one part to another or occuring simultaneously in all parts of a limb; duration and constancy; efforts to treat
2. Location or path: occur along expected distribution of a peripheral nerve
3. Associated manifestations: crying, decreased activities, sweating, muscle rigidity, tremor, impaired mental processes or concentration
4. Headache: see Chapter 5 (Head and Neck)

Gait Coordination

1. Balance: sensation of listing when walking to doorway
2. Falling: fall one way, backward, forwards, consistent direction; associated with looking high up; ataxia; legs just give way

Vertigo, Dizziness, Loss of Balance

1. Onset: sudden or gradual; any warnings; occurrence with exertion
2. Sensation: room spinning around (objective vertigo) or patient is spinning (subjective vertigo), nausea or vomiting, faintness, giddiness, lightheadedness, tinnitus
3. Associated symptoms: loss of consciousness, numbness or tingling of extremities, mood or mental changes occurring with position change (standing, moving head, looking high up), falling, facial expression change, vision changes, chest pain

Weakness or Numbness

1. Onset: with onset of or after activity, time before symptoms begin
2. Character: generalized or specific body area affected; occurs with onset of activity or after sustained activity
3. Associated symptoms: tingling, limb feels encased in tight bandage, pain, shortness of breath, stiffness of joints, spasms, muscle tension

Swallowing Difficulty

1. Excessive saliva, drooling
2. Problems with solids or liquids

Past Medical History

1. Trauma: head injury, spinal cord injury, localized injury, central nervous system insult, birth trauma, cerebrovascular accident
2. Meningitis, encephalitis, plumbism
3. Deformities, congenital anomalies
4. Cardiovascular, circulatory problem: hypertension, aneurysm
5. Neurologic disorder
6. Psychiatric counseling

Family History

1. Hereditary disorders: neurofibromatosis, Huntington's chorea, muscular dystrophy, Tay-Sach's disease
2. Psychiatric disorders, mental illness, alcoholism
3. Mental retardation
4. Epilepsy or seizure disorder, headaches
5. Alzheimer's disease
6. Learning disorders
7. Weakness or gait disorders
8. Medical or metabolic disorder: thyroid disease, hypertension, diabetes mellitus

INFANTS

1. Prenatal history: mother's health, medications taken, infections, exposure to TORCH viruses, feelings of well being, toxemia, bleeding, history of trauma or stress, persistent vomiting, hypertension, drug or alcohol use
2. Birth history: Apgar score, gestational age, birth weight, presentation, use of instruments, prolonged or precipitate labor, fetal distress
3. Respiratory status at birth: breathed immediately, need for oxygen, continuous apnea, cyanosis, resuscitative efforts, need for ventilator
4. Neonatal health: jaundice (from blood type incompatibility or breast feeding), infections, seizures, irritability, sucking and swallowing poorly coordinated
5. Congenital anomalies, multiple handicapping conditions

CHILDREN

1. Developmental milestones
   a. Age attained: smiling, head control in prone position, grasping, transferring, sitting, crawling, independent walking, toilet trained, similar pattern in siblings
   b. Loss of previously achieved function: change in the child's rate of development; progress occurred as expected until _____ age with slow progress after that; or has always been slow to do things
2. Speech and language: first words, intelligibility, quality of sounds, progression to phrases and sentences
3. Behavior: temper tantrums, breath-holding, hyperactivity, limited attention span, ability to separate from family and adjust to new situations
4. Performance of self-care activities: dressing, toileting, feeding
5. Health problems
   a. Headaches, unexplained vomiting, lethargy, personality changes
   b. Seizure activity: association with fever, frequency, duration, character of movement
   c. Any clumsiness, unsteady gait, progressive muscular weakness, or unexplained falling, problems going up and down stairs, getting up after lying down on floor
6. Personality and behavior patterns: changes related to any specific event, fever of unknown origin, trauma
7. Learning or school difficulties: associated with attention, interest, activity level, or ability to concentrate

OLDER ADULTS

1. Pattern of increased stumbling, falls, or decreased agility; safety modifications in home
2. Interference with performance of daily living tasks, social withdrawal, feelings about symptoms
3. Hearing loss, vision deficit, or anosmia
4. Changes in mental functions: cognitive, thought process, memory, sudden or gradual confusion
5. Development of tremor: exacerbated by anxiety, relieved by alcohol

Examination and Findings

EQUIPMENT

- Penlight
- Tongue blade
- Sterile needles
- Tuning forks, 200 to 400 Hz and 500 to 1000 Hz
- Familiar objects—coins, keys, paper clip
- Cotton wisp
- Reflex hammer
- Vials of aromatic substances—coffee, orange, ammonia, peppermint extract, oil of cloves
- Vials of solutions—glucose, salt, lemon or vinegar, and quinine—with applicators
- Test tubes of hot and cold water
- Denver Developmental Screening Test (for infants and children)

The neurologic system can be examined almost constantly while the rest of the body is explored. In fact, when the patient enters the room and you offer some suggestion as to where he or she might sit, the patient's response tells you a good deal about the functioning of the neurologic system. Assessment of mental state is implicit in taking a routine history, and your observation throughout the history and physical examination makes reasonably complete many aspects of the neurologic examination. By the time you begin to examine the neurologic status specifically, you should already be armed with clues on the system's state of health.

Because the neurologic examination is complex, the discussion is divided into five sections to give you an organizational approach. These sections include: mental status and speech patterns, cranial nerves, proprioception and cerebellar function, sensory function, and reflex function. Evaluation of muscle tone and strength, an integral part of the neurologic examination, is detailed in Chapter 16, Musculoskeletal System.

Mental Status and Speech Patterns

Mental status (cerebral function) is assessed throughout the physical examination by evaluating the patient's awareness, orientation, cognitive abilities, and affect. Observe the patient's physical appearance, behavior, and responses to questions asked during the history. Note any variations in response to questions of differing complexity. Speech should be clearly articulated. Questions should be answered appropriately with ideas expressed logically, relating current and past events.

The detailed examination listed below is rarely used in its entirety. The "Mini-Mental State," a standardized tool, may be used to quantitatively estimate cognitive function or to serially document cognitive changes. The more extensive examination should be conducted when problems are detected in an effort to relate disturbances to anatomic structures (Fig. 17-11).

Physical Appearance and Behavior

Grooming. Poor hygiene, lack of concern with appearance, or inappropriateness of dress for season, gender, and occasion in a previously well-groomed individual may indicate an emotional problem, psychiatric disturbance, or organic brain syndrome.

Fig. 17-11

"Mini-mental state" test, a standardized screening tool of mental status. A score greater than 20 is acceptable. A score of 20 or less is found in patients with dementia, delirium, schizophrenia, or an affective disorder.

Reprinted with permission from Journal of Psychiatric Research, vol. 12, Folstein et al.: "Mini-mental state": a practical method for grading the cognitive state of patients for the clinician. Copyright 1975. Pergamon Press, Ltd.

Patient.....................................
Examiner................................
Date ....

"MINI-MENTAL STATE"

Maximum Score	Score	

ORIENTATION

| 5 | ( ) | What is the (year) (season) (date) (day) (month)? |
| 5 | ( ) | Where are we: (state) (county) (town) (hospital) (floor). |

REGISTRATION

| 3 | ( ) | Name 3 objects: 1 second to say each. Then ask the patient all 3 after you have said them. Give 1 point for each correct answer. Then repeat them until he learns all 3. Count trials and record. |

Trials

ATTENTION AND CALCULATION

| 5 | ( ) | Serial 7's. 1 point for each correct. Stop after 5 answers. Alternatively spell "world" backwards. |

RECALL

| 3 | ( ) | Ask for the 3 objects repeated above. Give 1 point for each correct. |

LANGUAGE

| 9 | ( ) | Name a pencil, and watch (2 points) |

Repeat the following "No ifs, ands or buts." (1 point)

Follow a 3-stage command:

"Take a paper in your right hand, fold it in half, and put in on the floor" (3 points)

Read and obey the following:

CLOSE YOUR EYES (1 point)

Write a sentence (1 point)

Copy design (1 point)

_____ Total score

ASSESS level of consciousness along a continuum _____

Alert   Drowsy   Stupor   Coma

INSTRUCTIONS FOR ADMINISTRATION OF MINI-MENTAL STATE EXAMINATION

ORIENTATION

(1) Ask for the date. Then ask specifically for parts omitted, e.g., "Can you also tell me what season it is?" One point for each correct.

(2) Ask in turn "Can you tell me the name of this hospital?" (town, county, etc.). One point for each correct.

REGISTRATION

Ask the patient if you may test his memory. Then say the name of 3 unrelated objects, clearly and slowly, about one second for each. After you have said 3, ask him to repeat them. The first repetition determines his score (0-3) but keep saying them until he can repeat all 3, up to 6 trials. If he does not eventually learn all 3, recall cannot be meaningfully tested.

ATTENTION AND CALCULATION

Ask the patient to begin with 100 and count backwards by 7. Stop after 5 subtractions (93,86,79,72,65). Score the total number of correct answers.

If the patient cannot or will not perform this task, ask him to spell the word "world" backwards. The score is the number of letters in correct order. E.g. dlrow = 5, dlorw = 3.

RECALL

Ask the patient if he can recall the 3 words you previously asked him to remember. Score 0-3.

LANGUAGE

Naming: Show the patient a wrist watch and ask him what it is. Repeat for pencil. Score 0-2.

Repetition: Ask the patient to repeat the sentence after you. Allow only one trial. Score 0 or 1.

3-Stage command: Give the patient a piece of plain blank paper and repeat the command. Score 1 point for each part correctly executed.

Reading: On a blank piece of paper print the sentence "Close your eyes", in letters large enough for the patient to see clearly. Ask him to read it and do what it says. Score 1 point only if he actually closes his eyes.

Writing: Give the patient a blank piece of paper and ask him to write a sentence for you. Do not dictate a sentence, it is to be written spontaneously. It must contain a subject and verb to be sensible. Correct grammer and puncuation are not necessary.

Copying: On a clean piece of paper, draw intersecting pentagons, each side about 1 in., and ask him to copy it exactly as it is. All 10 angles must be present and 2 must intersect to score 1 point. Tremor and rotation are ignored.

Estimate the patient's level of sensorium along a continuum, from alert on the left to coma on the right.

Emotional Status. The patient should behave in a manner expressing appropriate concern with the visit. Note behavior that conveys carelessness, indifference, inability to sense emotions in others, loss of sympathetic reactions, unusual docility, rage reactions, or excessive irritability.

Body Language. Posture should be erect and the patient should make eye contact with you. Slumped posture and a lack of facial expression may indicate depression. Excessively energetic movements or constantly watchful eyes suggests tension, anxiety, or a metabolic disorder.

Cognitive Abilities

Cognitive functions are evaluated while the patient responds to your questions during history. Specific questions and specific tasks can provide detailed assessment of cognition.

State of Consciousness. The patient should be oriented to time, place, and person and be able to appropriately respond to questions and environmental stimuli. Time disorientation is associated with anxiety, depression, and organic brain syndrome. Place disorientation occurs with psychiatric disorders and organic brain syndromes. Person disorientation results from cerebral trauma, seizures, or amnesia.

Analogies. Ask the patient to describe simple analogies and then those more complex:

- What is similar about these objects: peaches and lemons; ocean and lake; pencil and typewriter?
- Complete this comparison: An engine is to an airplane as an oar is to a _____.
- What is different about these two objects: a magazine and a telephone book; a bush and a tree?

UNEXPECTED LEVELS OF CONSCIOUSNESS

Confusion	Inappropriate response to question
	Decreased attention span and memory
Lethargy	Drowsy, falls asleep quickly
	Once aroused, responds appropriately
Delirium	Confusion with disordered perceptions and decreased attention span
	Marked anxiety with motor and sensory excitement
	Inappropriate reactions to stimuli
Coma	Lowering of consciousness in stages
Stupor	Arousable for short periods to visual, verbal, or painful stimuli; simple motor or moaning responses to stimuli; slow responses
Light Coma	Simple motor or moaning response to painful stimuli
Deep Coma	Decerebrate posturing to painful stimuli

Adapted from Malasanos et al., 1986.

An adequate description should be given when the patient has average intelligence. An inability to describe similarities or differences may indicate a lesion of the left cerebral hemisphere.

Abstract Reasoning. Ask the patient to tell you the meaning of a fable, proverb, or metaphor, for example:
- A stitch in time saves nine.
- A bird in a hand is worth two in a bush.
- A rolling stone gathers no moss.

An adequate interpretation of the phrase should be given when the patient has average intelligence. An inability to give adequate explanation may indicate organic brain syndrome, brain damage, or lack of intelligence.

Arithmetic Calculations. Ask the patient to do simple arithmetic without paper and pencil.
- Subtract 7 from 50 and 7 from that answer, and so on until the answer is less than 10.
- Add 8 to 50, and 8 to that total, and so on, until the answer is near 100.

The calculations should be completed with few errors within a minute when the patient has average intelligence. Impairment of arithmetic skills is associated with depression and diffuse brain disease.

Writing Ability. The patient should write his or her name and address, or you can dictate a phrase. Omission or addition of letters, syllables, words, or mirror writing may indicate aphasia. If the patient cannot write, ask him or her to draw simple geometric figures (triangle, circle, square) and then figures such as a house or flower. Uncoordinated writing or drawing may indicate a cerebellar lesion or peripheral neuropathy.

Execution of Motor Skills. Ask the male patient to comb his hair or the female patient to put on her lipstick. Apraxia, an inability to complete a task unrelated to paralysis or lack of comprehension, may indicate a cerebral disorder.

Memory. Immediate recall is tested by asking the patient to listen and then repeat a sentence or series of numbers. Five to eight numbers forward or four to six number backwards can usually be repeated. Test recent memory by showing the patient three or four test objects, saying you will ask about them in a few minutes. Ten minutes later, ask the patient to list the objects. All objects should be remembered. Remote memory is tested by asking the patient about verifiable past events, such as his or her mother's maiden name, high school attended, or a subject of basic knowledge.

Impaired memory occurs in various neurologic or psychiatric disorders. Loss of immediate and recent memory with retention of remote memory suggests organic brain syndrome.

Attention Span. Ask the patient to follow a series of short commands or repeat a short story you relate. The patient should respond to directions appropriately. Easy distraction, confusion, negativism, and impairment of recent and remote memory may all indicate a decreased attention span. This may be related to fatigue, anxiety, or medication in an otherwise healthy patient.

Judgment. Determine the patient's reasoning skills by exploring these areas:
- How is the patient meeting social and family obligations?
- What are the patient's plans for the future? Do they seem appropriate?
- Have the patient provide solutions to hypothetical situations, such as: What would you do if you found a stamped envelope? If a policeman stopped you after driving through a red light?
- Explain fables or metaphors.

The patient should be able to evaluate the situation presented and provide an appropriate response. If the patient is meeting social and family obligations and adequately dealing with business affairs, judgment is considered intact. Impaired judgment may indicate mental retardation, emotional disturbance, or organic brain syndrome.

Emotional Stability

Emotional stability is evaluated when the patient does not seem to be coping well or does not have resources to meet his or her personal needs.

Mood and Feelings. Observe the mood and emotional expression from the patient's verbal and nonverbal behavior during the physical examination. Note any mood swings or behaviors indicating anxiety or depression.

Ask the patient how he or she feels right now, if feelings are a problem in daily life, and if there are times or experiences that are particularly difficult.

The patient should express appropriate feelings that correspond to the situation. Unresponsiveness, hopelessness, agitation, euphoria, irritability, or wide mood swings indicate disturbances in mood, affect, and feelings.

Thought Process and Content. During the examination, observe the patient's patterns of thinking, especially the appropriateness of sequence, logic, coherence, and relevance to the topics discussed. You should be able to follow the patient's thought processes, and the ideas expressed should be logical and goal directed.

Illogical or unrealistic thought processes, blocking (a pause in the middle of a thought, phrase, or sentence), or disturbance in the stream of thinking (repetition of a word, phrase, or behavior) indicate emotional disturbance or psychiatric disorder.

Disturbance in thought content is evaluated by asking the patient about obsessive thoughts related to making decisions, fears, or guilt. Does the patient ever feel like he or she is watched or followed, controlled or manipulated, or loses touch with reality? Does the patient compulsively repeat actions or check and recheck something to make sure it is done? Obsessive thought content or compulsive behavior that interferes with daily life or is disabling indicates mental dysfunction or psychiatric disorder.

Perceptual Distortions and Hallucinations. Determine if the patient perceives any sensations that are not caused by external stimuli (hears voices, sees vivid images or shadowy figures, smells offensive odors, feels worms crawling on skin).

Auditory and visual hallucinations are associated with psychiatric disorders, organic conditions, and psychedelic drug ingestion. Tactile hallucinations are most frequently associated with alcohol withdrawal.

Speech and Language Skills

Detailed evaluation of the patient's communication skills, both receptive and expressive, should be performed when the patient has difficulty communicating during the history. The patient's voice should have inflections, be clear and strong, and be able to increase in volume. Speech should be fluent and articulate, with clear expression of thoughts.

Voice Quality. Determine if there is any difficulty or discomfort in making laryngeal speech sounds. Dysphonia, a disorder of voice volume, quality, or pitch, suggests a problem with laryngeal innervation or disease of the larynx.

Articulation. Evaluate spontaneous speech for pronunciation, fluency, rhythm, and ease of expression. Abnormal articulation includes imperfect pronunciation of words, difficulty articulating a single speech sound, rapid-fire delivery, or speech with hesitancy, stuttering, repetitions, or slow utterances. Dysarthria, a defect in articulation, is associated with a motor deficit of the lips, tongue, palate, or pharynx. Cerebellar dysarthria, which is poorly coordinated, irregular speech with unnatural separation of syllables (scanning), is associated with multiple sclerosis.

Comprehension. The patient should follow simple instructions during the history and physical examination.

Coherence. The patient's intentions or perceptions should be clearly conveyed to you. Circumlocutions and perseveration (repetition of a word, phrase, or gesture) should not be present. Words or sentences that proceed in disorderly fashion (flight of ideas), jibberish, neologisms, echolalia, or utterances of unusual sounds are associated with psychiatric disorders.

Aphasia. Listen for an omission or addition of letters, syllables, and words or the misuse or transposition of words. Indications of aphasia include hesitations, omissions, inappropriate word substitutions, circumlocutions, creation of new words, and disturbance of rhythm of words in sequence. Aphasia can result from facial muscle or tongue weakness or neurologic damage to brain regions controlling speech and language.

Cranial Nerves

An evaluation of the cranial nerves is an integral part of the neurologic examination. Ordinarily, taste and smell are not evaluated unless a problem is suspected. Quite often patients will not recognize that they have lost hearing in some ranges, certain taste sensations, or some visual aspects. Thus when a sensory loss is suspected, it is necessary in testing the relevant cranial nerve to be compulsive about determining the extent of loss.

Examination of some cranial nerves are described in detail in other chapters. The optic (II), oculomotor (III), trochlear (IV), and abducens (VI) nerves are tested in Chapter 6 (Eyes), the acoustic nerve (VIII) in Chapter 7 (Ears, Nose, and Throat), and the spinal accessory nerve (XI) in Chapter 16 (Musculoskeletal System).

Cranial nerve function is expected to be intact, as described in Table 17-2 for each individual nerve. Unexpected findings indicate trauma or a lesion in the cerebral hemisphere or local injury to the nerve.

Olfactory (I)

Have available two or three vials of familiar aromatic odors. Use the least irritating aromatic substance first so that the patient's perception of weaker odors is not impaired. To make sure the patient's nasal passages are patent, you should alternately occlude each naris as the patient inspires and expires.

The patient's eyes should be closed and one naris occluded. As you hold an opened vial under the nose, the patient should take a deep inspiration for the odor to reach the upper nose and swirl around the olfactory mucosa (Fig. 17-12). Ask the patient to identify the odor. Repeat the process with the other naris occluded, using a different odor. Continue the process, comparing the patient's sensitivity and discriminatory ability from side to side, alternating the two or three odors. It is important to allow periods of rest between the offerings of different odors. Offering one odor after the other too quickly can confuse the olfactory sense.

The patient should be able to perceive an odor on each side, usually identifying it. Inflammation of the mucous membranes, allergic rhinitis, and excessive tobacco smoking may all interfere with the ability to distinguish odors. The sense of smell may diminish with age. Anosmia, loss of sense of smell or inability to discriminate odors, can be caused by trauma to the cribform plate or by an olfactory tract lesion.

Optic (II)

Visual acuity and visual fields are evaluated in Chapter 6, Eyes.

Oculomotor, Trochlear, and Abducens (III, IV, and VI)

Movement of the eyes through the six cardinal points of gaze, pupil size, shape, response to light and accommodation, and opening of the upper eyelids are all in Chapter 6, Eyes.

When assessing patients with severe, unremitting headaches, the experienced examiner evaluates movement of the eyes for the presence or absence of lateral gaze. The sixth cranial nerve is frequently one of the first functions to be lost in the presence of increased intracranial pressure.

Trigeminal (V)

Motor function is evaluated by observing the face for muscle atrophy, deviation of the jaw to one side, and fasciculations. Have the patient tightly clench the teeth as you palpate the muscles over the jaw evaluating tone (Fig. 17-13). Muscle tone over the face should be symmetric without fasciculations.

Three divisions of the nerve are evaluated for sharp, dull, and light touch sensation (Fig. 17-14). While the patient's eyes are closed, touch each side of the face at the scalp, cheek, and chin areas, alternately using the point and hub of the sterile

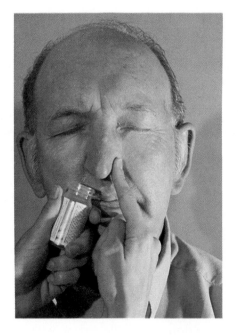

Fig. 17-12
Examination of the olfactory cranial nerve. Occlude one naris, hold the vial with aromatic odor under the nose, and ask the patient to deeply inspire. The patient should discriminate between odors.

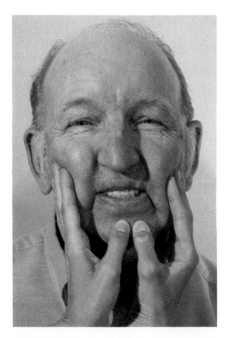

Fig. 17-13
Examination of the trigeminal cranial nerve for motor function. Have the patient tightly clench the teeth and palpate the muscles over the jaw for tone.

Fig. 17-14
Examination of the trigeminal cranial nerve for sensory function. Touch each side of the face at the scalp, cheek, and chin areas alternately, using no predictable pattern with,
A, the point and rounded edge of a paper clip and,
B, a brush. Ask the patient to discriminate between sensations.

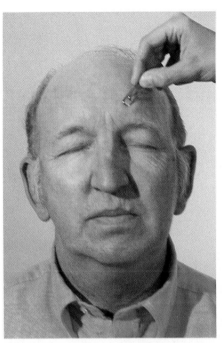

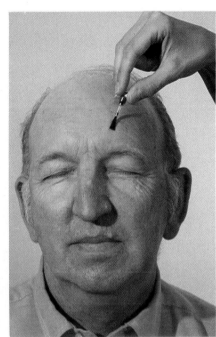

A

B

needle or a paper clip, making sure you use no predictable pattern. Ask the patient to report whether the sensation is sharp or dull. Then stroke the face in the same six areas with a cotton wisp or brush, asking the patient to tell when the stimulus is felt. A wooden applicator is used to test sensation over the buccal mucosa. There should be symmetric sensory discrimination over the face to all stimuli.

If sensation is impaired, use test tubes filled with hot and cold water to evaluate temperature sensation. Ask the patient to tell you if hot or cold is felt as you touch the same six areas of the face. Contrast the sensory discrimination with temperature to the other primary sensations.

To test the corneal reflex, have the patient look up and away from you, as you approach from the side. (Contact lenses, if used, should be removed.) Avoiding the eyelashes and the conjunctiva, lightly touch the cornea of one eye with a cotton wisp. Repeat the procedure on the other cornea. A symmetric blink reflex to corneal stimulation should occur. Patients who wear contact lenses may have diminished or absent reflex.

Facial (VII)

Motor function is evaluated by observing a series of expressions you ask the patient to make: raise the eyebrows, squeeze the eyes shut, wrinkle the forehead, frown, smile, show the teeth, purse the lips to whistle, and puff out the cheeks (Fig. 17-15). Observe for tics, unusual facial movements, and asymmetry of expression. Listen to the patient's speech and note any difficulties with enunciating labial sounds (*b, m,* and *p*). Muscle weakness is evidenced by one side of the mouth drooping, a flattened nasolabial fold, and lower eyelid sagging.

When evaluating taste, a sensory function of the cranial nerves VII and IX, have available the four solutions, applicators, and a card listing the tastes. Make sure the patient cannot see the labels on the vials. Ask the patient to keep the tongue protruded and to point out the taste perceived on the card. Apply one solution at a time

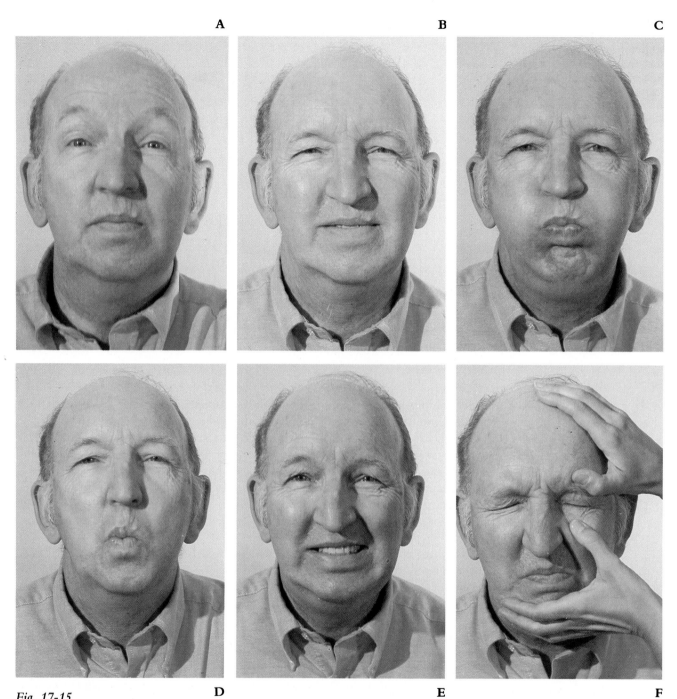

Fig. 17-15
Examination of the facial cranial nerve for motor function. Ask the patient to, **A,** wrinkle the forehead by raising the eyebrows; **B,** smile; **C,** puff out the cheeks; **D,** purse the lips and blow out; **E,** show the teeth; and **F,** squeeze the eyes shut.

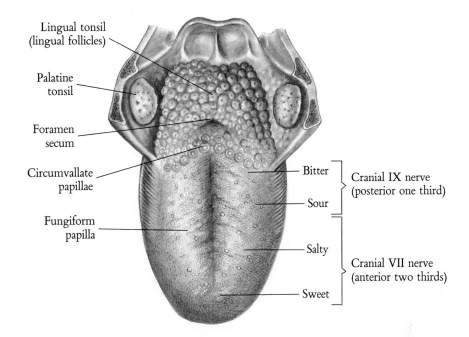

Fig. 17-16
Location of the taste bud regions tested for the sensory function of the facial and glossopharyngeal cranial nerves.

Lingual tonsil (lingual follicles)

Palatine tonsil

Foramen secum

Circumvallate papillae

Fungiform papilla

Bitter
Sour
} Cranial IX nerve (posterior one third)

Salty
Sweet
} Cranial VII nerve (anterior two thirds)

to the lateral side of the tongue in the appropriate tastebud region (Fig. 17-16). Alternate the solutions, using a different applicator for each. Offer a sip of water after each stimulus. Each solution is used on both sides of the tongue to identify taste discrimination. The patient should identify each taste bilaterally when placed correctly on the tongue surface.

Acoustic (VIII)

Hearing is evaluated with an audiometer or the simple screening tests described in Chapter 7 (Ears, Nose, and Throat). Vestibular function is not routinely tested.

Glossopharyngeal (IX)

The sensory function of taste over the posterior third of the tongue is tested during cranial nerve VII evaluation. The glossopharyngeal nerve is simultaneously tested during evaluation of the vagus nerve for nasopharyngeal sensation (gag reflex) and the motor function of swallowing.

Vagus (X)

To evaluate nasopharyngeal sensation, tell the patient you will be testing the gag reflex. Touch the posterior wall of the patient's pharynx with an applicator as you observe for upward movement of the palate and contraction of the pharyngeal muscles. The uvula should remain in the midline, and no drooping or absence of an arch on either side of the soft palate should be noted.

Motor function is evaluated by inspection of the soft palate for symmetry. Have the patient say "Ah," and observe the movement of the soft palate and uvula for asymmetry. If the vagus or glossopharyngeal nerve is damaged and the palate fails to rise, the uvula will deviate from the midline.

Have the patient sip and swallow water. This observation can be made while examining the thyroid. The patient should swallow easily, having no retrograde passage of water through the nose after the nasopharynx has closed off. Listen to the patient's speech, noting any hoarseness, nasal quality, or difficulty with guttural sounds.

Fig. 17-17
Examination of the hypoglossal cranial nerve.
A, Inspect the size, shape, symmetry, and fasciculations of the protruded tongue. **B,** Observe movement of the tongue from side to side.

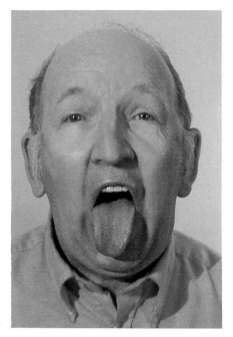
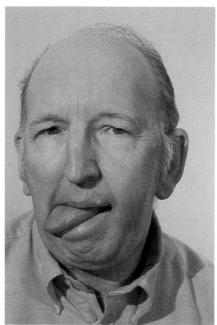

A   B

Spinal Accessory (XI)

The size, shape, and strength of the trapezius and sternocleidomastoid muscles are evaluated in Chapters 5 (Head and Neck) and 16 (Musculoskeletal System).

Hypoglossal (XII)

Inspect the patient's tongue while at rest on the floor of the mouth and while protruded from the mouth (Fig. 17-17). Note any fasciculations, asymmetry, atrophy, or deviation from the midline. Ask the patient to move the tongue in and out of the mouth, from side to side, curled upward as if to touch the nose, and curled downward as if to lick the chin. Test the tongue's muscle strength by asking the patient to push the tongue against the cheek as you apply resistance with an index finger. When listening to the patient's speech, no problems with lingual speech sounds *(l, t, d, n)* should be apparent.

Proprioception and Cerebellar Function

Coordination and Fine Motor Skills

Rapid Rhythmic Alternating Movements. Ask the seated patient to pat his or her knees with both hands, alternately turning up the palm and back of the hands, and increase the rate gradually (Fig. 17-18, *A* and *B*). As an alternate procedure, have the patient touch the thumb to each finger on the same hand, sequentially from the index finger to the little finger and back. Test one hand at a time, increasing speed gradually (Fig. 17-18, *B* and *C*).

Observe for stiff, slowed, nonrhythmic, or jerky clonic movements. The patient should smoothly execute these movements, maintaining rhythm with increasing speed.

Accuracy of Movements. The finger-to-finger test is performed with the patient's eyes open. Ask the patient to use the index finger and alternately touch his or her nose and your index finger (Fig. 17-19, *A* and *B*). Position your index finger about

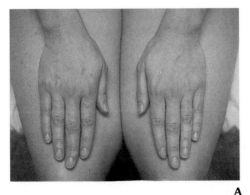
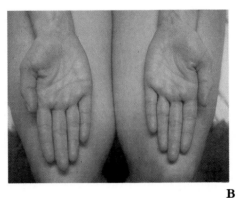
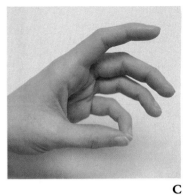

A   B   C

Fig. 17-18
Examination of coordination with rapid alternating movements. **A** and **B,** Pat the knees with both hands, alternately using the palm and back of the hand. **C,** Touch the thumb to each finger of the hand in sequence from index finger to small finger and back.

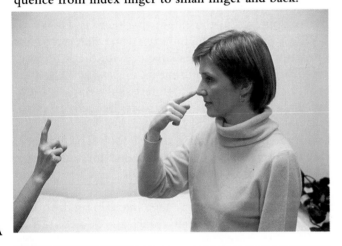
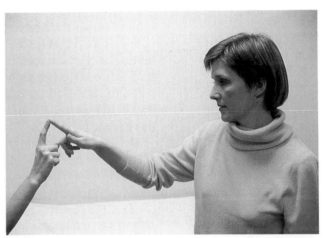

A   B

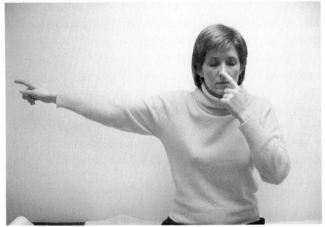
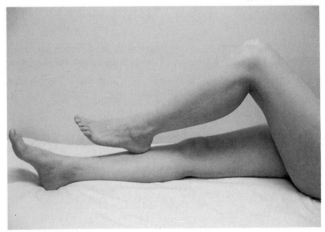

C   D

Fig. 17-19
Examination of fine motor function. The patient, **A** and **B,** alternately touches own nose and the examiner's index finger with the index finger of one hand; **C,** alternately touches own nose with the index finger of each hand; and **D,** runs the heel of one foot down the shin or tibia of the other leg.

18 in from the patient and change the location of your finger several times during the test. Repeat the procedure with the other hand. The movements should be rapid, smooth, and accurate.

To perform the finger-to-nose test, ask the patient to close the eyes and touch his or her nose with the index finger of each hand. Alternate the hands used and increase speed gradually (Fig. 17-19, C). Movement should be smooth, rapid, and accurate, even with increasing speed.

The heel-to-shin test is performed with the patient standing, sitting, or supine. Ask the patient to run the heel of one foot up and down the shin (from knee to ankle) of the opposite leg (Fig. 17-19, D). Repeat the procedure with the other heel. The patient should move the heel up and down the shin in a straight line, without irregular deviations to the side.

Balance

Equilibrium. Balance is initially evaluated with the Romberg test. Ask the patient (eyes open and then closed) to stand, feet together and arms at the sides (Fig. 17-20). Stand close, prepared to catch the patient if he or she starts to fall. Slight swaying movement of the body is expected, but not to the extent that there is danger of falling. Loss of balance, a positive Romberg sign, indicates cerebellar ataxia or vestibular dysfunction. If the patient staggers or loses balance with the Romberg test, postpone other tests of cerebellar function requiring balance.

To further evaluate balance, have the patient stand with feet slightly apart. Push the shoulders with enough effort to throw him or her off balance. Be ready to catch the patient if necessary. Recovery of balance should occur quickly.

Balance may also be tested with the patient standing on one foot. The patient's eyes should be closed with arms held straight at the sides. Repeat the test on the opposite foot. Balance on each foot should be maintained for 5 sec, but slight swaying is expected.

Have the patient (eyes open) hop in place first on one foot and then on the other (Fig. 17-21). Note any instability, a need to continually touch the floor with the opposite foot, or a tendency to fall. The patient should hop on each foot for 5 sec without loss of balance.

Gait. Observe the barefooted patient walk around the examining room or down a hallway, first with the eyes open and then closed. Observe the expected gait sequence, noting simultaneous arm movements (Fig. 17-22):

1. The first heel strikes the floor and then moves to full contact with the floor.
2. The second heel pushes off, leaving the ground.
3. Body weight is transferred from the first heel to the ball of its foot.
4. The leg swing is accelerated as weight is removed from the second foot.
5. The second foot is lifted and travels ahead of the weight-bearing first foot, swinging through.
6. The second foot slows in preparation for heel strike.

Note any shuffling, widely placed feet, toe walking, foot flop, leg lag, scissoring, loss of arm swing, staggering, or reeling. The patient should continuously sequence both stance and swing, step after step. The gait should have a smooth, regular rhythm and symmetric stride length. The trunk posture should sway with the gait phase, and arm swing should be smooth and symmetric. Fig. 17-23 and Table 17-3 describe unexpected gait patterns.

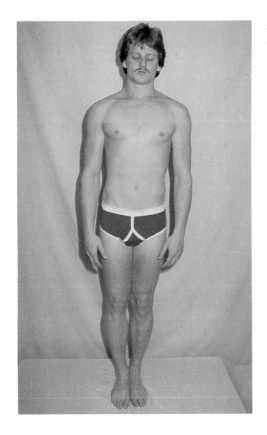

Fig. 17-20
Evaluating balance with
the Romberg test.

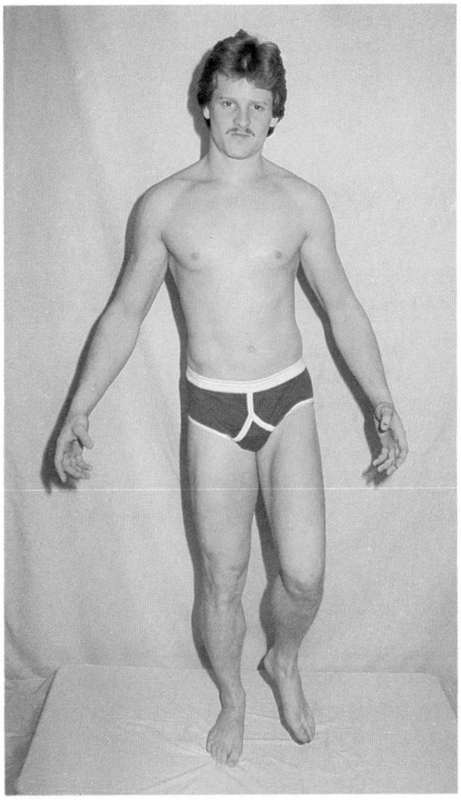

Fig. 17-21
Evaluation of balance with
the patient hopping in
place on one foot.

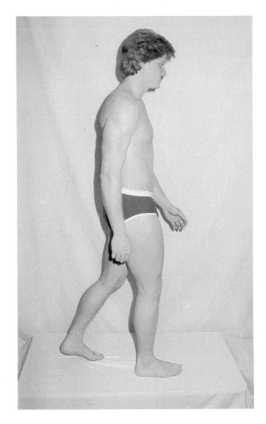

Fig. 17-22
Evaluation of gait. Note
the expected gait sequence
and arm movements.

Table 17-3
Characteristics of Unexpected
Gait Patterns

Gait Pattern	Characteristics
Spastic hemiparesis	The affected leg is stiff and extended with plantar flexion of the foot. Movement of the foot results from pelvic tilting upward on the involved side. The foot is dragged, often scraping the toe, or it is circled stiffly outward and forward (circumduction). The affected arm remains flexed, adducted, and does not swing.
Spastic diplegia (scissoring)	The patient uses short steps, dragging the ball of the foot across the floor. The legs are extended, and the thighs tend to cross forward on each other at each step.
Steppage	The hip and knee are elevated excessively high to lift the plantar flexed foot off the ground. The foot is brought down to the floor with a slap. The patient is unable to walk on the heels.
Dystrophic	The legs are kept apart and weight is shifted from side to side in a waddling motion. The abdomen often protrudes and lordosis is common.
Tabetic	The legs are positioned far apart, lifted high and forcibly brought down with each step. The heel stamps on the ground.
Cerebellar ataxia	The patient's feet are wide-based. Staggering and lurching from side to side is often accompanied by swaying of the trunk.
Sensory ataxia	The patient's gait is wide-based. The feet are thrown forward and outward, bringing them down first on heels then on toes. The patient watches the ground to guide his or her steps. A positive Romberg sign is present.
Dystonic	Jerky dancing movements appear nondirectional.
Ataxia	Uncontrolled falling occurs.

Adapted from Burns and Johnson, 1980.

Fig. 17-23
Unexpected gait patterns.
A, Spastic hemiparesis.
B, Spastic diplegia (scissoring). **C,** Steppage gait.
D, Cerebellar ataxia.
E, Sensory ataxia.

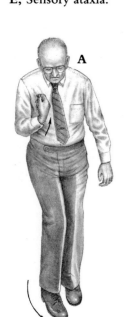
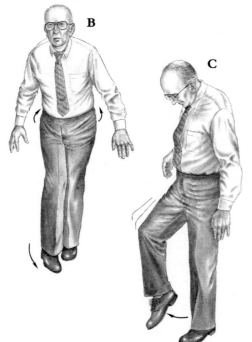
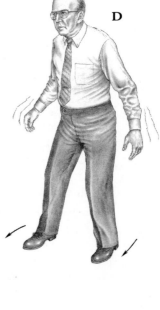
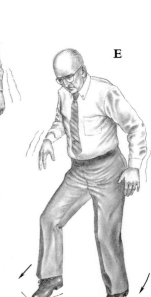
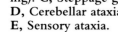

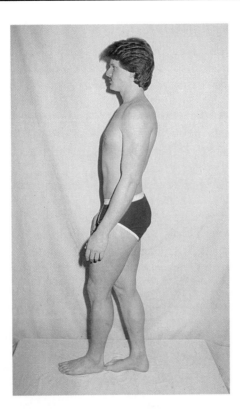

Fig. 17-24
Evaluation of balance with heel-toe walking on a straight line.

Heel-toe walking will exaggerate any unexpected finding in gait evaluation. Have the patient walk a straight line, first forward and then backward, with eyes open and arms at the sides. Direct the patient to touch the toe of one foot with the heel of the other foot (Fig. 17-24). Note any extension of the arms for balance, instability, a tendency to fall, or lateral staggering and reeling. Consistent contact between the heel and toe should occur, although slight swaying is expected.

Sensory Function

Both primary and cortical discriminatory sensation are evaluated by having the patient identify various sensory stimuli. For the complete neurologic examination, each sense is tested in each major peripheral nerve. These sites should be routinely evaluated during the physical examination: hands, lower arms, abdomen, feet, and lower legs. Sensory discrimination of the face is determined with cranial nerve evaluation.

Each sensory discrimination procedure is tested with the patient's eyes closed. Use minimal stimulation initially, increasing it gradually until the patient becomes aware of it. A stronger stimulus is needed over the back, buttocks, and heavily cornified areas, where lower levels of sensitivity occur. Test contralateral areas of the body, and ask the patient to compare perceived sensations, side to side. With each type of sensory stimulus, there should be:
- Minimal differences side to side
- Correct interpretation of sensations (hot/cold, sharp/dull)
- Discrimination of the side of the body tested
- Location of sensation and whether proximal or distal to the previous stimuli

If evidence of sensory impairment is found, map the boundaries of the impairment by the distribution of major peripheral nerves or dermatomes. Loss of sensation can indicate spinal tract, brainstem, or cerebral lesions.

Primary Sensory Functions

Superficial Touch. Touch the skin with a cotton wisp or with your fingertip, using light strokes. Do not depress the skin, and avoid stroking areas with hair (Fig. 17-25, *A*). Have the patient point to the area touched or tell you when the sensation is felt.

Superficial Pain. Alternating the point and hub of a sterile needle, touch the patient's skin in an unpredictable pattern. Allow 2 sec between each stimulus to avoid a summative effect (Fig. 17-25, *B*). Ask the patient to identify the sensation as sharp or dull and where it is felt.

Temperature and Deep Pressure. Only when superficial pain sensation is not intact are temperature and deep pressure sensation tests performed. Roll test tubes of hot and cold water alternately against the skin, again in no predictable pattern, to evaluate temperature sensation. Ask the patient to indicate which temperature is perceived and where it is felt. Deep pressure sensation is tested by squeezing the trapezius, calf, or biceps muscle. The patient should experience discomfort.

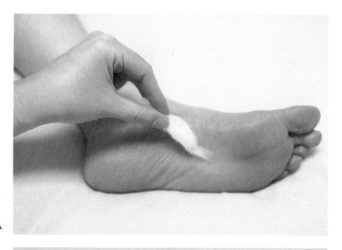

A

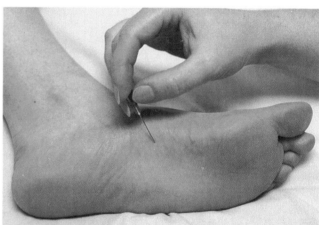

B

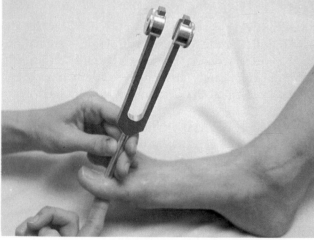

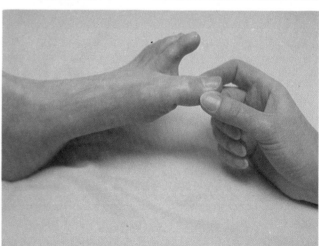

C

D

Fig. 17-25

Evaluation of primary sensory function. **A,** Superficial tactile sensation; use a light stroke to touch the skin with a cotton wisp or brush. **B,** Superficial pain sensation; use the point and hub of a sterile needle in a nonpredictable alternate pattern. **C,** Vibratory sensation; place the stem of a vibrating tuning fork against several bony prominences. **D,** Position sense of joints; hold the toe or finger by the lateral aspects in a raised or lowered position.

Vibration. Place the stem of a vibrating tuning fork (the tuning fork with lower Hz has slower decay of vibration) against several bony prominences, beginning at the most distal joints. The sternum, shoulder, elbow, wrist, finger joints, shin, ankle, and toes may all be tested (Fig. 17-25, *C*). A buzzing or tingling sensation should be felt. Ask the patient to tell you when and where the vibration is felt. Occasionally damp the tines to see if the patient distinguishes a difference.

Position of Joints. Hold the joint to be tested (great toe or finger) by the lateral aspects to avoid giving a clue about the direction moved. Beginning with the joint in neutral position, raise or lower the digit, and ask the patient to tell you which way it was moved. Return the digit to the neutral position before moving it another direction (Fig. 17-25, *D*). Repeat the procedure so the great toe of each foot and a finger on each hand is tested.

Cortical Sensory Functions

Cortical or discriminatory sensory functions test cognitive ability to interpret sensations associated with coordination abilities. Inability to perform these tests should make you suspicious of a lesion in the sensory cortex or the posterior columns of the spinal cord.

Stereognosis. With the patient's eyes closed, hand him or her a familiar object (key, coin) to identify by touch and manipulation (Fig. 17-26, *A*). Tactile agnosia, an inability to recognize objects by touch, suggests a parietal lobe lesion.

Fig. 17-26
Evaluation of a cortical sensory function. **A,** Stereognosis; patient identifies a familiar object by touch. **B,** Two-point discrimination; use two sterile needles, alternately place one or two points simultaneously on the skin, and ask the patient to determine if one or two sensations are felt. **C,** Graphesthesia; draw a letter or number on the body and ask the patient to identify it.

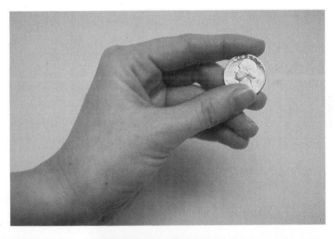

A

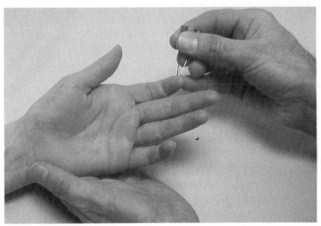

B

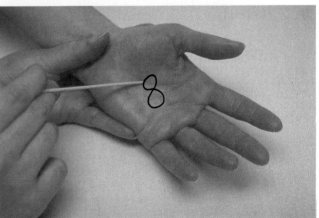

C

Table 17-4
The Minimal Distances of
Discriminating Two Points
by Body Location

Body Part	Minimal Distance (mm)
Tongue	1
Fingertips	2–8
Toes	3–8
Palms of hands	8–12
Chest and forearms	40
Back	40–70
Upper arms and thighs	75

From Malasanos et al., 1986.

Two-point discrimination. Use two sterile needles and alternate touching the patient's skin with one point or both points simultaneously at various locations over the body (Fig. 17-26, *B*). Find the distance at which the patient can no longer distinguish two points. Table 17-4 lists the minimal distances at which adults can discriminate two points on various parts of the body.

Extinction phenomenon. Simultaneously touch the cheek, hand, or other area on each side of the body with a sterile needle. Ask the patient to tell you how many stimuli there are and where they are. Both sensations should be felt.

Graphesthesia. With a blunt pen or an applicator stick, draw a letter or number on the palm of the patient's hand (Fig. 17-26, *C*). Other body locations may also be used. Ask the patient to identify the figure. Repeat the procedure with a different figure on the other hand. The letter or number should be readily recognized.

Point location. Touch an area on the patient's skin and withdraw the stimulus. Ask the patient to point to the area touched. No difficulty localizing the stimulus should be noted. This procedure is often performed simultaneously with superficial tactile sensation.

Reflexes

Both superficial and deep tendon reflexes are used to evaluate the function of specific spine segmental levels (Table 17-5).

Superficial Reflexes

With the patient supine, stroke each quadrant of the abdomen with the end of a reflex hammer or other pointed object. The upper abdominal reflexes are elicited by stroking upward and lower abdominal reflexes are elicited by stroking downward making a diamond pattern around the umbilicus (Fig. 17-27). A slight movement of the umbilicus toward each area of stimulation should be bilaterally equal. When abdominal reflexes are absent, either an upper or lower motor neuron disorder should be suspected.

Stroke the inner thigh of the male patient (proximal to distal) to elicit the cremasteric reflex. The testicle and scrotum should rise on the stroked side.

Deep Tendon Reflexes

Evaluation of deep tendon reflexes are performed with the patient relaxed, either sitting or lying down. Focus the patient's attention on an alternate muscle contraction, such as pulling clenched hands apart. Position the limb with slight tension on the tendon to be tapped. Palpate the tendon to locate the correct point for stimulation, rather than randomly tapping in the area. Hold the reflex hammer loosely

Table 17-5
Superficial and Deep Tendon Reflexes and their Corresponding Spine Segmental Level

Reflex	Spinal Level
Superficial	
Upper abdominal	T7, T8, and T9
Lower abdominal	T10 and T11
Cremasteric	T12, L1, and L2
Deep	
Biceps	C5 and C6
Brachioradial	C5 and C6
Triceps	C6, C7, and C8
Patellar	L2, L3, and L4
Achilles	S1 and S2
Plantar	L4, L5, S1, and S2

Adapted from Rudy, 1984.

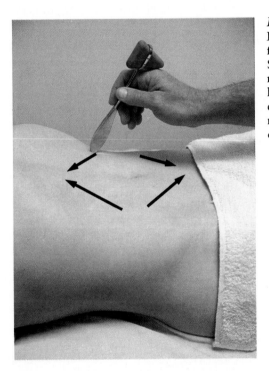

Fig. 17-27
Examination of the superficial abdominal reflexes. Stroke the upper abdominal area upwards and the lower abdominal area downwards to form a diamond around the umbilicus.

between your thumb and index finger, and briskly tap the tendon with a wrist-flicker movement.

Test each reflex, comparing responses on corresponding sides. Symmetric visible or palpable responses should be noted. Scoring of deep tendon reflex responses are shown in Table 17-6. Absent reflexes may indicate a neuropathy or lower motor neuron disorder, while hyperactive reflexes suggests an upper motor neuron disorder. The characteristics of upper and lower motor neuron disorders are listed in the box on p. 612.

Biceps Reflex. Flex the patient's arm up to 45 degrees at the elbow. Palpate the biceps tendon in the antecubital fossa (Fig. 17-28, *A*). Place your thumb over the tendon and your fingers over the biceps muscle. Strike your thumb, rather than the tendon directly, with the reflex hammer. Contraction of the biceps muscle causes visible or palpable flexion of the elbow.

Brachioradial Reflex. Flex the patient's arm up to 45 degrees and rest his or her forearm on your arm with the hand slightly pronated (Fig. 17-28, *B*). Strike the brachioradial tendon (about 1 to 2 in above the wrist) directly with the reflex hammer. Pronation of the forearm and flexion of the elbow should occur.

Triceps Reflex. Flex the patient's arm at the elbow up to 90 degrees and rest the patient's hand against the side of the body. Palpate the triceps tendon and strike it directly with the reflex hammer, just above the elbow (Fig. 17-28, *C*). Contraction of the triceps muscle causes visible or palpable extension of the elbow.

Patellar Reflex. Flex the patient's knee up to 90 degrees, allowing the lower leg to hang loosely. Support the upper leg with your hand, not allowing it to rest against the edge of the examining table. Strike the patellar tendon just below the patella (Fig. 17-28, *D*). Contraction of the quadriceps muscle causes extension of the lower leg.

Achilles Reflex. With the patient sitting, flex the knee and dorsiflex the ankle up to 90 degrees, holding the heel of the foot in your hand. Alternatively, the patient may kneel on a chair with the toes pointing toward the floor. Strike the Achilles tendon at the level of the ankle malleoli (Fig. 17-28, *E*). Contraction of the gastrocnemius muscle causes plantar flexion of the foot.

Clonus. Test for ankle clonus, especially if the reflexes are hyperactive. Support the patient's knee in partially flexed position and briskly dorsiflex the foot with your other hand, maintaining the foot in flexion (Fig. 17-28, *F*). No rhythmic oscillating movements between dorsiflexion and plantar flexion should be palpated. Sustained clonus is associated with upper motor neuron disease.

Table 17-6
Scale of Responses Used to Score Deep Tendon Reflexes

Grade	Deep Tendon Reflex Response
0	No response
1+	Sluggish or diminished
2+	Active or expected response
3+	More brisk than expected, slightly hyperactive
4+	Brisk, hyperactive, with intermittent or transient clonus

CLINICAL SIGNS OF MOTOR NEURON LESIONS

Upper Motor Neuron
Muscle spasticity, possible contractures
Little or no muscle atrophy
Hyperreflexia
Damage above level of brainstem will affect opposite side of body

Lower Motor Neuron
Muscle flaccidity
Loss of muscle tone
Muscle atrophy
Hyporeflexia or areflexia
Fasciculations
Changes in muscles supplied by that nerve, usually a muscle on the same side as the lesion

From Rudy, 1984.

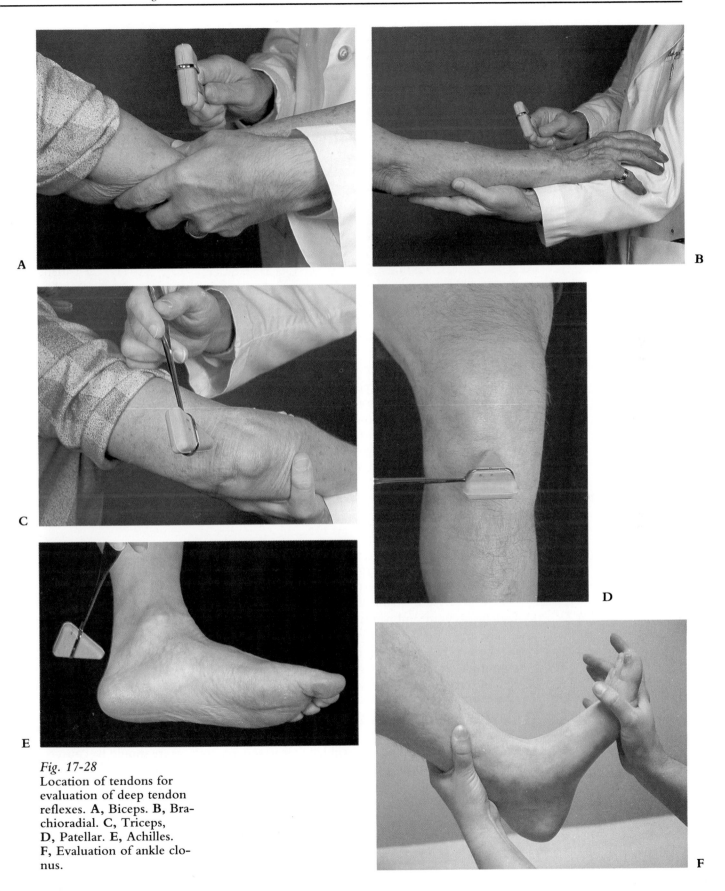

Fig. 17-28
Location of tendons for evaluation of deep tendon reflexes. **A**, Biceps. **B**, Brachioradial. **C**, Triceps, **D**, Patellar. **E**, Achilles. **F**, Evaluation of ankle clonus.

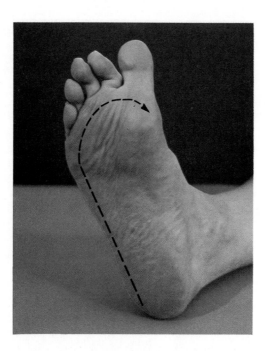

Fig. 17-29
Plantar reflex indicating the direction of the stroke and the Babinski sign—dorsiflexion of the great toe with or without fanning of the toes.

Plantar Reflex. Using a pointed object, stroke the lateral side of the foot from the heel to the ball, then curve across the ball of the foot to the medial side (Fig. 17-29). Observe for plantar flexion, fanning of the toes, or dorsiflexion of the great toe with or without fanning of the other toes.

The patient should have plantar flexion of all toes. Babinski's sign is present when there is dorsiflexion of the great toe with or without fanning of the other toes. This is an expected response in children under 2 years of age, but it indicates pyramidal tract disease in other individuals. However, the ticklish patient may respond with some degree of Babinski's sign.

INFANTS

We ordinarily begin to suspect neurologic problems in the young because they are *not* doing something we expect them to do, rather than because we find an abnormality on physical examination. As in so much else, the major clues are discovered with an accurate and painstaking history.

The infant's general behavior and level of consciousness are evaluated by observing the level of activity and responsiveness to environmental stimuli. Note whether the baby is lethargic, drowsy, stuporous, alert, active, or irritable. By 2 months of age, the infant should appear alert, quiet, and content and should recognize the face of a significant other.

By the time an infant is 2 to 3 months old, it is reasonable to expect that a careful examiner who devotes time to developing a relationship with the baby could coax a smile. If it is difficult or impossible to elicit a social smile, there should be concern about the child's immediate health and neurologic competence.

Drooling babies are ubiquitous. In the first year of life drooling is frequently attributed to teething. Past the age of 1 year, drooling becomes much less common; by age 2 it generally disappears. If it should persist, the examiner should be concerned about some neurologic handicap, perhaps mental retardation, or anomalies of the teeth or the upper gastrointestinal tract.

Table 17-7
Testing Procedures and Expected Behaviors for Indirect Cranial Nerve Evaluation in Newborns and Infants

Cranial Nerves	Procedures and Observations
CN II, III, IV, and VI	Optical blink reflex: shine a light at the infant's open eyes. Observe the quick closure of the eyes and dorsal flexion of the infant's head. No response may indicate poor light perception. Gazes intensely at close object or face. Focuses on and tracks an object with its eyes. Doll's eye maneuver: see CN VIII.
CN V	Rooting reflex: touch one corner of the infant's mouth. The infant should open its mouth and turn its head in the direction of stimulation. If the infant has been recently fed, minimal or no response is expected (Fig. 17-30). Sucking reflex: place your finger in the infant's mouth, feeling the sucking action. The tongue should push up against your finger with a fairly good rate. Note the pressure, strength, and pattern of sucking.
CN VII	Observe the infant's facial expression when crying. Note the infant's ability to wrinkle its forehead and the symmetry of the smile.
CN VIII	Acoustic blink reflex: loudly clap your hands about 30 cm from the infant's head; avoid producing an air current. Note the blink in response to the sound. No response after 2-3 days of age may indicate hearing problems. Infant will habituate to repeated testing. Moves eyes in direction of sound. Freezes position with high-pitched sound. Doll's eye maneuver: hold the infant under the axilla in an upright position, head held steady, facing you. Rotate the infant first in one direction and then in the other. The infant's eyes should turn in the direction of rotation and then the opposite direction when rotation stops. If the eyes do not move in the expected direction, suspect a vestibular problem or eye muscle paralysis.
CN IX and X	Swallowing and gag reflex.
CN XII	Coordinated sucking and swallowing ability. Pinch infant's nose; mouth will open and tip of tongue will rise in a midline position.

Adapted from Thompson et al., 1986.

Fig. 17-30
Elicitation of the rooting reflex. Touch the corner of the infant's mouth and observe for movement of the head and opening of the mouth on the side of the stimulation.

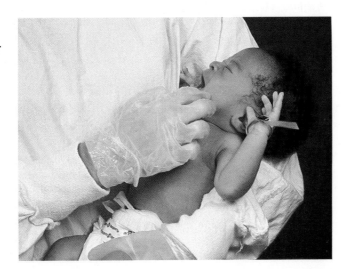

Because language has not yet developed, crying and other vocal sounds are evaluated. The infant's cry should be loud and angry, not high pitched or hoarse. A shrill or whiny high-pitched cry or cat-like screeching cry suggests a central nervous system deficit. Cooing and babbling are expected after 3 and 4 months of age, respectively. One or two words (mama, dada, bye-bye) should be distinct by 9 to 10 months of age.

The cranial nerves are not directly tested, but several observations made during the physical examination provide indirect evaluation (Table 17-7).

Table 17-8
Primitive Reflexes Routinely Evaluated: Procedure for Examination, Expected Findings, Time of Appearance and Disappearance

Reflex (Appearance)	Procedure and Findings
Palmar grasp (birth)	Making sure the infant's head is in midline, touch the palm of the infant's hand from the ulnar side (opposite the thumb). Note the strong grasp of your finger. Sucking facilitates the grasp. It should be strongest between 1 and 2 months of age and disappear by 3 months (Fig. 17-31, *A*).
Plantar grasp (birth)	Touch the plantar surface of the infant's feet at the base of the toes. The toes should curl downward. It should be strong up to 8 months of age (Fig. 17-31, *B*).
Moro (birth)	With the infant supported in semi-sitting position, allow the head and trunk to drop back to a 30-degree angle. Observe symmetric abduction and extension of the arms, fingers fan out and thumb and index finger form a C. The arms then adduct in an embracing motion followed by relaxed flexion. The legs may follow a similar pattern of response. The reflex diminishes in strength by 3 to 4 months and disappears by 6 months (Fig. 17-31, *C*).
Placing (4 days of age)	Hold the infant upright under its arms next to a table or chair. Touch the dorsal side of the foot to the table or chair edge. Observe flexion of the hips and knees and lifting of the foot as if stepping up on the table. Age of disappearance varies (Fig. 17-31, *D*).
Stepping (between birth and 8 weeks)	Hold the infant upright under the arms and allow the soles of the feet to touch the surface of the table. Observe for alternate flexion and extension of the legs, simulating walking. It disappears before voluntary walking (Fig. 17-31, *E*).
Tonic neck or "fencing" (by 2 to 3 months)	With the infant lying supine and relaxed or sleeping, turn its head to one side so the jaw is over the shoulder. Observe for extension of the arm and leg on the side to which the head is turned and for flexion of the opposite arm and leg. Turn the infant's head to the other side, observing the reversal of the extremities' posture. This reflex diminishes at 3 to 4 months of age and disappears by 6 months. Be concerned if the infant never exhibits the reflex or seems locked in the fencing position. This reflex must disappear before the infant can roll over or bring its hands to its face (Fig. 17-31, *F*).

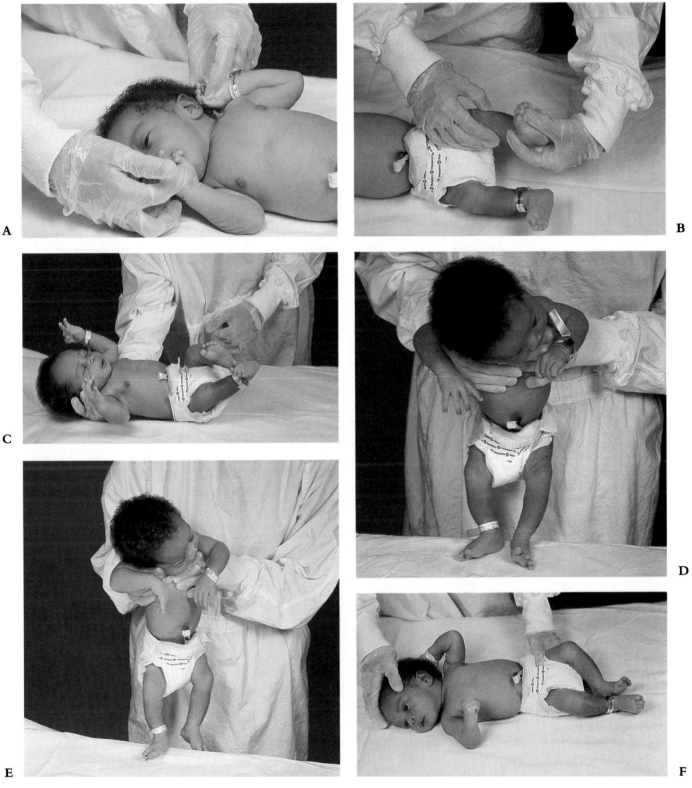

Fig. 17-31
Elicitation of the primitive reflexes. **A,** Palmar grasp. **B,** Plantar grasp. **C,** Moro reflex. **D,** Placing reflex. **E,** Stepping reflex. **F,** Tonic neck reflex. This illustration shows proper positioning of the head and neck, but this infant is too young for the reflex to be present.

Table 17-9
Less Commonly Evaluated Primitive Reflexes

Reflex (Appearance)	Procedure and Findings
Glabella (birth)	With your index finger briskly tap the bridge of the infant's nose (glabella) when its eyes are open. Observe the sudden symmetric blinking of the eyes. The infant will blink for the first 4 to 5 taps.
Galant's (trunk incurvature) (birth to 4 weeks)	Suspend the infant in prone position on one of your hands or on a flat surface. Stroke one side of the infant's back between the shoulders to the buttocks, about 4 to 5 cm from the spinal cord (Fig. 17-32). Observe for the curvature of the trunk toward the side stroked. Repeat on the other side.
Landau (birth to 6 months)	Suspend the infant in prone position on both of your hands so that the infant's legs and arms are extending over both sides of your hand. Observe the infant's ability to lift its head and extend its spine on a horizontal plane. The reflex diminishes by 18 months of age and disappears by 3 years.
Parachute (4 to 6 months)	Hold the infant suspended in prone position and slowly lower it head first toward a surface. Observe the infant extend its arms and legs as if to protect itself. This reflex should not disappear.
Neck righting (3 months, after tonic neck disappears)	With the infant supine, turn its head to the side. Observe the infant turning its whole body in the direction the head is turned.

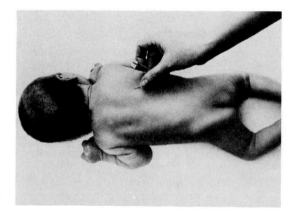
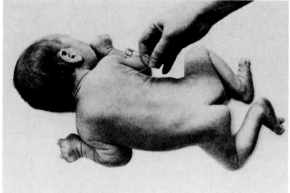

Fig. 17-32
Elicitation of Galant's reflex.
From Bobak and Jensen, 1984.

Observe the infant's spontaneous activity for symmetry and smoothness of movement. Coordinated sucking and swallowing is also a function of the cerebellum. Hands are usually held in fists for the first 3 months of life, but not constantly; after 3 months they begin to open for longer periods. Purposeful movement (reaching and grasping for objects) begins at about 2 months of age. This progresses to taking objects with one hand at 6 months, transferring objects hand to hand at 7 months, and a purposeful release by 10 months of age. There should be no tremors or constant overshooting of movements.

A withdrawal of all limbs from a painful stimulus provides a measure of sensory integrity. Other sensory function is not routinely tested.

The patellar tendon reflexes are present at birth, and the Achilles and brachioradial tendon reflexes appear at 6 months of age. When deep tendon reflexes are tested, the examiner should use a finger to tap the tendon, rather than the reflex hammer. In each case, the muscle attached to the tendon struck should contract. Interpret findings as for adults; however, one to two beats of ankle clonus are common.

The plantar reflex is routinely performed as described in the adult examination. A positive Babinski's sign, fanning of the toes and dorsiflexion of the great toe, is found until the infant is 24 months of age.

The posture and movement of the developing infant are routinely evaluated by primitive reflexes (Table 17-8) and are shown in Fig. 17-31. These reflexes appear and disappear in a sequence corresponding with central nervous system development. Symmetry and smoothness of response are important observations. Less commonly evaluated primitive reflexes are listed in Table 17-9 and shown in Fig. 17-32.

Muscle strength and tone are especially important to evaluate in the newborn and infant. Chapter 16, Musculoskeletal System, provides details related to this portion of the examination. Remember that the infant's neuromuscular development at the time of birth should be evaluated with the Dubowitz Clinical Assessment for gestational age (see Chapter 3, Growth and Measurement).

CHILDREN

The neurologic examination of the young child is done by observing the neuromuscular developmental progress and skills displayed during the examination. The Denver Developmental Screening Test (DDST) is a useful tool to determine if the child is developing as expected with fine and gross motor skills, language, and personal-social skills.

Observe the child's mood, communication pattern, preferences, and responsiveness to the parent. Evaluate the types of words and speech patterns used. The child's language and speech should be appropriate for age. Table 17-10 describes expressive language milestones. Articulation is a fine motor skill, and speech should be more clearly understood with advancing age. Articulation milestones may be evaluated with the Denver Articulate Screening Exam (DASE).

Memory testing may be attempted at about 4 years of age, if the child pays attention and is not too anxious. Expected memory skills vary with the age of the child. Test immediate recall by asking the child to repeat either numbers or words. A 4-year-old can repeat 3 digits or words, a 5-year-old can repeat 4 digits or words, and a 6-year-old can repeat 5 digits or words. Recent memory is not usually tested in children but may be done with modification. Show the child only 3 objects, and wait no longer than 5 minutes to ask the child to recall what objects were shown.

Table 17-10

Expressive Language Milestones for the Toddler between 12 and 36 Months of Age

Age (Months)	Expressive Language Milestones
12 to 15	Says 3-4 words appropriately, including names; uses flow of connected sounds that have inflection and seem like a sentence
15 to 18	Uses 10 words including names; makes requests by naming objects; begins to repeat words heard in adult conversations
18 to 24	Uses short sentences (3-4 words); uses pronouns but some syntax errors; tells full name; echoes last 2-3 words of a rhyme
24 to 36	Mother understands 90% of speech; uses noun-verb combinations with correct verb tense; repeats 3 numbers, given intervals

Adapted from Krajicek and Tomlinson, 1983.

Table 17-11

Cranial Nerve Examination Procedures for Young Children

Cranial Nerves	Procedures and Observations
CN II	If the child cooperates, the Snellen E or Picture Chart may be used to test vision.
	Visual fields may be tested, but the child may need the head immobilized.
CN III, IV, and VI	Have the child follow an object with the eyes, immobilizing the head if necessary. Attempt to move the object through the cardinal points of gaze.
CN V	Observe the child chewing a cookie or cracker, noting bilateral jaw strength.
	Touch the child's forehead and cheeks with cotton and watch the child bat it away.
CN VII	Observe the child's face when smiling, frowning, and crying.
	Ask the child to show his or her teeth.
	Demonstrate puffed cheeks and ask the child to imitate.
CN VIII	Observe the child turn to sounds such as a bell or whisper.
	Whisper a commonly used word behind the child's back and have him or her repeat the word.
	Perform audiometric testing.
CN IX and X	Elicit gag reflex
CN XI and XII	Instruct older child to stick out the tongue and shrug the shoulders or raise the arms.

Adapted from Bowers and Thompson, 1984.

Table 17-12
Activities for Evaluating Neurologic Soft Signs in Children, the Associated Soft Sign, and the Age at Which the Finding Should No Longer Be Observed

Activity	Soft Sign Findings	Latest Expected Age of Disappearance (Years)
Walking, running gait	Stiff-legged with a foot slapping quality, unusual posturing of the arms	3
Heel walking	Difficulty remaining on heels for a distance of 10 ft	7
Tip-toe walking	Difficulty remaining on toes for a distance of 10 ft	7
Tandem gait	Difficulty walking heel to toe, unusual posturing of arms	7
One-foot standing	Unable to remain standing on one foot longer than 5-10 sec	5
Hopping in place	Unable to rhythmically hop on each foot	6
Motor-stance	Difficulty maintaining stance (arms extended in front, feet together, and eyes closed), drifting of arms, mild writhing movements of hands or fingers	3
Visual tracking	Difficulty following object with eyes when keeping the head still; nystagmus	5
Rapid thumb-to-finger test	Rapid touching thumb to fingers in sequence is uncoordinated; unable to suppress mirror movements in contralateral hand	8
Rapid alternating movements of hands	Irregular speed and rhythm with pronation and supination of hands patting the knees	10
Finger-nose test	Unable to alternately touch examiner's finger and own nose consecutively	7
Right-left discrimination	Unable to identify right and left sides of own body	5
Two-point discrimination	Difficulty in localizing and discriminating when touched in one or two places	6
Graphesthesia	Unable to identify geometric shapes you draw in child's open hand	8
Stereognosis	Unable to identify common objects placed in own hand	5

Adapted from Smith and McNamara, 1984.

Older preschoolers will be more skilled with this test. Test remote memory by asking the child what he or she had for dinner the previous night, his or her address, or to recite a nursery rhyme.

Direct examination of cranial nerves requires some modifications in procedure according to the age of the child. Often a game is played to elicit the response. Table 17-11 describes the procedures.

Observe the young child at play, noting gait and fine motor coordination. The beginning walker exhibits a wide-based gait, while the older child walks with feet closer together, has better balance, and recovers easier when unbalanced. Observe the child's skill in reaching for, grasping, and releasing toys. No tremors or constant overshooting movements should be apparent.

Heel to toe walking, hopping, and jumping are all coordination skills that develop in the young child. They can be evaluated by modifying the skill tested into a game for the child. The DDST provides guidance for the ages at which you can expect these maneuvers to be accomplished.

Deep tendon reflexes are not routinely tested in a child who demonstrates appropriate development, because poor cooperation is often a problem. When reflexes are tested, use the same techniques described for adults; responses should be the same.

Evaluate light touch sensation by asking the child to close his or her eyes and point to where you touch or tickle. Have the child discriminate between rough and soft textures as an alternate procedure. Use the tuning fork to evaluate vibration sensation, asking the child to point to the area where the buzzing sensation is felt. Superficial pain sensation is not routinely tested in young children because of their fear of needles.

When checking cortical sensory integration, use geometric figures rather than numbers to evaluate graphesthesia. Draw each figure twice and ask the child if they are the same or different. (Make sure the child understands the terms *same* and *different*.) Some children will need a practice session with their eyes open to get good compliance with the examination.

Many of the techniques used in the adult neurologic examination are utilized for children, with some modifications for the child's level of understanding.

Because the child is still developing, there may be some unexpected findings in the school-age child that would be normal in younger children. These neurologic soft signs are nonfocal, functional neurologic findings that often provide subtle clues to an underlying central nervous system deficit or a neurologic maturation delay. Soft signs can be found in gross motor, fine motor, sensory, and reflex functional areas. Table 17-12 describes neurologic soft sign findings, and the age at which you should become concerned if still present. Children with multiple soft signs are often found to have learning problems.

OLDER ADULTS

Examination of the neurologic system of the older adult is identical to that of the adult. You may need to allow more time for performing maneuvers that require coordination and movement.

There is little evidence that the individual's personality changes with age, in the absence of other health problems. Paranoid thought is the most striking alteration in personality. Attempt to determine if the thought process is accurate or a paranoid ideation, keeping in mind that the incidence of abuse of the elderly is increasing.

Deterioration of intellectual function should not be found unless the patient has a disease of the central nervous system or a disease affecting it. Determine if any changes in cerebral function could be the consequence of cardiovascular, hepatic, renal, or metabolic disease. Medications can also impair central nervous system function, causing slowed reaction time, disorientation, confusion, loss of memory, tremors, and anxiety. Problems may develop because of the dosage, number, or interaction of medications prescribed or purchased over the counter.

Some problem solving skills deteriorate with aging, but this may be related to disuse. Skills involving vocabulary and inventories of available information are expected to remain at younger adult levels of performance. Recent memory deteriorates before remote memory. Most older adults comment that their remembrance of distant events actually improves.

The older adult has markedly diminished senses of smell and taste. Sweet and salty tastes are usually impaired first.

Gait with advancing age is characterized by short, uncertain steps. Shuffling may occur as speed, balance, and grace decrease with age. Legs may be flexed at the hips and knees (Fig. 17-33).

Tactile and vibratory sensation, as well as position sense, are often impaired in the older adult. This patient may need stronger stimuli to detect sensation.

Changes in deep tendon reflexes occur with aging. The older adult usually has less brisk or even absent reflexes, with response diminishing in the lower extremities before the upper extremities are affected. The Achilles and plantar reflexes may be absent or difficult to elicit in some older adults. The superficial reflexes may also disappear.

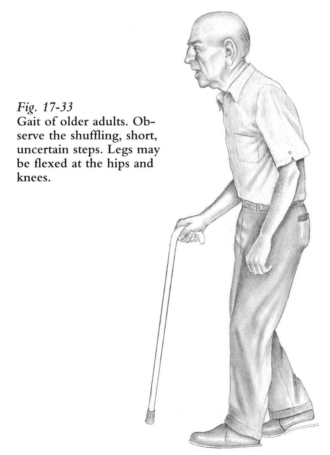

Fig. 17-33
Gait of older adults. Observe the shuffling, short, uncertain steps. Legs may be flexed at the hips and knees.

Common Abnormalities

Parkinson's Disease

Parkinson's disease is a progressive, degenerative neurologic disorder of unknown cause. Although more common in older adults, this disorder sometimes occurs in young adults. Symptoms begin with tremors at rest and with fatigue, disappearing with intended movement and sleep. Progression of symptoms is illustrated with tremor of the head, continued slowing of voluntary movements, and bilateral "pill-rolling" of the fingers. Muscular rigidity and resistance to passive motion interfere with walking and swinging the arms. The gait consists of more rapid, short, shuffling steps. Facial expression may be blank with widely opened eyes and a poor blink reflex. Speech becomes slowed, monotonous, slurred, and sometimes severely dysarthric. Difficulty swallowing and drooling with excess saliva may also occur. Symptoms of parkinsonism can also be caused by drugs, cerebral trauma, and carbon monoxide and manganese poisoning (Fig. 17-34).

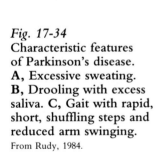

Fig. 17-34
Characteristic features of Parkinson's disease. A, Excessive sweating. B, Drooling with excess saliva. C, Gait with rapid, short, shuffling steps and reduced arm swinging.
From Rudy, 1984.

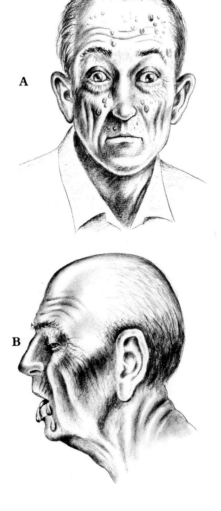

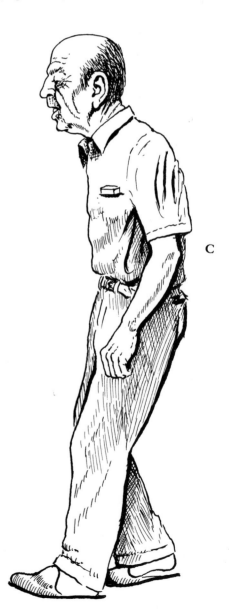

Multiple Sclerosis	A debilitating, degenerative neurologic disorder, multiple sclerosis is characterized by demyelinated plaques throughout the white matter of the central nervous system. The cause is unknown. The onset of symptoms occurs between 20 and 40 years of age. Acute episodes occur with symptoms varying in type	and severity over time. Periods of remission are common. An array of sensory and visual disturbances, slow, progressive, spastic weakness of the lower extremities, cerebellar ataxia, urinary incontinence, and euphoric affect may occur over time.
Myasthenia Gravis	A neuromuscular disease involving the lower motor neurons and muscle fibers, myasthenia gravis is believed to be autoimmune in origin, causing a defect in transmission at the neuromuscular junction. Symptoms may begin either be-	tween 20 and 30 years of age or in late middle age. It is characterized by weakness and abnormal fatigue of the muscles involved in ocular movement, facial expression, respiration, chewing, and swallowing.
Seizures	Seizures are spontaneous, involuntary, paroxysmal episodes of contraction in a group of muscles. No cause may be found, but in some cases seizures are	related to tumors, cerebrovascular disease, trauma, or metabolic disorders. They may be clonic, tonic, focal, unilateral, or bilateral.
Huntington's Chorea	An autosomal hereditary, progressive degenerative disease, Huntington's chorea is characterized by chorea and mental deterioration progressing to demen-	tia. Symptoms usually appear between 30 and 40 years of age, and death occurs about 15 years later.
Delirium Tremens	Delirium tremens is a psychotic reaction caused by withdrawal from excessive intake of alcohol over a period of time. Symptoms begin with loss of appetite, insomnia, and general restlessness. There is progression to agitation, ex-	citement, disorientation, mental confusion, hallucinations, acute fear and anxiety, coarse tremors of the extremities and tongue, and an increased metabolic response. Symptoms last 3 to 6 days and are followed by deep sleep.
Peripheral Neuropathy	Loss of discriminatory sensation can be related to a lesion in the posterior columns or sensory cortex or can be caused by a metabolic disorder such as diabetes	mellitus. Frequently both hands or feet are affected with all sensory modalities lost.
Meningitis	Inflammatory processes in the meninges are caused by bacteria and viruses. Signs and symptoms include fever, chills,	nuchal rigidity, headache, and vomiting, followed by alterations in consciousness.

CHILDREN

Cerebral Palsy

A group of nonprogressive neuromuscular disorders of abnormal muscle tone and coordination, cerebral palsy results from insult to the cerebellum, basal ganglia, or motor cortex. Signs include delayed gross motor development, alterations in muscle tone, and abnormalities of posture, motor performance, and reflexes. The degree of disability produced depends on the extent of neurologic damage. Some patients can expect near-normal levels of functioning.

Reye's Syndrome

Reye's syndrome is an acute encephalopathy accompanied by fatty degeneration of the liver. The prodromal stage consists of a viral illness, followed by the encephalopathic stage. Symptoms progress from lethargy and drowsiness with vomiting to behavioral changes with delirium, irrational behavior, disorientation, and combativeness. The use of aspirin in viral illnesses is thought to predispose a child to this disorder.

Mental Retardation

Significant subaverage general intellectual functioning, existing concurrently with deficits in adaptive behavior, is manifested during the developmental period. Signs and symptoms include delayed developmental milestones, inability to discriminate between two or more stimuli, impaired short-term memory, and lack of motivation.

Attention Deficit Disorder

A combination of behavior problems that interfere with the child's ability to learn include developmentally inappropriate inattention, impulsivity, and hyperactivity. Its onset occurs before 7 years of age and is not related to mental retardation or a psychiatric disorder.

OLDER ADULTS

Alzheimer's Disease

Alzheimer's disease causes mental deterioration (dementia) that is documented by a standard mental status test with evidence of deficits in two or more areas of cognition. There is progressive worsening of memory and other cognitive functions, no disturbance of consciousness, absence of systemic disorders or other brain diseases that in themselves could account for the deficits. It may begin in late middle age, but its incidence is greatest in women and in persons over 80 years of age. Risk factors for Alzheimer's disease are its occurrence in a parent or sibling, a history of serious head trauma, and the presence of trisomy 21 (Katzman, 1986).

Senile Dementia

Senile dementia is an organic brain syndrome in which mental function progressively deteriorates. Signs and symptoms include disorientation, mood swings, irritability, and impaired attention span, judgment, and recent memory. Senile dementia and Alzheimer's disease are often difficult to distinguish clinically.

Putting It All Together

General Guidelines

When you begin learning about a patient, you should not expect to proceed from A to Z on a rigid pathway. The material presented in this book is arranged by body systems, but the actual examination should be flexible while remaining disciplined.

Taking the history and performing the physical examination are so interrelated that they are not necessarily done in a particular sequence. The artistry of your effort arises from your ability to integrate the two procedures. Each of the steps in history and physical examination stands as a separate entity with its own sensitivity and specificity. You must understand each of those steps and how much valuable information can be gained from them. You will learn when to omit steps that will yield information of little value. This is not being sloppy; this is using clinical judgment in adapting to circumstance.

The physical examination is pragmatic and ritualistic—the "laying on of hands." The process not only teaches you much about the patient but also teaches the patient much about you, your personal discipline, your professional composure, and the respect you accord others. You must not forget that the patient usually seeks your help because of a problem and is in a dependent role. Almost all patients feel some unease, anxiety, or even fear. You can help allay these feelings simply by respecting the patient's unease. Your explanations of what you will do next reassures the patient and alleviates some of the anxiety. Always be honest about the possibility that a part of the examination may cause discomfort or pain; otherwise you risk losing the patient's trust. If either you or the patient feel the need to have a third person in the room, you must certainly act on it.

Always respect the patient's modesty. This does not mean that you do not ask the patient to undress, but rather that comfortable gowns and covers are available that can be shifted or removed from the area under examination while providing cover for other parts of the body. Doors and curtains should be closed.

The invasion of a stranger's sensibilities can be most distracting to the student. You will learn to carry yourself with a gentle calm and a balanced approach. Your professional concern will be reassuring to the patient, but you must avoid both inappropriate reassurance and premature expressions of concern over unexpected findings. Remember that while you examine the patient, he or she is also examining you, titrating his or her anxiety by your manner, your hesitations in speech, your changes in facial expression, your lingering over a part of the examination. In fact, many patients equate the gravity of the situation with the length of time you spend on part of the examination, whereas others equate length of time with thoroughness.

The patient should be told that you are a student and that you are apt to be a bit slower than the more experienced. You will naturally feel some pressure and uncertainty regarding your level of ability, but there is a half-life on this period of anxiety. Time, experience, and the appropriate observation of preceptors will help build the foundation for your self-confidence.

At the beginning, when you are unaccustomed to the sequence of an examination, rely on guides such as those in this book. But do not hesitate to develop your own sequence of observations. There is no such thing as a "complete" examination. The goal is to perform an examination in which your observations are appropriate to the circumstance. This varies with the nature of the complaint and the age and sex of the patient.

The examination of a patient of any age is subject to variation. Because there is no "best way," you should develop your own approach, one that feels comfortable for you and one that assures comfort for your patient. You need not take the history or perform the physical examination in the same sequence in which you will record them. Part of the history can be obtained while you are doing the physical examination, because as you discover certain findings you will require more details than the earlier history may have elicited.

Regardless of sequence there are certain guidelines that should never be ignored:

- Assure comfort for the patient and, to the extent possible, for yourself.
- Be gentle.
- The setting should be quiet (radios and TVs should be turned off), comfortable, and well lighted (without glare).
- Avoid distraction and interruption (the telephone should not be allowed into the history and examining room unless there is an emergency).
- Adapt to the patient's circumstance; a person in traction will offer a different challenge from the 7-month-old baby on the parent's lap.
- Be flexible and avoid rigid adherence to a particular sequence. However, be certain that by the end you have made all the necessary observations.
- An examining table should allow you access to the patient from every side and at a height that is convenient for both you and the patient. Because a table against the wall is an obstacle to examining the patient from every perspective, it is preferable to have the table away from the wall.
- Have the patient free of clothing but comfortably draped, paying attention to modesty at every age.
- Expose the part of the body to be examined appropriately and well, or you may lose *the* vital finding.
- Have your hands and stethoscope warm.
- Avoid using a too vigorous approach when examining tender areas.
- Talk with the patient but do not chatter. Explain as you go, anticipating the patient's concern about what comes next. Briefly state the reasons for examining an area and warn the patient of any discomfort it might incur.
- Never *order* the patient to do things. Say "please" and "thank you" (but not so endlessly so that the courtesy itself becomes obsequious). Occasionally ask if the patient is warm enough, comfortable enough, or has any questions.
- Gather information from the patient's attitude, demeanor, speech, and body. It is worrisome, for example, to find the patient apathetic, disinterested, unable to respond socially, or so overwhelmed by the problem that a smile cannot be elicited. This is as true for a 3-month-old baby as it is for an adult.

- Be objective and make no premature assumptions about what you find. Carefully describe first without diagnosing. For example, a lump in the neck may be a swollen node and not a cyst. Diagnosis can usually wait until after the examination is completed.
- Make quantitative measurements with a ruler. Don't use a piece of fruit or a nut for comparison.
- Always remember that physical findings are age-oriented and that their meanings will vary according to age.
- Be reassuring only when you can. Do not make promises that cannot be kept. The composure that allows you to be reassuring without overstating the case takes practice and time.
- Do not feel that you have to do it all in one sitting. If the situation requires it, you can allow the patient a chance for rest and return later to complete the examination.

Once you have obtained basic information on the patient, you need to make an assessment about the urgency of the situation, determine whether the principal problems are fresh or long-standing, decide which clues are most important, determine the extent of the problems and the number of body systems involved, and decide which of the possible clinical areas concerned are dominant.

At this point, you need to ask more questions and return to your physical examination. The clinical circumstance often requires repeated examination in order to understand the problem. You cannot assume that your initial list of clinical possibilities is all-inclusive. There may be an unusual presentation of a common problem or a common presentation of a rarity. There may be more than one disease process or a confounding emotional or social problem. There may be a new illness superimposed on an existing one. You must pay attention to all clues in an effort to explain all symptoms, signs, and abnormal findings.

HUMANS VERSUS MACHINES

There are a number of observations you can make better than machines:
- All that you can perceive by watching, listening, touching, and smelling
- The appearance of the patient, his or her vitality, the presence or absence of apathy, the sense of illness
- The patient's cognitive awareness

On the other hand, there are some things that machines can perform better:
- The size of masses *within* the body (an x-ray can better determine heart size; a CT scan or an MRI can better measure the size of masses throughout the body)
- An ECG tells more about cardiac arrythmias
- Endoscopy facilitates the discovery of lesions within the gastrointestinal tract
- Blood gases more accurately assess respiratory compromise

Finally, you need to discover where in that patient's realm you need to concentrate. In order to do this well, you must review all the systems and consider the whole range of pathophysiologic and psychosocial problems. You must go beyond the obvious to the obscure. Ultimately, you will have to challenge your conclusions by acting as your own devil's advocate or asking others to do so.

EQUIPMENT SUPPLIES FOR PHYSICAL EXAMINATION

Basic Materials

Cotton balls
Cotton applicator sticks
Examining gloves
Flashlight with transilluminator
Gauze squares
Lubricant
Marking pen
Measuring tape
Nasal speculum
Odorous substances
Ophthalmoscope
Otoscope with pneumatic bulb
Penlight
Percussion hammer
Ruler
Sharp and dull testing implements
Sphygmomanometer
Stethoscope with diaphragm and bell
Taste-testing substances
Thermometer
Tongue blades
Tuning forks
Vaginal speculum
Visual acuity screening charts for near and far vision

Materials for Gathering Specimens

Culture media
Glass slides
KOH (postassium hydroxide)
Occult blood testing materials
Pap smear spatula, fixative, and container
Saline
Sterile cotton-tipped applicators

Examination Sequence

As we have already said, there is no one right way to put together the parts of the physical examination so that the end product is an easily flowing process that minimizes the number of times the patient has to change positions and that conserves patient energy. The following is a suggested approach. In reality, this or any other approach may need to be adapted for a particular setting, patient condition, or patient disability.

General Inspection	Begin the inspection as you greet the patient on entering the room.
	  1. Skin color
	  2. Facial expression
	  3. Mobility
	    a. Use of assistive devices
	    b. Gait
	    c. Sitting, rising from chair
	    d. Taking off coat
	  4. Dress and posture
	  5. Speech pattern, disorders, foreign language
	  6. Difficulty hearing, assistive devices
	  7. Stature and build
	  8. Musculoskeletal deformities
	  9. Vision problems, assistive devices
	  10. Eye contact with examiner
	  11. Orientation, mental alertness
	  12. Nutritional state
	  13. Respiratory problems
	  14. Significant others accompanying patient

Patient Instructions	Instruct patient to empty bladder, remove clothing, and put on gown.

Measurements	1. Height
	2. Weight
	3. Distance vision: Snellen chart
	4. Vital signs
	  a. Temperature
	  b. Pulse
	  c. Respiration
	  d. Blood pressure in both arms

Patient Seated,
Wearing Gown

Patient is seated on examining table; examiner stands in front of patient.

HEAD AND FACE
1. Inspect skin characteristics
2. Inspect symmetry and external characteristics of eyes and ears
3. Inspect configuration of skull
4. Inspect and palpate scalp and hair for texture, distribution, and quantity of hair
5. Palpate facial bones
6. Palpate temporomandibular joint while patient opens and closes mouth
7. Palpate sinus regions; if tender transilluminate
8. Inspect ability to clench teeth, squeeze eyes tightly shut, wrinkle forehead, smile, stick out tongue, puff out cheeks (CN V, VII)
9. Test light sensation of forehead, cheeks, chin (CN V)

EYES
1. External examination
   a. Inspect eyelids, eyelashes, palpebral folds
   b. Determine alignment of eyebrows
   c. Inspect sclera, conjunctiva, iris
   d. Palpate lacrimal apparatus
2. Near vision screening: Rosenbaum chart (CN II)
3. Eye function
   a. Test pupillary response to light and accommodation
   b. Perform cover-uncover test and light reflex
   c. Test extraocular eye movements (CN III, IV, VI)
   d. Assess visual fields (CN II)
   e. Test corneal reflex (CN V)
4. Ophthalmoscopic examination
   a. Test red reflex
   b. Inspect lens
   c. Inspect disc, cup margins, vessels, retinal surface, vitreous humor

EARS
1. Inspect alignment
2. Inspect surface characteristics
3. Palpate auricle
4. Assess hearing with whisper test or ticking watch (CN VIII)
5. Perform otoscopic examination
   a. Inspect canals
   b. Inspect tympanic membranes for landmarks, deformities, inflammation
6. Perform Rinne and Weber tests

NOSE
1. Note structure, position of septum
2. Determine patency of each nostril
3. Inspect mucosa, septum, and turbinates with nasal speculum
4. Assess olfactory function: test sense of smell (CN I)

MOUTH AND PHARYNX

1. Inspect lips, buccal mucosa, gums, hard and soft palates, floor of mouth for color and surface characteristics
2. Inspect oropharynx: note anteroposterior pillars, uvula, tonsils, posterior pharynx, mouth odor
3. Inspect teeth for color, number, surface characteristics
4. Inspect tongue for color, characteristics, symmetry, movement (CN XII)
5. Test gag reflex and "ah" reflex (CN IX, X)
6. Perform taste test (CN VII)

NECK

1. Inspect for symmetry and smoothness of neck and thyroid
2. Inspect for jugular venous distention
3. Inspect and palpate range of motion; test resistance against examiner's hand
4. Test shoulder shrug (CN IX)
5. Palpate carotid pulses
6. Palpate tracheal position
7. Palpate thyroid
8. Palpate lymph nodes: pre- and postauricular, occipital, tonsillar, submaxillary, submental, superficial cervical chain, posterior cervical, deep cervical, supraclavicular
9. Auscultate carotid arteries and thyroid

UPPER EXTREMITIES

1. Observe and palpate hands, arms, and shoulders
   a. Skin and nail characteristics
   b. Muscle mass
   c. Musculoskeletal deformities
   d. Joint range of motion: fingers, wrists, elbows, shoulders
2. Assess pulses: radial, brachial
3. Palpate epitrochlear nodes

Patient Seated, Back Exposed

Patient is still seated on examining table. Gown is pulled down to the waist for males so the entire chest and back are exposed; back is exposed but breasts are covered for females. Examiner stands behind the patient.

BACK AND POSTERIOR CHEST

1. Inspect skin and thoracic configuration
2. Inspect symmetry of shoulders, musculoskeletal development
3. Inspect and palpate scapula and spine
4. Palpate and percuss costovertebral angle

LUNGS

1. Inspect respiration: excursion, depth, rhythm, pattern
2. Palpate for expansion and tactile fremitus
3. Palpate scapular and subscapular nodes
4. Percuss posterior chest and lateral walls systematically for resonance
5. Percuss for diaphragmatic excursion
6. Auscultate systematically for breath sounds: note characteristics and adventitious sounds

Patient Seated,
Chest Exposed

Examiner moves around to front of the patient. The gown is lowered in females to expose anterior chest.

ANTERIOR CHEST, LUNGS, AND HEART

1. Inspect skin, musculoskeletal development, symmetry
2. Inspect respirations: patient posture, respiratory effort
3. Inspect for pulsations or heaving
4. Palpate chest wall for stability, crepitence, tenderness
5. Palpate precordium for thrills, heaves, pulsations
6. Palpate left chest to locate apical impulse
7. Palpate for tactile fremitus
8. Palpate nodes: infraclavicular, axillary
9. Percuss systematically for resonance
10. Auscultate systematically for breath sounds
11. Auscultate systematically for heart sounds: aortic area, pulmonic area, second pulmonic area, apical area

FEMALE BREASTS

1. Inspect in the following positions: patient's arms extended over head, pushing hands on hips, hands pushed together in front of chest, patient leaning forward
2. Palpate breasts in all four quadrants, tail of Spence, over areolae; if breasts are large perform bimanual palpation
3. Palpate nipple; compress breasts to observe for discharge

MALE BREASTS

1. Inspect breasts and nipples for symmetry, enlargement, surface characteristics
2. Palpate breast tissue

Patient Reclining
45 Degrees

Assist the patient to a reclining position at a 45-degree angle. Examiner stands to the right side of the patient.

1. Inspect chest in recumbent position
2. Inspect jugular venous pulsations and measure jugular venous pressure

---

Patient Supine,
Chest Exposed

Assist the patient into a supine position. If the patient cannot tolerate lying flat, maintain head elevation at 30-degree angle. Uncover the chest while keeping abdomen and lower extremities draped.

FEMALE BREASTS

1. Inspect in recumbent position
2. Palpate systematically with patient's arm over head and arm at side

HEART

1. Palpate chest wall for thrills, heaves, pulsations
2. Auscultate systematically; you can turn patient slightly to left side and repeat auscultation

Patient Supine, Abdomen Exposed	Patient remains supine. Cover the chest with the patient's gown. Arrange draping to expose the abdomen from pubis to epigastrium.

ABDOMEN
1. Inspect skin characteristics, contour, pulsations, movement
2. Auscultate all quadrants for bowel sounds
3. Auscultate aorta, renal arteries, femoral arteries for bruits, venous hums
4. Percuss all quadrants for tone
5. Percuss liver borders and estimate span
6. Percuss left midaxillary line for splenic dullness
7. Lightly palpate all quadrants
8. Deeply palpate all quadrants
9. Palpate right costal margin for liver border
10. Palpate left costal margin for spleen
11. Palpate for right and left kidneys
12. Palpate midline for aortic pulsation
13. Test abdominal reflexes
14. Have patient raise head as you inspect abdominal muscles

INGUINAL AREA
Palpate for lymph nodes, pulses, hernias

EXTERNAL GENITALIA, MALES
1. Inspect penis, urethral meatus, scrotum, pubic hair
2. Palpate scrotal contents

Patient Supine, Legs Exposed	Patient remains supine. Arrange drapes to cover abdomen and pubis and to expose lower extremities.

FEET AND LEGS
1. Inspect for skin characteristics, hair distribution, muscle mass, musculoskeletal configuration
2. Palpate for temperature, texture, edema, pulses (dorsal pedis, posterior tibial, popliteal)
3. Test range of motion and strength of toes, feet, ankles, knees

HIPS
1. Palpate hips for stability
2. Test range of motion and strength of hips

Patient Sitting, Lap Draped	Assist the patient to a sitting position. Patient should have gown on with drape across lap.

MUSCULOSKELETAL
1. Observe patient moving from lying to sitting position
2. Note coordination, use of muscles, ease of movement

NEUROLOGIC

1. Test sensory function: dull and sharp sensation of forehead, paranasal sinus area, lower arms, hands, lower legs, feet
2. Test vibratory sensation of wrists, ankles
3. Test two-point discrimination of palms, thighs, back
4. Test stereognosis, graphesthesia
5. Test fine motor function, coordination, and position sense of upper extremities
   a. Touch nose with alternating index fingers
   b. Rapidly alternate fingers to thumb
   c. Rapidly move index finger between own nose and examiner's finger
6. Test fine motor function, coordination, and position sense of lower extremities
   a. Run heel down tibia of opposite leg
   b. Alternately and rapidly cross leg over knee
7. Test deep tendon reflexes and compare bilaterally: biceps, triceps, brachioradial, patellar, Achilles
8. Test Babinski reflex bilaterally

Patient Standing

Assist patient to a standing position. Examiner stands next to patient.

SPINE

1. Inspect and palpate spine as patient bends over at waist
2. Test range of motion: hyperextension, lateral bending, rotation of upper trunk

NEUROLOGIC

1. Observe gait
2. Test proprioception and cerebellar function
   a. Romberg test
   b. Walk heel to toe
   c. Stand on one foot then the other with eyes closed
   d. Hop in place on one foot then the other
   e. Do deep knee bends

ABDOMINAL/GENITAL

Test for inguinal and femoral hernias

Female Patient, Lithotomy Position

Assist female patients into lithotomy position and drape appropriately. Examiner is seated.

EXTERNAL GENITALIA

1. Inspect pubic hair, labia, clitoris, urethral opening, vaginal opening, perineal and perianal area, anus
2. Palpate labia and Bartholin's glands; milk Skene's glands

INTERNAL GENITALIA
1. Perform speculum examination
    a. Inspect vagina and cervix
    b. Collect Pap smear and other necessary specimens
2. Perform bimanual palpation to assess for characteristics of vagina, cervix, uterus, adnexae
3. Perform rectovaginal examination to assess rectovaginal septum, broad ligaments
4. Perform rectal examination
    a. Assess anal sphincter tone and surface characteristics
    b. Obtain rectal culture if needed
    c. Note characteristics of stool when gloved finger is removed

Male Patient, Bending Forward

Assist male patients in leaning over examining table or into knee-chest position. Examiner is behind patient.
1. Inspect sacrococcygeal and perianal areas
2. Perform rectal examination
    a. Palpate sphincter tone and surface characteristics
    b. Obtain rectal culture if needed
    c. Palpate prostate gland and seminal vesicles
    d. Note characteristics of stool when gloved finger is removed

• • •

The conclusion of the examination is another point for review and reflection. It gives the patient an opportunity to hear your findings, your interpretations to the extent that you can give them, and to ask questions.

If the patient is examined in a hospital bed, remember to put everything back in order when you are finished. Make sure the patient is comfortably settled in an appropriate manner, bed sides up if the clinical condition warrants, and buttons and buzzers within easy reach.

INFANTS

Newborns

The newborn is at greater risk and has a better potential for health than patients of other ages. The Apgar score, taken at 1 and 5 minutes of age, provides a major clue to the baby's in utero, intrapartum, and immediate postnatal experience. This score is essentially a measure of the vital signs. A low score is evidence of difficulty. A depressed heart rate, respiratory difficulty, loss of muscle tone, and increased reflex irritability all indicate trouble. Of all these observations, color is the least reliable because most new babies have blue fingers and toes. You should note that the Apgar score does not address problems that are suggested by increased irritability, tachypnea, or tachycardia. Nor should it be interpreted as an actual quantitative measure. Still, it is a readily available measure of combined objective and subjective observations and allows communication from one observer to the next over time.

Since menstrual histories are often inaccurate, more objective means of estimating gestational age are required. The following observations are helpful in determining gestational age: Before 36 weeks, only one or two transverse creases are present on the sole of the foot, the breast nodule is less than 3 mm in diameter, no cartilage is present in the helix of the ear, and the testes are seldom in the scrotum, which has few or no rugae. By 40 weeks, many creases are present on the sole, the breast nodule exceeds 4 mm, cartilage is present in the helix of the ear, and the testes have descended into the scrotum, which is covered with rugae. Increasing muscle tone with a posture of predominantly flexed extremities is another sign of increased maturity.

The premature infant often has brief periods of apnea lasting up to 20 seconds. Respiratory distress is indicated by an increased rate, grunting, retraction of intercostal and subcostal spaces and suprasternal notch, seesaw sinking of the chest with rising abdomen in contrast to the normal synchronous motions, and flaring of the nostrils.

Major congenital anomalies are usually obvious, but there are exceptions. Some life-threatening problems such as diaphragmatic hernia may not be quite readily apparent. When confronting a new baby, your index of suspicion must be high and your search for clues must extend into intrauterine life, the mother's immediate postnatal experience, and the family history. The difficulty and mode of labor and delivery will have meaning and need exploration. If the mother has fever 1 or 2 days after delivery or if she is found to have herpetic lesions about the mouth or genitalia, the infant's health may be adversely affected. Her use of drugs—prescribed, over-the-counter, or illicit—will often have an impact on the baby. Most medications are safe but some have teratogenic effects; sedatives and anticonvulsants can have a worrisome impact on the baby's state of consciousness; frequent use of narcotics will cause the baby to go through withdrawal. Problems with earlier pregnancies may be relevant to the newborn's intrauterine life. The fate of siblings may forbode the fate of your present patient.

With a baby, as with patients at every age, it is important to look first. You can learn a lot before touching the patient, without abruptly handling or invading with an instrument. Note the baby's degree of awareness or apathy; the posture and whether unusual flaccidity, tension, or spasticity is present; skin color; and unexpected gross deformities or distortions of facies. The wide-eyed, responsive, eager infant with a strong suck is reassuring. Note the presence or absence of spontaneity in the baby's behavior.

When you begin the physical examination, palpate the head and fontanels, then the extremities and abdomen, and finally the rest of the baby. Use a gentle touch that will not obscure unusual findings. Chest percussion is generally of little value because of the relatively small chest, especially in the premature infant, and the examiner's relatively large hands and fingers. However, an abdomen distended from intestinal obstruction may resonate on percussion.

Older Infants

The examination of the newborn and infant vary somewhat from each other in sequence. Modifications in the examination of each are made when the infant is sleeping or awake at the beginning of the examination. As with adults, there is no single way to sequence the examination of infants. It is important to develop a sequence that is comfortable for you, while ensuring the cooperation of the infant for as much of the examination as possible. This is usually helped by reserving all invasive procedures until the end.

Take advantage of opportunities presented throughout the examination. The sleeping infant presents a wonderful opportunity to auscultate the heart, lungs, and abdomen, as well as a chance to observe the infant's position at rest. The crying infant can be evaluated for lustiness of cry, tactile fremitus, lung excursion, and facial symmetry; the mouth and pharynx can be assessed for integrity of the soft palate and cranial nerves IX, X, and XII. Observe the infant during feeding to evaluate sucking and swallowing coordination, cranial nerve XII, and alertness and responsiveness. A crying infant may keep his or her eyes tightly shut, but the parent can stand and hold the infant over the shoulder, allowing you to stand behind the parent. At this point, the child will often stop crying for a moment and open the eyes. If you are poised with flashlight, you can quickly make some assessment. Similarly, the crying infant—and older children, too—will still need to take a breath, and you can be ready to listen to the heart each time a breath is taken. Over several intervals of breathing, you can hear much of the heart and lung sounds. Taking advantage of these opportunities often means you will change the sequence of the examination to suit the moment.

Physical Examination

The following is a guideline for the examination sequence of the newborn or young infant. The infant's temperature, weight, length, and head circumference are usually measured first. Weight, length, and head circumference are plotted on a growth curve for the infant's age. Newborns may have the Dubowitz Assessment of Gestational Age done before or during the examination.

GENERAL INSPECTION. Inspect the undressed supine newborn on a warming table or the infant on a parent's lap.
1. Positioning or posture at rest: symmetry and size of extremities, the newborn's assumption of in utero position, flexion of extremities or flaccid or spastic appearance, any difference in positioning between upper and lower extremities
2. Voluntary movement of extremities
3. Skin: color; meconium staining and vernix in newborn
4. Presence of tremors
5. Any apparent anomalies
6. Face: symmetry of features, spacing and position of features
7. Configuration and movement of the chest
8. Shape of the abdomen, movement with respiration

CHEST, LUNGS, AND HEART
1. Focused inspection: chest structure, symmetry of expansion with respiration; presence of retractions, heaves, or lifts
2. Note quality of respirations, count the rate
3. Inspect the breasts for nipple and tissue development
4. Palpate chest and precordium: locate apical impulse (point of maximal impulse), note any thrills, note tactile fremitus in crying infant
5. Auscultate entire anterior and lateral chest for breath sounds; note any bowel sounds
6. Auscultate each cardiac listening area for S_1 and S_2, splitting, murmurs
7. Count the apical pulse rate
8. Percussion is rarely performed

ABDOMEN

1. Focused inspection of shape and configuration: note scaphoid or distended appearance
2. Inspect the umbilicus, count the vessels, note oozing of blood; if the stump has fallen off, inspect area for lesions, erythema, drainage, foul odor
3. Auscultate each quadrant for bowel sounds
4. Lightly palpate all areas: note size of liver, muscle tone, bladder, spleen tip
5. Palpate more deeply for kidneys, any masses, note any muscle rigidity or tenseness
6. Percuss each quadrant
7. Check skin turgor
8. Palpate the femoral pulses and for inguinal lymph nodes

HEAD AND NECK. Inspection and palpation can be done preceding or simultaneously with use of invasive instrument.

1. Inspect shape of the head: note molding, swelling, scalp electrode site, hairline
   a. Palpate the head: fontanels, sutures, areas of swelling or asymmetry; measure fontanels in two dimensions
   b. Measure head circumference
   c. Transilluminate newborn's skull
2. Inspect ears
   a. Shape and alignment of auricles; patency of auditory canals; pits, sinuses
   b. Otoscopic examination
3. Inspect eyes: swelling of eyelids and discharge, size, shape, position, epicanthal folds, conjuctivae, pupils
   a. Pupillary response to light
   b. Corneal light reflex
   c. Red reflex, ophthalmoscopic examination
   d. Inspection of eye movement: nystagmus, tracking a light or following a moving picture or face
4. Inspect nose: flaring, discharge, size, shape
   a. Inspect nasal mucosa, alignment of septum
   b. Check patency of choanae, observe respiratory effort while alternately occluding each naris; if any doubt about patency, pass a small feeding tube through each naris to the stomach
5. Inspect mouth: lips, gums, hard and soft palate; size of tongue; excessive secretions in the newborn, drooling in the infant; presence of teeth, lesions
   a. Palpate mouth: insert gloved small finger into mouth, palpate hard and soft palates with fingerpad, evaluate suck
   b. Stimulate gag reflex
   c. Stroke each side of mouth to evaluate rooting reflex
6. Lift infant's trunk, allowing head to fall back and rest against the table, slightly hyperextended
   a. Inspect and palpate the position of the trachea
   b. Inspect for alignment of head with neck
   c. Inspect for webbing, excess skin folds
   d. Palpate for masses, thyroid, muscle tone
   e. Palpate lymph nodes: anterior and posterior cervical, preauricular, postauricular, submental, sublingual, tonsillar, supraclavicular

    f. Palpate the clavicles for integrity, crepitus

    g. Lift infant and test Moro reflex with a sudden dropping motion

7. Inspect neck with infant again supine

    a. Rotate head to each side for passive range of motion

    b. Observe tonic neck reflex for asymmetry

    c. Observe neck righting reflex in older infants

UPPER EXTREMITIES

1. Inspect and palpate arms
2. Move arms through range of motion
3. Palpate brachial or radial pulses; compare quality and timing with femoral pulses
4. Open the hands: inspect nails and palmar and phalangeal creases; count fingers
5. Place a finger in infant's palms to evaluate palmar grasp reflex
6. Keeping fingers in infant's hands, pull the infant slowly to sitting position, evaluate grasp and arm strength; evaluate head control
7. Measure blood pressure

LOWER EXTREMITIES

1. Inspect the legs and feet for alignment and skin folds
2. Palpate the bones and muscles of each leg
3. Move legs through range of motion, adduct and abduct the hips
4. Palpate the dorsalis pedis pulses
5. Count the toes
6. Elicit the plantar, patellar, and Achilles reflexes

GENITALS AND RECTUM

1. Females: inspect external genitalia noting size of clitoris, any discharge, hymenal opening, any ambiguity of structures
2. Males
    a. Inspect placement of urethral opening without retracting the foreskin
    b. Inspect scrotum for rugae and presence of contents; note any ambiguity of structures
    c. Palpate scrotum for the testes, presence of hernia or hydrocele
    d. Transilluminate the scrotum when a mass other than testes is noted
    e. Observe voiding for strength of stream
3. Inspect rectum; assess sphincter tone; if newborn has not passed meconium within 24 hours of birth, evaluate rectal patency with a soft catheter

NEUROLOGIC.
Hold the infant upright facing you with your hands under the axillae.

1. Observe for the sunset sign as the baby's eyes open
2. Perform the doll's eyes maneuver
3. Evaluate general body strength: without gripping the infant's chest, keep your hands under the infant's axillae, and note whether the baby slips through your hands or maintains its position
4. Elicit the stepping reflex
5. Elicit the placing reflex

BACK. Position the newborn prone on the warming table or have the parent hold the infant upright over the shoulder.
1. Inspect spine: observe for alignment, symmetry of muscle development, any masses, tufts of hair, dimples, lesions, defects over lower spine
2. Palpate each spinal process for defect
3. Auscultate posterior chest for breath sounds, any heart sounds
4. Inspect symmetry of gluteal folds

BEHAVIOR. Throughout examination of the newborn, note its alertness, ability to quiet or console itself, and how it responds to handling. Throughout examination of the infant, note its alertness, its responsiveness to the parent, ability of the parent to sense the infant's need for consoling.
1. Note the quality of crying, presence of stridor or hoarseness
2. Note the response to voices or noise: quieting, stopping movement, turning toward sounds

CHILDREN

Most infants and children will be accompanied by one or more parents or parent surrogates. For children who are small enough, the parent's lap is a splendid examining table. It is helpful when taking the history to keep child and parent together and to observe the nature of their interaction. How they feel about each other is conveyed through the parent's touching, soothing, and reassuring gestures and the child's response. An excessive parental response indicates a smothering relationship. On the other hand, if these interactions are absent and the child does not look to the parent for help, the family dynamic is devoid of warmth and affection. Take note of the obvious and subtle ways in which children and parents communicate with each other, and record what you learn.

With the young of any age, you will often take a history and do a physical examination at the same time. These need not be in a rigid sequence, and the complaint and degree of illness can govern your approach to integration. In general, however, you may prefer to start with the history while making overtures to the child to establish some reassuring contact before you actually begin examination. A gentle pat (always with warm hands), a few pleasant words, or playing with the child can often win cooperation. A few relaxed moments—and patience—can break the ice. Children do not know your routine. You are often a stranger, and the environment may be frightening. Not every child will be smiling and happy about an examination.

It usually does not pay to rush, and sometimes it pays not to be too persistent. It is always important to be thorough, but rarely is it necessary to be "complete" in doing a physical examination and taking a history. Unless the matter is urgent, defer some of your inquiries and observations to when the child is more relaxed and less afraid of you. It takes time, after all, to develop friendship and to establish trust.

General inspection of the toddler and preschooler begins as the child enters the examining room. The temperature, weight, and length are usually taken earlier. Offer toys or paper and pencil to entertain the child, to develop rapport, and to evaluate development, motor, and neurologic status. Use the Denver Developmental Screening Test to evaluate language, motor coordination, and social skills. Evaluate mental status as the child interacts with you and with the parent.

TIPS FOR EXAMINING A YOUNG CHILD

- Restraining a child with wrappings and adults looming over the examining table increase the child's apprehension and decrease cooperation. If the child's arms must be restrained and the head kept still to look at the ears, for example, it is usually better to do this on the parent's lap.
- Postpone using the tongue blade until the end of the examination. If the tongue blade must be used, ease the tendency to gag by moistening it first with warm water.
- Allow a young child to "blow out" your flashlight as one way of gaining familiarity with your instruments. Offer your flashlight, otoscope, or stethoscope as a toy (they really will not break), or draw a doll's face on a tongue blade. There are times when you might get down on the floor with the child, or use your own lap as an examining table. You will not sacrifice your dignity; anything goes (within bounds of propriety) to get the information you need.
- Enlist the help of the child if he or she is ticklish. Place your hand on top of the child's hand to gently probe the abdomen or the axilla. The diaphragm of your stethoscope can also serve as a probe.
- Take the opportunity to hold and feed a young baby. This increases your understanding of the child and helps establish rapport.
- If the child is uncomfortable or uncooperative, be patient. You can stop and come back to the child at a later time when calm is restored to complete the examination.

The following sequence is intended only as a guideline to get you started. Take advantage of opportunities the child presents during the examination to make your observations. You will find that the sequence of examination will vary with each child.

Child Playing	The child playing on the floor offers an opportunity to evaluate both the musculoskeletal and neurologic systems while developing a rapport with the child.

1. Observe the child's spontaneous activities
2. Ask the child to demonstrate some skills: throwing a ball, building block towers, drawing geometric figures, coloring
3. Evaluate gait, jumping, hopping, range of motion
4. Muscle strength: observe the child climb on the parent's lap, stoop, and recover

Child on Parent's Lap   Performing the examination on the parent's lap usually enhances the child's participation. Begin with the child sitting and undressed except for the diaper or underpants.

HEAD AND NECK
1. Inspect head
   a. Shape, alignment with neck, hairline, position of auricles
   b. Palpate anterior fontanel for size; head for sutures, depressions; hair for texture
2. Measure head circumference
3. Inspect neck for webbing, voluntary movement
4. Palpate neck: position of trachea, thyroid, muscle tone, lymph nodes

CHEST, HEART, AND LUNGS
1. Inspect chest for respiratory movement, size, shape, precordial movement, deformity, nipple and breast development
2. Palpate anterior chest, locate point of maximal impulse, note tactile fremitus in the talking or crying child
3. Auscultate anterior, lateral, and posterior chest for breath sounds; count respiratory rate
4. Auscultate all cardiac listening areas for S_1 and S_2, splitting, and murmurs; count apical pulse rate

UPPER EXTREMITIES
1. Inspect arms for movement, size, shape; observe use of the hands; inspect hands for number and completeness of fingers, palmar creases
2. Palpate radial pulses
3. Elicit biceps and triceps reflexes when child cooperates
4. Take blood pressure at this point or later, depending on child's attitude

LOWER EXTREMITIES. Child may stand for much of part of the examination.
1. Inspect legs for movement, size, shape, alignment, lesions
2. Inspect feet for alignment, longitudinal arch, number of toes
3. Palpate dorsalis pedis pulse
4. Elicit plantar reflex and, if cooperative, the Achilles and patellar reflexes

Child Supine,   1. Inspect abdomen
Diaper Loosened   a. Auscultate for bowel sounds
                            b. Palpate: identify size of the liver, any other organs or masses palpable
                            c. Percuss
                         2. Palpate the femoral pulses, compare to radial pulses
                         3. Palpate for lymph nodes
                         4. Inspect the external genitalia
                         5. Males: palpate scrotum for descent of testes and other masses

Child Standing   1. Inspect spinal alignment as the child bends slowly forward to touch toes
                         2. Observe posture from anterior, posterior, and lateral views
                         3. Observe gait

Child Returns to Parent's Lap

Only as a last resort should you restrain the child for the fundoscopic, otoscopic, and oral examination. Lessen the fear of this aspect of the examination by permitting the child to handle the instruments, blow out the light, or use them on a doll or the parent. Attempt to gain the child's cooperation, even if it takes more time. It will be worth the effort as future visits will be more pleasant for the child.

1. Inspect eyes: corneal light reflex, red reflex, extraocular movements, fundoscopic examination
2. Otoscopic examination
3. Inspect nasal mucosa
4. Inspect mouth and pharynx

By the time the child is school age, it is usually possible to use an examination sequence very similar to that for adults.

OLDER ADULTS

The process of physical examination is the same for older adults as it is for younger adults. However, special considerations may be necessary. Many older patients have difficulty assuming some of the positions, particularly the lithotomy and knee-chest positions. Sometimes all that is needed is a little extra assistance and patience on your part, but otherwise you may need to utilize alternate positioning. The quality of clinical data is not necessarily compromised by having the patient lie on the side rather than assume a knee-chest position, for example. Your skill, thoroughness, and willingness to take whatever time is necessary are far more important in yielding accurate clinical data.

YOUR FUTURE RESPONSIBILITIES

As with all patients, those who are dying need your respect and attention. When we are face to face with death, we often cope by attempting to avoid it. We tend not to visit with the patient who is dying as often as with the patient we know will live. We are reluctant to confront the fact of dying, whether because of our own personal fears or because we unconsciously feel we have failed in our healing role. If you learn to understand your own feelings about death, you will be better equipped to care for the dying.

Learn to accept that the dying patient needs you as much as other patients. Talk with them, share with them. Never hesitate to participate in chit-chat. But become comfortable with being quiet and filling the silent spaces with the touch of a hand.

Above all, do not back away from the patient. This avoidance behavior denies them an assumptive world, the world that they had hoped for and may not have. We usually lack the wisdom to know precisely when that world will be truly denied, and backing away is a sign that hope is lost. Your attention and honest discussion offers hope without denial.

Time is a central issue in examining older patients. Time may be needed to develop the patient's trust and subsequent cooperation. A hurried pace or an impatient manner can create tension that may fluster or confuse an older patient. In neurologic testing reaction time may be longer or may require more intense stimuli.

As in the history, functional assessment is an important part of examining the older adult. Initial observation and interaction can provide a wealth of information regarding the individual's independent functional capacity. Watch how the patient walks, and observe the ability to follow instructions, remove clothes, and maneuver to the examining table. In doing this you will obtain information related to mobility, balance, fine motor skills (for example, unbuttoning clothes), and range of motion. In addition, you may gather some clues as to perceptual abilities and mental status.

Postexamination Decision Making

After you have acquired the information you need from the history and physical examination and any necessary laboratory tests, the process of arriving at a diagnosis continues. You must think about the range of possibilities, from the common to the rare. Common problems often have unusual presentations; the rare disease often has a common chief complaint.

One of your most important contributions is your sensitivity, which you must always keep operative. As you look for the hidden clue to a problem, you must also stay attuned to the slight variations in more obvious signs and symptoms. Such variations may have important implications that are not at first obvious. Clinical acumen develops from a sensitivity to the meaning of events and from your ability to intermingle the precise and the probable.

One of the cliches of medicine is that all findings should be unified into one diagnosis. Not always. More than one disease process can exist in the same person, an acute illness can be imposed over a chronic one, and a chronic disease can cycle through remission and relapse endlessly. You must be sure that all of the information is logically explained by your ultimate conclusions. You must explore the possibilities of error by accounting for *all* symptoms and signs and *all* abnormalities in any of the tests you have done.

Illness is almost always a multifaceted invasion of life. You may not be able to easily explain it all on a pathophysiologic level, because the physical is inseparable from the emotional. Therefore, you must not be misled into believing that a physical diagnosis and appropriate management will necessarily solve a problem. You must consider all the elements that might affect the patient's problems, from the physical to the emotional, social, and economic. This understanding is what distinguishes medicine as an art.

You cannot assume that patients will behave predictably or that they will invariably respond to your suggestions and instructions. We define adherence to our instructions as *compliance*. There is some arrogance in the inference that we order and the patient must respond. Still, compliance is one measure of your interaction with patients. The controlling factors include the nature of the relationship you have developed, your success in communicating the basics of the patient's condition, and the clarity of your instructions to the patient. Equally important factors are the patient's ability to understand the problem and the value the patient places on resolving the problem. For example, your primary concern may be a patient's hypertension, whereas the patient's main worry may be an alcoholic spouse. There are also times when a patient's refusal to comply may be appropriate. Always ask that the patient repeat the instructions to you so you can be sure he or she understands. This can also help you discover if there may be a problem with compliance.

Obviously most interactions with patients are unique, and you must be adaptable and flexible—particularly when your first efforts may be halting. Not always easy! You will at times be sorely tried, particularly when you are worried, rushed, and tired. If you are to be successful, you must also understand the biases you bring to each interaction with the patient. You will respond differently to children and the aged, to men and women, to blacks and whites, to rich and poor. You must know why and how.

Finally, you must be disciplined enough to pursue complete information, even when the solution seems obvious—for sometimes the obvious is wrong—and courageous enough to make the decision for urgency when the data are incomplete.

Dealing with the total patient—the physical, emotional, and social needs—is not an easy task, but you can succeed if you follow a disciplined course and learn how to be flexible within that course, guided by it, but not imprisoned by it.

Recording Information

After collecting the history and completing the physical examination, it is time to condense, organize, and record the collected raw data. The information in the patient's record enables you and your colleagues to care for the patient by identifying health problems, making diagnoses, planning appropriate care, and monitoring the patient's responses to treatment.

Appropriate medical terminology and a traditional organizational style make the record more readily understood by your colleagues. The patient's record is only as good as the accuracy, depth, and detail provided.

A customary organization of information from the interview and physical examination is used by most health professionals. Health agencies often incorporate the information in standardized forms or systems of recording. Following this customary outline of information enables all health professionals in the agency to use the patient information more efficiently.

Remember that the patient's record is a legal document, and any information contained in it may be used in court. It is your responsibility to present the data legibly, accurately, and in a manner that is representative of the examination. Any portion of the examination that has been deferred or omitted should be so noted, rather than neglecting to mention particular findings. It is appropriate in some circumstances to defer a portion of an examination, and stating the reason for that deferral is useful. A clear, exact record of your assessment, analysis of the problem, and a management plan is vital to your protection should there ever be a question relevant to your care of the patient.

As you begin to examine patients, it is often difficult to determine how to cluster information that will lead to a diagnosis. As a result, all collected information is initially part of the puzzle. With experience, you will be able to identify appropriate groupings of information, enabling you to better organize and synthesize the raw data. If you form a conclusion about the patient's problem too quickly, you might omit some necessary information from the patient's record. Your first attempts to write a complete history and physical examination will be lengthy, perhaps disorganized, but clinical experience will eventually lead to a more concise and organized record.

General Guidelines

It is certainly permissible to take brief notes about the patient's concerns and your findings during the course of the interview and physical examination. You should record certain data as you obtain it, specifically the vital signs and any measurements. However, do not try to record all the data during the visit, because writing must not detract your attention from the patient.

New information related to a previously discussed topic may emerge later in the interview or examination. Postponement of recording will sharpen your interviewing skills, but it also enables you to gather, reflect, and organize all the data appropriately before making the record final.

Your recall of information is limited, however, so recording should be completed as soon as possible after the examination. Avoid going on to other patients before completing the first patient's record. While this is sometimes unavoidable, you can easily become confused about which patient had a particular finding, or even forget to record an important finding.

It is important to be concise because of the volume of information collected during the examination. Use an outline form to avoid the repetition of phrases, such as "Patient states. . .". Abbreviations and symbols may be used judiciously and sparingly, but take care to use only those acceptable in your setting. Inappropriate abbreviations may be confusing to other health professionals. Similarly, avoid the use of words such as normal, good, poor, and negative, because these words are open to various interpretations by other examiners.

Document what you observe and what the patient tells you, rather than what you interpret or infer. Use direct quotes from the patient when a description is particularly vivid. Keep subjective and symptomatic data in the history, making sure none gets woven into the physical findings. Physical examination findings should be the result of your observation and interpretation of the patient's description. For example, when a patient complains of pain (a symptom) during palpation, you should note "tenderness" (a sign) in the record or report the patient's reaction to pain by crying, withdrawal, rigid posturing, or facial expression.

Description of Findings

It is as important to record expected findings, both subjective and objective, as it is to record the unexpected. Any physical finding that can change with age, disease, or pathology should be described in its present state. Detectable changes can then be better documented in the future. Details of a patient's history and examination are lost if not recorded, and clues about health changes over time would be unavailable.

Subjective Data

One way to record expected findings is to indicate the absence of symptoms—for example, "no vomiting, diarrhea, or constipation."

Unexpected findings should be described by their quality or character. Indicating the presence of pain without providing characteristics (timing, location, severity, quality) is not useful, either for future comparison or for determining the extent of the present problem. The severity of pain may be recorded on a scale of 1 to 10, with 0 being no pain and 10 the most pain ever felt by the patient. The severity of pain may also be described by its interference with activity. Note whether the patient is able to continue regular activity in spite of pain, or if it is necessary to decrease or stop all activity until pain subsides.

Objective Data   Relate physical findings to the processes of inspection, palpation, auscultation, and percussion, making clear the process of detection in the event confusion may occur. For example, "no masses on palpation" may be stated when recording abdominal findings. Details about expected objective findings should be included as well, such as, "tympanic membranes pearly gray, translucent, light reflex and bony landmarks present, good mobility bilaterally." Similarly, accurate description of unexpected objective findings should also be provided. Suggestions for recording the character and quality of objective findings follow.

LOCATION OF FINDINGS. Use topographic and anatomic landmarks to add precision to your description of findings. Indicating the liver span measurement at the midclavicular line enables future comparison, since measurement at this location can be replicated. The location of the apical impulse is commonly described by both a topographic landmark (the midsternal line) and an anatomic landmark (a specific intercostal space)—for example, "the apical impulse is 4 cm from the midsternal line at the fifth intercostal space."

In some cases, location of a finding on or near a specific structure (tympanic membrane, rectum, vaginal vestibule) may be described by its position on a clock. It is important that others recognize the same landmarks for the 12 o'clock reference point. For rectal findings use the anterior midline, and for vaginal vestibule findings (Bartholin's glands, episiotomy scar) use the clitoris.

INCREMENTAL GRADING. Findings that vary by degrees are customarily graded or recorded in an incremental scale format. Pulse amplitude, heart murmur intensity, muscle strength, and deep tendon reflexes are findings often recorded in this manner. Additionally, retinal vessel changes and prostate size are sometimes graded in a similar manner. See the chapters where these examination techniques are discussed for the grading system used to describe the findings.

ORGANS, MASSES, AND LESIONS. For organs or any type of mass, such as an enlarged lymph node, or skin lesion, various characteristics noted by inspection and palpation are described.
- Texture or consistency: smooth, soft, firm, nodular, granular, fibrous.
- Size: record in centimeters on two diameters, plus height if the lesion is elevated. Future changes in the lesion size can then be detected with assurance. This is more precise than comparing the lesion's size to fruit or nuts, which have different dimensions.
- Shape or configuration: annular, linear, tubular, elliptical, etc.
- Mobility: moves freely under skin or fixed to overlying skin.
- Tenderness
- Induration
- Heat
- Color: hyper- or hypopigmentation, redness or erythema, or the specific color of the lesion.
- Location
- Other characteristics: may include oozing, bleeding, discharge, scab formation, scarring, and excoriation.

DISCHARGE. Regardless of the orifice, discharge is described by color and consistency (clear, serous, mucoid, white, green, yellow, purulent, bloody or sanguinous), odor, and amount (minimal, moderate, copious).

ILLUSTRATIONS. Drawings can sometimes provide a better description than words and should be used when appropriate. You do not have to be an artist to communicate information. Illustrations are particularly useful in describing the origin of pain and where it radiates; the size, shape, and location of a lesion; and the comparison of findings in extremities, such as pulse amplitude and deep tendon reflex response.

Organizing the Data

The History

The patient's history, especially for an initial visit, provides a comprehensive data base. Information should be recorded appropriately in specific categories, usually in a particular sequence. The following organized sequence, which includes the appropriate information to record, will guide you in writing a comprehensive, narrative, traditional medical history.

IDENTIFYING INFORMATION. Patient's name, identification number, age, marital status, address, phone numbers, occupation, and date of visit. For children and dependent adults, make sure the names of parents or next of kin are noted. Health agencies often have forms with headings where this information is recorded. Make sure adequate identifying information is noted on each page of the record.

SOURCE AND RELIABILITY OF INFORMATION. Historian's identity: patient or the person's relationship to the patient. Indicate when the old record is used. State your judgment about the reliability of the historian's information.

CHIEF COMPLAINT. Reason the patient sought health care, stated in the patient's own words or paraphrased. Restate the information only if it makes the complaint more clear, making sure it is a statement of symptoms, not a premature diagnosis.

PRESENT ILLNESS. List and describe current symptoms of the chief complaint and their appearance chronologically in reverse order. Add the absence of certain symptoms you might expect from the pattern of the complaint.

Pertinent information from the review of systems, family history, and personal/social history should be noted with the findings. When more than one problem is identified, address each problem in a separate paragraph. Include the following details of symptom occurrence:

Time Intervals. Time of day, duration, and changes in symptoms over time.
Character or Quality. Severity, location, and nature, as for pain.
Association with Certain Events. Eating, activity, rest, etc.
Treatments. Those attempted and the outcome.
Interference with Daily Living

MEDICAL HISTORY. List and describe each of the following with dates of occurrence and any specific information available:

Hospitalizations and Illnesses. Surgery, injuries and disabilities, major childhood and adult illnesses.
Previous Health Care. Including past health examinations, immunizations, laboratory studies, obstetric care.

Current Health Habits or Risk Factors. Exercise, smoking, alcohol, salt, weight control.

Current Medications. Both prescriptions and over-the-counter, dosage and schedule.

Allergies. Especially to drugs, previous transfusion reactions, and to other substances.

FAMILY HISTORY. Information about the age and health of family members may be presented in narrative or genogram form.

Family Members. Include parents, grandparents, aunts and uncles, siblings, spouse, and children. For deceased family members, note the age at time of death and cause, if known.

Major Health or Genetic Disorders. Include hypertension, cancer, cardiac, respiratory, renal, cerebrovascular, or thyroid disorders, asthma or other allergic manifestations, blood dyscrasias, psychiatric difficulties, tuberculosis, diabetes mellitus, hepatitis, or other familial disorders.

PERSONAL/SOCIAL HISTORY. The information included in this section varies according to the concerns of the patient and the influence of the health problem on the patient's life.

Cultural Background

Family Structure. Who is at home, stresses, personal problems, events of a typical day, sources of strength, and the impact of the health problem or response to illness.

Educational and Economic Status

Environment. Home, school, work, structural barriers if handicapped, community services utilized.

REVIEW OF SYSTEMS. Organize in a general head-to-toe sequence, and include an impression of each symptom. Expected or negative findings are usually recorded as the absence of symptoms or problems. When unexpected or positive findings are stated by the patient, include details from further inquiry, as you would in the present illness. The following categories of information are generally included, but the sequence may vary:

- General overview
- Nutrition
- Integumentary
- Head, eyes, ears, nose, sinuses, mouth, and throat (HEENT)
- Neck
- Breast
- Cardiovascular
- Respiratory
- Endocrine
- Immunologic
- Hematologic
- Lymphatic
- Gastrointestinal
- Genitourinary
- Musculoskeletal
- Neurologic
- Psychiatric

List each system separately, rather than running all information together. See Chapter 1 for the range of information to include in each category. The detailed review of system-related history included in each chapter will help you write a more complete summary of problems noted by the patient.

Even though you make inquiries about symptoms and problems at the patient's level of understanding, use medical terminology to record your findings. Your agency may have a time-saving form listing important symptoms for each body system, which allows you to circle positive findings and add pertinent details.

The Physical Findings

The objective data are usually recorded by body systems and anatomic location. Begin with a general statement about the overall health status of the patient. All observations of physical signs should be described in the appropriate body system or region, usually organized in a sequence from head to toe. Take care to describe findings in detail, rather than make diagnostic statements.

List each anatomic location or body system as a separate category, using the groupings customary for your agency. The findings generally included in each category are listed below.

GENERAL STATEMENT
Age, race, sex, general appearance
Nutritional status, weight and height
Vital signs: temperature, pulse rate, respiratory rate, blood pressure
Communication skills, behavior, awareness, orientation, and cooperation with examination

SKIN
Color, integrity, texture, temperature, hydration
Presence of edema, excessive perspiration, unusual odor
Presence and description of lesions (inflammation, tenderness, induration, discharge, parasites, trauma)
Hair texture and distribution
Nail configuration, color, texture, condition, presence of clubbing

HEAD
Size and contour of head, scalp appearance
Distribution and texture of hair
Symmetry and spacing of facial features
Presence of edema or puffiness

EYES
Visual acuity, visual fields
Appearance of orbits, conjunctivae, sclerae, eyelids, eyebrows
Extraocular movements, pupillary shape, consensual response to light and accommodation, corneal light reflex, cover-uncover test
Ophthalmoscopic findings of cornea, lens, retina, optic disc, macula, retinal vessel size, caliber, and arteriovenous (AV) crossings

EARS

Configuration, position, and alignment of auricles

Otoscopic findings of canals (cerumen, discharge, foreign body) and tympanic membranes (integrity, color, landmarks, and mobility)

Hearing: Weber and Rinne tests, other stimuli

NOSE

Appearance of external nose, nasal patency

Presence of discharge, crusting, flaring, polyp

Appearance of turbinates, alignment of septum

Presence of sinus tenderness or swelling

Discrimination of odors

MOUTH AND THROAT

Number, occulsion, and condition of teeth; presence of dental appliances

Appearance of lips, tongue, buccal and oral mucosa, and floor of mouth (color, moisture, surface characteristics, symmetry)

Appearance of pharynx, tonsils, palate

Symmetry and movement of tongue, soft palate, and uvula; gag reflex

Discrimination of taste

Voice quality

NECK

Mobility, suppleness, and strength

Position of Trachea

Thyroid size, shape, tenderness

Presence of masses

CHEST

Size and shape of chest, anteroposterior diameter, symmetry of movement with respiration

Presence of retractions, use of accessory muscles

BREASTS

Symmetry, presence of masses, scars, tenderness, thickening, discharge, or dimpling

CARDIAC

Anatomic location of apical impulse

Rate, rhythm, amplitude, contour, and symmetry of apical impulse and pulse in extremities

Blood pressure: comparison between extremities; with position change

Palpation findings: pulsations, thrills, heaves, or lifts

Auscultation findings: characteristics of S_1 and S_2 (location, intensity, pitch, timing, splitting, systole, and diastole)

Presence of murmurs, clicks, snaps, S_3 or S_4 (timing, location, radiation, intensity, pitch, quality)

PERIPHERAL VASCULAR
Jugular vein distension and pressure measurement
Presence of bruits over carotid, temporal, renal, and femoral arteries, abdominal aorta
Temperature, color, hair distribution, skin texture, nail beds of lower extremities
Presence of edema, swelling, vein distension, Homans' sign, or tenderness of lower extremities

RESPIRATORY
Respiratory rate, depth, regularity, quietness or ease of respiration
Palpation findings: symmetry and quality of tactile fremitus
Percussion findings: quality and symmetry of percussion notes, difference in diaphragm level on inspiration and expiration
Auscultation findings: characteristics of breath sounds (vesicular, bronchial, bronchovesicular, adventitious), phase and location where audible
Characteristics of cough
Presence of friction rub, egobronchophony, whispered pectoriloquy, or bronchophony

ABDOMEN
Shape, contour, visible aorta pulsations
Auscultation findings: bowel sounds in all quadrants, their character
Palpation findings: organs, feces, masses, location, size, contour, consistency, tenderness
Percussion findings: areas of different percussion notes, costovertebral angle (CVA) tenderness

MALE GENITALIA
Appearance of external genitalia, circumcision status, location and size of urethral opening, discharge, lesions, distribution of pubic hair
Palpation findings: penis, testes, epididymii, vas deferens, contour, consistency, tenderness
Presence of hernia or scrotal swelling

FEMALE GENITALIA
Appearance of external genitalia, distribution of pubic hair
Palpation findings: tenderness, scarring, discharge
Vaginal speculum findings: appearance of vaginal mucosa, cervix, discharge
Bimanual findings: size, tenderness of uterus, adnexae, and ovaries

RECTUM
Rectal wall contour, tenderness
Prostate size, contour, consistency
Sphincter control, presence of hemorrhoids, fissures, skin tags
Color and consistency of stool

LYMPHATIC
Presence of lymph nodes in neck, epitroclear, axillary, or inguinal areas
Size, shape, tenderness, mobility, consistency, discreteness

MUSCULOSKELETAL
Alignment of extremities and spine, symmetry of body parts
Symmetry of muscle mass and strength, grading of strength
Range of motion, passive and active; presence of pain with movement
Appearance of joints; presence of deformities, tenderness, or crepitus

NEUROLOGIC
Cranial nerves: specific findings for each or specify those tested, if findings are recorded in head and neck sections
Cerebellar and motor function: gait, balance, coordination with rapid alternating motions
Sensory function, symmetry
Superficial and deep tendon reflexes: symmetry, grade
Mental status: thought processes, cognitive function, speech and language, mental status examination score

INFANTS

The organizational structure for recording the history and physical examination of newborns and infants is the same as for adults. The recorded information varies from the adult's primarily because of the developmental status of the infant. With the newborn you focus on their transition to extrauterine life and the detection of any congenital anomalies. Specific additions to the history and physical examination are listed below.

History

PRESENT ILLNESS. For newborns, include the details of the mother's pregnancy and any events occurring since birth. For older infants, record as for adults.

Details of Pregnancy. Weeks gestation, prenatal care, mother's illnesses, x-rays, drugs taken, bleeding, hypertension, diabetes, weight gained, planned pregnancy, complications of pregnancy.

Infant's Status at Birth. Respiratory status, color, Apgar scores if known; nutrition; nursery care needed.

MEDICAL HISTORY. None for newborns. Older infants should have prenatal and neonatal events added to this category, unless this information is directly related to the present problem.

PERSONAL/SOCIAL HISTORY. Focus on the newborn's and infant's family structure, number of siblings, presence of both parents, stresses of new infant in family, arrangements for infant care, and mother's plans to return to work.

FAMILY HISTORY. Focus on congenital anomalies and hereditary disorders in the family.

GROWTH AND DEVELOPMENT. Placement of this information is variable by agency or according to the purpose of the examination. For the infant with no growth or development problems, it may be recorded as history, review of systems, or stand alone. When a problem with growth or development is apparent, the information will be recorded in the present illness. Pass or failure of the Denver Developmental Screening Test (DDST) would be recorded with objective data.

Developmental Milestones. List with age attained.

Current Motor and Interaction Abilities. Specify current attainments unless the DDST is used, in which case this information is repetitive.

NUTRITION. Placement of this information varies by agency, appearing in the present illness, review of systems, or standing alone.

Breast Fed. Note the frequency, use of supplemental feedings and vitamins; mother's diet, fluid intake, concern with milk supply, any problems with nipple soreness, cracking, infections.

Formula Fed. Note the specific formula, preparation method, concentration and amount of water added, frequency fed, amount per feeding, total ounces per day, juice or water, vitamins.

Solid Foods. Age cereal and other foods introduced; specifics about feeding methods, amount, food preparation; response of infant to foods.

Physical Findings

GENERAL

Age in hours, days, weeks or months, sex, race

Gestational age

Length, weight, and head circumference with percentiles; for newborns note percentiles for gestational age

Infant state during examination (irritable, crying, sleeping, alert, quiet)

SKIN

Color, texture, presence of lanugo or vernix, Mongolian spot, nails

Presence of hemangiomas, nevi, telangiectasia, milia

HEAD

Shape, molding, forceps or electrode marks

Fontanel sizes, swelling

Transillumination

EYES

Red reflex, corneal light reflex, follows object with eyes

Swelling of lids, discharge

EARS

Shape and alignment of auricles, skin tags or pits

Startle to noise or response to voice

NOSE

Patency of nares, nasal flaring, discharge.

MOUTH

Palate and lip integrity

Presence and number of teeth

Strength of sucking, coordinated sucking and swallowing

NECK

Head position, neck control

Presence of masses, webbing, excess skin folds

CHEST

Symmetry of shape, circumference

Breast swelling or discharge

CARDIAC

No variations in manner of recording. However, peripheral vascular findings are often integrated in this section.

RESPIRATORY

Abdominal or thoracic breathing

Presence of retractions (intercostal, supraclavicular, substernal), presence of grunting or stridor

Quality of cry

ABDOMEN

Number of umbilical arteries and veins, stump dryness, color, odor

Any bulging or separation of abdominal wall

Apparent peristaltic waves

MALE GENITALIA

Appearance of penis, scrotum, position of urethra

Location of testes: descended, descendable, do not descend, not palpable

Urinary stream

Presence of hernia or hydrocele

FEMALE GENITALIA

Appearance of labia, presence of discharge.

RECTUM

Perforate, sphincter control

Character of meconium or stool, if observed

Presence of pilonidal dimple

MUSCULOSKELETAL

Alignment of limbs and spine

Presence of joint deformity, fixed or flexible; integrity of clavicles

Symmetry of movement in all extremities, hip abduction

Number of fingers and toes, webbing or extra digits, palmar creases

NEUROLOGIC

Presence and symmetry of primitive reflexes

Consolability, presence of tremors or jitteriness

Gross and fine motor development

CHILDREN AND ADOLESCENTS

As during infancy, some adaptations in recorded history reflect the developmental progress of the child. Such modifications in recording the child's history are described below.

PAST MEDICAL HISTORY. Prenatal and neonatal history is less important as the child gets older. Birth weight and major neonatal problems are generally included in the history of the initial examination until the child reaches school age. If a health problem can be related to birth events, more detail is recorded, often summarized from old records as the mother's recall will be a factor in getting accurate information.

PERSONAL/SOCIAL HISTORY. Record how the child gets along with parents, siblings, and other children; his or her behavior in group situations; and any evidence of family problems.

For older children record school performance: grade level, progress, adjustment to school, and the parent's attitude toward education. Note any habits of the child, such as nail biting or thumb sucking, and hobbies, sports participation, clubs, and temperament.

For adolescents add peer group activities, sexual activity, and concerns with identity and independence.

GROWTH AND DEVELOPMENT. For toddlers and young children, list motor and language milestones attained, age toilet trained, and age weaned from bottle.

The physical findings are recorded in the same format used for adults and infants. Some additional notations related to development include the following:

Breast. For females record the Tanner stage of breast development.

Genitalia. Record the Tanner stage of pubic hair and genital development as appropriate.

Neurologic. Findings should indicate developmental expectations of mental status, cerebellar function, cranial nerves, and deep tendon reflexes.

OLDER ADULTS

The organizational structure, again, does not vary from that recorded for other adults. A few modifications in aspects of the history and physical examination are made, primarily in personal social information.

PERSONAL/SOCIAL HISTORY. Identify the older adult's abilities to perform activities of daily living, such as meal preparation, dressing, walking, and engaging in meaningful activities. The community and family support systems should be noted as well.

GENERAL ASSESSMENT. Note the difficulty or need for extra time in assuming positions for the physical examination procedures.

The Problems and Diagnoses

Once the collected subjective and objective information has been organized, review all unexpected findings in the physical examination. Identify areas of concern, both those you detect and those the patient expresses. In many cases, the physical examination provides confirmation of problems identified during the interview.

A problem may be defined as *anything* that will require further evaluation (by laboratory tests or consultants) or attention. A problem may be related to any of the following:

- A firmly established diagnosis
- New findings related to a previous diagnosis
- New findings of unknown origin
- Unusual findings revealed by laboratory tests
- Personal or social difficulties

Using clinical judgment, make every effort to state problems as specifically as possible. To do this, cluster all collected subjective and objective information related to the same body system or body region. This includes symptoms expressed by the patient and physical findings, both expected and unexpected. Next, consider the underlying pathophysiology of the problem, be it physical, social, or emotional. Note the absence of a finding you would expect with a presumed diagnosis or an unexpected finding that does not fit the pattern of a presumed diagnosis. In each case, these might be important clues.

Review collected data repeatedly. Decide if the patient's complaints are related to the pattern of expected and unexpected findings. Think through all of the patient's nonverbal communication, attempting to determine if there is any information you may have neglected to ask or possibly not understood. Make every effort to integrate all of the subjective and objective findings to identify a problem or diagnosis, even those that do not appear at first to fit an established diagnosis. Then try to relate the problems you have identified to a pathologic, pathophysiologic, or psychopathologic process. Simply stated, this is the process of clinical decision-making.

Your ability to make clinical decisions will, of course, mature with practice and experience. As you gain experience, you will collect, analyze, evaluate, and synthesize information all at once, relating it to the chief complaint or your initial impression of the problem. Be cautious about doing this too quickly. Do not let your first thoughts narrow the focus of your questions during the history. The first thought will not always be the best one.

List your impression of the patient's diagnoses or problems at their most precise level. Avoid stating the problem as a tentative diagnosis or diagnostic guess. Do not use the term *rule out* in your list of problems, even when you do not have a diagnosis. It is much better to state the problem as you recognize it. The section of the patient's record in which the plan or evaluation notes are written may be used to discuss and plot further assessment to determine the diagnosis. Give yourself every opportunity to do this. While it is important to be concise, it is more important to be complete.

The Management Plan

Your plan to address and care for each of the patient's problems is the proposed management. Make sure you develop the plan jointly with the patient, relating it to the patient's reason for seeking health care.

The proposed management plan is usually written in a list and may include the following:

- Laboratory studies to be obtained and why
- Consultations requested and why
- Medications or appliances prescribed
- Special care to be provided (such as nursing, physical therapy, respiratory therapy)
- Surgery
- Diet modification
- Activity modification
- Follow-up visit schedule
- Goals for patient education

In addition to the above list of items, the plan may include the urgency of the problem, pathophysiology of the problem, and possible pathophysiologic relationship between problems.

Follow-Up Visits

Visits subsequent to the comprehensive health examination are often recorded in a more brief format, since the entire patient data base should not be repeated. In some circumstances, it may be necessary to make a lengthy repetition of subjective and objective data. A summary of changes in symptoms for each of the patient's problems, as well as the patient's cooperation and response to prescribed treatment, are recorded in the section on present illness. Only new or previously uncollected data should be added to other categories of the history. Physical findings for body systems related to the diagnoses or problems are recorded. Frequently the examination of other body systems has been deferred, unless in your judgment a complete physical examination was needed. The problem list and plan format are unchanged, unless there is need for revision because of new problems or because old problems have lower priority or are resolved.

In settings using the problem-oriented system of medical recording rather than the traditional medical record format, visits subsequent to the comprehensive health examination are recorded in a SOAP note format (acronym for Subjective, Objective, Analysis, Plan). Each SOAP note is tied to a specific problem found on the patient's problem list, which contains all health problems and diagnoses identified with their date of recognition and resolution.

The SOAP note contains an update of subjective and objective data, relevant only to one problem or to a new patient complaint. Progression or improvement in symptoms and physical findings, or new findings that differ from the last comprehensive examination, are specifically noted. If more than one problem is addressed during the visit, a separate SOAP note is written for each.

The analysis statement is a revised statement about the problem or diagnosis, either a refined diagnosis or progression of the disorder. This is followed by the plan, listing appropriate management for the current status of the patient's problem.

Sample Records

Ambulatory Adult

IDENTIFYING INFORMATION
Martha Smith, 55 years old, married   Date: 10-30-86
841 Foxtrail Drive   ID #: 54970B
St. Louis, MO 63146
555-6423
Registered Nurse

SOURCE AND RELIABILITY OF INFORMATION
Self—very reliable
Old record

CHIEF COMPLAINT. Time for annual examination. Has noticed pain in hands when doing needle work.

PRESENT ILLNESS. Pain and stiffness in hands, began about 6 months ago but seems to be increasing in severity and with shorter time of activity. Pain now occurs after 15 minutes of needlepoint or crocheting. Usually resolves with rest. Some stiffness in morning but does not currently interfere with ability to perform all job and household activities. Uses aspirin (650 mg q 4 hrs) when pain does not resolve with rest; good relief. No other joint pain or stiffness.

MEDICAL HISTORY

Hospitalizations and Illnesses. Hysterectomy for fibroids in 1975, usual childhood illnesses, no major adult illness, auto accident 1984 without major injury.

Previous Health Care. Annual physical, Td booster 5 years ago, oral polio vaccine 1972, dental care q 6 months, vision exam q year, Pap smear and mammogram 6 months ago, 2 pregnancies (1953 and 1956), vaginal delivery without complications.

Current Health Habits. Walks dog daily about ½ mile, 15 lb weight gain in last 2 years with varying success in dieting, no smoking, 2 to 3 glasses wine on weekends, 2 to 3 cups coffee and 1 glass iced tea daily.

Allergies. Hayfever in spring, no food or drug allergies known, no reaction to blood transfusions.

Current Medications. Aspirin 650 mg q 4 hours for pain when needed, Allerest for hay fever as needed, no prescription drugs.

FAMILY HISTORY. See genogram below. No history of cancer, tuberculosis, or respiratory, renal, thyroid, or psychiatric disorders.

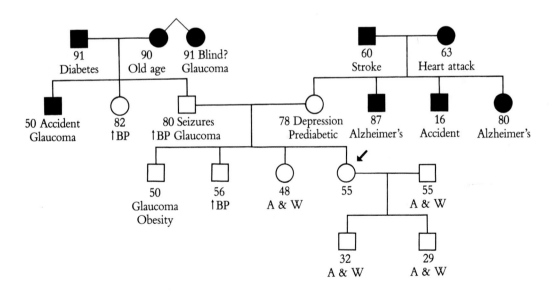

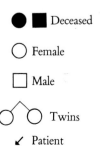

● ■ Deceased

○ Female

□ Male

○╱╲○ Twins

↙ Patient

PERSONAL/SOCIAL HISTORY. Lives with husband, a psychologist in private practice, in 3-bedroom home in good neighborhood. Works as RN in hospital clinic 3 days a week. Has 2 sons, both married with 2 children each. Visits each at least once a month. Both parents still living, in retirement home in town, visits them 2 to 3 times a week. Active in church and local arts and craft group. Needlepoint and crocheting main hobbies.

REVIEW OF SYSTEMS

General. Considers self in good health, feels her life is productive.

Nutrition. Would like to lose 15 lbs, currently 155 lbs, 5′6″, diets sporadically, uses 1200 calorie diabetic exchange lists, usually has good results when she persists, does own grocery shopping and cooking, rarely fries foods, binges on ice cream when traveling.

Integumentary. Several flat nevi, no change in appearance noted, bathes daily without special skin preparations, washes hair once a week, permanent and colored, nails short, crack and split frequently.

Head. Periodic headaches, no more than once a month, related to tension, pain up neck and back of head, relieved by aspirin.

Eyes. Wears glasses for reading, no pain, swelling, tearing, or halos around lights. Sees optometrist yearly.

Ears. No change in hearing noted; no dizziness, sensitivity to noise, or pain; some pressure and popping in ears when hay fever symptoms occur, resolves with Allerest.

Nose and Sinuses. Hay fever in spring, postnasal drip, no problem with sense of smell.

Mouth and Throat. No sore throats, hoarseness, change in voice, no dental appliances, no difficulty eating or chewing food, brushes and flosses daily.

Neck. No tenderness or stiffness currently, has had muscle spasm in past, some pain with auto accident 2 years ago, no enlarged lymph nodes noted.

Breast. No pain, tenderness, or nipple discharge; breast-self exam done when she remembers, about every 2 months; had mammogram 6 months ago; no history of masses.

Cardiovascular. No difficulty performing regular activities, no shortness of breath or chest pain, last BP 126/82; no pain, tenderness, discoloration, temperature change, or swelling in extremities; wears support hose for work, some varicose veins.

Respiratory. No history of asthma, bronchitis, or pneumonia; no breathing difficulties, cough, or pain.

Endocrine. No history of changes in thyroid, skin, hair, or temperature preference; no polydipsia or polyuria.

Immunologic. No frequent illnesses or recurrent infections.

Hematologic. Denies bleeding, excess bruising, anemia, blood transfusion.

Lymphatic. No known lymph node enlargement.

Gastrointestinal. No diarrhea, constipation, blood in stool, or emesis; has bowel movement every other day, brown, formed, no pain; hemorrhoids during pregnancies only; indigestion occasionally after eating fried or rich foods, resolves with Gelusil. Uses no laxatives, tries to add bulk to daily food intake.

Genitourinary. Voids 5-6 times a day, light yellow, no change in odor or color, no complaint of nocturia or dysuria, good control of stream; no history of sexually transmitted disease; no known genital lesions, discharge, pain, itching, dyspareunia; satisfied with sexual activity.

Musculoskeletal. No weakness, twitching, or pain other than in hands; no history of backache, fracture.

Neurologic. No problems with walking, balance, or sensations; no known changes in cognitive functioning; expresses concern with family history of Alzheimer's and her possibility of developing the disorder.

Psychiatric. Coping well with stress of older parents requiring increasing care; no history of long-term depression; gets depressed and anxious occasionally about growing old, but feels this does not interfere with her ability to work or lead a productive life.

PHYSICAL EXAMINATION

General. 55-year-old white female, alert, cooperative, well groomed, communicates well, makes eye contact, and expresses appropriate concern throughout history.

T 98.4° F, P 72, R 18

BP 130/76 sitting L arm, 134/80 supine L arm

Wt. 66.2 kg (150 lb), Ht. 165 cm (5′5″), about 50th percentile weight for height, medium frame

Skin. Pink, soft, moist, good turgor, no lesions or tenderness; nailbeds pink without clubbing, uniform thickness; hair with silky texture, thinning on crown, female distribution.

Head. Scalp without lesions or tenderness; symmetric, well-spaced facial features.

Eyes. Brows, lids, and lashes intact; no tearing; conjunctiva pink without discharge; pupils react equally to light and accommodation; extraocular movements intact; visual field equals examiner's, red reflex present, discs with well-defined border bilaterally; AV ratio 2:5, no crossing changes noted; cornea, lens, and vitreous clear; retina pink; macula present; Snellen 20/20 each eye without glasses; near vision 20/40 each eye without glasses, 20/20 with glasses.

Ears. Auricles in good alignment, without lesions, masses, or tenderness; canals with small amount dry cerumen; tympanic membranes gray, translucent; light reflex and bony landmarks present; no perforations. Rinne—air conduction > bone conduction bilaterally; Weber—no lateralization, repeats whispered words at 2 ft bilaterally.

Nose and Sinuses. Septum slightly to left of midline, patent bilaterally, mucosa pink and moist, no polyps or discharge; correctly identified coffee, chocolate, and orange odors bilaterally; no sinus tenderness with palpation or percussion.

Mouth and Throat. Buccal mucosa pink and moist, no lesions, 28 teeth in good repair, no movement, gingiva slightly spongy, tongue in midline without fibrillation, no lesions, uvula midline with elevation of soft palate, gag reflex intact, pharynx clear without erythema, no hoarseness, clearly enunciates words; correctly identified sweet, salty, and sour tastes bilaterally.

Neck. Trachea midline, freely moveable, thyroid lateral borders palpable, no enlargement or nodules noted, no palpable lymph nodes, full range of motion and good strength.

Chest and Lungs. AP diameter < lateral; muscle and respiratory effort symmetric, equal excursion, tactile fremitus symmetric, resonant percussion throughout, 4 cm excursion bilaterally, vesicular breath sounds throughout without adventitious sounds, even, quiet breathing.

Breasts. Moderate size, L slightly > R, nodular, granular consistency bilaterally, nipples erect without discharge, areolas equal size with Montgomery tubercles, no palpable axillary nodes, no dimpling.

Cardiovascular. Apical impulse barely palpable at 5th intercostal space, 4 cm from midsternal line, no heaves, lifts or thrills, S_1 and S_2 heard without splitting, no murmurs, S_1 heard best at base, S_2 heard best at apex, apical impulse timed with radial pulse, pulse regular rhythm, smooth contour.

Peripheral Vascular. Jugular venous pressure at sternal angle with 30-degree elevation; no carotid, renal, or abdominal bruits; no edema, swelling, or tenderness in lower extremities; Homans' sign negative; lower extremities warm, pink with symmetric hair distribution.

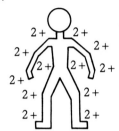

Abdomen. Rounded, faded scar from umbilicus to symphysis pubis; aorta midline with no visible pulsation; bowel sounds heard in all quadrants; tympanic percussion tones over epigastrium, remainder dull to percussion; liver span 6 cm at R midclavicular line by percussion; spleen percussed at L midaxillary line; liver, spleen, and kidney not palpable; no tenderness on palpation; no CVA tenderness; superficial abdominal reflexes intact.

Genital/Rectal. Deferred. Gyn exam 6 months ago.

Lymphatic. No palpable lymph nodes in neck, axillary, epitroclear, or inguinal areas.

Musculoskeletal. Heberden's nodes at distal interphalangeal joints on both hands; good mobility of hands but tenderness when making a tight fist bilaterally; no swelling, heat, or redness noted. Remainder of muscles appear symmetric, full range of active and passive motion, spine and extremities in good alignment, slight kyphosis.

Neurologic. Mini-mental status score = 26; coordinated, smooth gait; negative Romberg's sign; balance, rapid alternating movements, sensory functioning, and cranial nerves I-XII intact; Babinski negative bilaterally, no clonus.

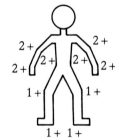

IMPRESSION
Osteoarthritis of hands
Family history of Alzheimers'—current mental status good
Otherwise in good health

MANAGEMENT PLAN
Ibuprofen 300 mg tid
Use no aspirin or aspirin products for other discomfort
Heat and rest for joint pain as necessary
Routine blood and urine studies
Maintain current health habits—breast self-examination every month, regular health and dental examinations
Return for physical in 1 year or sooner if arthritis discomfort or limitation of movement increases

FOLLOW-UP VISIT 6 MONTHS LATER

Chief Complaint. Pain in hands increasing.

Subjective. Initial relief of pain in hands with ibuprofen, 300 mg tid, able to resume needlework activities, but in last month more stiffness in hands in AM and pain with needlework after short time. She finds it difficult to rest hands as this interferes with other daily activities.

Objective. Heberden's nodes in distal interphalangeal joints both hands, Bouchard's nodes in proximal interphalangeal joints right hand, no swelling or heat present, tenderness on palpation, limitation of flexion in R hand, cannot make fist without pain; no tenderness, heat, limited motion of other joints

Analysis. Degenerative osteoarthritis

Plan.

Ibuprofen 400 mg qid
Consultation with arthritis specialist
Limit time doing needlework
Consider finding hobby requiring less intensive use of fingers
Return for annual exam in 6 months

Infant

IDENTIFYING INFORMATION

Tom Mitchell, 7-month-old male   Date: 11-3-86
Mother: Anne Mitchell   ID# 49076M
749 Delta Circle, Apt. 5   DOB: 3-25-86
Baltimore, MD 21205
555-9307

SOURCE AND RELIABILITY OF INFORMATION

Mother, reliable

CHIEF COMPLAINT. Needs immunizations

PRESENT ILLNESS. No illnesses or concerns at present. Cold last month resolved without fever or sequelae. Overdue for third shot.

MEDICAL HISTORY

Prenatal. Full-term infant, birth weight 7 lb 9 oz, 21 in, mother healthy throughout pregnancy, no x-rays, prescription drugs, or health problems. Began care in third month, vaginal vertex delivery after 10 hours labor, spinal anesthesia, awake for delivery, baby breathed immediately, in regular nursery, home with mother on third day.

Health Care. Has attended well baby clinic since birth, goes to Dr. Green or hospital clinic for illness. DPT 6-1-86, 8-8-86; OPV 6-1-86.

NUTRITION. Breast fed since birth, feeds 3 times a day, uses supplemental feeding of Similac, 8 oz., 2 times a day in effort to begin weaning, seems content. Started cereal and fruit at 5 months of age, now introducing vegetables and meat. Give about 2 tbs each of cereal and fruit in AM and 2 tbs each of vegetable and meat in PM. Takes 3 oz juice and 3 oz water and teething cookies a day. Eats eagerly. Gives ADC vitamins with iron.

PERSONAL/SOCIAL. Lives with parents and brother in 2-bedroom apartment, fair neighborhood, father employed as machinist, mother worked as secretary until Tom's birth, to return to work part time next week in temporary secretarial pool. MGM to care for Tom during day while she works. Live close to grandparents, many family events, attend church fairly regular. Money has been tight for last few months, but family has met major expenses. Tom was planned child, has been pleasure to family, some sibling rivalry with older son, father helps occasionally in care of infant, more in care of older son.

FAMILY HISTORY. Grandparents all living: MGF 55 years with hypertension, MGM 51 years A & W, PGF 60 years with myocardial infarction 2 years ago, PGM 58 with hypertension; mother 32 years and father 34 years, both healthy; aunts and uncles A & W, 1 brother 4 years old with asthma. No known diabetes, cancer, tuberculosis, renal, seizure, psychiatric, or hereditary disorders.

GROWTH AND DEVELOPMENT. Sitting without support for 2 weeks, reaches for objects, passes object hand to hand, babbles and coos, uses walker, has started scooting on floor, rolled over at 3 months.

REVIEW OF SYSTEMS

General. Happy infant, easy temperament, cries only when hungry or wet.

Integument. Slight jaundice after birth, never enough to be treated, birthmark on back, fingernails fully formed.

Head and Neck. Holds head up well, turns head in all directions.

Eyes. Seems to follow mother around room with eyes, no crossed eyes noted, no tearing, redness, or discharge noted.

Ears. No infections, turns head toward loud noise or family member speaking.

Nose. One cold with clear to whitish discharge from nose, lasted 1 week, saw doctor, given nose drops and Triaminic Syrup.

Mouth and Throat. 2 teeth, no difficulty sucking or swallowing.

Chest and Lungs. No problems breathing, noisy breathing with cold.

Cardiovascular. No known heart murmur, has never turned blue, does not tire easily with feeding, no excess perspiration.

Hematologic/Immunologic. No bleeding, bruises, no known anemia, has only had one cold, no swollen glands.

Gastrointestinal. No vomiting or diarrhea; spits up small amount of milk after feeding formula; bowel movement 2 times a day, light brown, mushy.

Genitourinary. Circumcised; good urine stream, 10 wet or dirty diapers a day, no odor to urine; had hydrocele at birth, not noted 2 months ago.

Musculoskeletal. Moves all extremities, stands with support, left foot turned in at birth, seems straight now, ready to buy first hard sole shoes.

Neurologic. No seizures or tremors noted.

PHYSICAL EXAMINATION

General. 7-month-old black male, alert, happy, playful, responsive, and easily consoled by mother.

T 37.1° C, P 100, R 26, BP 90/62 L arm

Wt 9.0 kg, 75%, Length 70 cm, 50%, Head Circ. 45 cm, 50%

Skin. Soft, smooth, light brown, good turgor, Mongolian spot over buttocks, cafe au lait spot 2 × 4 cm over R scapula, no lesions, nailbeds pink.

Head. Normocephalic, anterior fontanel 1 × 2 cm, flat, posterior fontanel closed, scalp without lesions, sparse fine hair, facial features symmetric, well spaced.

Eyes. Conjunctivae pink without discharge, no excess tearing, PERRLA, follows object with eyes 180 degrees, no epicanthal folds, blinks to bright light, corneal light reflex symmetric, red reflex present bilaterally, discs visualized with clear margins, retina pink.

Ears. Auricles well formed, good alignment with outer eye canthus; tympanic membranes pink, light reflex and bony landmarks present, good mobility bilaterally; turns head to noise and mother's voice.

Nose. No discharge, nasal mucosa pink, nares patent bilaterally.

Mouth and Throat. Buccal mucosa pink and moist; 2 lower incisors present, 2 upper incisors erupting; palate intact, uvula midline and soft palate rises symmetrically with crying, pharynx without erythema; drooling saliva, sucks and swallows well.

Neck. Trachea midline; thyroid not palpable; supple, full passive range of motion; no palpable masses or lymph nodes.

Chest and Lungs. Symmetric shape and expansion with respiration, no retractions, equal fremitus with crying, lungs clear to auscultation, even smooth respirations.

Cardiovascular. Apical impulse at 4th ICS, 3 cm from midsternal line; no heaves or thrills; S_1 heard loudest at apex, S_2 heard loudest at base, splitting of S_2 with inspiration, no murmurs; radial and femoral pulses strong and equal.

Abdomen. Soft, nontender, rounded, umbilical ring open 2 cm with hernia, bowel sounds heard all quadrants, liver palpable 1 cm below right costal margin at R midclavicular line, spleen and kidney not palpable, no other masses palpable, tympany percussed at epigastrium, dullness over remainder of abdomen.

Genitalia. Circumcised, urethral opening on tip of glans, both testes descended, no hernia or hydrocele noted, voids with good stream, urine pale yellow.

Rectal. Good sphincter control, no fissures or cracks.

Lymphatic. Few shotty anterior cervical lymph nodes, 1 cm in diameter, no other lymph nodes palpable.

Musculoskeletal. Spine and extremities in good alignment, full hip abduction bilaterally, muscle development symmetric, slight inward twisting of tibia bilaterally, 5 digits each hand and foot, weight bearing with support.

Neurologic. Good grasp, suck, head control, patellar and bicep deep tendon reflexes 2+ and Babinski positive bilaterally, no clonus, cranial nerves II-XII intact.

IMPRESSION
Healthy 7-month-old needing immunizations.
Mild internal tibial torsion, bilateral.
Umbilical hernia.

MANAGEMENT PLAN
DPT #3, OPV #2
Anticipatory guidance: nutrition, safety, fostering growth and development, shoes
Re-evaluate tibial torsion and umbilical hernia at 12 months of age
Hematocrit and hemoglobin

References

Alexander, M.M., and Brown, M.S.: Pediatric history taking and physical, diagnosis for nurses, ed. 2, New York, 1979, McGraw-Hill, Inc.

Andreoli, K.G., et al., editors: Comprehensive cardiac care: a text for nurses, physicians, and other health practitioners, ed. 5, St. Louis, 1983, The C.V. Mosby Co.

Andres, R., et al.: Principles of geriatic medicine, New York, 1985, McGraw-Hill Book Co.

Apple, D.J., and Rabb, M.F.: Ocular pathology: clinical applications and self-assessment, ed. 3, St. Louis, 1985, The C.V. Mosby Co.

Arenberg, D.: Estimates of age change on the Benton Visual Retention Test (BVRT), J. Gerontol. 37:87, 1982.

Arthritis Foundation Clinical Slide Collection on the Rheumatoid Diseases, Copyright 1972, The Foundation.

Athreya, B.H.: Clinical methods in pediatric diagnosis, New York, 1980, Van Nostrand Reinhold Co., Inc.

Ausband, J.R.: Ear, nose, and throat disorders, ed. 2, New Hyde Park, N.Y., 1982, Medical Examination Publishing Co., Inc.

Avery, M., and Taeusch, H.: Schaffer's diseases of the newborn, ed. 5, Philadelphia, 1984, W.B. Saunders Co.

Barness, L.A.: Manual of pediatric physical diagnosis, ed. 5, Chicago, 1981, Yearbook Medical Publishers, Inc.

Barsky, A.J.: Hidden reasons some patients visit doctors, Ann. Intern. Med. 94:492-498, 1981.

Bates, B.: A guide to physical examination, ed. 3, Philadelphia, 1983, J.B. Lippincott Co.

Battaglia, F.C., and Lubchenco, L.C.: J. Pediatr. 71:159, 1967.

Beckman, H.B., and Frankel, R.M.: The effect of physician behavior on the collection of data, Ann. Intern. Med. 101:692-696, 1984.

Behrman, R.E., and Vaughn, V.C.: Nelson's textbook of pediatrics, ed. 12, Philadelphia, 1983, W.B. Saunders Co.

Bellack, J.P., and Bamford, P.A.: Nursing assessment, a multidisciplinary approach, Belmont, Calif., 1984, Wadsworth, Inc.

Berne, R.M., and Levy, M.N.: Physiology, St. Louis, 1983, The C.V. Mosby Co.

Bernbeck, R., and Sinios, A.: Neuro-orthopedic screening in infancy, schedules, examinations, and findings, Baltimore, 1978, Urban & Schwarzenberg, Inc. (Translated by K. Eckstein.)

Birrell, J.F., editor: Logan Turner's diseases of the nose, throat and ear, ed. 9, Boston 1982, PSG Publishing Co., Inc.

Bluestone, C.D., and Shurin, P.A.: Middle ear disease in children: Pathogenesis, diagnosis, and management, Ped. Clin. NA, 21:379, May 1974.

Bobak, I.M., and Jensen, M.D.: Essentials of maternity nursing, St. Louis, 1984, The C.V. Mosby Co.

Bonadonna, G., editor: Cancer investigation and management Vol. 1, Breast cancer: diagnosis and management, New York, 1984, John Wiley & Sons, Inc.

Bowers, A.C., and Thompson, J.M.: Clinical manual of health assessment, ed. 2, St. Louis, 1984, The C.V. Mosby Co.

Brashear, H.R., Jr., and Raney, R.B.: Shands' handbook of orthopaedic surgery, ed. 9, St. Louis, 1978, The C.V. Mosby Co.

Brook, C.G.D.: Growth assessment in childhood and adolescence, Oxford, 1982, Blackwell Scientific Publications, Inc.

Buckler, J.M.H.: A reference manual of growth and development, Oxford, 1979, Blackwell Scientific Publications, Inc.

Bull, T.R.: A colour atlas of E.N.T. diagnosis, London, 1974, Wolfe Medical Publications, Ltd.

Bullock, B.L., and Rosendahl, P.P.: Pathophysiology: adaptations and alterations in function, Boston, 1984, Little Brown & Co., Inc.

Bunch, W.H.: Common deformities of the lower limb, Pediatr. Nurs. 5(4):18, 1979.

Burack, R.C., and Carpenter, R.R.: The Predictive value of the presenting complaint, J. Fam. Pract. 16:749-754, 1983.

Burns, K.R., and Johnson, P.J.: Health assessment in clinical practice, Englewood Cliffs, N.J., 1980, Prentice-Hall, Inc.

Burroughs Wellcome Co., Research Triangle Park, N.C.

Caldarelli, D.D., editor: Pediatric otolaryngology: new directions in therapy, New Hyde Park, N.Y., 1983, Medical Examination Publishing Co., Inc.

Carotenuto, R., and Bullock, J.: Physical assessment of the gerontologic client, Philadelphia, 1980, F.A. Davis Co.

Caufield, C.: A developmental approach to hearing screening in children, Pediat. Nurs. 4(2):39, 1978.

Centers for Disease Control: Chlamydia trachomatis infection, MMWR 34(suppl. 35) Aug. 23, 1985.

Chow, M.P., et al.: Handbook of pediatric primary care, ed. 2, New York, 1984, John Wiley & Sons, Inc.

Church, J.A., Allen, J.R., and Steihm, E.R.: New scarlet letter(s), J. Pediatr. Psychol. 38:793, 1980.

Committee on Maternal Nutrition, Food and Nutrition Board, National Research Council, National Academy of Sciences: Maternal nutrition and the course of pregnancy, Washington, D.C., 1970, The Committee.

Costa, R.J., et al.: Enduring dispositions in adult males, J. Pers. Soc. Psychol. 38:793, 1980.

Crouch, J.E., and McClintic, J.R.: Human anatomy and physiology, ed. 2, New York, 1976, John Wiley & Sons, Inc.

Cutler, P.: Problem solving in clinical medicine: from data to diagnosis, ed. 2, Baltimore, 1985, Williams & Wilkins.

DeAngelis, C.: Pediatric primary care, ed. 3, Boston, 1984, Little, Brown & Co., Inc.

De Groot, L.J., et al.: The thyroid and its diseases, New York, 1984, John Wiley & Sons, Inc.

Delancy, V., and North, C.: Skin assessment, Top. Clin. Nurs. 5(2):5-10, July 1983.

REFERENCES

DePalma, A.F.: Surgery of the shoulder, ed. 3, Philadelphia, 1983, J.B. Lippincott.

DeWeese, D.D., and Saunders, W.H.: Textbook of otolaryngology, ed. 6, St. Louis, 1982, The C.V. Mosby Co.

Diagnostic picture tests in clinical medicine, vol. 4, London, 1984, Wolfe Medical Publications, Ltd.

Diamond, S., and Dalessio, D.: The practicing physician's approach to headache, Baltimore, 1982, Williams & Wilkins.

DiSaia, P.J., and Creasman, W.T.: Clinical gynecologic oncology, ed. 2, St. Louis, 1984, The C.V. Mosby Co.

Donaldson, D.D.: Atlas of the eye: the crystalline lens, vol. V, St. Louis, 1976, The C.V. Mosby Co.

Dubowitz, L.M.S., et al.: J. Pediatr. **77**:1, 1970.

Dyken, P.R., and Miller, M.D.: Facial features of neurologic syndromes, St. Louis, 1980, The C.V. Mosby Co.

Ebersole, P., and Hess, P.: Toward healthy aging, ed. 2, St. Louis, 1985, The C.V. Mosby Co.

Edmonson, A.S., and Crenshaw, A.H., editors: Campbell's operative orthopedics, ed. 6, St. Louis, 1980, The C.V. Mosby Co.

Elias, E., and Hawkins, C.: Lecture notes on gastroenterology, Oxford, 1985, Blackwell Scientific Publications, Inc.

Eliopoulos, C., editor: Health assessment of the older adult, Menlo Park, 1984, Addison-Wesley Publishing Co., Inc.

Ezrin, D., Godden, J.O., and Volpe, R.: Systematic endocrinology, ed. 2, New York, 1979, Harper & Row, Publishers.

Fanaroff, A.A., and Martin, R.J.: Behrman's neonatal-perinatal medicine: diseases of the fetus and infant, ed. 3, St. Louis, 1983, The C.V. Mosby Co.

Fitzsimmons, V.: The aging integument: a sensitive and complex system, Top. Clin. Nurs. **5**(2): 32-38, July 1983.

Fleming, J.: Common dermatologic conditions in children, Am. J. Mat. Child Nurs. **16**, Sept.-Oct. 1981.

Folstein, M.F., Folstein, S.E., and McHugh, P.R.: "Mini-mental state": a practical method for grading the cognitive state of patients for the clinician, J. Psychiatr. Res. **12**:189, 1975.

400 Self-assessment picture tests in clinical medicine, London, 1984, Wolfe Medical Publications, Ltd.

Frankel, R.M.: From sentence to sequence: understanding the medical encounter through microinteractional analysis, discourse, Process **7**:135-170, 1984.

Frasier, S.D.: Growth disorders in children, Pediatr. Clin. North Am. **26**(1):3, 1976.

Frisancho, A.R.: New standards of weight and body composition by frame size and height for assessment of nutritional status of adults and the elderly, Am. J. Clin. Nutr. **40**:808, 1984.

Frisancho, A.R., and Flegel, P.N.: Elbow breadth as a measure of frame size for US males and females, Am. J. Clin. Nutr. **37**:311, 1983.

Gallager, H.S., et al.: The breast, St. Louis, 1978, The C.V. Mosby Co.

Gardner, H.L., and Kaufman, R.H.: Benign diseases of the vulva and vagina, St. Louis, 1969, The C.V. Mosby Co.

Garoon, O., et al.: Ophthalmology **87**:1128, 1980.

G.I. series: Physical examination of the abdomen, Chapter 2, Palpation, Richmond, Virginia, 1981, A.H. Robins Co.

Gibbons, M.B.: Circumcision: the controversy continues, Pediatr. Nurs. **10**(2):103-109, Mar.-April 1984.

Goodman, R.M., and Gorlin, R.J.: Atlas of the face in genetic disorders, ed. 2, St. Louis, 1977, The C.V. Mosby Co.

Gorlin, R., et al.: Syndromes of the head and neck, New York, 1976, McGraw-Hill Book Co.

Guyton, A.: Human physiology and mechanisms of diseases, ed. 3, Philadelphia, 1982, W.B. Saunders Co.

Guzzetta, C.E., and Dossey, B.M.: Cardiovascular nursing: body-mind tapestry, St. Louis, 1984, The C.V. Mosby Co.

Habif, T.: Clinical dermatology: a color guide to diagnosis and therapy, St. Louis, 1985, The C.V. Mosby Co.

Halstead, C.L., et al.: Physical evaluation of the dental patient, St. Louis, 1982, The C.V. Mosby Co.

Harvey, A.M., et al.: The principles and practice of medicine, Norwalk, Conn., 1984, Appleton-Century-Crofts.

Hawkins, J., and Gorvine, B.: Postpartum nursing: health care of women, New York, 1985, Springer Publishing Co., Inc.

Herzog, L.W.: Prevalence of lymphadinophosis of the head and neck in infants and children, Clin. Pediatr. **22**:485, 1983.

Hillman, R.S., et al.: Clinical skills: interviewing, history taking, and physical diagnosis, New York, 1981, McGraw-Hill Book Co.

Hoekelman, R.A., et al.: Principles of pediatrics: health care of the young, New York, 1978, McGraw-Hill Book Co.

Hogstel, M.: Skin care for the aged, J. Gerontol. Nurs. **9**:8, 1983.

Hughes, J.G.: Synopsis of pediatrics, ed. 6, St. Louis, 1984, The C.V. Mosby Co.

Jolly, H.: Diseases of children, ed. 4, Oxford, 1981, Blackwell Scientific Publications, Ltd.

Judge, R., Zuidema, G., and Fitzgerald, F.: Clinical diagnosis, ed. 4, Boston, 1982, Little, Brown & Co., Inc.

Kampmeier, R.H., and Blake, T.M.: Physical examination in health and disease, ed. 4, Philadelphia, 1970, F.A. Davis Co.

Katzman, R.: Alzheimer's disease, N. Engl. J. Med. **314**:964, 1986.

Kaye, D., and Rose, L.F., editors: Fundamentals of internal medicine, St. Louis, 1983, The C.V. Mosby Co.

Keith, N.M., Wagner, H.P., and Barker, N.W.: Some different types of essential hypertension: their course and prognosis, Am. J. Med. Sci. **197**:337, 1939.

Kelley, W.N., et al.: Textbook of rheumatology, ed. 2, Philadelphia, 1985, W.B. Saunders Co.

Ketenjian, A.Y.: Muscular dystrophy: diagnosis and treatment, Orthop. Clin. North Am. **9**(1):25, January 1978.

Kiene, R.H., and Johnson, K.A. In American Academy of Orthopedic Surgeons: Symposium on the foot and ankle, St. Louis, 1983, The C.V. Mosby Co.

Klenerman, L., editor: The foot and its disorders, ed. 2, Oxford, 1982, Blackwell Scientific Publications, Ltd.

Korones, S.B.: High-risk newborn infants: the basis for intensive nursing care, ed. 4, St. Louis, 1986, The C.V. Mosby Co.

Krajicek, M.J., and Tomlinson, A.T.: Detection of developmental problems in children, ed. 2, Baltimore, 1983, University Park Press.

Kraytman, M.: The complete patient history, New York, 1979 McGraw-Hill Book Co.

Larsson, L., and Karlsson, J.: Isometric and dynamic endurance as a function of age and skeletal muscle characteristics, Acta Physiol. Scand. **104**:129, October 1978.

Lloyd-Davies, R.W., Gow, J.G., and Davies, D.R.: Color atlas of urology, London, 1983, Wolfe Medical Publications, Ltd.

Lowrey, G.H.: Growth and development of children, ed. 8, Chicago, 1986, Year Book Medical Publishers, Inc.

Lubchenco, L.C., et al.: J. Pediatr. **37**:403, 1966.

Lubinsky, M.: Neonatal assessment for anomalies and syndromes, Pediatr. Basics **37**:1, 1984.

Mahan, L.K., and Rees, J.M.: Nutrition in adolescence, St. Louis, 1984, Times Mirror/Mosby College Publishing.

Malasanos, L., et al.: Health assessment, ed. 3, St. Louis, 1986, The C.V. Mosby Co.

Mancall, E.L.: Essentials of the neurologic examination, ed. 2, Philadelphia, 1981, F.A. Davis Co.

Mann, R.A., editor: Surgery of the foot, ed. 5, St. Louis, 1986, The C.V. Mosby Co.

Mazur, T.: Ambiguous genitalia: detection and counseling, Pediatr. Nurs. **9**(6):417-422, Nov.-Dec., 1983.

Mazzaferri, E.L.: Endocrinology case studies, ed. 2, Flushing, N.Y., 1975, Medical Examination Publishing Co., Inc.

McDonald, R.E., and Avery, D.R.: Dentistry for the child and adolescent, ed. 4, St. Louis, 1983, The C.V. Mosby Co.

McKusick, V.A.: Heritable disorders of connective tissues, ed. 4, St. Louis, 1972, The C.V. Mosby Co.

Medcom: Selected topics in ophthalmology, Medcom Clinical Lecture Guides, Garden Grove, Calif., 1983, Medcom, Inc.

Milford, L.: The hand, ed. 2, St. Louis, 1982, The C.V. Mosby Co.

Moore, K.L.: The developing human: clinically oriented embryology, ed. 2, Philadelphia, 1977, W.B. Saunders Co.

Mott, S., Fazekas, N., and James, S.: Nursing care of children and families, Menlo Park, Calif., 1985, Addison-Wesley Publishing Co., Inc.

Mountcastle, V.B.: Medical physiology, ed. 14, St. Louis, 1980, The C.V. Mosby Co.

National Center for Health Statistics: NCHS growth charts, 1976, Monthly Vital Statistics Report, vol. 25, no. 3, suppl. 9 (HRA) 76-1120, Health Resources Administration, Rockville, Maryland, June, 1976.

Nellhaus, G.: Head circumference from birth to eighteen years, Pediatrics **41**:106, 1968.

Newell, F.W.: Ophthalmology, principles and concepts, ed. 6, St. Louis, 1986, The C.V. Mosby Co.

Owen, G.M.: Measurement, recording, and assessment of skin-fold thickness in childhood and adolescence: a report of a small meeting, Am. J. Clin. Nutr. **35**:629, 1982.

Parsons, C., editor: Diagnosis of breast disease, Baltimore, 1983, University Park Press.

Peck, E.B., and Ullrich, H.D.: Children and weight: a changing perspective, Berkley, Calif., 1985, Nutrition Communications Associates.

Pfeifer, M.A., et al.: Differential changes of autonomic nervous function with age in man, Am. J. Med. **75**:249, 1983.

Pipes, P.: Nutrition in infancy and childhood, ed. 3, St. Louis, 1985, The C.V. Mosby Co.

Potter, P.M., and Perry, A.G.: Basic nursing, St. Louis, 1987, The C.V. Mosby Co.

Prior, J.A., et al.: Physical diagnosis: the history and examination of the patient, ed. 6, St. Louis, 1981, The C.V. Mosby Co.

Pritchard, J.A., MacDonald, P.C., and Gant, N.F.: Williams obstetrics, ed. 17, Norwalk, Conn., 1985, Appleton-Century-Croft.

Raskin, N., and Appenzeller, K.O.: Headache. In Smith, L.H., Jr., editor: Major problems in internal medicine, Philadelphia, 1980, W.B. Saunders Co.

Roter, D.L.: Patient participation in the patient-provider interaction: the effects of patient question asking on the quality of interaction, satisfaction and compliance. In Wolf, G.A., editor: Collecting data from patients, Baltimore, 1977, University Park Press.

Rudy, E.B.: Advanced neurological and neurosurgical nursing, St. Louis, 1984, The C.V. Mosby Co.

Ryan, N.: Recurrent abdominal pain among school-aged children, Am. J. Mat. Child Nurs. **11**:102-106, Mar.-April 1986.

Sapar, J.R.: Headache disorders—current concepts and treatment strategies, Boston, 1983, PSG Publishing Co., Inc.

Saunders, W.H., et al.: Nursing care in eye, ear, nose and throat disorders, ed. 4, St. Louis, 1979, The C.V. Mosby Co.

Scanlon, J.W., et al.: A system of newborn physical examination, Baltimore, 1979, University Park Press.

Scherzer, A.L., and Tscharnuter, I.: Early diagnosis and therapy in cerebral palsy, New York, 1982, Marcel Dekker, Inc.

Schneider, H.A., et al.: Nutritional support of medical practice, New York, 1977, Harper & Row, Publishers.

Schneiderman, H.: The review of systems, an important part of comprehensive examination, Postgrad. Med. **71**:151-158, June 1982.

Sculco, T.P., editor: Orthopedic care of the geriatric patient, St. Louis, 1985, The C.V. Mosby Co.

Silen, W.: Cope's early diagnosis of the acute abdomen, ed. 16, New York, 1983, Oxford University Press.

Silverman, A., and Roy, C.: Pediatric clinical gastroenterology, ed. 3, St. Louis, 1983, The C.V. Mosby Co.

Silverman, W.A., and Andersen, D.H.: A controlled clinical trial of effects of water mist on obstructive respiratory signs, death rates, and necropsy findings among premature infants, Pediatrics **17**:1, 1956.

Smith, D.W.: Growth and its disorders, Philadelphia, 1977, W.B. Saunders Co.

Sprague, J.: Vision screening. ed. 2. In Krajicek, M., and Tomlinson, A.I.T., editors: Detection of developmental problems in children, Baltimore, 1983, University Park Press.

Staheli, L.T.: Torsional deformity, Pediatr. Clin. North Am. **24**(4):799, 1977.

Stein, H.A., and Slatt, B.J.: The ophthalmic assistant: fundamentals and clinical practice, ed. 4, St. Louis, 1983, The C.V. Mosby Co.

Steinberg, F.U., editor: Care of the geriatric patient, ed. 6, St. Louis, 1983, The C.V. Mosby Co.

Stewart, W.D., Danto, J.L., and Maddin, S.: Dermatology: diagnosis and treatment of cutaneous disorders, St. Louis, 1978, The C.V. Mosby Co.

Swaiman, K.F., and Wright, F.S.: The practice of pediatric neurology, ed. 2, St. Louis, 1982, The C.V. Mosby Co.

Swanson, A.B.: Flexible implant arthroplasty in the hand and extremities, St. Louis, 1973, The C.V. Mosby Co.

Tanner, J.M.: Foetus into man: physical growth from conception to maturity, Cambridge, Mass., 1978, Harvard University Press.

Tanner, J.M.: Growth at adolescence, ed. 2, Oxford, 1962, Blackwell Scientific Publications, Ltd.

Tanner, J.M., and Davies, P.S.W.: Clinical longitudinal standards for height and height velocity for North American children, J. Pediatr. **107**:317, 1985.

Tanner, J.M., and Whitehouse, R.H.: Clinical longitudinal standards for height, weight, height velocity, weight velocity, and the stages of puberty, Arch. Dis. Child. **51**:170, 1976.

Thompson, J.M., et al.: Clinical nursing, St. Louis, 1986, The C.V. Mosby Co.

Trauner, D.A.: Childhood neurological problems: a textbook for health professionals, Chicago, 1979, Year Book Medical Publishers, Inc.

Trevor-Roper, P.D., and Curran, P.V.: The eye and its disorders, ed. 2, Oxford, 1984, Blackwell Scientific Publications, Ltd.

Urdang, L., editor: Mosby's medical and nursing dictionary, St. Louis, 1983, The C.V. Mosby Co.

Varney, H.: Nurse-midwifery, ed. 2, Boston, 1986, Blackwell Scientific Publications, Inc.

Walsh, P.C., et al.: Campbell's urology, ed. 5, Philadelphia, 1986, W.B. Saunders Co.

Waring, W.W., and Jeansonne, L.O.: Practical manual of pediatrics, ed. 2, St. Louis, 1982, The C.V. Mosby Company.

Wasserman, R.C., and Inui, T.S.: Systematic analysis of clinician-patient interaction: a critique of recent approaches with suggestions for future research. Med. Care **21**:279-93, 1983.

Whaley, L.F., and Wong, D.L.: Nursing care of infants and children, ed. 2, St. Louis, 1983, The C.V. Mosby Co.

Willson, J.R., Carrington, E.R., and Ledger, W.J.: Obstetrics and gynecology, ed. 7, St. Louis, 1983, The C.V. Mosby Co.

Wilson, J.D., and Walsh, P.C.: In Harrison, J.H., et al.: Campbell's urology, ed. 4, Philadelphia, 1979, W.B. Saunders Co.

Wolf, G.A.: Collecting data from patients, Baltimore, 1977, University Park Press.

Wong, D.L., and Whaley, L.F.: Clinical handbook of pediatric nursing, St. Louis, 1981, The C.V. Mosby Co.

Wood, N.K., and Goaz, P.W.: Differential diagnosis of oral lesions, ed. 3, St. Louis, 1985, The C.V. Mosby Co.

Wynn-Davies, R.: Heritable disorders in orthopedics, Orthop. Clin. North Am. **9**(1):3, 1978.

Zelle, R.S., and Coyner, A.B.: Developmentally disabled infants and toddlers: assessment and intervention, Philadelphia, 1983, F.A. Davis Co.

Ziegel, E.E., and Cranley, M.S.: Obstetric nursing, ed. 8, New York, 1984, Macmillan Publishing Co.

Glossary

abduction movement of the limbs toward the lateral plane or away from the axial line of a limb.

accommodation adjustment of the eye for various distances through modification of the lens curvature; negative accommodation is adjustment for far vision by relaxation of ciliary muscle; positive accommodation is adjustment for near vision by contraction of ciliary muscle.

acini cells milk-producing alveoli located in the glandular tissue of the breast.

adduction movement of the limbs toward the medial plane of the body or toward the axial line of a limb.

adenitis inflammation of a lymph node or a group of lymph nodes.

adnexae appendages; adnexae uteri are the structures adjacent to the uterus including the ovaries, fallopian tubes, and uterine ligaments.

adventitious accidental or acquired, not natural or hereditary; located away from the usual place.

alveolar ridge bony prominence of the maxilla and mandible that supports the teeth or dentures.

amblyopia reduced vision in an eye that appears structurally normal and without detectable cause when examined, including inspection with an ophthalmoscope.

anesthesia partial or complete loss of sensation.

aneurysm a balloon-like swelling of the wall of an artery, vein, or heart; generally the result of a congenital defect in the wall or degenerative disease or infection (e.g., atherosclerosis or syphilis); dissecting aneurysm is longitudinal splitting of the arterial wall from hemorrhage.

angle of Louis (sternal angle) the angle between the manubrium and the body of the sternum.

annulus a ring or circular structure; tympanic annulus is a fibrous ring around the tympanic membrane that looks whiter and denser than the membrane itself.

anosmia absence of the sense of smell.

anthropometry measurement of the size, weight, and proportions of the human body.

apex beat the visible or palpable pulsation made by the apex of the left ventricle as it strikes the chest wall in systole; usually located in the fifth left intercostal space, several centimeters to the left of the median line (midsternal line).

aphakia a condition in which part or all of the crystalline lens of the eye is absent, usually because of surgical removal for the treatment of cataracts.

aphasia impairment of language function in which speech or writing is not understood (receptive or sensory), words cannot be formed (expressive), or a combination of both.

apical pertaining to the apex or the area of the apex (top or tip) of a body, organ, or part.

appropriate for gestational age a weight classification of newborns associated with better health outcomes, the weight falling between the 10th and 90th percentiles on the intrauterine growth curve for the newborn's calculated gestational age.

apnea a temporary halt to breathing.

apraxia inability to execute a skilled or learned motor act, not related to paralysis or lack of comprehension; caused by a lesion in the cerebral cortex.

arrhythmia a deviation from the expected rhythm of the heart.

arteriovenous fistula a pathologic direct communication between an artery and a vein without an intervening capillary bed.

arteriovenous shunt the passage of blood directly from an artery to a vein, without an intervening capillary network.

articulation the ability to pronounce speech sounds, words, and thoughts clearly and fluently; the junction of two or more bones; contact of the occlusal surfaces of the teeth.

ascites abnormal intraperitoneal accumulation of serous fluid.

asterixis postural tremor characterized by nonrhythmic, flapping movements of wide amplitude; extended wrist or fingers suddenly and briefly flex and then return to their original position.

astigmatism an abnormal condition in which the light rays cannot be focused clearly in a point on the retina because of an irregular curvature of the cornea or lens.

ataxia impaired ability to coordinate muscular movement, usually associated with staggering gait and postural imbalance.

atelectasis incomplete expansion of the lung, either congenital or acquired.

athetosis slow, twisting, writhing movements with larger amplitude than chorea that commonly involve the hands.

atrioventricular valve refers to the tricuspid or mitral valves.

Austin Flint murmur a presystolic murmur, not unlike that of mitral stenosis, best heard at the apex of the heart; caused by aortic insufficiency.

autonomic nervous system the portion of the nervous system that regulates involuntary functions supporting life; divided into the sympathetic and parasympathetic nervous systems.

baroreceptor sensory nerves within the walls of the atria, vena cava, aortic arch, and carotid sinus that monitor blood pressure change.

barrel chest increased anteroposterior diameter of the chest, often with some degree of kyphosis; commonly seen with COPD.

Bartholin's glands (vestibular glands) mucus-secreting glands located posteriolaterally to the vaginal opening.

biferious pulse an arterial pulse with two palpable peaks, the second stronger than the first, but not markedly so; detected in instances of decreased arterial tension.

bifurcated having two branches, tines, or prongs.

bigeminal pulse a pulse in which two beats occur in rapid succession so that they seem coupled and distinct from the succeeding set of two. Each set is separated by a longer interval.

borborygmi rumbling, gurgling, tinkling noises heard on auscultation of the abdomen as a result of hyperactive intestinal peristalsis.

bossing bulging of the frontal areas of the skull; associated with prematurity and rickets.

boutonnière deformity fixed flexion of the proximal interphalangeal joint associated with hyperextension of the distal interphalangeal joint.

bradycardia a heart rate less than 60.

bradypnea slower than expected respiratory rate.

bronchial breathing harsh breathing characterized by prolonged high-pitched expiration with a tubular quality; frequently heard when lung tissue is consolidated.

bronchial fremitus adventitious pulmonary or voice sounds palpable over the chest or audible to the ear.

bronchiectasis persistent dilation of bronchi or bronchioles as a consequence of inflammatory disease, obstruction, or congenital abnormality.

bronchiolitis (bronchopneumonia) inflammation of the bronchioles, caused by bacteria or viruses.

bronchogenic originating from the bronchi.

bronchophony an exaggeration of vocal resonance emanating from a bronchus surrounded by consolidated lung tissue.

bronchovesicular pertaining to bronchial tubes and alveoli.

bruit an unexpected audible swishing sound or murmur over an artery or vascular organ.

bruxism compulsive unconscious grinding of the teeth.

bubo inflammation and swelling of one or a group of lymph nodes, particularly in the groin or axilla, often accompanied by suppuration.

buccal mucosa mucous membrane inside the mouth.

bundle of His a small band of modified heart muscle fibers that originates at the atrioventricular node, passes through the right atrioventricular junction to the interventricular septum where the fibers divide into right and left branches and enter the respective ventricles; this bundle carries the atrial contractual rhythm to the ventricles; an interruption results in some degree of heart block.

bunion abnormal prominence of the medial aspect of the first metatarsal head, with bursa formation, resulting in lateral or valgus deviation of the great toe.

bursa disk-shaped, fluid-filled synovial sacs that develop at points of friction around joints, between tendons, cartilage, and bone; they decrease friction and promote ease of motion.

canthus the angle at the medial or lateral margin of the eyelid; the medial canthus opens into a small space containing openings to the lacrimal duct.

caput succedaneum an edematous swelling of the scalp of the newborn resulting from labor.

cardiac cycle the complete sequence of cardiac action occurring from one heart beat to the next, including both systole and diastole.

cardiac impulse the thrust of the ventricles against the chest wall as a result of cardiac contraction.

cardiac output the amount of blood ejected by the heart, usually stated in liters per minute calculated by stroke volume × number of heart beats per unit of time.

cardiac reserve the heart's ability to respond to demands that exceed ordinary circumstances.

carrying angle the angle at which the humerus and radius articulate.

cellulitis inflammation of soft or connective tissue that causes a watery exudate to spread through the tissue spaces.

cephalhematoma a subperiosteal hemorrhage, usually benign, along one of the cranial bones; it generally results from birth trauma.

cheilitis inflammation and cracking of the lips.

choanae a pair of posterior openings between the nasal cavity and the nasopharynx.

chordee ventral curvature of the penis caused by a fibrous band of tissue; often associated with hypospadias or gonorrhea.

choreiform movements brief, rapid, jerky, irregular, and involuntary movements that occur at rest or interrupt normal coordinated movements; most often involve the face, head, lower arms, and hands.

choroid the thin, highly vascular membrane covering the posterior five sixths of the eye between the retina and sclera.

ciliary body the thickened part of the vascular tunic of the eye that joins the iris with the anterior portion of the coroid.

circumcorneal around the cornea.

circumduction circular movement of a limb (e.g., the shoulder) or the eye.

circumlocution the use of pantomime, nonverbal expressions, or word substitutions to avoid revealing that a word has been forgotten.

clonus rapidly alternating involuntary contraction and relaxation of skeletal muscles.

coarctation constriction, stricture, stenosis, or narrowing, as of the aorta.

cochlea a coiled bony structure within the inner ear; it contains the organ of Corti and perforations for the passage of the cochlear division of the auditory nerve.

cognition the mental process of knowing, thinking, learning, and judging.

colic gradual onset of pain that increases in crescendo fashion until it reaches a peak of severity, then slowly subsides.

colostrum yellow, milky secretion from the breast that precedes the onset of true lactation; composed primarily of serum and white blood cells.

concha a structure that is shell-shaped; the deep cavity in the auricle of the external ear containing the auditory canal meatus.

conductive hearing loss reduction in hearing acuity relating to interference of sound being transmitted through the outer and middle ear.

conjunctivitis inflammation of the conjunctiva caused by infectious agents or by allergies.

consolidation solidification of part of the lung into a firm, dense mass, particularly when the alveoli fill with fluid as a result of inflammation.

contracture permanent fixed flexion of a joint resulting from atrophy and shortening of muscles or from loss of skin elasticity.

coryza rhinitis; inflammation of the nasal mucous membranes, accompanied by swelling of the mucosa and nasal discharge.

craniotabes an unusual softness of the skull in infants with hydrocephalus and rickets; the skull feels brittle and has a ping pong ball snapping sensation when firmly pressed.

crepitus a crinkly, crackling, grating feeling or sound in the joints, skin, or lungs; the quality of sound is simulated by Rice Krispies in milk; the quality of touch is somewhat simulated by rubbing hair between the fingers.

croup an inflammation of the larynx, causing swelling of the vocal chords and sometimes severe obstruction; characterized by harsh, difficult breathing and a hoarse cough; usually occurs in young children.

cryptorchidism failure of one or both testicles to descend into the scrotum.

cyanosis a bluish or purplish color (may range from slight to intense) of the skin and mucous membranes because of insufficient oxygen levels in the blood.

deafness partial or complete loss of hearing.

decerebrate posturing rigid extension of all four extremities with hyperpronation of the forearms and plantar flexion of the feet.

dermatome the area of skin innervated by a single posterior spinal nerve.

development the process of growth and differentiation; the acquisition of function associated with cell differentiation and maturation of individual organ systems.

dextrocardia location of the heart in the right hemithorax, either by displacement from disease or congenital mirror-image reversal.

diastole that time between two contractions of the heart when the muscles relax, allowing the chambers to fill with blood; diastole of the atria precedes that of the ventricles; diastole alternates, usually in a regular rhythm, with systole.

dicrotic notch the notch in a pulse tracing between two elevations for each pulse beat.

dicrotic pulse a pulse characterized by two peaks, the second usually weaker than the first.

diplopia double vision caused by defective function of the extraocular muscles or a disorder of the nerves that innervate the muscles.

dizziness (vertigo) sensation of an inability to maintain normal balance in a standing or sitting position.

dorsiflexion backward bending or flexion of a joint.

dysarthria defective articulation secondary to a motor deficit involving the lips, tongue, palate, or pharynx.

dyspareunia difficult or painful sexual intercourse.

dysphagia difficulty in swallowing.

dyspnea difficult and labored breathing, shortness of breath.

dysrhythmia unexpected variation in the regular rhythm of the heart.

ecchymosis (bruise) discoloration of the skin or mucous membrane as the result of hemorrhage into subcutaneous tissue.

echolalia automatic and meaningless repetition of another's words or phrases.

edema excessive accumulation of fluid in the cells, tissues, or serous cavities of the body.

edentulous without teeth.

effusion loss of fluid from the blood vessels or lymphatics into the tissues or a body cavity.

ejection murmur a diamond-shaped systolic murmur occupying most but not necessarily all of systole; produced by the ejection of blood into the aorta or pulmonary artery.

electrocardiogram (ECG) a graphic record of the heart's electrical currents obtained with an electrocardiograph.

embolism obstruction of an artery by a blood clot or foreign matter.

emphysema pathologic accumulation of air in tissue or organs, especially the lungs.

endocardium the innermost membrane lining the heart cavities that is continuous with the lining of the blood vessels; its slippery surface eases the flow of blood.

epicardium the inner visceral layer of the serous pericardium lying directly on the heart, forming the outermost layer of the heart wall.

epigastrium the upper central region of the abdomen between the costal margins and a line drawn horizontally across the lowest costal margin.

epispadias a congenital defect resulting in the urethra opening on the dorsum of the penis.

epulis a tumor on the gingiva.

esotropia (cross-eye) the inward or nasal deviation of an eye.

eustachian tube the cartilaginous and bony passage between the nasopharynx and the middle ear that allows equalization of air pressure between the inner ear and external pressure.

exotrophia (walleye) the outward or temporal deviation of an eye.

extension movement that increases the angle between two adjoining bones to 180 degrees, bringing a limb toward a straight line.

external rotation lateral turning of a limb.

exudate fluid that has escaped from tissue or capillaries, usually after injury or inflammation, typically containing protein and white blood cells.

facies expression or appearance of the face; often used to describe characteristic expressions of disease states or congenital anomalies.

fasciculation a localized, uncoordinated twitching of a single muscle group innervated by a single motor nerve filament; it is visible or palpable.

fibrosis the formation of excessive connective tissue as an attempt to repair damage or as a reaction to foreign material, resulting in scarring and thickening.

flaccid muscles that are weak, soft, flabby, and lacking expected muscle tone.

flank the posterior part of the body below the ribs and above the ilium.

flatulence the presence of excessive air or gases in the stomach or intestines, causing abdominal distention and resulting in rectal passage.

flexion movement that decreases the angle between two articulating bones, bending the limb.

floater one or more spots that appear to drift in front of the eye; caused by a shadow cast on the retina by vitreous debris or separation of the vitreous humour from the retina.

fluctuant a wavelike motion that is felt when a structure containing liquid is palpated.

flutter a rapid vibration or pulsation that impedes appropriate function.

fontanels membranous spaces at the juncture of an infant's cranial bones that later ossify.

foramen ovale the communication between the two atria of the fetal heart; if it remains patent, blood shunts between the atria after birth, usually from left to right.

Fordyce's spots ectopic sebaceous glands of the buccal mucosa appearing as small yellow-white raised lesions.

fornix arched structure; vaginal fornix is the recess between the cervix and the vaginal wall; although one continuous structure, the vaginal fornix is anatomically divided into the anterior, posterior, and lateral fornices.

fourchette ridges of tissue formed by the fusion of the labia minora at the posterior aspect of the vulva.

fovea centralis a tiny pit in the center of the macula lutea that is the area of clearest vision, permitting light to fall on the cones; it appears as an oval yellow spot on the retina and is free of blood vessels.

fremitus a tremor vibration in any part of the body, detectable on palpation.

frenulum, lingual band of tissue that attaches the ventral surface of the tongue to the floor of the mouth.

friction rub a sound audible through the stethoscope, resulting from the rubbing of opposed, inflamed serous surfaces.

gestational age fetal age of a newborn, calculated from the number of completed weeks since the first day of the mother's last menstrual period to the date of birth.

gingivae gums of the mouth.

glaucoma an abnormal condition of elevated pressure within an eye resulting from obstruction of the outflow of aqueous humor.

goiter cystic or fibrous enlargement of the thyroid gland, often related to thyroid dysfunction.

graphesthesia the ability to recognize symbols, shapes, numbers, and letters traced on the skin.

helix the prominent outer rim of the auricle of the ear.

hemangioma a benign tumor of newly formed blood vessels that may occur anywhere in the body, most readily noticed in the skin and subcutaneous tissues.

hemodynamic pertaining to the movement of blood and other aspects of the circulation.

hemoptysis coughing up blood or blood-stained sputum from the respiratory tree.

hernia protrusion of an organ or tissue through an abnormal opening.

hilus of the lung a hollow depression on the mediastinal surface of each lung, which is the point of entry of the bronchus, blood vessels, nerves, and lymphatics.

hirsutism excessive hair growth, especially an adult male pattern of hair distribution in women; usually related to heredity, hormonal dysfunction, porphyria, or medications.

holodiastolic occupying all of diastole.

holosystolic occupying all of systole.

Homans' sign pain or discomfort behind the knee or in the calf when the ankle is gently dorsiflexed while the knee is flexed; it suggests thrombosis of the leg veins.

hyperesthesia unusual increased sensitivity to sensory stimuli, such as touch or pain.

hyperextension a position of maximum extension.

hyperkeratosis overgrowth of the corneous layer of the skin or the cornea.

hyperkinesia excessive muscular activity; hyperactivity.

hyperopia (farsightedness) a refractive error in which light rays entering the eye are focused behind the retina.

hyperpnea respiration that is deeper and more rapid than expected.

hyperresonance greater than expected resonance that is lower pitched in response to percussion of the chest wall or abdomen.

hyperthyroidism excessive activity of the thyroid gland with an increase in thyroid secretion.

hyperventilation a state in which an increased amount of air enters the lungs, usually a result of deep and rapid breathing; if severe, it leads to alkalosis with the excessive loss of carbon dioxide.

hypokinesia abnormally diminished muscular activity.

hypospadias a congenital defect in which the urethra opens on the ventral surface of the penis rather than on the glans.

hypotension a condition in which arterial blood pressure is lower than expected.

hypothyroidism diminished activity of the thyroid gland with consequent reduction of thyroid hormone.

incus one of the three ossicles of the middle ear, lying between the malleus and stapes.

induration excessive hardening or firmness of any body site.

infarction an acute interruption to the blood supply of a part of the body by thrombi, emboli, extrinsic pressure, or twisting of blood vessels resulting in tissue death at the involved site.

infrapatellar fat pad the soft tissue palpable in front of the joint space on either side of the patellar tendon.

intermittent claudication cramping pain and limping commonly in the calf brought on by walking; caused by ischemia of the muscles, usually from atheroma that narrow the leg's arteries.

internal rotation   medial turning of a limb.

intertriginous   an area where opposing skin surfaces touch and may rub, such as skin folds in the axillae, groin, inner thighs, and beneath large breasts.

introitus   the vaginal opening.

isthmus   a narrow band of tissue connecting the two lateral lobes of the thyroid.

joint instability   an unusual increase in joint mobility.

jugular pulse   a pulsation in the jugular vein resulting from waves transmitted from the right side of the heart via circulating blood.

keratin   a scleroprotein that is the primary constituent of epidermis, hair, and nails.

Kiesselbach's plexus   a convergence of small, fragile arteries and veins located superficially on the anterosuperior portion of the nasal septum.

Koplik's spots   small red spots with bluish-white centers on the buccal mucosa opposite the molar teeth, appearing in the prodromal stage of measles.

kyphosis   a posterior curvature of the thoracic spine.

lactation   the production and secretion of milk from the breasts.

large for gestational age (LGA)   a weight classification of newborns associated with poorer health outcomes, the weight falling above the 90th percentile on the intrauterine growth curve for the infant's calculated gestational age.

leukoplakia   circumscribed, firmly attached, thick white patches on the tongue and other mucous membranes, often occurring as a precancerous growth.

lobule   a small lobe; the soft, lower, pendulous portion of the auricle of the ear.

lordosis   accentuation of the lumbar curvature of the spine.

lymphangioma   a tumor composed of lymphatic vessels that vary in size, are often dilated, and lined with normal endothelium.

lymphangitis   inflammation of lymph vessels from bacterial infection of an extremity, characterized by fine red streaks running from the extremity toward the groin or axilla.

lymphedema   swelling, particularly of subcutaneous tissues, caused by obstruction of the lymphatic system and accumulation of interstitial fluid.

macroglossia   excessively large tongue.

malleus   one of the three ossicles of the middle ear, connected to the tympanic membrane.

malocclusion   inappropriate contact between the teeth of the upper and lower jaw.

McBurney's point   in acute appendicitis, extreme sensitivity over the appendix, approximately 2 in. above the right anterosuperior iliac spine, on a line between that spine and the umbilicus.

meconium   first stools of the newborn; viscous, sticky, dark green, usually sterile and odorless.

mediastinum   the space in the thoracic cavity behind the sternum and between the two pleural sacs; contains the remaining thoracic organs and structures.

menarche   the first menstruation and initiation of cyclic menstrual function.

meninges   one of three layers (dura mater, pia mater, and arachnoid) that enclose the brain and spinal cord.

midaxillary line   a vertical line drawn midway between the anterior and posterior axillary folds.

midclavicular line   a vertical line drawn through the midpoint of the clavicle.

midsternal line   a vertical line drawn through the middle of the sternum.

miosis   contraction of the pupil to less than 2 mm in diameter.

mitral valve   the heart valve between the left atrium and left ventricle consisting of two cusps; it allows blood to flow into the ventricle and prevents back flow.

Montgomery's tubercles   enlarged sebaceous glands located on the areola of the breast.

mucopurulent   an exudate that contains both pus and mucus.

murmur   a heart sound audible with the stethoscope, generated by disruptions in the passage of blood within the heart or blood vessels.

Murphy's sign   pain on inspiration during palpation of the liver and gallbladder that causes the patient to stop inspiration; usually a sign of gallbladder disease.

muscle tone   level of tension or consistency of muscle mass.

myalgia   tenderness or pain in muscle.

myocardium   the middle and thickest of the three layers of the wall of the heart, consisting of cardiac muscle.

myopia   (nearsightedness) a condition resulting from a refractive error in which light rays entering the eye are brought into focus in front of the retina.

myxedema   a condition caused by hypothyroidism characterized by dry, waxy skin, coarse hair, intolerance to cold, cognitive impairment, and slowing of the relaxation phase of deep tendon reflexes.

nasal polyp   boggy, dependent mucosa that is rounded, elongated, and projects into the nasal cavity.

nasopharynx   the portion of the pharynx extending from the posterior nares to the level of the soft palate.

neurogenic   arising from or caused by the nervous system.

nevus   a circumscribed skin lesion that is presumed to be genetic; the excess or deficient tissue may involve epidermal or connective tissue, nerve elements, or vascular elements; the nevus may be pigmented or nonpigmented.

nocturia   urination at night; the individual is awakened from sleep by the need to void.

nuchal rigidity   resistance to flexion of the neck, seen in individuals with meningitis.

nystagmus   involuntary rhythmic movements of the eyes; the oscillations may be horizontal, vertical, rotary, or mixed.

oncotic pressure   the pressure difference between the osmotic pressure of blood and that of tissue fluid or lymph; an important force in maintaining balance between blood and surrounding tissues.

oropharynx   division of the pharynx extending from behind the soft palate dorsally to the upper edge of the epiglottis.

orthostatic   referring to an upright body position; orthostatic edema develops after standing; orthostatic hypotension occurs when the patient stands erect.

ossification   the formation of bone.

otorrhea   discharge, especially a purulent one, from the ear.

palpebral fissures   the elliptical opening between the upper and lower eyelids.

palpitation   beating of the heart so vigorous that the patient is aware of it; causes include exertion, emotional stress, hyperthyroidism, and various heart diseases.

papillae   small nipple-shaped projections; papillae on the dorsal portion of the tongue contain the taste buds.

papilledema   edema of the optic disc resulting in loss of definition of the disc margin; the cause is often increased intracranial pressure.

parasternal   situated close to or beside the sternum.

parasympathetic nervous system   the division of the autonomic nervous system responsible for the protection, conservation, and restoration of body resources.

parenchyma   the functional cells of an organ, as distinguished from the supporting connective tissue framework.

paresthesia   unusual sensation such as numbness, tingling, or burning.

parietal   referring to inner walls of any body cavity.

paroxysm   a sudden sharp spasm, convulsion, or attack; a sudden relapse of disease.

peak height velocity   the time during pubescence at which the tempo of growth is greatest.

peau d'orange   dimpling of the skin that gives it the appearance of the skin of an orange.

pectoriloquy   a striking transmission of voice sounds through the pulmonary structures, so that they are clearly audible through the stethoscope; commonly occurs from lung consolidation.

pectus carinatum   (pigeon chest) forward protrusion of the sternum.

pectus excavatum   (funnel chest) depression of the sternum.

pedunculated   having a stalk or stem that acts as a means of connection.

pericardium   the fibroserous membrane covering the heart and roots of the great vessels.

perineum   the region between the thighs, in the female between the vulva and the anus and in the male between the scrotum and the anus.

peristalsis   the wavelike motion by which the alimentary tract propels its contents.

petechiae   purple or red pinpoint spots on the skin as the result of minute hemorrhages into the dermal or submucosal layers.

Peyer's patches   collections of closely packed lymphoid follicles, forming elevations on the mucous membrane of the small intestine.

philtrum   the vertical groove on the upper lip.

photophobia   abnormal sensitivity to light; the condition is prevalent in albinism and disorders of the conjunctiva and cornea.

pica   a craving to eat non-food substances such as dirt, clay, or starch; may occur with some nutritional deficiency states, pregnancy, or mental disorders.

pilonidal   pertaining to the sacrococcygeal area.

pitch   a quality of sound that typifies its highness or lowness of tone, as determined by the frequency of vibrations.

plantar flexion   extension of the foot so that the forepart is lower than the ankle.

pleura   the serous membranes covering the lungs (visceral pleura) and lining the inner aspect of the pleural cavity (parietal pleura).

pleural cavity   the potential space between the usually closely opposed parietal and visceral layers of the pleura.

pleurisy   inflammation of the pleura, often associated with pneumonia.

plumbism   lead poisoning.

pneumothorax   accumulation of air or gas in the pleural space.

polydactyly   extra digits on the hands or feet.

postauricular   behind the auricle of the ear.

posterior axillary line   a vertical line drawn inferiorly from the posterior axillary fold.

postterm infant   an infant born after 41 completed weeks of gestation.

postural hypotension   (orthostatic hypotension) the presence of low blood pressure when the patient stands erect.

preauricular   in front of the auricle of the ear.

precordium   that area of the thorax situated over the heart.

prepuce   the foreskin of the penis.

presbyopia   hyperopia and impaired near vision from loss of lens elasticity, generally developing during middle age.

preterm infant   an infant born prior to 37 weeks gestation.

prodromal event   an early sign or warning of a developing disorder.

prognathism   protrusion of the jaws, causing malocclusion of the teeth.

pronate   the act of assuming a prone position; applied to the hand, the act of turning the palm backward or downward by medially rotating the forearm; applied to the foot, turning the medial edge of the foot lower and outward by eversion and abduction of the tarsal and metatarsal joints.

proprioception   the sensation of position and muscular activity originating from within the body, which provides awareness of posture, movement, and changes in equilibrium.

proptosis, proptotic   bulging or protrusion of an organ, such as the eyes.

pruritus   an itching sensation producing the urge to scratch.

ptosis   prolapse of an organ or part; drooping of the upper eyelid.

pubarche   beginning growth of pubic hair, breasts, and genitals.

pulmonary pressure   the blood pressure in the pulmonary artery.

pulmonary valve   the valve at the junction of the pulmonary artery and right ventricle consisting of three half-moon–shaped cusps; it prevents blood from regurgitating into the ventricle.

pulse   the palpable, rhythmical expansion and contraction of an artery, the result of an increased thrust of blood into the circulation each time the heart contracts; it is readily felt in the arterial component of the systemic circulation and also occurs in veins (e.g., jugular vein) and highly vascular organs (e.g., liver).

punctum   the tiny aperture in the margin of each eyelid that opens into a lacrimal duct.

purpura   brownish-red or purple discolorations on the skin as the result of hemorrhage into the tissue; also a group of disorders characterized by purpura.

pyrosis   epigastric burning sensation; heartburn.

QRS complex   the central deflections of the electrocardiogram representing the activity of the ventricles.

rale   a general term for an unexpected sound heard on auscultation of the chest; sometimes used to denote crepitus heard on auscultation.

regurgitation   an abnormal backward flowing, e.g., the blood between the chambers of the heart or between the great vessels and the heart.

retrognathia   position of the jaws behind the frontal plane of the forehead.

rhonchus   a dry, coarse rale in the bronchial tubes heard on auscultation of the chest, the result of partial obstruction; a sonorous rhonchus is low-pitched; a sibilant rhonchus is high-pitched and squeaky.

rigidity   a condition of hardness and inflexibility.

saccular   pouched; shaped like a sac.

scapular line   a vertical line drawn through the inferior angle of the scapula.

sclerosis   hardening or induration of body tissues, which can be the result of inflammation, particularly when it is prolonged.

scoliosis   lateral curvature of the spine.

scotoma   a loss of vision in a defined area in one or both eyes; shimmering film appearing as an island in the visual field, often occurring as a prodromal symptom.

scrotal raphe   the line of union of the two halves of the scrotum; often more highly pigmented than the surrounding tissue.

sebum   a thick substance secreted by the sebaceous glands that consists of fat and epithelial debris.

semilunar valve   refers to the pulmonic or aortic valves.

sensorineural hearing loss   reduction in hearing acuity related to a defect in the inner ear or damage to the eighth cranial nerve.

sessile   attached by a base rather than a stalk; a sessile lesion adheres closely to the surface of the skin or mucosa (see *pedunculated*).

shunt, left to right   referring to a diversion of blood from the left side of the heart to right (e.g., from a septal defect) or from the systemic to pulmonary circulation (e.g., from a patent ductus arteriosus).

sibilant   having the character of a hiss or whistle.

sign   an objective finding perceived by the examiner.

sinus arrhythmia   an irregularity of the heart rhythm caused by interference in the impulses arising from the sinoatrial node.

sinus rhythm   the expected regular cardiac rhythm stimulated by the sinoatrial node.

Skene's glands   (paraurethral glands) mucous-secreting glands that open onto the vestibule on each side of the urethra.

small for gestational age (SGA)   a weight classification of newborns associated with poorer health outcomes, the weight falling below the 10th percentile on the intrauterine growth curve for the infant's calculated gestational age.

smegma   the secretion of sebaceous material by the glans penis and the desquamation of epithelial cells from the prepuce; it appears as a cheesy white material.

spasm   involuntary contraction of a muscle or group of muscles, interfering with normal function of that particular muscle group.

spastic   increased muscle tone, spasms, or uncontrolled contractions of skeletal muscles causing stiff, awkward movements.

sprain   traumatic injury to the tendons, muscles, or ligaments around a joint.

stapes   one of the three ossicles of the middle ear, connected to the inner ear.

steatorrhea   frothy, foul-smelling fecal matter that floats because of its high fat content; associated with malabsorption syndromes.

stellate   shaped like a star; arranged in a rosette.

stereognosis   the ability to recognize objects by the sense of touch.

striae   streaks or lines; skin striae result from weakening of the elastic tissue associated with pregnancy, weight gain, rapid growth periods, and high levels of corticosteroids.

stridor   a harsh, high-pitched sound during respiration caused by laryngeal or tracheal obstruction.

stroke volume   the amount of blood pumped out of one ventricle of the heart as the result of a single contraction.

stroma   the supportive connective tissue framework of an organ as distinguished from the functional tissue (parenchyma).

sty   a purulent infection of a meibomian gland of the eyelid, often caused by a staphylococcal organism.

subcutaneous emphysema   the presence of air or gas beneath the skin.

subjective data   that information collected during the interview from the patient or a significant other.

subluxation   partial or incomplete dislocation.

sulcus   a shallow groove or depression on the surface of an organ (e.g., the median sulcus of the prostate gland separating the two lateral lobes).

supernumerary nipples   extra nipples usually not associated with underlying glandular tissue located along the embryonic mammary ridge.

supinate   to assume a supine position; applied to the arm, the act of turning the palm forward or upward by laterally rotating the forearm; applied to the foot, the act of raising the medial margin of the foot.

sutures   a fibrous joint in which the bones are closely approximated, as between the infant's cranial bones permitting expansion of the skull for brain growth.

swan neck deformity   hyperextension of the proximal interphalangeal joint with fixed flexion of the distal interphalangeal joint.

sympathetic nervous system the division of the autonomic nervous system that activates responses to physiologic or psychologic stress.

symptom the subjective indication of disease perceived by the patient.

syndactyly webbing between the digits of the hand or feet.

systole the part of the cardiac cycle during which the heart contracts, particularly the ventricles, resulting in a forceful flow of blood into both the systemic and pulmonary circulations.

tachycardia rapid beating of the heart at a rate over 100 per minute.

tachypnea rapid, usually shallow, breathing.

tactile fremitus a tremor or vibration in any part of the body detected by palpation.

tail of Spence upper outer tail of the breast that extends into the axilla.

term infant an infant born between 37 and 41 weeks gestation.

terminal hair the pigmented coarse hair that grows on the scalp, axilla, pubis, and in males the face.

thelarche the beginning of female pubertal breast development.

thrill a palpable vibration or tremor resulting from a cardiac murmur or a disruption in vascular blood flow.

thrombophlebitis inflammation of the wall of a vein associated with thrombus formation.

thrombosis the formation or presence of a blood clot within a blood vessel or within one of the cavities of the heart.

thyrotoxicosis a disease caused by excessive quantities of thyroid hormones.

tic an involuntary movement or spasm of a small group of muscles that may be aggravated by stress or anxiety; sometimes momentarily controllable.

tinnitus an auditory sensation in the absence of sound heard in one or both ears, such as ringing, buzzing, hissing, or clicking.

tonus expected state of muscle tone, maintained by partial contraction or alternate contraction and relaxation of neighboring muscle fibers in a group of muscles.

tophus a chalky deposit of uric acid crystals around joints or on the external ear; associated with gout.

tragus the cartilaginous projection of the ear anterior to the auditory canal meatus.

tremor rhythmic, purposeless, quivering movements resulting from involuntary alternately contracting and relaxing of opposing muscle groups.

tricuspid valve a heart valve between the right atrium and right ventricle, consisting of three cups, that allows blood to flow to the ventricle and prevents back flow.

turbinates extensions of the ethmoid bone located along the lateral wall of the nose, covered by erectile mucous membrane.

tympanic membrane (eardrum) a membranous structure separating the external ear from the middle ear.

umbo landmark on the tympanic membrane created by the attachment of the tympanic membrane to the malleus.

valgus an abnormal position in which part of a limb is twisted outward away from the midline.

varicosity an unnaturally swollen, often tortuous, blood or lymph vessel.

varus an abnormal position in which part of a limb is twisted inward toward the midline.

vascular referring to blood vessels.

vasoconstriction a narrowing in the caliber of a blood vessel.

vasomotor referring to control over the dilation and constriction of blood vessels.

vasopressor stimulating contraction of the muscular tissues of the capillaries and arteries, causing a rise in blood pressure.

vellus hair the soft, nonpigmented hair that covers the body.

velocity of growth the rate of growth or change in growth measurements over a period of time.

venous hum a continuous musical murmur heard on auscultation over the major veins at the base of the neck, particularly when a patient is anemic, upright, and looking to the contralateral side; also heard in the healthy individual, particularly the young.

venous thrombosis thrombosis of a vein.

ventilation the movement of air into and out of the lungs, resulting in the exchange of gases between the lungs and the air.

vertigo sensation of dizziness, either oneself or external objects whirling around oneself.

vesicular breath sounds expected breathing sounds when the patient is healthy and free of respiratory embarrassment, usually soft and with harsh vocal fremitus; the vibration felt on palpation of the chest wall, the result of spoken sound.

vestibular function balance.

vestibule the almond-shaped area enclosed by the labia minora laterally, extending from the clitoris to the fourchette anteroposteriorly.

Virchow's node (signal or sentinel node) a firm supraclavicular lymph node, particularly on the left, so enlarged that it is palpable.

virilization the process by which a female acquires male secondary sexual characteristics, usually as a result of adrenal dysfunction.

vulva (pudendum) the visible external female genitalia consisting of the mons pubis, labia, clitoris, vaginal orifice, vestibule, and vestibular glands.

water-hammer pulse full, forcible impulse and immediate collapse, providing a jerking sensation; characteristic of aortic regurgitation.

webbing skin folds in the neck from the acromion to the mastoid; associated with chromosomal anomalies.

whispered pectoriloquy the transmission of a whisper in the same way as that of more readily audible speech, commonly detected when the lung is consolidated by pneumonia (see *pectoriloquy*).

whoop the noisy spasm of inspiration that terminates the paroxysms of coughing, characteristic of pertussis (whooping cough); caused by a sudden, sharp increase in tension of the vocal chords.

winged scapula an outward prominence of the scapula caused by disruption of its nerves or muscles.

Appendix A

Conversion Tables

Length					Weight			
In	*cm*	*cm*	*In*		*lb*	*kg*	*kg*	*lb*
1	2.54	1	0.4		1	0.5	1	2.2
2	5.08	2	0.8		2	0.9	2	4.4
4	10.16	3	1.2		4	1.8	3	6.6
6	15.24	4	1.6		6	2.7	4	8.8
8	20.32	5	2.0		8	3.6	5	11.0
10	25.40	6	2.4		10	4.5	6	13.2
20	50.80	8	3.1		20	9.1	8	17.6
30	76.20	10	3.9		30	13.6	10	22
40	101.60	20	7.9		40	18.2	20	44
50	127.00	30	11.8		50	22.7	30	66
60	152.40	40	15.7		60	27.3	40	88
70	177.80	50	19.7		70	31.8	50	110
80	203.20	60	23.6		80	36.4	60	132
90	228.60	70	27.6		90	40.9	70	154
100	254.00	80	31.5		100	45.4	80	176
150	381.00	90	35.4		150	66.2	90	198
200	508.00	100	39.4		200	90.8	100	220

1 in = 2.54 cm
1 cm = 0.3937 inch

1 lb. = 0.454 kg
1 kg. = 2.204 lb

Appendix B

Abbreviations

A & P	Anterior and posterior; auscultation and percussion
A & W	Alive and well
abd	Abdomen; abdominal
a̅c	Before meals
ADL	Activities of daily living
AJ	Ankle jerk
AK	Above knee
ANS	Autonomic nervous system
AP	Anteroposterior
bid	Twice a day
BK	Below knee
BP	Blood pressure
BPH	Benign prostatic hypertrophy
BS	Bowel sounds; breath sounds
c̅	With
CC	Chief complaint
CHD	Childhood disease; congenital heart disease; coronary heart disease
CHF	Congestive heart failure
CNS	Central nervous system
c/o	Complains of
COPD	Chronic obstructive pulmonary disease
CV	Cardiovascular
CVA	Costovertebral angle; cerebrovascular accident
CVP	Central venous pressure
Cx	Cervix
D & C	Dilatation and curettage
D/C	Discontinued
DM	Diabetes mellitus
DOB	Date of birth
DOE	Dyspnea on exertion
DTRs	Deep tendon reflexes
DUB	Dysfunctional uterine bleeding
Dx	Diagnosis
ECG, EKG	Electrocardiogram; electrocardiograph
EENT	Eye, ear, nose, and throat
ENT	Ear, nose, and throat
EOM	Extraocular movement
FB	Foreign body
FH	Family history
FROM	Full range of motion
FTT	Failure to thrive
Fx	Fracture
GB	Gallbladder
GE	Gastroesophageal
GI	Gastrointestinal
GU	Genitourinary
GYN	Gynecologic
HA	Headache
HCG	Human chorionic gonadotropin
HEENT	Head, eyes, ears, nose, and throat
HPI	History of present illness
Hx	History
ICS	Intercostal space
IOP	Intraocular pressure
IUD	Intrauterine device
IV	Intravenous
JVP	Jugular venous pressure
KJ	Knee jerk
KUB	Kidneys, ureters, and bladder
lat	Lateral
LCM	Left costal margin
LE	Lower extremities
LLL	Left lower lobe (lung)
LLQ	Left lower quadrant (abdomen)
LMD	Local medical doctor
LMP	Last menstrual period
LOC	Loss of consciousness; level of consciousness
LS	Lumbosacral; lumbar spine
LSB	Left sternal border
LUL	Left upper lobe (lung)
LUQ	Left upper quadrant (abdomen)

M	Murmur		**Pt**	Patient
MAL	Midaxillary line		**PVC**	Premature ventricular contraction
MCL	Midclavicular line			
MGF	Maternal grandfather		**q**	Every
MGM	Maternal grandmother		**qd**	Every day
MSL	Midsternal line		**qh**	Every hour
MVA	Motor vehicle accident		**qod**	Every other day
NA	No answer; not applicable		**RCM**	Right costal margin
N & T	Nose and throat		**REM**	Rapid eye movement
N & V	Nausea and vomiting		**RLL**	Right lower lobe (lung)
NKA	No known allergies		**RLQ**	Right lower quadrant (abdomen)
NPO	Nothing by mouth		**RML**	Right middle lobe (lung)
NSR	Normal sinus rhythm		**ROM**	Range of motion
			ROS	Review of systems
OD	Oculus dexter; right eye		**RSB**	Right sternal border
OM	Otitis media		**RUL**	Right upper lobe (lung)
OS	Oculus sinister; left eye		**RUQ**	Right upper quadrant (abdomen)
OTC	Over the counter			
OU	Oculus uterque; both eyes		**s̄**	Without
			SCM	Sternocleidomastoid
p̄	After		**SQ**	Subcutaneous
P & A	Percussion and auscultation		**Sx**	Symptoms
p̄c	After meals			
PE	Physical examination		**T & A**	Tonsillectomy and adenoidectomy
PERRLA	Pupils equal, round, react to light and accommodation		**TM**	Tympanic membrane
			TPR	Temperature, pulse, and respiration
PGF	Paternal grandfather			
PGM	Paternal grandmother		**UE**	Upper extremities
PI	Present illness		**URI**	Upper respiratory infection
PID	Pelvic inflammatory disease		**UTI**	Urinary tract infection
PMH	Past medical history			
PMI	Point of maximum impulse; point of maximum intensity		**WD**	Well developed
			WN	Well nourished
PMS	Premenstrual syndrome			
prn	As necessary		**x**	Times; by (size)

Index